Brain Theory and Neural Networks

Brain Theory and Neural Networks

Editor: John Dalvi

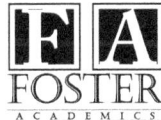

FA FOSTER
ACADEMICS

www.fosteracademics.com

www.fosteracademics.com

FA
FOSTER
ACADEMICS

Cataloging-in-Publication Data

Brain theory and neural networks / edited by John Dalvi.
    p. cm.
Includes bibliographical references and index.
ISBN 978-1-63242-529-4
1. Brain. 2. Neurology--Philosophy. 3. Neural networks (Neurobiology). I. Dalvi, John.
QP376 .B73 2018
612.82--dc23

Foster Academics,
118-35 Queens Blvd., Suite 400,
Forest Hills, NY 11375, USA

ISBN 978-1-63242-529-4 (Hardback)

Contents

Preface

The main aim of this book is to educate learners and enhance their research focus by presenting diverse topics covering this vast field. This is an advanced book which compiles significant studies by distinguished experts in the area of analysis. This book addresses successive solutions to the challenges arising in the area of application, along with it; the book provides scope for future developments.

A biological neural network passes information between receptors and effectors by using electrical impulses. Neural networks are a collection of neurons that allow the body to process various stimuli and respond to them. Signals passed between neurons are either inhibitory or excitatory, and an action potential is initiated when the excitatory signals reach threshold potential. This book is compiled in such a manner, that it will provide in-depth knowledge about the theory and practice of brain theory and neural networks. With state-of-the-art inputs by acclaimed experts of this field, this book targets students and professionals.

It was a great honour to edit this book, though there were challenges, as it involved a lot of communication and networking between me and the editorial team. However, the end result was this all-inclusive book covering diverse themes in the field.

Finally, it is important to acknowledge the efforts of the contributors for their excellent chapters, through which a wide variety of issues have been addressed. I would also like to thank my colleagues for their valuable feedback during the making of this book.

Editor

Modulatory Effect of Acupuncture at Waiguan (TE5) on the Functional Connectivity of the Central Nervous System of Patients with Ischemic Stroke in the Left Basal Ganglia

Junqi Chen[1]¶, Jizhou Wang[2]¶, Yong Huang[3]*, Xinsheng Lai[4]*, Chunzhi Tang[4], Junjun Yang[4], Junxian Wu[5], Tongjun Zeng[6], Shanshan Qu[3]

1 Department of Rehabilitation, The Third Affiliated Hospital of Southern Medical University, Guangzhou, China, 2 The First Clinical Medical School, Southern Medical University, Guangzhou, China, 3 School of Traditional Chinese Medicine, Southern Medical University, Guangzhou, China, 4 School of Acupuncture and Rehabilitation, Guangzhou University of Traditional Chinese Medicine, Guangzhou, China, 5 Department of Acupuncture and Moxibustion, Shantou Central Hospital, Shantou, China, 6 The First People's Hospital of Shunde, Foshan, China

Abstract

Objective: To study the influence of acupuncture at Waiguan (TE5) on the functional connectivity of the central nervous system of patients with ischemic stroke.

Methods: Twenty-four patients with ischemic stroke in the left basal ganglia were randomized based on gender to receive TE5 acupuncture (n = 12) or nonacupoint acupuncture (n = 12). Each group underwent sham acupuncture and then verum acupuncture while being scanned with functional magnetic resonance imaging. Six regions of interest (ROI) were defined, including bilateral motor, somatosensory, and bilateral basal ganglia areas. The functional connectivity between these ROIs and all voxels of the brain was analyzed in Analysis of Functional NeuroImages(AFNI) to explore the differences between verum acupuncture and sham acupuncture at TE5 and between TE5 acupuncture and nonacupoint acupuncture. The participants were blinded to the allocation.

Result: The effect of acupuncture on six seed-associated networks was explored. The result demonstrated that acupuncture at Waiguan (TE5) can regulate the sensorimotor network of the ipsilesional hemisphere, stimulate the contralesional sensorimotor network, increase cooperation of bilateral sensorimotor networks, and change the synchronization between the cerebellum and cerebrum. Furthermore, a lot of differences of effect existed between verum acupuncture and sham acupuncture at TE5, but there was little difference between TE5 acupuncture and nonacupoint acupuncture.

Conclusion: The modulation of synchronizations between different regions within different brain networks might be the mechanism of acupuncture at Waiguan (TE5). Stimulation of the contralesional sensorimotor network and increase of cooperation of bilateral hemispheres imply a compensatory effect of the intact hemisphere, whereas changes in synchronization might influence the sensorimotor function of the affected side of the body.

Trial Registration: Chinese Clinical Trial Registry ChiCTR-ONRC-08000255

Editor: Cornelis Jan Stam, VU University Medical Center, Netherlands

Funding: This study was supported by National 973 Program of China (no.: 2006CB504505), National 973 Program of China (no.: 2012CB518504) and Third Key Subject of the '211 Project' of Guangdong Province. The funders had no role in study design, data collection and analysis, decision to publish, or preparation of the manuscript.

Competing Interests: The authors have declared that no competing interests exist.

* E-mail: nfhy@fimmu.com (YH); lai1023@163.com (XSL)

꒐ These authors contributed equally to this work.

¶ These authors joint senior authors on this work.

Introduction

Acupuncture is one of the most widely used alternative treatments whose curative effect has been recognized and approved by the World Health Organization [1]. In traditional Chinese medicine, it is believed that acupuncture can affect the energy flow through the body which in turn modulates functions of the whole body system. However, the mechanism of its effect has not been well characterized to date. Clinical and experimental studies suggest that the modulatory effect of acupuncture might be mediated via the central and peripheral nervous systems [2,3].

Functional magnetic resonance imaging (fMRI) is an efficient, noninvasive method of studying the mechanism by which acupuncture affects the central nervous system (CNS). Many fMRI studies indicated that acupuncture can activate or deactivate certain areas of the brain related to a corresponding disease or function [4–12]. Meanwhile, its effect seems to be relevant to the regulation of brain networks, such as the default mode network, sensorimotor network, amygdala-associated network, and vision network [6,13–15]. Distinct from the conventional fMRI, functional connectivity MRI (fcMRI) can be used to detect the temporal correlation of the blood oxygen level–dependent (BOLD) signals of spatially remote brain regions. The connectivity of two areas, including functional connectivity and effective connectivity, depicts the cooperation pattern of these areas. Functional connectivity is the pattern of statistical dependency resulting from the nonlinear dynamics of neurons and neuronal populations within the neuroanatomical substrate [16], which reflects the existence and the strength of the connectivity between remote brain regions.

Patients with stroke in the basal ganglia have significant deficiency in the sensorimotor function of the contralesional side of their body. To date, researchers have found several relevant changes in the CNS of these patients, such as changes in the effective connectivity of core motor areas [17]. Recovery seems to be related to the extent of connectivity between the ipsilesional primary motor area and contralesional postcentral gyrus, change in the topological structure, centrality of the ipsilesional primary sensorimotor area, recruitment of bilateral somatosensory association areas and contralesional SII, and activation of the contralesional cerebellum [18,19]. Similarly, the abnormal function of many regions of the brain is also crucial in the deficiency in somatosensory function [20–22]. The sensorimotor function is regulated by complex functional networks formed by the neuronal populations of the cortex and subcortex [23]. Thus, ischemic stroke lesions may affect the functional network architecture in both hemispheres [24–28] and break the balance of the network, which in turn causes the deficiency in sensorimotor function.

Acupuncture is one of the most important treatments for stroke rehabilitation. Several studies demonstrated that acupuncture not only regulates the functional state and connectivity of sensorimotor areas of normal people [9,14,29] but also affects the functional state of the bilateral sensorimotor cortex of stroke patients [30,31].

TE5 is an important traditional acupuncture point common in the treatment of stroke-related motor, neurological and autonomic nerve problems in clinical practice [32]. We hypothesize that acupuncture at TE5 has a specific influence on the functional networks, including sensorimotor areas, of the CNS to improve the sensorimotor function of the body [33].

Twenty-four patients with ischemic stroke in the left basal ganglia were recruited to investigate this hypothesis. Data extracted from fMRI were assessed with seed-based analysis to discover the differences between TE5 verum acupuncture and nonacupoint acupuncture and between TE5 verum acupuncture and TE5 sham acupuncture. Results of this study elucidate the specific influence of acupuncture at TE5 on sensorimotor networks.

Methods

Subject

The study was carried out during October 2008 and August 2010 in the Imaging Center of Nanfang Hospital, Guangzhou, China. Twenty-four patients admitted to the First Affiliated Hospital of Guangzhou University of Chinese Medicine and matching the diagnostic criteria of ischemic stroke in ICD-9 434 and ICD-8 433 [34] were screened based on the following inclusion criteria: ischemic stroke in the left basal ganglia that occurred more than a month ago but less than a year, significant right hemiplegia (the score of the muscle strength of the upper limb and the lower limb ≤4), stable condition and receiving usual treatment (including antiplatelet medicine like aspirin and clopidogrel, and lipid-lowering drugs like statins et al.), right handedness, naive to acupuncture or not being treated by acupuncture for at least 4 weeks, no severe aphasia, no previous neurological or psychiatric disease, and no coagulation or other severe diseases. The experimental protocol was approved by the Ethical Committee of the First Affiliated Hospital of Guangzhou University of Chinese Medicine. This study was registered on the Chinese Clinical Trial Registry (http://www.chictr.org, ChiCTR-ONRC-08000255). All patients signed a written informed consent.

The participants were randomly (using random number table) divided into two groups of 12: Waiguan (TE5) group and nonacupoint group. Each group underwent sham acupuncture and then verum acupuncture.

Experiment Design

The fMRI brain scan was conducted on a 3.0-T whole-body scanner (GE Signa) with a standard head coil. The participants were prevented from experiencing auditory and visual activities via earplugs and eyeshades, respectively. The scanning procedure (Fig. 1) began after the participants rested on the bed for 5 min. The participants in each group were given sham acupuncture stimulus and then verum acupuncture while being simultaneously scanned. Each stimulus lasted for 6 min and 30 s. The two stimuli had an interval lasting for 6 min and 2 s, which was considered sufficient for restoring the sensitivity of cutaneous sensory receptor. The participants were blinded as to which stimulus was given to them; they were only aware of receiving acupuncture. The experiment operator, data analyst, and researcher were strictly separated from each other.

Verum Acupuncture Stimulation

TE5 is located on the dorsal aspect of the forearm at midpoint of the interosseous space between the radius and the ulna, 2 cun proximal to the dorsal wrist crease, whereas the nonacupoint is medial to TE5 at midpoint between the two meridians, i.e. triple energizer meridian and small intestine meridian (Fig. 2). During stimulation, a sterile silver needle 0.30 mm in diameter and 40 mm in length (tube purchased from Dongbang AcuPrime Co. and needle from Zhongyan Taihe Co., Beijing, China) was inserted vertically into the skin at a depth of 15±2 mm. The needle was twisted for ±180° evenly at a frequency of 60 circles per min after the needling sensation (de qi), i.e., the feeling of increased resistance to further insertion, was assured by the acupuncturist.

Sham Acupuncture Stimulation

In this study, sham acupuncture served as the tactile control. Tactile stimulation has been widely used as a noninvasive control for acupuncture neuroimaging studies. The procedure involved pushing the end of the needle with its tip out of the tube within 1 mm and touching the skin.

Acupuncture was conducted manually by an experienced acupuncturist. During experimental stimulation, the subjects were required to keep quiet and remain calm without speaking.

fMRI Scan

After the patients rested on the bed for 5 min, 3D anatomy images were collected with a T1-weighted 3D gradient echo-pulse

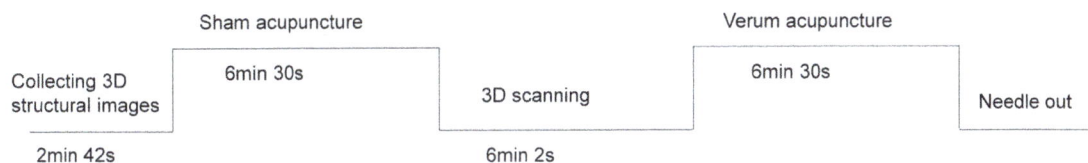

Figure 1. Stimulation and scanning pattern.

fast spin sequence, with axial view T1 fluid-attenuated-inversion-recovery scan. The exact scanning parameters were as follows: TR = 2.3 s, TE = 21 ms, TI = 920 ms, slice thickness = 6.0 mm, gap = 1.0 mm, 20 layers for a total of 2 min and 45 s, field of view (FOV) = 240×180 mm^2, matrix = 320×256, number of excitations (NEX) = 2, echo train length = 9, and band width = 50. During the acupuncture stimulation, BOLD functional images were collected with a T2-weighted single-shot, gradient-recalled echo-planar imaging sequence. The exact scanning parameters were as follows: TR = 3 s, TE = 20 ms, flip angle = 90°, FOV = 240×240 mm^2, slice thickness = 6.0 mm, slice gap = 1.0 mm, matrix = 96×96, NEX = 1, phase per location = 130, and 2600 phases per 6 min and 30s.

Data Analysis

The preprocessing steps were implemented in AFNI (Cox, 1996; http://afni.nimh.nih.gov/afni). The functional images from each run were aligned, slice timing corrected, temporally standardized, space smoothed (6 mm full width at half maximum Gaussian kernel), and transformed into Talairach space (Talairach and Tournoux, 1988).

For each subject, we analyzed the functional connectivity using the average activity of a seed region defined by the anatomical template in AFNI to find other voxels in the brain that behaved similarly. The ROIs (seeds) selected were areas related to motor ability [Brodmann area (BA) 4 and BA6], sensations (BA1, BA2, BA3, BA5, and BA7), and basal ganglia area. The objective was to find the changes in correlations between these regions and other parts of the brain, which might affect the function of motor ability and sensations. The low-frequency BOLD correlations (0.01 Hz to 0.1 Hz) or functional connectivity between the time series of a given seed and that of all voxels in the brain was partially correlated by Pearson correlation analysis with covariance of head motion and time series from white matter and cerebrospinal fluid. Individual correlation coefficient maps for both the acupuncture and tactile conditions were generated and transformed to Fisher's z-distribution for group-level analysis. All the resultant t-maps were set to the threshold level of P<0.05. Multiple-comparison error was corrected with Monte Carlo simulation.

Results

Baseline Data

Two participants from the Waiguan (TE5) group and one participant from the nonacupoint group were excluded for significant movement during the scan, and three participants from the nonacupoint group were excluded for spoiled data (Fig. 3). No significant difference was found in the baseline data of the remaining 18 participants (Table 1).

Functional Connectivity

The different effects of TE5 verum acupuncture, TE5 sham acupuncture, and nonacupoint acupuncture on six seed-associated networks were observed through seed-based analysis (Table 2 and Fig. 4).

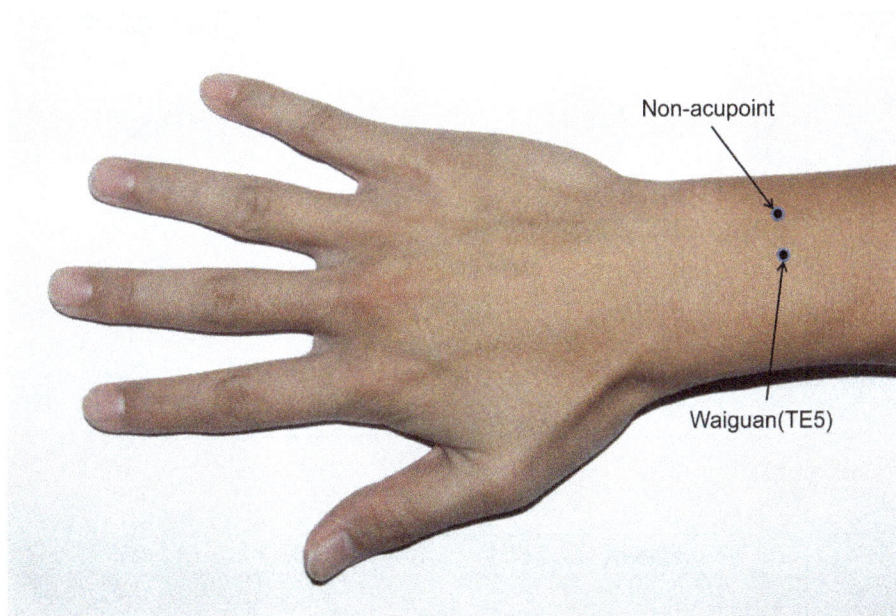

Figure 2. *Waiguan* and nonacupoint on the right forearm.

Table 1. Baseline data.

Items	Waiguan (TE5) (n = 10)	Nonacupoint (n = 8)	Statistics	P
Gender (M/F, n)	9/1	7/1		1*
Age	56.10±5.53	58.50±7.05	t = −0.811	0.429
Duration, months	5.30±3.71	3.38±3.29	t = 1.148	0.268
CSS score	18.20±4.02	17.13±4.76	t = 0.520	0.611
Hypertension (Yes/No, n)	9/1	6/2		0.559*
Diabetes mellitus (Yes/No, n)	2/8	1/7		1*

The P values with "*" were obtained using Fisher's Exact Test, whereas the rest were the result of independent samples t-test.

The correlation between the left precuneus and the left motor area was stronger under acupuncture than under the tactile control. Greater correlation was found between the left precuneus and the left somatosensory area, the latter being the seed. Stronger correlation was found between the left basal ganglia area and the right middle frontal gyrus, with the former being the seed.

The three seed-associated networks of the ROIs in the right hemisphere were more complicated than that in the left hemisphere. The correlation between the right motor area and the left postcentral gyrus, right middle frontal gyrus, and left thalamus was stronger under acupuncture than under the tactile control. Meanwhile, the correlation between the right somatosensory area and the bilateral postcentral gyrus and left putamen was stronger under acupuncture than under the tactile control. The right cerebellum and cerebellar culmen had greater connectivity with the right basal ganglia, whereas the left cerebellum had weaker correlation with the right motor and somatosensory areas.

Unlike the many differences demonstrated in the comparison of TE5 verum acupuncture and TE5 sham acupuncture stated before, only the left thalamus and left cuneus showed greater connectivity with the right motor area and right basal ganglia, respectively, when TE5 verum acupuncture was compared with nonacupoint acupuncture. Interestingly, stronger connectivity between left thalamus and right motor area was also aroused by verum acupuncture relative to sham acupuncture.

Discussion

Specific Effects of TE5 Acupuncture Compared with TE5 Sham Acupuncture

First, the left precuneus showed stronger connectivity with both the left motor area and left somatosensory area. Anatomical connectivity exists between the precuneus and the sensorimotor cortex and subcortex [35]. A clinical study indicated that

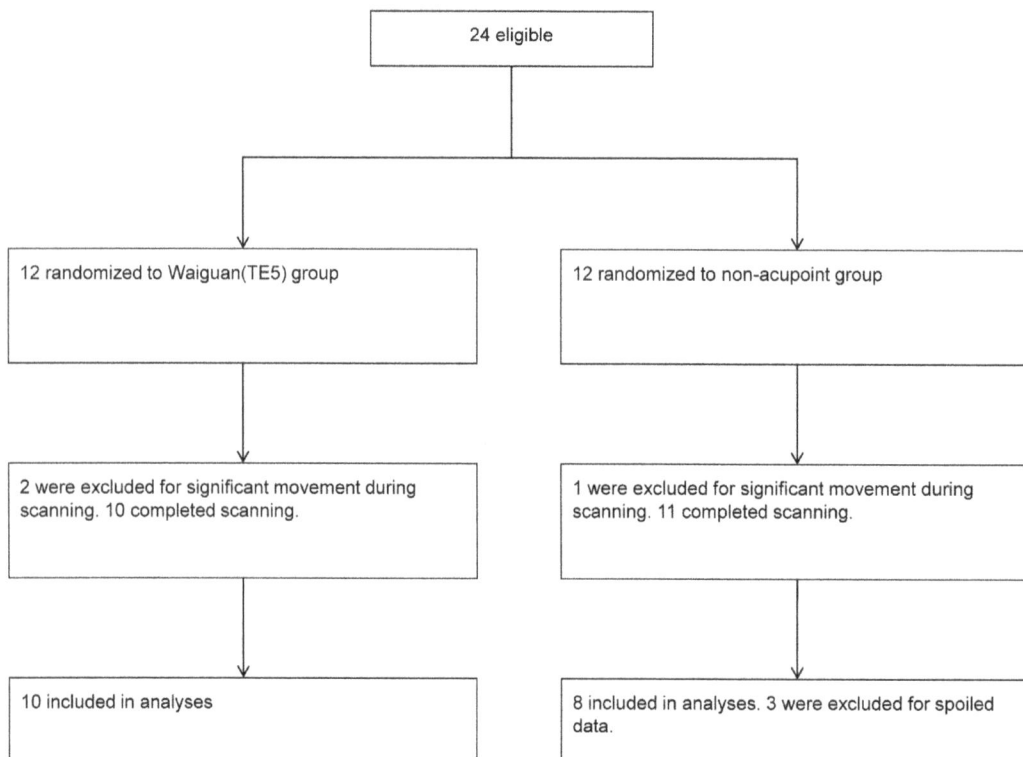

Figure 3. Consort flow diagram.

Table 2. Localization of the acupuncture specific effects by comparing TE5 verum acupuncture (Group A) vs. TE5 sham acupuncture (Group B) and TE5 verum acupuncture (Group A) vs. nonacupoint acupuncture (Group C).

ROI	Group A vs. Group B							Group A vs. Group C						
	Anatomical structures	BA	X	Y	Z	vox	t	Anatomical structures	BA	X	Y	Z	vox	t
Left motor area	Left precuneus	7	−10	−40	47	69	3.5							
Left somatosensory area	Left precuneus	5,7	−1	−37	47	48	5.2							
	Right paracentral lobule	4*	23	−37	50	33	3.5							
Left basal ganglia area	Right middle frontal gyrus	6	32	5	50	53	4.2							
Right motor area	Left postcentral gyrus	3	−25	−31	50	133	4.2	Left thalamus	N/A	−16	−22	5	31	3.8
	Left thalamus	N/A	−16	−25	8	66	4							
	Right middle frontal gyrus	6	32	−7	47	40	5.8							
	Left cerebellar	N/A	−19	−79	−34	38	−4.4							
Right somatosensory area	Right postcentral gyrus	3	20	−31	50	121	4.4							
	Left postcentral gyrus	3	−28	−31	50	69	3.5							
	Left putamen	N/A	−31	−16	8	50	4							
	Left cerebellar	N/A	−19	−79	−34	44	−7.2							
Right basal ganglia area	Right cerebellar	N/A	5	−55	−25	113	4.9	Left cuneus	18	−10	−85	17	41	5.2
	Cerebellar culmen	N/A	2	−34	−1	47	5.2							
	Left lingual gyrus	18	−25	−79	−4	44	−3.1							

Abbreviation: BA, Brodmann area; Vox, voxel (represents the number of voxels); N/A, not available (means that the peak voxel was out of the BA zone). The BA area marked by "*"was corrected by a neurological physician.

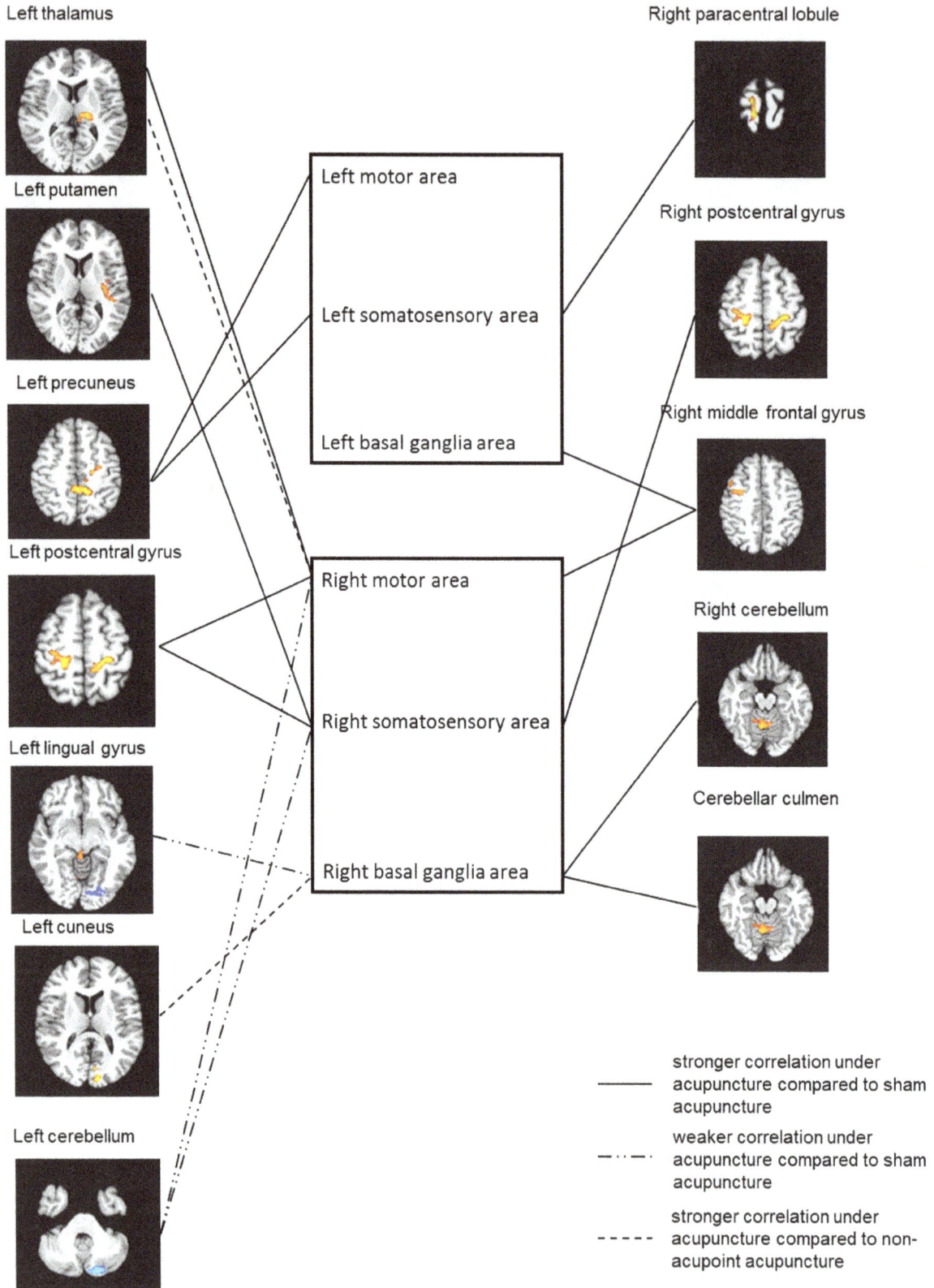

Figure 4. Differences of seed associated networks between ROIs from the left hemisphere and the right hemisphere. Full line represents stronger correlation under acupuncture compared with sham acupuncture, whereas the "dash–dot–dot" line represents weaker correlation. Dash line stands for weaker correlation compared with nonacupoint acupuncture (P<0.05, multiple comparison error corrected using Monte Carlo simulation). Regions of the left hemisphere and right hemisphere that had significant differences in correlation with seeds are placed on left side and right side, respectively, and ROIs in the same box are from the same hemisphere.

acupuncture can activate regions of ipsilesional hemisphere, which is correlated with the extent of rehabilitation [31]. Taking the anatomical connectivity and this clinical study into account, we hypothesize that acupuncture at TE5 can change the functional connectivity among ipsilesional neuronal populations of sensorimotor cortexes and subcortexes, leading to the modulation of the sensorimotor network, which might have a positive effect on the recovery of the affected side of the body. In addition, the precuneus was also found to have strong correlation with other brain regions [11], implying that the precuneus affects the efficiency of acupuncture.

Second, the correlation between the right sensorimotor areas and the left somatosensory area (left postcentral gyrus), right somatosensory area (right postcentral gyrus), right motor area [right middle frontal gyrus (BA6, premotor area)], and left basal ganglia area (left thalamus, left putamen) was stronger under acupuncture than under sham acupuncture. Meanwhile, a clinical study suggested that the regions activated or deactivated by acupuncture at TE5 of the affected forearm are mainly the components of the contralesional hemisphere [30]. Hence, the modulatory effects of acupuncture at TE5 might be attributed to the enhancement of compensatory process by the redistribution of functions to the sensorimotor areas of the contralesional hemisphere and to the increase in the cooperation of functioning between the bilateral sensorimotor areas. Our results were similar to those of Johansen-Berg [36,37] and Grefkes [17], who indicated that the sensorimotor areas of the contralesional hemisphere might have a role in modulating the function of the affected side of the body. Moreover, Grefkes et al. also found that the contralesional M1 of patients with stroke in the left basal ganglia was not only significantly activated while moving the affected limb but also exerted a negative influence on the ipsilesional M1. This result was not observed in healthy people. According to these studies, the negative influence can be attributed to the abnormal coupling between bilateral M1 caused by the damage of basal ganglia. Our analysis methods are different from theirs. Hence, ensuring whether or not the change in connectivity between the bilateral sensorimotor areas implies a modulatory effect on the coupling of these areas warrants further study.

Moreover, the connectivity between the left cerebellar cortex and the right motor area was weaker. The left cerebellum and the right motor area cooperate to control the left limb. Therefore, the result might reflect a decrease in the modulation of the sensorimotor function of the left limb. Meanwhile, the cerebella medial zone and the right cerebellar intermediate zone, which regulate the tension and cooperation of the body and proximal limb muscles and modulate the motor function of the right distal limb muscle, respectively, were more correlated with the right basal ganglia under acupuncture than under the tactile control. This result implies that the cooperation possibly aroused by the acupuncture between the right basal ganglia area and the right cerebellum might have a modulatory effect on the sensorimotor function of the right side (affected side) of the body. Moreover, the correlation between the right basal ganglia and the cerebellar culmen might regulate the sensorimotor function of both sides. Similar to our study, some clinical studies found that the functional recovery of patients improves with more activity in the contralesional cerebellum and with weaker centrality of the ipsilesional cerebellum [18,38]. Nevertheless, the reasons behind why the correlations between the cerebellum and other sensorimotor areas did not show significant differences need further study. In general, acupuncture at the right TE5 of stroke patients attenuates the cooperation of the right hemisphere and the left cerebellum responsible in modulating the sensorimotor function of the

unaffected limb while enhancing the cooperation of the right hemisphere and the right cerebellar to promote the regulation of the sensorimotor function of the right side (affected side) body.

Finally, a difference in correlation was also found between the visual cortex and the ROI, apart from the one between the sensorimotor function-associated areas and ROIs. Lingual gyrus is a part of the visual cortex, which also has functions in word comprehension and in the regulation of emotion and motor ability. Hence, the weaker correlation between these areas implies an attenuated cooperation on these functions with the use of acupuncture. However, a clinical study reported that acupuncture at TE5 can activate the bilateral occipital lobe compared with the baseline; however, the activation is not significant relative to that of tactile stimulation [30]. One reason that could account for this result is the different stimulation patterns of the verum and sham acupuncture on the visual cortex, such that distinction was found in its connectivity with the right basal ganglia, but not in activity. However, further studies are needed to investigate the exact benefit of this difference for the rehabilitation of stroke patients.

Specific Effects of TE5 Acupuncture Compared with Nonacupoint Acupuncture

Only the left thalamus and the left cuneus exhibited greater connectivity with the right motor area and the right basal ganglia, respectively, when TE5 acupuncture was compared with nonacupoint acupuncture. The stronger correlation between the left thalamus and the right motor areas implies an enhancement in the compensatory effect of the right intact sensorimotor areas. Interestingly, stronger connectivity between the left thalamus and the right motor area was also observed when TE5 acupuncture was compared with sham acupuncture. Thus, it can be a relatively specific effect of acupuncture at TE5. As stated above, the difference in the correlation between the left cuneus and the right basal ganglia might have resulted from the distinct stimulation pattern on the visual cortex and the augmented correlation under acupuncture when compared with nonacupoint acupuncture. When referring to the comparison between acupuncture and sham acupuncture, the correlation between the left visual cortex and the right basal ganglia was attenuated by acupuncture. This seemingly conflict needs to be clarified in further study with more exact data.

We propose the fact that little difference was found between the two groups might be related to the location of the nonacupoint. Locating the acupoint and the nonacupoint is rather arbitrary, and the surface area and spatial structure of an acupoint vary with the acupoint [39–41]. Thus, stimulating the nonacupoint and TE5 might have similar effects since these two points were close to each other, and the small difference in location might contribute to the differences in functional connectivity. Another possibility is that the nonacupoint is a new acupoint that might have a similar effect because it is situated close to TE5. Moreover, the fact that little difference was found might proceed from the analysis of acupuncture's instant effects. Acupuncture's long lasting effects have been demonstrated by many researchers. Hence more difference might be found if these effects were measured [42]. Although nonacupoint is commonly used as a control, investigating how to design a nonacupoint to reflect the actual effect of acupuncture is necessary to avoid the influence of nervous tissue, connective tissue, and other anatomic structures.

Characteristics of Connectivity Difference

Differences in connectivity were observed in several pairs of brain regions when TE5 acupuncture was compared with TE5 sham acupuncture and nonacupoint acupuncture (Table 2 and

Fig. 4). A pair of brain regions consisted of an ROI and another brain region. Most of the ROIs within these pairs were from the right hemisphere, whereas the other parts of the pairs were mainly areas of the left hemisphere and the left cerebellum. This type of distribution pattern implies that the main effect of acupuncture at TE5 of stroke patients might be the enhancement of the association between the two hemispheres, which cooperate to modulate the sensorimotor function of the affected side. Moreover, it could also be a sign of increasing the compensatory effect of the unaffected side of the brain.

Limitations

The sample size of our study was relatively small, and all participants were diagnosed of ischemic stroke in the left basal ganglia. We were unable to distinguish the exact regions of stroke. Therefore, our results only gave a preview on the mechanism of the effect of acupuncture on the CNS of patients with left basal ganglia ischemic stroke. In addition, the functional connectivity only refers to the correlation of the BOLD signal of two distinct brain regions, which indirectly reflects the correlation or cooperation of the neuronal activities. However, the correlation cannot indicate the effect passage of the neural function. Hence, further studies on the topic should use effective connectivity or graph theory, which is effective in revealing the direction of neural function, to enhance our understanding of the effect of acupuncture at TE5. We only focused on the connectivity between ROIs and all the voxels of the brain. Thus, the connectivity between the voxels that showed significant change in correlation with ROIs and the connectivity between regions other than the chosen ROIs and all voxels of the whole brain were not studied. Acupuncture is known to have a long lasting effect [13,15,43], and this characteristic was not investigated in this study. Further studies are warranted to explore the sustained effects of acupuncture on functional connectivity and its correlation with function recovery.

The commonly used TE5 sham acupuncture and nonacupoint acupuncture served as controls. However, previous research indicated that sham acupuncture and nonacupoint acupuncture have certain curative effects [44,45]. Therefore, the present study also neglected the connectivity, which did not show significant difference between groups that might influence the effect of acupuncture. A more suitable control needs to be adopted to reflect the exact effects of acupuncture.

Conclusion

The present study found that acupuncture helps regulate the functional connectivity between the sensorimotor areas of intra-hemisphere and inter-hemispheres as well as between the cerebellum and cerebrum. Results indicate that the compensatory effect of the intact sensorimotor network of contralesional hemisphere might be enhanced. The cooperation of the sensorimotor network of the ipsilesional hemisphere might be augmented. The impact on the functional connectivity between the cerebellum and cerebrum might also be important for the acupuncture's effects. The modulation of synchronizations between different regions within different brain networks might be the mechanism of acupuncture at Waiguan (TE5). A number of limitations were discussed.

Supporting Information

Checklist S1   Stricta checklist.

Protocol S1   Trial protocol.

Acknowledgments

We would like to give our sincere appreciation to all the participants and their families, and to Prof. Yanping Chen and Dr. Shanshan Tang for the technical support from the Imaging Center of Nanfang Hospital, China.
   Patient consent: Obtained.
   Ethical approval: The Ethical Committee of the First Affiliated Hospital of Guangzhou University of Chinese Medicine.

Author Contributions

Conceived and designed the experiments: YH XSL. Performed the experiments: JQC. Analyzed the data: SSQ. Wrote the paper: JQC JZW. Enrolled subjects: CZT JJY. Integrated all experiment data: TJZ JXW.

References

1. (1998) NIH Consensus Conference. Acupuncture. JAMA 280: 1518–1524.
2. Cheng XN (2000) Chinese Acupuncture and Moxibustion. Beijing: People's Medical Publishing House.
3. Han JS (2003) Acupuncture: neuropeptide release produced by electrical stimulation of different frequencies. Trends Neurosci 26: 17–22.
4. Liu P, Qin W, Zhang Y, Tian J, Bai L, et al. (2009) Combining spatial and temporal information to explore function-guide action of acupuncture using fMRI. J Magn Reson Imaging 30: 41–46.
5. Clauch JD, Chan ST, Nixon EE, Qiu WQ, Sporko T, et al. (2012) Commonality and specificity of acupuncture action at three acupoints as evidenced by FMRI. Am J Chin Med 40: 695–712.
6. Zhang Y, Liang J, Qin W, Liu P, von Deneen KM, et al. (2009) Comparison of visual cortical activations induced by electro-acupuncture at vision and nonvision-related acupoints. Neurosci Lett 458: 6–10.
7. Hui KK, Napadow V, Liu J, Li M, Marina O, et al. (2010) Monitoring acupuncture effects on human brain by FMRI. J Vis Exp.
8. Huang W, Pach D, Napadow V, Park K, Long X, et al. (2012) Characterizing acupuncture stimuli using brain imaging with FMRI–a systematic review and meta-analysis of the literature. PLoS One 7: e32960.
9. Liu J, Qin W, Guo Q, Sun J, Yuan K, et al. (2011) Divergent neural processes specific to the acute and sustained phases of verum and SHAM acupuncture. J Magn Reson Imaging 33: 33–40.
10. Feng Y, Bai L, Ren Y, Chen S, Wang H, et al. (2012) FMRI connectivity analysis of acupuncture effects on the whole brain network in mild cognitive impairment patients. Magn Reson Imaging 30: 672–682.
11. Liu P, Zhang Y, Zhou G, Yuan K, Qin W, et al. (2009) Partial correlation investigation on the default mode network involved in acupuncture: an fMRI study. Neurosci Lett 462: 183–187.
12. Hsu SF, Chen CY, Ke MD, Huang CH, Sun YT, et al. (2011) Variations of brain activities of acupuncture to TE5 of left hand in normal subjects. Am J Chin Med 39: 673–686.
13. Qin W, Tian J, Bai L, Pan X, Yang L, et al. (2008) FMRI connectivity analysis of acupuncture effects on an amygdala-associated brain network. Mol Pain 4: 55.
14. Hui KK, Marina O, Clauch JD, Nixon EE, Fang J, et al. (2009) Acupuncture mobilizes the brain's default mode and its anti-correlated network in healthy subjects. Brain Res 1287: 84–103.
15. Dhond RP, Yeh C, Park K, Kettner N, Napadow V (2008) Acupuncture modulates resting state connectivity in default and sensorimotor brain networks. Pain 136: 407–418.
16. Sporns O, Chialvo DR, Kaiser M, Hilgetag CC (2004) Organization, development and function of complex brain networks. Trends Cogn Sci 8: 418–425.
17. Grefkes C, Nowak DA, Eickhoff SB, Dafotakis M, Kust J, et al. (2008) Cortical connectivity after subcortical stroke assessed with functional magnetic resonance imaging. Ann Neurol 63: 236–246.
18. Wang L, Yu C, Chen H, Qin W, He Y, et al. (2010) Dynamic functional reorganization of the motor execution network after stroke. Brain 133: 1224–1238.
19. Askim T, Indredavik B, Vangberg T, Haberg A (2009) Motor network changes associated with successful motor skill relearning after acute ischemic stroke: a longitudinal functional magnetic resonance imaging study. Neurorehabil Neural Repair 23: 295–304.
20. Dinomais M, Groeschel S, Staudt M, Krageloh-Mann I, Wilke M (2012) Relationship between functional connectivity and sensory impairment: red flag or red herring? Hum Brain Mapp 33: 628–638.

21. Gao JH, Parsons LM, Bower JM, Xiong J, Li J, et al. (1996) Cerebellum implicated in sensory acquisition and discrimination rather than motor control. Science 272: 545–547.
22. O'Reilly JX, Beckmann CF, Tomassini V, Ramnani N, Johansen-Berg H (2010) Distinct and overlapping functional zones in the cerebellum defined by resting state functional connectivity. Cereb Cortex 20: 953–965.
23. Breakspear M, Terry JR, Friston KJ (2003) Modulation of excitatory synaptic coupling facilitates synchronization and complex dynamics in a biophysical model of neuronal dynamics. Network 14: 703–732.
24. Grefkes C, Fink GR (2011) Reorganization of cerebral networks after stroke: new insights from neuroimaging with connectivity approaches. Brain 134: 1264–1276.
25. Hummel F, Celnik P, Giraux P, Floel A, Wu WH, et al. (2005) Effects of non-invasive cortical stimulation on skilled motor function in chronic stroke. Brain 128: 490–499.
26. Murase N, Duque J, Mazzocchio R, Cohen LG (2004) Influence of interhemispheric interactions on motor function in chronic stroke. Ann Neurol 55: 400–409.
27. He BJ, Snyder AZ, Vincent JL, Epstein A, Shulman GL, et al. (2007) Breakdown of functional connectivity in frontoparietal networks underlies behavioral deficits in spatial neglect. Neuron 53: 905–918.
28. Nomura EM, Gratton C, Visser RM, Kayser A, Perez F, et al. (2010) Double dissociation of two cognitive control networks in patients with focal brain lesions. Proc Natl Acad Sci U S A 107: 12017–12022.
29. Fang J, Jin Z, Wang Y, Li K, Kong J, et al. (2009) The salient characteristics of the central effects of acupuncture needling: limbic-paralimbic-neocortical network modulation. Hum Brain Mapp 30: 1196–1206.
30. Huang Y, Chen JQ, Lai XS, Tang CZ, Yang JJ, et al. (2013) Lateralisation of cerebral response to active acupuncture in patients with unilateral ischaemic stroke: an fMRI study. Acupunct Med.
31. Schaechter JD, Connell BD, Stason WB, Kaptchuk TJ, Krebs DE, et al. (2007) Correlated change in upper limb function and motor cortex activation after verum and sham acupuncture in patients with chronic stroke. J Altern Complement Med 13: 527–532.
32. Maciocia G (1994) The practice of Chinese medicine: the treatment of diseases with acupuncture and Chinese herbs. Edinburgh, UK: Churchill Livingstone. 342–385 p.
33. Liu B, Liu X, Chen J, Long Y, Chen ZG, et al. (2009) Study on the effects of acupuncture at acupoint and non-acupoint on functional connectivity of different brain regions with functional magnetic resonance imaging. Zhongguo Zhen Jiu 29: 981–985.
34. (1999) MONICA Manual.
35. Cavanna AE, Trimble MR (2006) The precuneus: a review of its functional anatomy and behavioural correlates. Brain 129: 564–583.
36. Johansen-Berg H, Dawes H, Guy C, Smith SM, Wade DT, et al. (2002) Correlation between motor improvements and altered fMRI activity after rehabilitative therapy. Brain 125: 2731–2742.
37. Johansen-Berg H, Rushworth MF, Bogdanovic MD, Kischka U, Wimalaratna S, et al. (2002) The role of ipsilateral premotor cortex in hand movement after stroke. Proc Natl Acad Sci U S A 99: 14518–14523.
38. Small SL, Hlustik P, Noll DC, Genovese C, Solodkin A (2002) Cerebellar hemispheric activation ipsilateral to the paretic hand correlates with functional recovery after stroke. Brain 125: 1544–1557.
39. Leibing E, Leonhardt U, Koster G, Goerlitz A, Rosenfeldt JA, et al. (2002) Acupuncture treatment of chronic low-back pain – a randomized, blinded, placebo-controlled trial with 9-month follow-up. Pain 96: 189–196.
40. Fink MG, Kunsebeck HW, Wippermann B (2000) Effect of needle acupuncture on pain perception and functional impairment of patients with coxarthrosis. Z Rheumatol 59: 191–199.
41. Molsberger AF, Manickavasagan J, Abholz HH, Maixner WB, Endres HG (2012) Acupuncture points are large fields: the fuzziness of acupuncture point localization by doctors in practice. Eur J Pain 16: 1264–1270.
42. Li Y, Liang F, Yang X, Tian X, Yan J, et al. (2009) Acupuncture for treating acute attacks of migraine: a randomized controlled trial. Headache 49: 805–816.
43. Zhong C, Bai L, Dai R, Xue T, Wang H, et al. (2012) Modulatory effects of acupuncture on resting-state networks: a functional MRI study combining independent component analysis and multivariate Granger causality analysis. J Magn Reson Imaging 35: 572–581.
44. Moffet HH (2009) Sham acupuncture may be as efficacious as true acupuncture: a systematic review of clinical trials. J Altern Complement Med 15: 213–216.
45. Wang JJ, Wu ZC (2009) [Thinking about the conclusion of no difference between the acupuncture and sham-acupuncture in the clinically therapeutic effects on migraine abroad]. Zhongguo Zhen Jiu 29: 315–319.

2

Neural Substrate of Initiation of Cross-Modal Working Memory Retrieval

Yangyang Zhang[1,9], Yang Hu[2,9], Shuchen Guan[1], Xiaolong Hong[1], Zhaoxin Wang[2], Xianchun Li[1]*

1 School of Psychology and Cognitive Science, East China Normal University, Shanghai, P. R. China, 2 Institute of Cognitive Neuroscience, East China Normal University, Shanghai, P. R. China

Abstract

Cross-modal working memory requires integrating stimuli from different modalities and it is associated with co-activation of distributed networks in the brain. However, how brain initiates cross-modal working memory retrieval remains not clear yet. In the present study, we developed a cued matching task, in which the necessity for cross-modal/unimodal memory retrieval and its initiation time were controlled by a task cue appeared in the delay period. Using functional magnetic resonance imaging (fMRI), significantly larger brain activations were observed in the left lateral prefrontal cortex (*l*-LPFC), left superior parietal lobe (*l*-SPL), and thalamus in the cued cross-modal matching trials (CCMT) compared to those in the cued unimodal matching trials (CUMT). However, no significant differences in the brain activations prior to task cue were observed for sensory stimulation in the *l*-LPFC and *l*-SPL areas. Although thalamus displayed differential responses to the sensory stimulation between two conditions, the differential responses were not the same with responses to the task cues. These results revealed that the frontoparietal-thalamus network participated in the initiation of cross-modal working memory retrieval. Secondly, the *l*-SPL and thalamus showed differential activations between maintenance and working memory retrieval, which might be associated with the enhanced demand for cognitive resources.

Editor: Andrea Antal, University Medical Center Goettingen, Germany

Funding: This work was supported by (1) National Natural Science Foundation of China (No. 31000501, http://www.nsfc.gov.cn/) and (2) Shanghai Pujiang Program (No. 11PJC044, http://www.stcsm.gov.cn/gk/ywgz/bssx/kyjh/76.htm). The funders had no role in study design, data collection and analysis, decision to publish, or preparation of the manuscript.

Competing Interests: The authors have declared that no competing interests exist.

* Email: xcli@psy.ecnu.edu.cn

9 These authors equally contributed to this work.

Introduction

Working memory is a central cognitive function at the interface of perception and action [1]. It allows humans and animals to use information that is not currently available in the environment. It is necessary for complex cognitive tasks such as language comprehension, learning, decision making and reasoning [2]. Fuster and Alexander (1971) first found that prefrontal neurons displayed persistent discharges during the delay period of a delayed-response task only when monkeys successfully maintained the memoranda [3]. The persistent delay activities are selective depending on the features of the memoranda, such as the spatial location [4], object identity [5] and haptic sensation [6]. Such sustained delay activity has been considered to be the neuronal basis for working memory. Memory cells have been repeatedly observed in prefrontal cortex [7], inferior temporal cortex [8], posterior parietal cortex [9] and subcortical structures [10,11]. Therefore, working memory is associated with a broad network in the brain.

In many cases, working memory requires integration/interaction of different senses [12]. When monkeys were trained to remember a tone of a certain pitch and then choose the color associated with it after delay period, most of prefrontal neurons activated selectively to tones responded to colors according to the association between tone and color. This finding revealed

neuronal responses to a tone in prefrontal cortex were correlated with their subsequent reaction to the associated color, while this correlation faltered in error trials [13]. It suggests that PFC is a member of neural networks related to cross-modal associations. More recently, sensory cortices (such as visual cortex and superior temporal syrus) displayed gradually increased activations as subjects learned both an auditory-visual and visuo-auditory paired-association learning tasks. However, these regions did not significantly change their activations as participants acquired a visuo-visual unimodal association task [14]. The findings indicate some sensory cortices are also involved in cross-modal working memory. A recent PET study also revealed that visual cortex of subjects who had previously been exposed to the audiovisual stimuli showed increased activation after presenting with auditory component of audiovisual events, while visual cortex of naive subjects did not significantly change the responses to auditory components [15]. These findings suggest that cross-modal working memory could be represented by the co-activation of the multiple cortical areas in the brain. In order to elucidate how brain initiates memory retrieval of long-term memory, Naya et al. (1996) trained monkeys to perform a pair-association task (PA task) or conventional delayed matching-to-sample (DMS) task according to a color switch in the middle of the delay period [16]. They

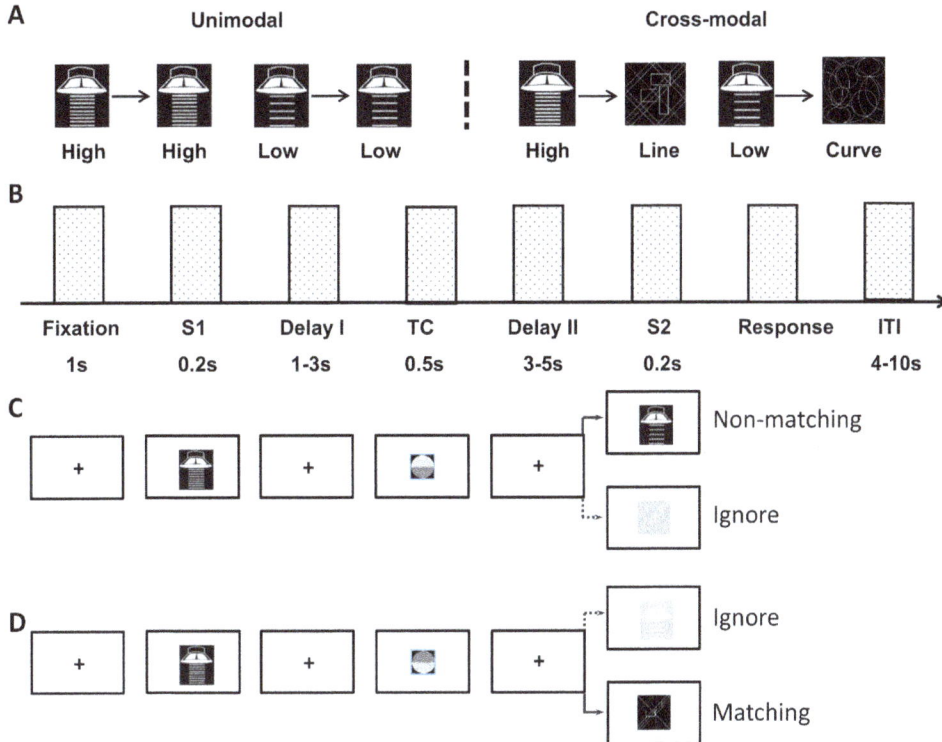

Figure 1. The schematic illustration for the cued matching tasks. *A*: The matching stimuli in the unimodal working memory task (*left*, high tone - high tone and low tone - low tone) and the crossmodal working memory task (*right*, high tone - line and low tone - curve); *B*: The events in a cued matching task trial. The solid arrows after task cue indicate the attended stimulus and the dashed arrows indicate the ignored stimulus according to the feature of task cue. *C*: the cued unimodal matching task (CUMT): S1 (high tone or low tone) with a duration of 200 ms is followed by a TC (a cycle with light-gray in upper half, 500 ms), the auditory (high or low tone) and visual (line or curve) stimuli are simultaneously presented for 200 ms after the Delay II, the participants are asked to attend the auditory stimulus and ignore the visual stimulus, finally they have to report whether the auditory S2 matches the S1 by pressing a button as correctly and quickly as possible. *D*: the cued crossmodal matching task (CCMT): the sequences of the CCMT are identical to the CUMT except that the task cue is the cycle with dark-gray in upper half. The participants are asked to attend the visual stimulus and ignore the auditory stimulus, and report whether the visual S2 matches auditory S1 by pressing a button.

found that many neurons in anterior inferotemporal cortex (AIT) showed increased discharges just after color switch in the PA task compared to the DMS task. They proposed AIT was involved in the initiation of memory retrieval of long-term memory. However, the neural basis of initiation of cross-modal working memory retrieval remains unknown.

Many pieces of evidence have revealed that different networks in the brain are involved in maintenance and manipulation components of working memory. D'Esposito et al (1999) required participants to retain a sequence of letters (maintenance trial) and reorder the sequence in alphabetical order (manipulation trial) during the delay period of delayed response task. They found that Dorsolateral prefrontal cortex (DLPFC) and ventrolateral pre-frontal cortex (VLPFC) enhanced their activations during delay period, but DLPFC displayed significantly higher delay activity in manipulation trials [17]. Therefore, DLPFC exhibit greater recruitment in transformation of information held in working memory. In another fMRI study, Glahn et al (2002) reported superior frontal sulcal area was involved in maintenance spatial information while DLPFC was involved in manipulation of internal representations [18]. However, manipulations in those studies just happened within one kind of modality of information, such as spatial and visual information. Then, which and how brain regions control retaining and manipulating the internal represen-tations held in working memory between different modalities still keep unknown so far.

In the present study, we developed a cued matching task in which the necessity for cross-modal/unimodal memory retrieval and their initiation time were controlled by a task cue appeared in the delay period. Participants were asked to hold sample stimulus (S1, auditory stimulus) in mind till appearance of task cue, then retrieve the associated sensory information (auditory or visual stimulus) according to the task cue, and finally decide whether the attended modality of simultaneous combination of auditory and visual stimuli matched S1 by pressing a button. The cued cross-modal matching trial (CCMT) and unimodal matching trial (CUMT) were presented in a random order in each block. By using this task, we first examined the neural substrates of initiation of cross-modal working memory retrieval by comparison of responses to task cues in CCMT trials with those in CUMT trials. We anticipated that task cue elicited greater activation in frontoparietal network in CCMT trials than in CUMT trials. We secondly investigated whether the differential networks of main-tenance and manipulation processes of cross-modal working memory differed from that of unimodal working memory by comparison of activations between intention period (time gap between sample stimulus and task cue) and memory retrieval period (time gap between task cue and matching stimuli).

Materials and Methods

Participants

Ethics Statement. Ethical approval was obtained from the East China Normal University Internal Review Board. All participants signed their written consent forms before experiment and got certain amount of financial reward as compensation for their time after experiment.

Participants. Twenty healthy college students (8 Women, 22–26 years old) participated in this study. All subjects were in good health with no history of psychiatric or neurological diseases. All of them had normal or corrected-to-normal (with contact lenses) visual acuity and could detect the range of auditory frequencies used in our experiment when presented monaurally.

Stimuli

Auditory stimulus. Two tones with a frequency of either 2 KHz or 0.5 KHz with duration of 200 ms (Fig. 1A) were used as auditory stimuli, and presented dichotically through magnetically compatible headphones.

Visual stimulus. Visual stimuli consisting of either line or curve were randomly generated by Matlab7.0 program (Fig. 1A). Each visual stimulus had a size of 2° visual angle with a duration of 200 ms.

Task cue. Task cue was a cycle with light-gray in half and dark-gray in the other (Fig. 1). The one with lower dark-gray indicated the ongoing trial was a cued unimodal (auditory-auditory) working memory trial (CUMT) (Fig. 1C). The one with upper dark-gray indicated the ongoing trial was a cued cross-modal (auditory-visual) working memory trial (CCMT) (Fig. 1D). Task cues of CCMT and CUMT were randomly presented in each block. Prior to scanning, all subjects were required to learn the meanings of the task cues.

Cued matching task

In the cued matching task, subjects performed a CUMT trial or CCMT depending on task cue trial-to-trial (Fig. 1). They were instructed to retrieve the associated sensory information (auditory or visual stimulus) immediately after task cue, and finally decided whether the attended modality of simultaneous combination of auditory and visual stimuli matched S1 according to task cue by pressing a button (i.e., "1" for matching, "2" for non-matching). Subjects completed 4 blocks of the cued matching task, and each block had 16 CCMT trials and 16 CUMT trials. Each block lasted for 6.8 min, and the inter-block interval was approximately 1 min. Thus the total session lasted for approximately 30 min for each subject. The order of the four blocks was counterbalanced across participants.

The cued unimodal matching trial (CUMT, Fig 1B&C). Each trial began with S1 (auditory stimulus, high tone or low tone) with the duration of 200 ms followed by a Delay-I (Duration of 1 s∼3 s with a step of 0.5 s). Participants were asked to memorize the feature of S1 during Delay-I. The task cue (a cycle with dark-gray in lower half) appeared for 500 ms at the end of Delay-I, participants were asked to retrieve the association between S1 and S2 during Delay-II (Duration of 3 s∼5 s with a step of 0.5 s). At the end of Delay-II, combination of auditory (high or low tone) and visual (line or curve) stimuli as S2 were presented for 200 ms, participants were required to attend the auditory stimulus and ignore the visual stimulus, finally to report whether the auditory S2 matched the S1 by pressing a button as correctly and quickly as possible (i.e., high tone-high tone and low tone-low tone).

The cued cross-modal matching trial (CCMT, Fig 1B&D). The procedures of CCMT were identical to CUMT except (1) task cue (a cycle with dark-gray in upper half) and (2) the matching stimuli (high tone-line and low tone-curve). The participants were asked to attend the visual stimulus and ignore the auditory stimulus, and to report whether the visual S2 matches auditory S1 by pressing a button.

Image acquisition

Imaging data were collected by a 3 T Siemens Trio MR scanner equipped with a head volume coil, with one anatomical run and four functional runs in total. The high-resolution structural image (matrix = 256×256, FOV = 240×240 mm^2, slice thickness = 1 mm, TR = 1900 ms, TE = 3.43 ms, flip angle = 7°) for each participant was recorded using 3D MRI sequences for anatomical co-registration and normalization. Functional MRI data were obtained using a T2*-weighted echo planar imaging (EPI) sequence (FOV = 240×240 mm^2, matrix = 64×64, in-plane resolution = 3.75×3.75 mm^2, thickness = 4 mm, without gap, TR = 2000 ms, TE = 30 ms, flip angle = 90°).

Image analysis

Data from 3 participants were excluded from further data analysis because of failure to accomplish the task, low behavioral performance (accuracy <70%) or serious head movements (> 2 mm), respectively. Functional MRI data were analyzed by SPM8 (http://www.fil.ion.ucl.ac.uk/spm, Welcome Department of Cognitive Neurology). EPI data were first corrected for the order of slice acquisition and then realigned to the first volume within a series to correct for head motion. Next, the structural image was co-registered to the mean EPI data, segmented and generated normalized parameters to MNI space. All EPI data were then normalized to the MNI space with a resolution of $2\times2\times2$ mm^3 and smoothed with an 8-mm FWHM (full width half maximum) Gaussian kernel. High-pass temporal filtering with a cut-off of 128 s was also carried out to remove low-frequency drifts.

Whole-brain analysis. In the first level analysis, 6 task-related regressors (i.e. unimodal S1, cross-modal S1, unimodal task cue, cross-modal task cue, auditory S2 and visual S2 convolved with the canonical hemodynamic response function (HRF) were included in a general linear model (GLM), which also included 6 additional estimated parameters of head movement to rule out the effect of head motion. Statistical parameter estimates from each participant were then put into the second-level analysis based on the random-effect to allow population inference. One-sample T-test was adopted to compare the activation pattern either between different sensory modalities during the same processing phase (e.g. unimodal task cue *v.s.* cross-modal task cue) or between different processing phases in the same sensory modality (e.g. task cue *v.s.* S1). The results were reported with a voxel-wise threshold of $p < 0.001$ (uncorrected) with a spatial extent threshold of $k = 20$.

Region-of-Interest (ROI) analysis. To further explore the activity of the task-related regions across conditions, ROI analysis was also performed via MarsBar (http://marsbar.sourceforge.net). Three ROIs was defined based on the clusters showing responses to cross-modal task cue (*v.s.* unimodal task cue) in the previous whole-brain analysis with a voxel-wise threshold of $p < 0.001$ (uncorrected). The maximal MNI coordinates of these ROIs were listed as follows: left lateral prefrontal cortex (*l*-LPFC, BA 9; x/y/z = −42/10/32), left superior parietal lobule (*l*-SPL, BA 7; x/y/z = −26/−56/44), and thalamus (x/y/z = −12/−22/12). For each ROI, the percentage signal change and fitted time course in each condition of each participant was extracted, which were then put into SPSS 16.0 (Chicago, IL) for further analysis.

Results

Behavioral performance

The averaged correct rate and reaction time in those correct trials were analyzed for both the cued unimodal matching trials (CUMT) and the cued cross-modal matching trials (CCMT). The correct rates were closed to 90% in both trials, and did not show significant difference between CUMT and CCMT trials (Fig. 2A, $p>0.05$, student t-test). The reaction times in the CCMT condition was statistically shorter than that in the CUMT condition (Fig. 2B, 480.7 ms $v.s.$ 690 ms, $p<0.001$, student t-test). We did not find significant gender difference in correct rates ($t_{(15)}=0$, $p=1$) or reaction times ($t_{(15)}=1.29$, $p=0.22$). Our behavioral results revealed that cross-modal association facilitated the retrieval of memorized information.

Neuroimaging results

Whole brain analysis. To elucidate which brain areas were involved in the initiation of cross-modal working memory retrieval, the activations in whole brain induced by the task cues were first contrasted between the CCMT and CUMT conditions (Table 1). The activations in left lateral prefrontal cortex (l-LPFC, BA9), left posterior parietal cortex, including superior parietal lobe (l-SPL, BA7) and inferior parietal lobe (l-IPL, BA40), and thalamus in the CCMT condition were significantly greater compared to that in the CUMT condition (Table 1 and Fig. 3A, $p<0.001$, uncorrected). However, fewer regions were found to have significantly

greater task cue related activity in the CUMT condition than that in the CCMT condition (Fig. 3B).

The ROI analysis. Next, we functionally define ROIs in l-LPFC (Fig. 4A), l-SPL (Fig. 4C) and the left/right thalamus (Fig. 4E). The percentages of signal change produced by task cue in the CCMT trials were much higher than that in the CUMT trials in l-LPFC (Fig. 4B *right, student t-test, p<0.001*), l-SPL (Fig. 4D *right, student t-test, p<0.001*) and thalamus (Fig. 4F *right, student t-test, p<0.001*) areas. However, responses to S1 in both l-LPFC and l-SPL were not significantly different between CUMT and CCMT conditions (Fig. 4B&D). The responses in thalamus induced by task cue displayed in the opposite pattern during Delay-I (Fig. 4F).

All these data indicated that the network consisting of l-LPFC, l-SPL and thalamus might be associated with initiation of cross-modal working memory retrieval.

Comparisons of activations between S1 stimulation and task cue

In order to examine the differential activations in these brain areas related to the maintenance of sample stimulus (S1) and initiation of working memory retrieval in the cued matching task, we compared the activations produced by task cue with the activations induced by S1 for each cued matching task. The activation of l-LPFC after S1 was not different from that after task cue onset in both CUMT and CCMT conditions (Fig. 4B, *student t-test, p>0.05*). However, the response to task cue in l-SPL was significantly higher than that to S1 in both CUMT (Fig. 4D, *student t-test, p<0.01*) and CCMT condition (Fig. 4D, *student t-test, p<0.001*). Thalamus showed reduced reactivation after task cue compared to S1 in the cued unimodal matching task (Fig. 4F, *student t-test, p<0.01*) while it did not show any difference in the cued cross-modal matching task (Fig. 4F, *student t-test, p>0.05*). Therefore, the memory maintenance and working memory retrieval might facilitate by different brain networks, especially in posterior parietal lobe and thalamus. More interestingly, the differential activation of posterior parietal lobe and thalamus in cross-modal working memory was different from those in unimodal working memory.

Discussion

The main purpose of the present study was to investigate how the brain initiated cross-modal working memory retrieval based on task cue appeared in the middle of delay period of a cued matching task by event-related fMRI methods. We found that greater activation generated by task cues in several brain regions in cross-modal condition than that in unimodal condition, including l-LPFC (BA9), l-SPL (BA7) and bilateral thalamus. However, no difference of responses to sample stimulus (S1, auditory stimulus) was found between cross-modal and unimodal conditions. Our data indicated these brain areas might be related to the initiation of cross-modal working memory retrieval. Secondly, differential activations during Delay-II (time gap between task cue and S2) versus Delay-I (time gap between S1 and task cue) between cross-modal condition and unimodal condition were observed in both l-SPL and thalamus. These data indicated the differential network underlying the maintenance and memory retrieval of working memory in cross-modal working memory differed from that in unimodal working memory, which could be associated with different levels of demand for cognitive resources.

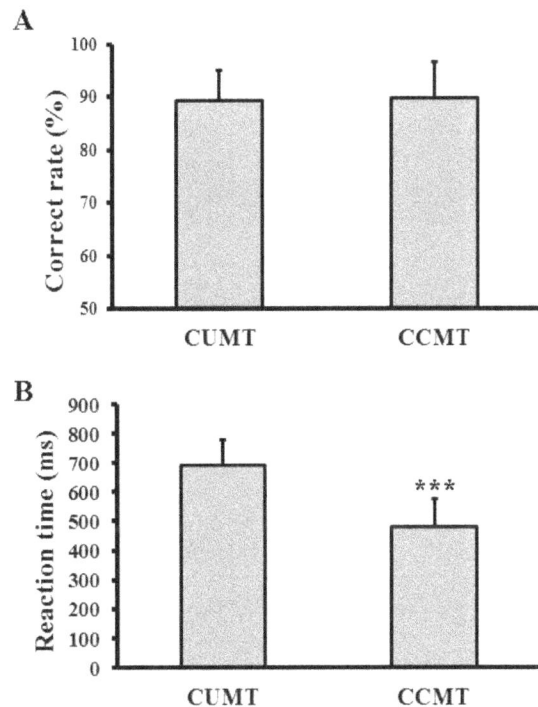

Figure 2. The behavioral performance of the cued matching task. *A*: Correct rate; *B*: Reaction time. CUMT indicates the cued unimodal matching trial. CCMT indicates the cued cross-modal matching trial. The error bars mean the standard deviations; ***$p<$ 0.001 (student t-test).

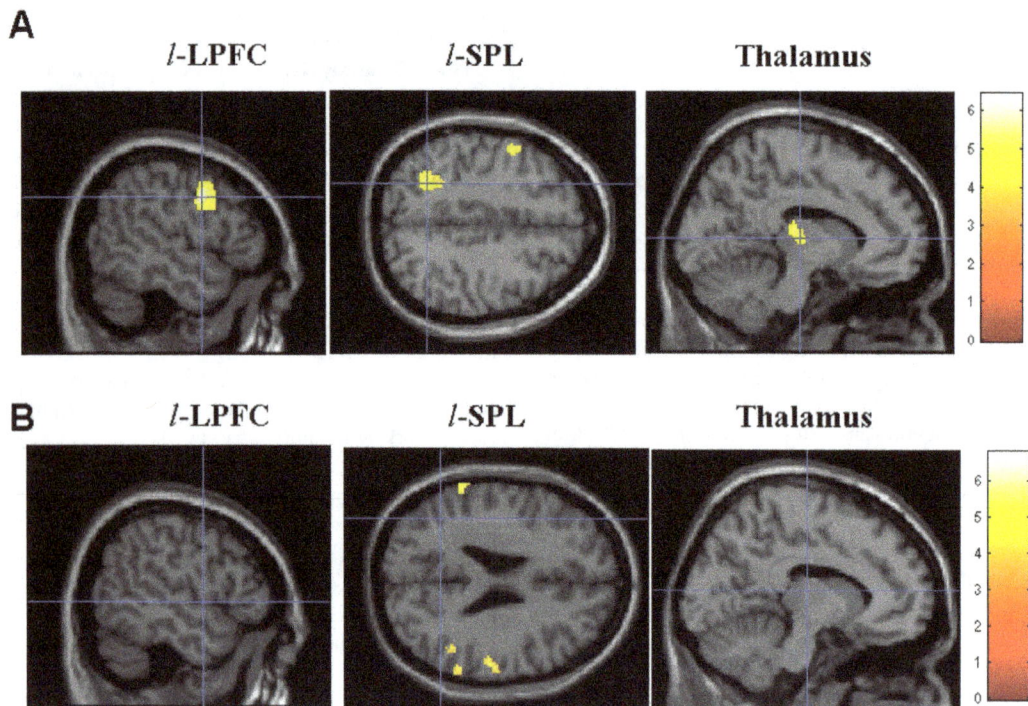

Figure 3. Brain regions related to initiation of cross-modal working memory retrieval ($p<0.001$, uncorrected, k = 100). *A*: the areas displaying stronger activities in CCMT trials compared to the CUMT trials; *B*: the areas displaying stronger activities in CUMT trials compared to the CCMT trials. *l*-LPFC (X = −50): left lateral prefrontal cortex; *l*-SPL (Z = 44): left superior parietal lobe; Thalamus(X = −10).

The frontoparietal network and initiation of cross-modal working memory retrieval

The flexibility of human or animal behavior depends on the ability to choose appropriate actions according to not only the sensory information at hand but also the information retrieved from memory. In present study, participants were required to recognize the feature of sample stimulus (high or low tone) and keep it in mind during delay-I period, which was mainly related to maintenance of working memory. Then, they were asked to retrieve and expect the associated auditory stimulus in CUMT trials or visual stimulus in CCMT trials during Delay-II period, which might be mainly related to working memory retrieval. Therefore, the cognitive components during delay-I should be identical between the CCMT and CUMT trials, while cognitive components during delay-II period in CCMT trials should differ from those in CUMT trials, which was associated with initiation of cross-modal working memory retrieval controlled by task cue. Our neuroimaging results showed that frontoparietal network consisting of *l*-LPFC and *l*-SPL did display much stronger activations during Delay-II period in CCMT trials compared to in the CUMT trials while similar activations of those areas during delay-I period were obtained between these two conditions. Therefore, we proposed that the frontoparietal loops participated in the initiation of cross-modal working memory retrieval when participants performed a cued matching task. In our follow-up experiment, the S1 in the cued matching task was changed into visual stimulus (line or curve). When participants performed new cued matching task, we found that those brain areas also show greater responses to task cue in CCMT trials than in CUMT trials (data did not show here). Therefore, our data indicated that network related to initiation of cross-modal memory retrieval was independent of the modality of sample sensory information in the cued matching task.

Using single-cell recording method, several lines of evidence suggest that neuronal activity in prefrontal cortex to an identical stimulus could significantly vary as a function of which portion of that stimulus must be attended [5], the specific motor response associated with it [19] and task context [20]. Accumulating evidence has demonstrated dorsolateral prefrontal cortex is rich with rule-dependent neurons [21]. In a recent fMRI study, Chiu et al (2011) reported that a network of dorsal frontoparietal regions (left middle frontal gyrus and left inferior and superior parietal lobule) exhibited distinct patterns for race and gender discriminations of face, suggesting that these regions may represent abstract goals during high-level categorization tasks [22]. When participants performed the different stimulus-response mapping tasks according to the instruction cue (screen color) indicating which rule should be applied, Woolgar et al (2011) demonstrated that a network of frontoparietal regions (including LPFC and IPS) was associated with representation of task-relevant information [23].

The PPC is also known to play a crucial role in the integration of different modalities of stimuli [24]. When subjects were instructed to perform motion discrimination task under the simultaneous presentation of visual stimulus and tactile stimulus, the left SPL was more prominently activated under the congruent event conditions than under incongruent conditions [25], which indicating SPL involves in cross-modal integration among different sensory modalities. Using intracranial recording [26] and EEG/ERP recording [27] on humans, the SPL had been showed greater activation to multisensory stimuli than that to the sum of responses to each uni-sensory stimulus. Shomstein and Yantis (2004) demonstrated that posterior parietal and superior prefrontal cortices exhibited transient increased activity produced by the initiation of voluntary attention shifts between vision and audition [28]. These findings revealed that posterior parietal and superior

Table 1. Summary of brain areas showing greater activation to task cue in CCMT than CUMT conditions ($p < 0.001$, uncorrected, k = 20).

Brain areas	t	k	Hemisphere	MNI Coordinate		
				x	y	z
Middle/Inferior Frontal Gyrus	6.44	419	L	-42	10	32
Superior Parietal Lobule	5.23	266	L	-26	-58	44
Thalamus	5.22	160	L/R	-12	-22	12
Inferior Parietal Lobule/Sub-Gyral	4.16	79	L	-44	-36	42
Middle Frontal Gyrus	4.21	55	L	-32	0	58
Lingual Gyrus	4.27	46	L	-20	-90	-2
Insula	4.54	43	R	32	-24	22
Cingulate Gyrus	5.74	28	R	8	2	29
Middle Frontal Gyrus	4.20	25	R	28	-6	48

CUMT indicates the cued unimodal matching trial, CCMT indicates the cued cross-modal matching trial.

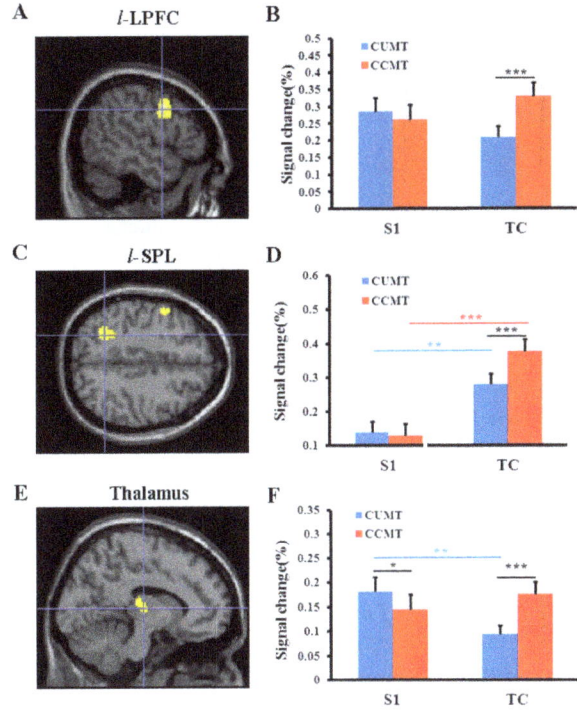

Figure 4. The ROI analysis of Brain activations to S1 stimulus and task. *A and B* (*l*-LPFC, X = −50): left lateral prefrontal cortex; *C and D* (*l*-SPL, Z = 44): left superior parietal lobe; *E and F* (Thalamus, X = −10); *S1*: the first stimulus (high tone or low tone) in the cued matching task; *TC*: the task cue in the cued matching task; Error bars corresponded to the standard error of mean; *p < 0.05, **p < 0.01, ***p < 0.001 (student t-test).

prefrontal cortices played an important role in the control of cross-modal shifts of attention.

All findings above suggested that the PFC and PPC might participate in maintaining rule information in cognition task. In present study, left frontoparietal network including *l*-LPFC and *l*-SPL showed stronger response to the task cues in the cross-modal matching trials compared to the unimodal matching trials while no differential responses to S1 were found between two conditions. In addition, the activation patterns were not observed in right side of the brain. These finding suggests that left frontoparietal network might play a more important role in the initiation of cross-modal working memory retrieval compared to right lateralization of brain. This finding is consistent with previous studies, such as, Tanabe et al (2005) reported that stronger left-lateralized activation than right-side of brain when subjects completed the visuo-auditory cross-modal association learning task [14]. The finding in our study was also consistent with the idea that auditory working memory activated left lateral prefrontal cortex and left parietal cortex [15].

Thalamus and initiation of cross-modal working memory

Converging evidence by anatomical multiple tracing methods have demonstrated there exists widely distributed thalamocortical and corticothalamic connections between different sensory and motor cortical areas and thalamic nuclei [29], which suggests the thalamus could act as a relay in multisensory processing [30]. In particular, the medial pulvinar nucleus (PuM) contains neurons projecting to the auditory cortex, the somatosensory cortex, the visual cortex, and the premotor cortex [31]. Previous studies on monkeys revealed that neurons in PuM could respond to visual stimuli [32] and auditory stimuli [33]. Therefore, the PuM is considered as the main candidate (although other thalamic nuclei may also play a role) to represent an alternative to corticocortical loops by which information can be transferred between cortical areas belonging to different sensory and sensorimotor modalities. Komura et al (2005) reported when rat performed an auditory spatial discrimination task, about 15% of neurons in the auditory thalamic nuclei displayed significantly higher discharges after simultaneous presentation of auditory and visual stimuli in the same side of animal than the sum of the unimodal responses [34]. Therefore, thalamus takes part in multisensory integration in addition to relay of sensory information through the cortico-thalamo-cortical route [35]. Using cued matching task in our present study, we found that thalamus displayed much stronger activation to task cue in CCMT trials compared to that in CUMT trials. These data indicated that thalamus might play an important role in the initiation of cross-modal memory retrieval, meanwhile we also provided the evidence for functional role of thalamus in multisensory integration. In our present study, we did not find any significant differential activation in hippocampus after appearance of task cue. Lot of evidence has shown that hippocampus is very important for acquision of memory [36,37] and working memory [38], few study has been found so far to support hippocampus plays very important role in cross-modal working memory. Our present findings indicate again that hippocampus plays much less important role than fronto-parietal network in some higher functions (such task switching, decision making, initiation of cross-modal working memory and so on).

Previous studies have demonstrated that dyslexia [39] and autism [40] patients display a significant deficit in integration of multisensory information. The deficit in the integration of letters and speech sounds is one of causes of reading and spelling failure in dyslexia [39]. Our data provided neurofunctional evidence for potential training approach to improvements of symptoms by increased activation of brain areas related to initiation of cross-modal association.

References

1. Linden DE (2007) The working memory networks of the human brain. Neuroscientist 13: 257–267.
2. Baddeley A (2010) Working memory. Curr Biol 20: R136–140.
3. Fuster JM, Alexander GE (1971) Neuron activity related to short-term memory. Science 173: 652–654.
4. Funahashi S, Bruce CJ, Goldman-Rakic PS (1989) Mnemonic coding of visual space in the monkey's dorsolateral prefrontal cortex. J Neurophysiol 61: 331–349.
5. Rainer G, Asaad WF, Miller EK (1998) Selective representation of relevant information by neurons in the primate prefrontal cortex. Nature 393: 577–579.
6. Wang L, Li X, Hsiao SS, Bodner M, Lenz F, et al. (2012) Persistent neuronal firing in primary somatosensory cortex in the absence of working memory of trial-specific features of the sample stimuli in a haptic working memory task. J Cogn Neurosci 24: 664–676.
7. Curtis CE, D'Esposito M (2003) Persistent activity in the prefrontal cortex during working memory. Trends Cogn Sci 7: 415–423.
8. Fuster JM, Jervey JP (1982) Neuronal firing in the inferotemporal cortex of the monkey in a visual memory task. J Neurosci 2: 361–375.
9. Constantinidis C, Steinmetz MA (1996) Neuronal activity in posterior parietal area 7a during the delay periods of a spatial memory task. J Neurophysiol 76: 1352–1355.
10. Watanabe Y, Funahashi S (2004) Neuronal activity throughout the primate mediodorsal nucleus of the thalamus during oculomotor delayed-responses. II. Activity encoding visual versus motor signal. Journal of Neurophysiology 92: 1756–1769.
11. Hikosaka O (2007) Basal ganglia mechanisms of reward-oriented eye movement. Ann N Y Acad Sci 1104: 229–249.
12. Stein BE, Huneycutt WS, Meredith MA (1988) Neurons and Behavior - the Same Rules of Multisensory Integration Apply. Brain Research 448: 355–358.
13. Fuster JM, Bodner M, Kroger JK (2000) Cross-modal and cross-temporal association in neurons of frontal cortex. Nature 405: 347–351.

Differential neural responses to maintenance and memory retrieval in between cross-modal and unimodal working memory

Accumulating evidence has shown that dissociated frontoparietal networks in the brain were related to short-term maintenance and manipulation processes in spatial [18] and object working memory [17]. Moreover, schizophrenic patients performed worse than healthy controls when faced with manipulation as compared to only maintenance [41]. Mohr et al (2006) found that higher fMRI signal during the delay period of the maintenance task was observed in right superior frontal gyrus and right rostral medial frontal gyrus, while the precuneus and inferior parietal lobles displayed stronger activations during delay period of the manipulation task [42]. In our study, we proposed that main cognitive process should be maintenance of the sensory information during the Delay-I, while one of most important cognition after task cue was the retrieval of the matching stimulus based on task cue, which could be related to memory retrieval (or manipulation of working memory). Our neuroimaging result showed that much higher activations in l-SPL after task cue compared to Delay-I in both unimodal working memory and cross-modal working memory. Therefore, our data also suggest that l-SPL played a more important role in the manipulation than maintenance of working memory. More interestingly, we also found the similar dissociation in thalamus. We proposed that PPC and thalamus might be the members of the neural networks encoding different components of working memory.

Acknowledgments

We thank Prof. Xiuyan Guo and Prof. Yi Hu for their comments.

Author Contributions

Conceived and designed the experiments: XCL. Performed the experiments: YYZ YH XLH. Analyzed the data: YYZ YH SCG ZXW. Wrote the paper: SCG XCL.

14. Tanabe HC, Honda M, Sadato N (2005) Functionally segregated neural substrates for arbitrary audiovisual paired-association learning. Journal of Neuroscience 25: 6409–6418.
15. Zangenehpour S, Zatorre RJ (2010) Crossmodal recruitment of primary visual cortex following brief exposure to bimodal audiovisual stimuli. Neuropsychologia 48: 591–600.
16. Naya Y, Sakai K, Miyashita Y (1996) Activity of primate inferotemporal neurons related to a sought target in pair-association task. Proc Natl Acad Sci U S A 93: 2664–2669.
17. D'Esposito M, Postle BR, Ballard D, Lease J (1999) Maintenance versus manipulation of information held in working memory: an event-related fMRI study. Brain Cogn 41: 66–86.
18. Glahn DC, Kim J, Cohen MS, Poutanen VP, Therman S, et al. (2002) Maintenance and manipulation in spatial working memory: Dissociations in the prefrontal cortex. Neuroimage 17: 201–213.
19. Asaad WF, Rainer G, Miller EK (1998) Neural activity in the primate prefrontal cortex during associative learning. Neuron 21: 1399–1407.
20. Warden MR, Miller EK (2007) The representation of multiple objects in prefrontal neuronal delay activity. Cereb Cortex 17 Suppl 1: i41–50.
21. Cole MW, Etzel JA, Zacks JM, Schneider W, Braver TS (2011) Rapid transfer of abstract rules to novel contexts in human lateral prefrontal cortex. Front Hum Neurosci 5: 142.
22. Chiu YC, Esterman M, Han Y, Rosen H, Yantis S (2011) Decoding task-based attentional modulation during face categorization. J Cogn Neurosci 23: 1198–1204.
23. Woolgar A, Thompson R, Bor D, Duncan J (2011) Multi-voxel coding of stimuli, rules, and responses in human frontoparietal cortex. Neuroimage 56: 744–752.
24. Lloyd D, Morrison I, Roberts N (2006) Role for human posterior parietal cortex in visual processing of aversive objects in peripersonal space. J Neurophysiol 95: 205–214.

25. Nakashita S, Saito DN, Kochiyama T, Honda M, Tanabe HC, et al. (2008) Tactile-visual integration in the posterior parietal cortex: a functional magnetic resonance imaging study. Brain Res Bull 75: 513–525.

26. Molholm S, Sehatpour P, Mehta AD, Shpaner M, Gomez-Ramirez M, et al. (2006) Audio-visual multisensory integration in superior parietal lobule revealed by human intracranial recordings. J Neurophysiol 96: 721–729.

27. Moran RJ, Molholm S, Reilly RB, Foxe JJ (2008) Changes in effective connectivity of human superior parietal lobule under multisensory and unisensory stimulation. Eur J Neurosci 27: 2303–2312.

28. Shomstein S, Yantis S (2004) Control of attention shifts between vision and audition in human cortex. J Neurosci 24: 10702–10706.

29. Cappe C, Morel A, Barone P, Rouiller EM (2009) The Thalamocortical Projection Systems in Primate: An Anatomical Support for Multisensory and Sensorimotor Interplay. Cerebral Cortex 19: 2025–2037.

30. Cappe C, Rouiller EM, Barone P (2012) Cortical and Thalamic Pathways for Multisensory and Sensorimotor Interplay. In: Murray MM, Wallace MT, editors. The Neural Bases of Multisensory Processes. Boca Raton (FL).

31. Viaene AN, Petrof I, Sherman SM (2011) Synaptic properties of thalamic input to layers 2/3 and 4 of primary somatosensory and auditory cortices. J Neurophysiol 105: 279–292.

32. Gattass R, Oswaldo-Cruz E, Sousa AP (1979) Visual receptive fields of units in the pulvinar of cebus monkey. Brain Res 160: 413–430.

33. Yirmiya R, Hocherman S (1987) Auditory- and movement-related neural activity interact in the pulvinar of the behaving rhesus monkey. Brain Res 402: 93–102.

34. Komura Y, Tamura R, Uwano T, Nishijo H, Ono T (2005) Auditory thalamus integrates visual inputs into behavioral gains. Nature Neuroscience 8: 1203–1209.

35. Sherman SM, Guillery RW (2011) Distinct functions for direct and transthalamic corticocortical connections. J Neurophysiol 106: 1068–1077.

36. Travis SG, Huang Y, Fujiwara E, Radomski A, Olsen F, et al. (2014) High field structural MRI reveals specific episodic memory correlates in the subfields of the hippocampus. Neuropsychologia 53: 233–245.

37. Ramirez S, Tonegawa S, Liu X (2013) Identification and optogenetic manipulation of memory engrams in the hippocampus. Front Behav Neurosci 7: 226.

38. Meck WH, Church RM, Olton DS (2013) Hippocampus, time, and memory. Behav Neurosci 127: 655–668.

39. Blau V, van Atteveldt N, Ekkebus M, Goebel R, Blomert L (2009) Reduced neural integration of letters and speech sounds links phonological and reading deficits in adult dyslexia. Curr Biol 19: 503–508.

40. Foss-Feig JH, Kwakye LD, Cascio CJ, Burnette CP, Kadivar H, et al. (2010) An extended multisensory temporal binding window in autism spectrum disorders. Exp Brain Res 203: 381–389.

41. Hill SK, Griffin GB, Miura TK, Herbener ES, Sweeney JA (2010) Salience of working-memory maintenance and manipulation deficits in schizophrenia. Psychol Med 40: 1979–1986.

42. Mohr HM, Goebel R, Linden DE (2006) Content- and task-specific dissociations of frontal activity during maintenance and manipulation in visual working memory. J Neurosci 26: 4465–4471.

3

How Art Changes Your Brain: Differential Effects of Visual Art Production and Cognitive Art Evaluation on Functional Brain Connectivity

Anne Bolwerk[1,2], Jessica Mack-Andrick[3], Frieder R. Lang[4], Arnd Dörfler[5], Christian Maihöfner[1,2]*

1 Department of Neurology, University Hospital Erlangen, Erlangen, Germany, 2 Department of Physiology and Pathophysiology, Friedrich-Alexander-University Erlangen-Nürnberg, Erlangen, Germany, 3 Education Department of the Museums in Nuremberg, Nuremberg, Germany, 4 Institute of Psychogerontology, Friedrich-Alexander-University Erlangen-Nürnberg, Nuremberg, Germany, 5 Department of Neuroradiology, University Hospital Erlangen, Erlangen, Germany

Abstract

Visual art represents a powerful resource for mental and physical well-being. However, little is known about the underlying effects at a neural level. A critical question is whether visual art production and cognitive art evaluation may have different effects on the functional interplay of the brain's default mode network (DMN). We used fMRI to investigate the DMN of a non-clinical sample of 28 post-retirement adults (63.71 years ±3.52 SD) before (T0) and after (T1) weekly participation in two different 10-week-long art interventions. Participants were randomly assigned to groups stratified by gender and age. In the visual art production group 14 participants actively produced art in an art class. In the cognitive art evaluation group 14 participants cognitively evaluated artwork at a museum. The DMN of both groups was identified by using a seed voxel correlation analysis (SCA) in the posterior cingulated cortex (PCC/preCUN). An analysis of covariance (ANCOVA) was employed to relate fMRI data to psychological resilience which was measured with the brief German counterpart of the Resilience Scale (RS-11). We observed that the visual art production group showed greater spatial improvement in functional connectivity of PCC/preCUN to the frontal and parietal cortices from T0 to T1 than the cognitive art evaluation group. Moreover, the functional connectivity in the visual art production group was related to psychological resilience (i.e., stress resistance) at T1. Our findings are the first to demonstrate the neural effects of visual art production on psychological resilience in adulthood.

Editor: Yong He, Beijing Normal University, Beijing, China

Funding: This work was supported by the STAEDTLER Foundation. The funder had no role in study design, data collection and analysis, decision to publish, or preparation of the manuscript.

Competing Interests: The authors have declared that no competing interests exist.

* Email: christian.maihoefner@uk-erlangen.de

Introduction

Recent research on visual art has focused on its psychological and physiological effects, mostly in clinical populations. It has shown that visual art interventions have stabilizing effects on the individual by reducing distress, increasing self-reflection and self-awareness, altering behaviour and thinking patterns, and also by normalizing heart rate, blood pressure, or even cortisol levels [1], [2], [3], [4], [5]. The extent to which visual art may also affect the functional neuroanatomy of the healthy human brain remains an open question.

A few fMRI studies have addressed the neural correlates of novel visual form production or have focused on the aesthetic experiences of visual artwork, the activation of the reward circuit by visual art perception for example [6]. Distinct brain areas of a certain resting state network, the default mode network (DMN), are thought to be associated with cognitive processes such as introspection, self-monitoring, prospection, episodic and autobiographic memory, and comprehension of the emotional states and intentions of others [7], [8], [9]. The DMN is characterized by positive and negative connectivity between the dorsal and ventral medial prefrontal cortex (MPFC), the medial parietal cortex (posterior and anterior cingulate cortex (PCC; ACC), precuneus (preCUN)), and the inferior parietal cortex during rest [7], [10], [11], [12]. Given the resource enhancing effects of visual arts, we hypothesized that participation in 10-week-long visual art groups may result in psychological changes and may alter the functional interplay of the DMN. Therefore, we used fMRI to investigate the DMN of a non-clinical sample of 28 post-retirement adults before (T0) and after (T1) participating in a visual art production group (8 female, 6 males, mean age 63.50 years ±3.80 SD) or in a cognitive art evaluation group (7 female, 7 males, mean age 63.93 years ±3.34 SD). The participants were randomly assigned to groups, which were stratified by gender and age. The cognitive art evaluation group served as a means of controlling for other possible alternative explanations of changes in the visual art production intervention that may have been related to group interaction, art reception, and cognitive activity, group activity and cognitive activity were thus considered to be present in both intervention groups. Transition into retirement has been found to be associated with well-being, stress experience, and health conditions [13]. The effects of job characteristics and pre-retirement resources on the well-being of retirees are also well documented [14]. Not much is known, however, about the possible effects of post-retirement activity on the stabilization of well-being [15]. Typically, normal ageing is accompanied by changes in brain physiology that involve neural degeneration but by compensatory mechanisms as well [16]. Therefore, we expected that post-retirement adults would be susceptible to the stabilizing effects of receiving artistic training. To understand the psychological relevance of functional changes, we assessed psychological resilience, i.e. stress resistance. Psychological resilience is conceptualized as a protective personality characteristic that allows individuals to control negatives effects of stress and thus enables a successful and healthy functioning even in stressful life conditions [17], [18]. Its neural correlates are thought to be located in the MPFC, which forms a core component of the DMN [19]. To test our results regarding functional connectivity in the DMN, we used the visual cortex (VisCx) as a control site. Due to the pivotal role of the primary sensory and motor cortices (S1/M1) in sensory and motor processing, we also studied the functional connectivity of S1/M1 at rest.

Materials and Methods

Experimental Design

From February through April 2011, 28 participants were recruited via advertisements in local newspapers. The study included participants who were between the ages of 62 and 70 (± 2 years) and who had been retired for at least 3 months but no longer than 3 years. The participants also needed to have sufficient time available over a period of 10 weeks for attending the art class interventions. Excluded from participation were professional visual artists and art historians, as well as people suffering from serious physical or mental disorders or taking psychotropic drugs. Table 1 shows the epidemiologic data. All participants completed a psychological examination and an fMRI measurement on 2 occasions: at pre-intervention (T0) and at post-intervention 10 weeks later (T1). The psychological examination consisted of the brief German version of the Resilience Scale (RS-11) by Wagnild & Young (1993) which is a valid and reliable instrument for measuring the individuals' capacity of stress resistance in elderly participants [18], [20], [21]. Participants rated their accordance of 11 resilience items on a 7-point Likert scale ranging from 1 (never) to 7 (always). Before the fMRI measurement, all participants were instructed to keep their eyes closed during the scan, to be relaxed but to not fall asleep. After the functional measurement the participants were asked if they followed the instructions. All participants were informed about the procedures of the study and gave informed written consent in line with the Declaration of Helsinki. The study was approved by the local ethics committees of the University of Erlangen-Nuremberg.

Art Interventions

Two different art interventions took place, each lasting two hours and occurring once a week for 10 weeks in the Germanisches Nationalmuseum and in the rooms of the Art Education Department of the Museums in Nuremberg (Germany). The two interventions were based on different methodological concepts. In the visual art production group the participants actively created art, and in the cognitive art evaluation group the participants cognitively evaluated pieces of art. The concept of visual art production intervention focused on discovering and developing the participant's own creativity. A visual artist trained as an art educator introduced different artistic methods and materials used in drawing and painting, and the participants were then able to experiment with different materials and techniques. Each participant was encouraged to produce visual art and find their own personal form of artistic expression. Each session

adhered closely to a precisely defined schedule, which included a sequence of thematic foci such as blind or fast drawing, drawing in the space/room, drawing still lives and figures, drawing with music, using colours, and composition. In the cognitive art evaluation group participants considered, analysed, and interpreted selected paintings and sculptures, in dialogue with a qualified art historian. The art historian helped encourage group discussion by providing expert background information and explaining associations between the work of art and everyday experiences. In each session the pre-defined schedule was strictly adhered to, and participants were required to consider two pieces of art that involved universal human concerns such as age, youth, love, lust, violence, the experience of nature, or faith. Such methodological concepts might improve the art experience [22], [23], [24].

FMRI Data Acquisition

Echoplanar images were collected on a 3 Tesla MRI scanner (Trio, Siemens Healthcare, Erlangen, Germany) using the standard head coil in the following order: First, a T1-weighted three-dimensional magnetization prepared rapid acquisition gradient-echo sequence (MPRAGE) scan (voxel size $= 1.0 \times 1.0 \times 1.0$ mm^3) was recorded for the individual brain anatomy and lasted 8 min and 21 s. Then, for each participant the time-series of 150 whole-brain images were obtained with a gradient-echo, echo-planar scanning sequence (EPI; TR 3 s, time to echo 40 ms, flip angle 90°; field of view 220×220 mm, acquisition matrix 128×128, 24 axial slices, slice thickness 4 mm, and gap 1 mm). The functional MRI data scan lasted 7 min and 30 s.

FMRI Data Analysis

Data analysis, registration, and visualization were performed with Brain Voyager QX version 1.10 (Brain Innovation, Maastricht, Netherlands). Data-motion-correction was implemented by the installed software package (Siemens, syngo MR B15) of the scanner. Afterwards, the data were motion corrected using sinc interpolation. Preprocessing also included Gaussian spatial (full width at half maximum (FWHM) =4 mm) and temporal (FWHM =3 volumes) smoothing of the functional data to reduce artefacts. The functional data were then linear-interpolated to $3.0 \times 3.0 \times 3.0$ mm^3 resolution and transformed into a standard stereoactic coordinate system of Talairach & Tournoux (1988). By using a Talairach daemon after analysis, we were able to locate the relevant brain regions of activations of functional connectivity [25]. Since the removal of the global signal as a further preprocessing step is very controversial, the global signal was included [26]. Anatomical data of each participant were averaged for group analysis. A z-transformation of the functional volume time course for each participant was applied to account for different baseline signal levels. Functional connectivity maps of the DMN, VisCX and S1/M1 were calculated using a seed voxel correlation analysis (SCA). After extracting the individual signal time course of each participant from three defined regions of interests (ROIs, 10×10×10 mm^3; PCC/preCUN; x = ±6, y = −54, z = 3, S1/M1; x = −32, y = −30, z = 44, VisCx; x = ±6, y = −72, z = 1) the signal time course was correlated with the signal time course of every other brain voxel. Due to the association of hemispheric specialization and creative thinking, the PCC/preCUN coordinates were located in both hemispheres [27]. The PCC/preCUN has been used in previous studies to explore the functional connectivity of the DMN [28], [29], [30]. The coordinates of S1/M1 were determined from an fMRI-study by Maihöfner et al. (2007) [31]. The coordinates of the VisCx were determined from an fMRI-study by Malinen et al. (2010) in which they investigated the functional connectivity in the DMN

Table 1. Epidemiologic data.

		Visual art production	Cognitive art evaluation	Total
Number of participants		14	14	28
Age		63.50 ($\pm$3.80 SD)	63.93 ($\pm$3.34 SD)	63.71 ($\pm$3.52 SD)
Sex	Female	8	7	15
	Male	6	7	13
Handedness	Right- handed	11	13	24
	Left- handed	1	1	2
	Ambidextrous	2	0	2
Education	Low	5	0	5
	Middle	6	5	11
	High	3	9	12
Retired since	0–12 months	9	6	15
	12–24 months	2	3	5
	24–36 months	3	5	8
Number of attendances	6 sessions	0	1	1
	7 sessions	2	3	5
	8 sessions	1	3	4
	9 sessions	5	3	8
	10 sessions	6	4	10

and used the VisCx to validate their findings [32]. Using the general linear model (GLM) the individual analysis resulted in a t-statistic map. Subsequently, connectivity analysis at the group level was performed. To identify significant group-related differences, group-level contrast maps were calculated between the connectivity maps of the ROIs. Paired-t-tests were used to compare the unsigned connectivity maps of T0 and T1 in each group. Connectivity maps were thresholded at $P<0.0001$ (after Bonferroni correction, two-tailed) and visualized at $9.5<T>15.5$. Group-level contrast maps ($T1>T0$) were determined by a ($q<0.001$) FDR corrected threshold. The resulting contrast maps of t-values were visualized at $3.22<T>8.00$. In all group analyses, a minimum cluster size of 108 mm^3 (4 voxels) was applied. The cluster size criterion was used as a conservative measure to minimize false positive activations due to type 1 errors [33]. The corresponding p-values at the cluster level were corrected for multiple comparisons.

Statistical Analysis

Epidemiological and psychological data were analysed using SPSS v.18.0.0 (SPSS, Inc., Chicago, IL). The epidemiological data are presented as mean $\pm$ SD and the psychological data as mean $\pm$ SEM. For a comparison of T0 and T1 in each group, we performed Wilcoxon signed-rank tests due to the small sample size in each group. Statistical significance was assumed for $P<0.05$ (see Text S1 for details). To measure correlations between the functional connectivity of the right and left PCC/preCUN and the psychological resilience, an analysis of covariance (ANCOVA), as implemented in the Brain Voyager, was performed. The resilience score at T1 of the visual art production group served as a covariate of interest. The ANCOVA was performed using a random-effects analysis. Correlation maps were thresholded at $P<0.05$ (uncorrected) and were visualized at $0.53<T>1.00$. At cluster level, values of $P<0.05$ (uncorrected) were considered to be statistically significant. A minimum cluster size of 108 mm^3 (4

voxel) was applied which was used as a conservative measure to minimize false positive activations due to type 1 errors [33].

Results

Psychological Examination

We found a significant improvement ($P=0.013$) in psychological resilience from pre-intervention (T0) (60.64 points $\pm$1.71 SEM) to post-intervention (T1) (63.50 points $\pm$1.47 SEM) in the visual art production group. In the cognitive art evaluation group, in contrast, no significant improvement ($P=0.195$) in psychological resilience from T0 (62.57 points $\pm$2.32 SEM) to T1 (64.79 points $\pm$1.80 SEM) was found (see Table 2).

Default Mode Network (DMN)

For the identification of the DMN by a seed voxel correlation analysis (SCA), we chose a region of interest (ROI) in the PCC/preCUN as described in the methods. Figure 1 shows brain areas with significant functional connectivity to the right and left PCC/preCUN at T0 and T1 (see Table S1 for details). Generally, we were able to identify the DMN in the visual art production group at both points in time (see Figure 1A). The common brain areas included the frontal cortices (BA 6, 8, 9, 10, 45, and 46) with extension across the middle and superior temporal gyri (MTG, BA 21; STG, 22) to the inferior parietal lobule (IPL, BA 39; PCC, BA 31) in both hemispheres. At T1 several DMN areas showed significant bilateral increases in functional connectivity of the left and right PCC/preCUN to the premotor cortex (BA 6), prefrontal cortex (BA 8, 9, 10, 46), to the superior and inferior parietal lobules (SPL, BA 7; IPL, BA 39, 40), PCC (BA 23, 30, 31), and to the MTG and STG (BA 21, BA 22) compared to T0. The cognitive art evaluation group presented similar findings at T0 as the visual art production group (see Figure 1B). At T1, however, the cognitive art evaluation group had only significantly greater functional connectivity from the right PCC/preCUN to SPL (BA

Table 2. Psychological resilience.

Group	n	Pre-intervention	Post-intervention	P-value
Visual art production	14	60.64 (±1.71 SEM)	63.50 (±1.47 SEM)	0.013*
Cognitive art evaluation	14	62.57 (±2.32 SEM)	64.79 (±1.80 SEM)	0.195

*significant at 0.05.

7) and to PCC (BA 31) compared to T0. No improvements were found for the left PCC/preCUN at T1 compared to T0.

Visual Cortex (VisCx)

To validate our findings regarding the functional connectivity of the DMN, we chose a ROI in the visual cortex. The functional connectivity of VisCx at rest included the occipital and parietal cortices. No functional connectivity pattern like the DMN was observed in the visual art production group or in the cognitive art evaluation group (see Figure 2 and Table S2 for details).

Sensorimotor Cortex (S1/M1)

For our investigation of the functional connectivity of the sensorimotor cortex at rest, a ROI around the S1/M1 was chosen.

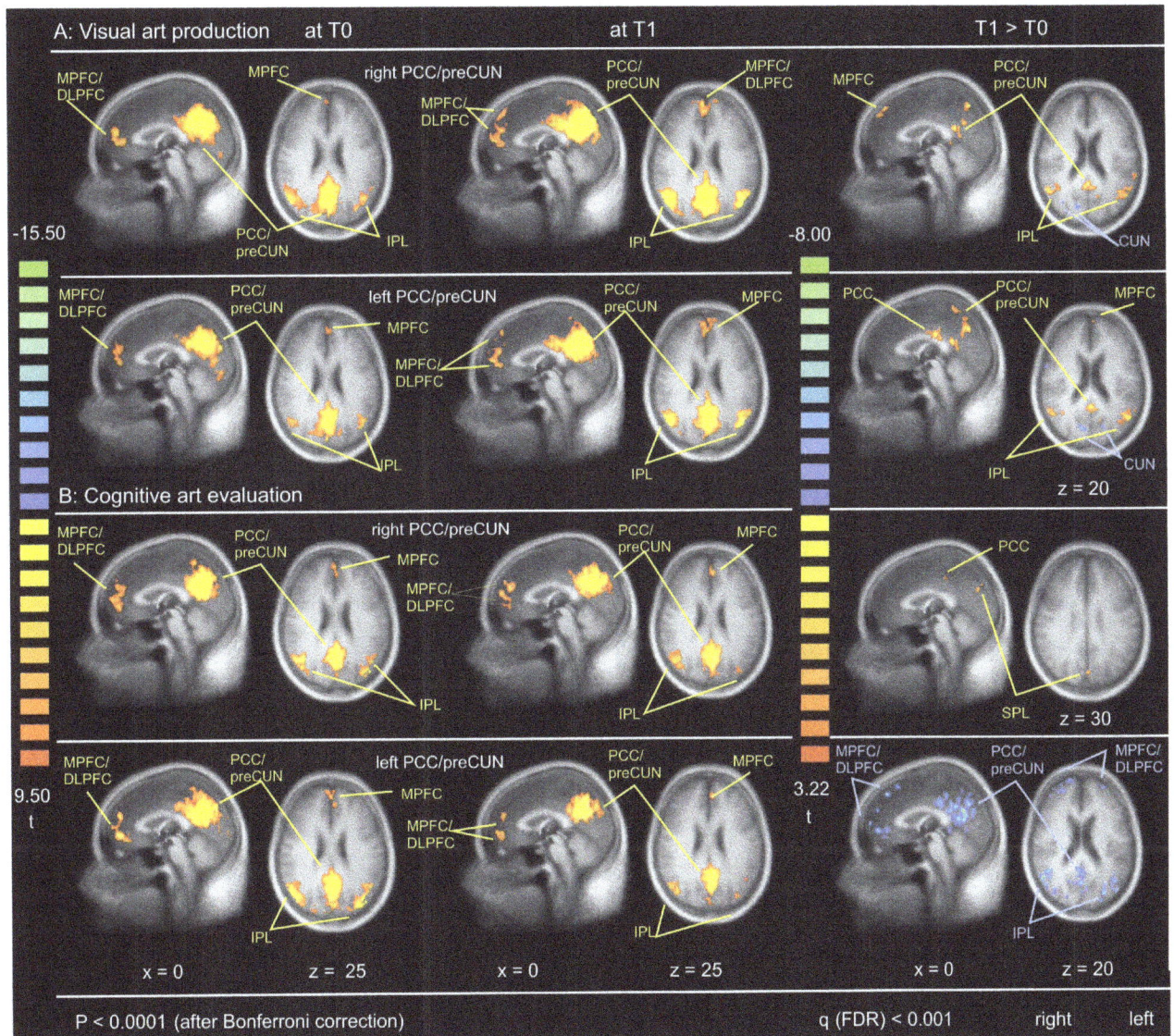

Figure 1. The default mode network (DMN). Brain regions that show significant functional connectivity of the PCC/preCUN in: (**A**) visual art production group (**B**) cognitive art evaluation group at pre-intervention (T0), post-intervention at 10 weeks (T1), and contrast T1 (red) >T0 (blue). PCC/preCUN used in each group is shown on the left and right sides.

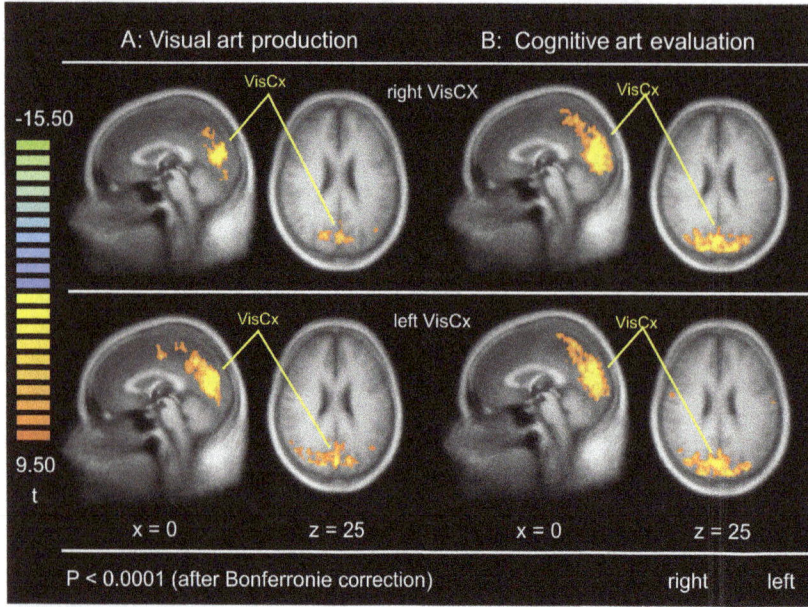

Figure 2. The visual cortex (VisCx). Brain regions that show significant functional connectivity of VisCx in: (**A**) visual art production group (**B**) cognitive art evaluation group. VisCx used in each group is shown on the left and right sides.

Due to the majority of right-handed participants (85.71%), we located the ROI in the left hemisphere. Handedness was measured with the German version of the Edinburgh Handedness Inventory (see Table 1) [34]. In both groups at T0 the SCA showed intraregional connectivity within S1/M1 with bilateral diffuse functional connectivity to the cingulate cortex, to the right S1/M1, and to the IPL. At T1 both groups showed significantly stronger intraregional connectivity of S1/M1 and less connectivity with other regions compared to T0 (see Figure 3 and Table S3 for details).

DMN and Resilience

In order to link the psychological resilience with the functional connectivity of the DMN in the visual art production group, we applied an ANCOVA (see Figure 4 and Table S4 for details). A statistically significant correlation (greater resilience in relation to greater PCC/preCUN functional connectivity) was noted for the frontal cortices (BA 6, r = 0.60; BA 8, r = 0.62; BA 9, r = 0.63; BA 10, r = 0.60; BA 45, r = 0.60; BA 47, r = 0.60). In addition, we found that greater resilience was associated with greater functional connectivity of the DMN with STG and MTG (BA 22, r = 0.63; BA 21, r = 0.59). In contrast, a negative correlation (greater

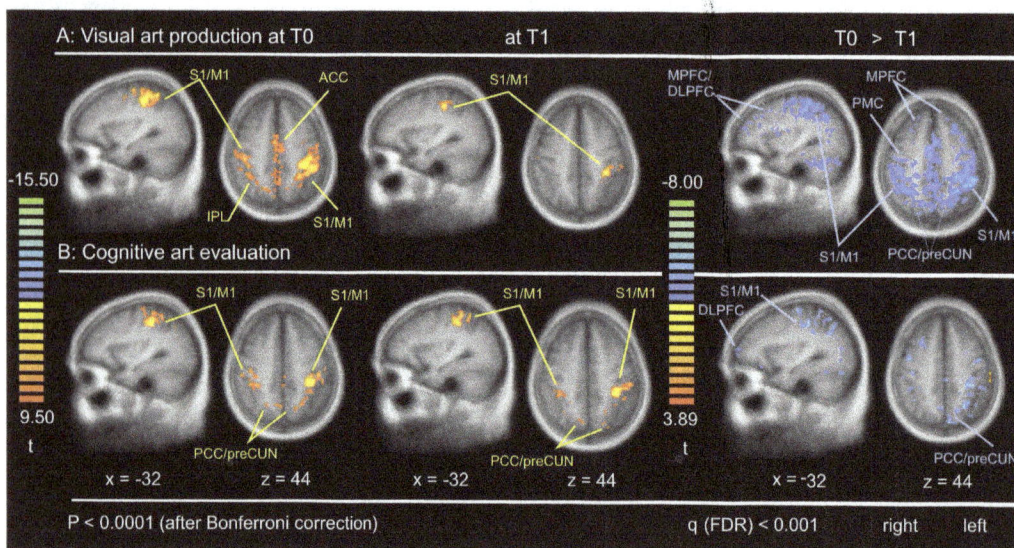

Figure 3. The sensorimotor cortex (S1/M1). Brain regions that show significant functional connectivity of S1/M1 in: (**A**) visual art production group (**B**) cognitive art evaluation group at pre-intervention (T0), post-intervention at 10 weeks (T1), and contrast T0 (blue) >T1 (red). S1/M1 used in each group is shown on the left side.

resilience in relation to less DMN functional connectivity) was observed for the parietal cortex (BA 40, r = −0.60; BA 31, r = −0.58; BA 23, r = −0.57).

Discussion

In the current study we used fMRI to investigate whether visual art production and cognitive art evaluation had different effects on the functional interplay of the DMN in a non-clinical sample of 28 post-retirement adults. Our findings demonstrate that training in a visual art production group enhances functional connectivity of the DMN, particularly between the parietal and frontal cortices. No such effects were observed in a cognitive art evaluation intervention group.

DMN

Recent fMRI studies on various neuropsychiatric disorders [35], [36], [37] as well as on chronic pain have demonstrated disruptions in the temporal and spatial properties of functional connectivity at rest [32], [38], [39]. Moreover, normal ageing also seems to affect the intrinsic activity and connectivity of the DMN [29], [40], [41], [42], [43], [44]. Age-related alterations in the DMN are proposed to result in less effective functional interactions between brain regions. Damoiseaux & colleagues (2008), for example, found that non-clinical samples of older participants (compared to younger participants) had less connectivity between the superior and middle frontal cortex, PCC, and the superior parietal gyrus [44]. Consistent with this finding, Sambataro & colleagues (2010) observed an age-related reduction in the connectivity between PCC and the MPFC, which was correlated with poor working memory performance [40]. Our study also included an older non-clinical sample and showed particular

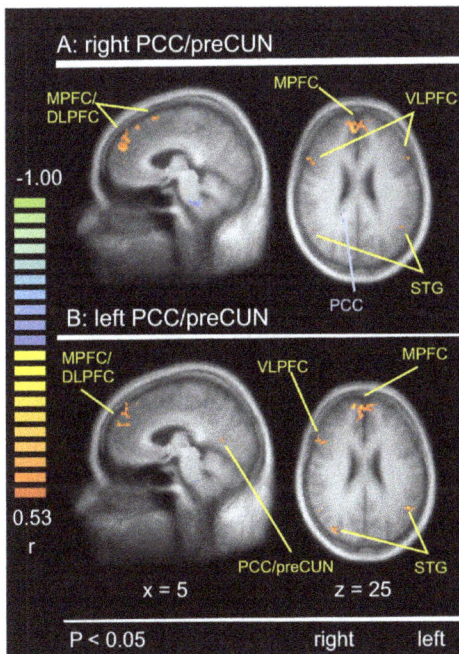

Figure 4. Analysis of covariance (ANCOVA). Covariations between DMN and resilience in the visual art production group at post-intervention (T1). Red – positive correlation; Blue – negative correlation. (**A**) Covariation between right PCC/preCUN and resilience at T1 (**B**) Covariation between left PCC/preCUN and resilience at T1.

improvement in the connectivity of the PCC/preCUN to the bilateral frontal cortices after producing visual art.

In contrast, no hard evidence of improved connectivity derives from the cognitive art evaluation group. The functional connectivity of the right PCC/preCUN showed only weak improvements between T0 and T1, and the left PCC/preCUN showed no change at all. The improvements included stronger connectivity to SPL and PCC. Generally, the evaluative reception of artwork is an aesthetic experience, in which the parietal regions of the brain, especially the SPL, are associated with visuo-spatial exploration and attention [45]. Furthermore, the improvements of only the right PCC/preCUN may result from hemispheric specialization in creative activities. Despite distinct empirical evidence, a recent meta-analysis by Mihov et al. (2010) demonstrated a relative dominance of the right hemisphere during abstract thinking, i.e., creative thinking, which was required in the cognitive art evaluation group [27]. Generally, functional studies suggest that the parietal and frontal cortices play key roles in creative activities [46]. It should be considered that the cognitive art evaluation group had higher education levels than the visual art production group. One could argue that this fact might contribute to possible habituations effects. However, as stated in the method section, we included participants who had no previous education in visual art and were no professional visual artists or art historians. Consequently, the participants had all the same starting point in contact with visual art at the beginning of the interventions.

The question of why the two groups demonstrated different changes in functional connectivity at rest remains open. The improvements in the visual art production group may be partially attributable to a combination of motor and cognitive processing. Other recent fMRI studies have demonstrated enhancements in the functional connectivity between the frontal, posterior, and temporal cortices after the combination of physical exercises and cognitive training [42], [47]. The participants in our study were required to perform the cognitive tasks of following, understanding, and imitating the visual artist's introduction. Simultaneously, the participants had to find an individual mode of artistic expression and maintain attention while performing their activity. Although we cannot provide mechanistic explanations, the production of visual art involves more than the mere cognitive and motor processing described. The creation of visual art is a personal integrative experience - an experience of "flow," - in which the participant is fully emerged in the creative activity [48].

Resilience and Functional Connectivity

The psychological relevance of the reported findings is illustrated by the statistically significant correlation between functional connectivity of PCC/preCUN in the prefrontal lobes and psychological resilience at T1 in the visual art production group. In general, regions of the prefrontal cortex, particularly BA 8, 9, and 10, are robustly activated during introspection [8]. Several fMRI studies have shown that MPFC activations are associated with the use of cognitive strategies to reduce negative emotional experience – suggesting that the MPFC is responsible for the successful cognitive regulation of emotions [49]. Moreover, increased activation of the anterior MPFC is correlated with a greater self-awareness, as a recent fMRI study by Jang and colleagues has demonstrated [50]. Our findings also point to greater activations and correlations to the anterior MPFC. This may indicate increased self-awareness, as a result of the methodological approaches applied in the visual art production intervention. The visual art production intervention involved the development of personal expression and attentional focus on self-related experience during art creation. Another interesting finding is a statistically significant correlation between resilience and functional connectivity of the PCC/preCUN in MTG and STG at T1. The medial temporal lobes play a central role in memory processing [51]. Thus, such associations point to enhanced memory processing, which is indeed required when stored knowledge is connected with new information to produce creative works [52]. Moreover, the lack of significant improvement in resilience in the cognitive art evaluation group strengthens the suggestion that visual art production has an impact on psychological resilience.

Sensorimotor Cortex

We found that the visual art production group at T1 had significantly stronger intraregional connectivity in S1/M1 and less connectivity with other brain regions compared to T0. The cognitive art evaluation group also showed stronger interregional connectivity at T1. However, the changes were less strong than in the visual art production group. Obviously, the increased intraregional connectivity demonstrates an improved specificity and differentiation of S1/M1 at rest. The loss of specialization in certain regions of the brain, with reduced distinctiveness or differentiation at the neural level, is generally thought to represent a compensational strategy of the ageing brain [42], [53]. Furthermore, our results strengthen the suggestion that the changes observed in functional connectivity were induced by the intervention.

Prospect

Our findings imply that the production of visual art improves effective interaction between brain regions of the DMN and increases the specificity and differentiation of S1/M1 at rest. Moreover, the improvements are associated with better resilience scores, meaning that our results may have important implications for preventive and therapeutic interventions. By the year 2030 one-fifth of Americans will be 65 or older, which will mean a greater number of challenging health conditions [54]. Our results revealed that visual art production leads to improved interaction, particularly between the frontal and posterior and temporal brain regions, and thus may become an important prevention tool in managing the burden of chronic diseases in older adults. In the

context of therapeutic intervention, further research is required to investigate whether improvements in disrupted functional connectivity of the DMN are associated with positive consequences for cognitive, emotional, and behavioural functions in various clinical disorders.

Supporting Information

Table S1   Regions of functional connectivity depicted in Fig. 1.

Table S2   Regions of functional connectivity depicted in Fig. 2.

Table S3   Regions of functional connectivity at rest depicted in Fig. 3.

Table S4   Correlation between functional connectivity and resilience depicted in Fig. 4.

Text S1   Estimation of missing data with an analysis of regression.

Acknowledgments

We would like to thank Pirko Julia Schröder, Sylvie Ludwig, Jutta Gschwendtner, Teresa Bischoff, & Steffi Nikol for designing and conducting the art interventions. We would also like to thank Jennifer Scheel & Martina Ott for their invaluable help with data assessment. The present work was performed by Anne Bolwerk in fulfillment of the requirements of the Friedrich-Alexander-University Erlangen-Nürnberg (FAU) for obtaining the degree "Dr. rer. biol. hum".

Author Contributions

Conceived and designed the experiments: AB JMA FL AD CM. Performed the experiments: AB JMA CM. Analyzed the data: AB JMA FL CM. Contributed reagents/materials/analysis tools: JMA FL AD CM. Wrote the paper: AB JMA FL CM.

References

1. Stuckey HL, Nobel J (2010) The Connection Between Art, Healing, and Public Health: A Review of Current Literature. Am J Public Health 100: 254–263.
2. Cohen GD, Perlstein S, Chaplin J, Kelly J, Firth KM, et al. (2006) The Impact of Professionally Conducted Cultural Programs on the Physical Health, Mental Health, and Social Functioning of Older Adults. Gerontologist 46: 726–734.
3. Leckey J (2011) The therapeutic effectiveness of creative activities on mental well-being: a systematic review of the literature. J Psychiatr Ment Health Nurs 18: 501–509.
4. Geue K, Goetze H, Buttstaedt M, Kleinert E, Richter D, et al. (2010) An overview of art therapy interventions for cancer patients and the results of research. Complement Ther Med 18: 160–170.
5. Clow A, Fredhoi C (2006) Normalisation of salivary cortisol levels and self-report stress by a brief lunchtime visit to an art gallery by London City workers. J Holist Health 3: 29–32.
6. Lacey S, Hagtvedt H, Patrick VM, Anderson A, Stilla R, et al. (2011) Art for reward's sake: Visual art recruits the ventral striatum. Neuroimage 55: 420–433.
7. Buckner RL, Vincent JL (2007) Unrest at rest: Default activity and spontaneous network correlations. Neuroimage 37: 1091–1096.
8. Gusnard DA, Akbudak E, Shulman GL, Raichle ME (2001) Medial prefrontal cortex and self-referential mental activity: Relation to a default mode of brain function. PNAS 98: 4259–4264.
9. Raichle ME (2006) The Brain's Dark Energy. Science 314: 1249–1250.
10. Fox MD, Raichle ME (2007) Spontaneous fluctuations in brain activity observed with functional magnetic resonance imaging. Nat Rev Neurosci 8: 700–711.
11. Raichle ME, MacLeod AM, Snyder AZ, Powers WJ, Gusnard DA, et al. (2001) A default mode of brain function. PNAS 98: 676–682.
12. Damoiseaux JS, Rombouts SARB, Barkhof F, Scheltens P, Stam CJ, et al. (2006) Consistent resting-state networks across healthy subjects. PNAS 103: 13848–13853.
13. Fehr R (2012) Is retirement always stressful? The potential impact of creativity. Am Psychol 67: 76–77.
14. Herzog RA, House JS, Morgan JN (1991) Relation of work and retirement to health and well-being in older age. Psychol Aging 6: 202–211.
15. Marshall VW, Clarke PJ, Ballantyne PJ (2001) Instability in the Retirement Transition: Effects on Health and Well-Being in a Canadian Study. Res Aging 23: 379–409.
16. Goh JO, Park DC (2009) Neuroplasticity and cognitive aging: The scaffolding theory of aging and cognition. Restor Neurol Neurosci 27: 391–403.
17. Windle G (2010) The Resilience Network. What is resilience? A systematic review and concept analysis. Rev Clin Geronto 21: 1–18.
18. Wagnild GM, Young HM (1993) Development and psychometric evaluation of the Resilience Scale. J Nurs Meas 1: 165–178.
19. Maier SF, Watkins LR (2010) Role of the medial prefrontal cortex in coping and resilience. Brain Res 1355: 52–60.
20. Schumacher J, Leppert K, Gunzelmann T, Strauß B, Brähler E (2005) The Resilience Scale - A questionnaire to assess resilience as a personality characteristic. Die Resilienzskala - Ein Fragebogen zur Erfassung der psychischen Widerstandsfähigkeit als Personmerkmal. Z Klin Psychol Psychiatr Psychother 53: 16–39.
21. Leppert K, Gunzelmann T, Schuhmacher J, Strauss B, Brähler E (2005) Resilience as a protective personality characteristic in the elderly. Psychother Psychosom Med Psychol. 55: 365–9.
22. Packer J (2008) Beyond Learning: Exploring Visitors' Perception of the Value and Benefits of Museum Experience. Curator 51: 33–54.

23. Silverman LH (2010) The Social Work of Museums, London and New York: Routledge.
24. Peez G (2002) Qualitative empirische Forschung in der Kunstpädagogik. Methodologische Analysen und praxisbezogene Konzepte zu Fallstudien über ästhetische Prozesse, biografische Aspekte und soziale Interaktion in unterschiedlichen Bereichen der Kunstpädagogik.Norderstedt: Books on Demand.
25. Talairach J, Tournoux P (1988) Co-Planar Stereotaxic Atlas of the Human Brain. New York: Thieme Medical Publishers.
26. Murphy K, Birn RM, Handwerker DA, Jones TB, Bandettini PA (2009) The impact of global signal regression on resting state correlations: are anti-correlated networks introduced? Neuroimage 44: 893–905.
27. Mihov KM, Denzler M, Förster J (2010) Hemispheric specialization and creative thinking: A meta-analytic review of lateralization of creativity. Brain Cog 72: 442–448.
28. Pyka M, Burgmer M, Lenzen T, Pioch R, Dannlowski U, et al. (2011) Brain correlates of hypnotic paralysis - a resting-state fMRI study. Neuroimage 56: 2173–2182.
29. Andrews-Hanna JR, Snyder AZ, Vincent JL, Lustig C, Head D, et al. (2007) Disruption of Large-Scale Brain Systems in Advanced Aging. Neuron 56: 924–935.
30. Grady CL, Protzner AB, Kovacevic N, Strother SC, Afshin-Pour B, et al (2010). A Multivariate Analysis of Age-Related Differences in Default Mode and Task-Positive Networks across Multiple Cognitive Domains. Cereb Cortex 20: 1432–1447.
31. Maihöfner C, Baron R, De Col R, Binder A, Birklein F, et al. (2007) The motor system shows adaptive changes in complex regional pain syndrome. Brain 130: 2671–2687
32. Malinen S, Vartiainen N, Hlushchuk Y, Koskinen M, Ramkumar P, et al. (2010) Aberrant temporal and spatial brain activity during rest in patients with chronic pain. PNAS 107: 6493–6497.
33. Maihöfner C, Handwerker HO (2005) Differential coding of hyperalgesia in the human brain: A functional MRI study. Neuroimage 28: 996–1006.
34. Oldfield RC (1971) The assessment and analysis of handedness: the Edingburg inventory. Neuropsychologia 9: 97–113.
35. Williamson P (2007) Are Anticorrelated Networks in the Brain Relevant to Schizophrenia? Schizophr Bull 33: 994–1003.
36. Kennedy DP, Redcay E, Courchesne E (2006) Failing to deactivate: Resting functional abnormalities in autism. PNAS 103: 8275–8280.
37. Greicius MD, Flores BH, Menon V, Glover GH, Solvason HB, et al. (2007) Resting-State Functional Connectivity in Major Depression: Abnormally Increased Contributions from Subgenual Cingulate Cortex and Thalamus. Biol Psychiatry 62: 429–437.
38. Baliki MN, Geha PY, Apkarian AV, Chialvo DR (2008) Beyond Feeling: Chronic Pain Hurts the Brain, Disrupting the Default-Mode Network Dynamics. J, Neurosci 28: 1398–1403.
39. Cauda F, Sacco K, Duca S, Cocito D, D'Agata F, et al. (2009) Altered Resting State in Diabetic Neuropathic Pain. PLoS ONE 4: e4542.
40. Sambataro F, Murty VP, Callicott JH, Tan H-Y, Das S, et al. (2010) Age-related alterations in default mode network: Impact on working memory performance. Neurobiol Aging 31: 839–852.
41. Hampson M, Driesen NR, Skudlarski P, Gore JC, Constable RT (2006) Brain Connectivity Related to Working Memory Performance. J Neurosci 26: 13338–13343.
42. Voss MW, Prakash RS, Erickson KI, Basak C, Chaddock L, et al. (2010) Plasticity of brain networks in a randomized intervention trial of exercise training in older adults. Front Aging Neurosci 2: 1–7.
43. Wu J-T, Wu H-Z, Yang C-G, Chen W-X, Zhang H-Y, et al. (2011) Aging-related changes in the default mode network and its anti-correlated networks: A resting-state fMRI study. Neurosci Lett 504: 62–67.
44. Damoiseaux JS, Beckamnn CF, Arigita EJS, Barkhof F, Scheltens P, et al. (2008) Reduced resting-state brain activity in the "default network" in normal aging. Cereb Cortex 18: 1856–1864.
45. Corbetta M, Shulman GL (2002) Control of goal-directed and stimulus-driven attention in the brain. Nat Rev Neurosci 3: 201–215.
46. Jung RE, Segall JM, Jeremy Bockholt H, Flores RA, Smith SM, et al. (2010) Neuroanatomy of creativity. Hum Brain Mapp 31: 398–409.
47. Voss MW, Erickson KI, Prakash RS, Chaddock L, Malkowski E, et al. (2010) Functional connectivity: A source of variance in the association between cardiorespiratory fitness and cognition? Neuropsychologia 48: 1394–1406.
48. Csikszentmihalyi M (1996) Creativity, flow and the psychology of discovery and invention. New York: Harper Perennial.
49. Wager TD, Davidson ML, Hughes BL, Lindquist MA, Ochsner KN (2008) Prefrontal-Subcortical Pathways Mediating Successful Emotion Regulation. Neuron 59: 1037–1050.
50. Jang JH, Jung WH, Kang D-H, Byun MS, Kwon SJ, et al. (2011) Increased default mode network connectivity associated with meditation. Neurosci Lett 487: 358–362.
51. Eichenbaum H, Yonelinas AP, Ranganath C (2007) The Medial Temporal Lobe and Recognition Memory. Annu Rev Neurosci 30: 123–152.
52. Fink A, Benedek M, Grabner RH, Staudt B, Neubauer AC (2007) Creativity meets neuroscience: Experimental tasks for the neuroscientific study of creative thinking. Methods 42: 68–76.
53. Park DC, Reuter-Lorenz P (2009) The Adaptive Brain: Aging and Neurocognitive Scaffolding. Annu Rev Psychol 60: 173–196.
54. He W, Sengupta M, Velkoff VA, DeBarros KA (2005) 65+ in the United States: 2005. Current Population Reports. Washington (DC): US Department of Commerce/US Department of Health and Human Services.

4

Time Delay and Long-Range Connection Induced Synchronization Transitions in Newman-Watts Small-World Neuronal Networks

Yu Qian[1,2,3]*

1 Nonlinear Research Institute, Baoji University of Arts and Sciences, Baoji, China, 2 Center for Systems Biology, Soochow University, Suzhou, China, 3 State Key Laboratory of Theoretical Physics, Institute of Theoretical Physics, Chinese Academy of Sciences, Beijing, China

Abstract

The synchronization transitions in Newman-Watts small-world neuronal networks (SWNNs) induced by time delay τ and long-range connection (LRC) probability P have been investigated by synchronization parameter and space-time plots. Four distinct parameter regions, that is, asynchronous region, transition region, synchronous region, and oscillatory region have been discovered at certain LRC probability $P = 1.0$ as time delay is increased. Interestingly, desynchronization is observed in oscillatory region. More importantly, we consider the spatiotemporal patterns obtained in delayed Newman-Watts SWNNs are the competition results between long-range drivings (LRDs) and neighboring interactions. In addition, for moderate time delay, the synchronization of neuronal network can be enhanced remarkably by increasing LRC probability. Furthermore, lag synchronization has been found between weak synchronization and complete synchronization as LRC probability P is a little less than 1.0. Finally, the two necessary conditions, moderate time delay and large numbers of LRCs, are exposed explicitly for synchronization in delayed Newman-Watts SWNNs.

Editor: Matjaz Perc, University of Maribor, Slovenia

Funding: This work was supported by the National Natural Science Foundation of China (Grant Nos. 11105003), and the Natural Science Foundation of the Education Bureau of Shaanxi Province of China (Grant No. 2013JK0619). The funders had no role in study design, data collection and analysis, decision to publish, or preparation of the manuscript.

Competing Interests: The author has declared that no competing interests exist.

* E-mail: qianyu0272@163.com

Introduction

Synchronization phenomena are common in nature and can be extensive observed in various realistic systems, especially in neuronal networks, biological systems and ecological systems [1,2]. Synchronization has been widely studied both theoretically and experimentally for decades. Several kinds of synchronization have been discovered in theoretical researches, such as complete synchronization, weak synchronization, lag synchronization, phase synchronization and generalized synchronization [3–7]. Complete synchronization indicates the coincidence of states of coupling systems, $\mathbf{X}_1(t) = \mathbf{X}_2(t)$ [3]. Lag synchronization described in Ref. [5] means the coincidence of shifted in time states of two systems, $\mathbf{X}_1(t + \tau_0) = \mathbf{X}_2(t)$. Experimental studies have shown that synchronous oscillations can emerge in many special areas of brain, especially in olfactory system or hippocampal region [8–10]. In recent years, synchronization in neuronal networks and brain systems has attracted much attention. Synchronous oscillations in these systems are related to some specific and important physiological functions, such as olfaction [11], visual perception [12], cognitive processes [13], and information processing [14].

Recently "small-world" network has been proposed by Watts and Strogatz, which takes into account both local and long-range interactions [15]. It is found that the existence of a small fraction of long-range connections (LRCs) can essentially change the features of the given systems [16–19]. These LRCs do exist in neuronal networks and do play crucial roles in deciding the specific physiological functions. The interactions from the long-range connected neurons must be time delayed due to the finite propagation velocities in the conduction of signals along neuron axons [20]. And the effects of time delays on self-organized spatiotemporal dynamics in neuronal systems have been extensively investigated. Lots of interesting phenomena have been discovered in recent decades [21–36]. For example, Dhamala et al. have investigated the enhancement of neural synchrony by time delay [21]. Ko et al have found that time delay can destabilize synchronous states and induce near-regular wave states [23]. Significantly, Wang et al. have discovered that time delays can enhance the coherence of spiral waves [27], tame desynchronized bursting [28], induce stochastic resonances [29] and synchronization transitions [30–32], and can cause synchronous bursts [33] and complex synchronous behavior [34]. Moreover, Yu et al. have demonstrated the synchronization transitions in delayed neuronal networks with hybrid synapses [35,36]. Although remarkable advances have been achieved in the field of delayed neuronal networks, the underlying mechanisms behind time delay induced spatiotemporal dynamic and related synchronization transitions are far from being fully understood. In addition, the lag synchronization, to our knowledge, has not been identified in delayed neuronal network. These are the tasks we aim to explore.

In this paper we extend the subject by systematically investigating time delay and long-range connection induced synchronization transitions in Newman-Watts small-world neuronal networks (SWNNs). By introducing synchronization parameter and plotting spatiotemporal patterns, four distinct parameter regions, i.e., asynchronous region, transition region, synchronous region and oscillatory region, have been found at certain LRC probability $P = 1.0$. Interestingly, desynchronization and oscillating behaviour of the order parameter are observed in oscillatory region. More importantly, the mechanisms of synchronous oscillations and the transition from non-synchronization to complete synchronization are discussed. Moreover, we consider the spatiotemporal patterns obtained in delayed Newman-Watts SWNNs are the competition results between long-range drivings (LRDs) and neighboring interactions. A new order parameter, LRD proportion, is used to verify our point of view. And the four distinct parameter regions can also be revealed by LRD proportion clearly. In addition, for moderate time delay, the synchronization of neuronal network can be enhanced remarkably by increasing LRC probability. Furthermore, lag synchronization has been found between weak synchronization and complete synchronization as LRC probability P is a little less than 1.0. And the mechanism is revealed. Finally, the two necessary conditions, moderate time delay and large numbers of LRCs, are exposed explicitly for synchronization in delayed Newman-Watts SWNNs.

Mathematical Model and Setup

We start from a one-dimensional (1D) regular ring that comprises $N = 100$ identical excitable Bär-Eiswirth neurons[37] with periodic boundary condition, and each neuron has two nearest neighbors. The evolvement of the 1D neuronal network is governed by the following equations:

$$\frac{du_i(t)}{dt} = -\frac{1}{\epsilon} u_i(t)[u_i(t)-1]\left[u_i(t)-\frac{v_i(t)+b}{a}\right] + D[u_{i-1}(t)+u_{i+1}(t)-2u_i(t)], \tag{1}$$

$$\frac{dv_i(t)}{dt} = f[u_i(t)] - v_i(t), \tag{2}$$

where $i = 1,2,\ldots,N$. The function $f[u_i(t)]$ takes the form: $f[u_i(t)] = 0$ for $u_i(t) < \frac{1}{3}$; $f[u_i(t)] = 1 - 6.75u_i(t)[u_i(t)-1]^2$ for $\frac{1}{3} \le u_i(t) \le 1$; and $f[u_i(t)] = 1$ for $u_i(t) > 1$. Here variables u and v are the activator and inhibitor variables, respectively. The small relaxation parameter ϵ represents the time ratio between activator u and inhibitor v. The dimensionless parameters a and b denote the activator kinetics with b effectively controlling the excitation threshold. D is the coupling intensity which decides the interaction strength between neighboring neurons. The system parameters are kept throughout this paper as $a = 0.84$, $b = 0.07$, $\epsilon = 0.04$ and $D = 0.5$. Therefore, the local dynamics can describe typical excitability of neurons where u represents the membrane potential, v is the somatic inhibitory current. The diffusive couplings simulates electrical conjunction interaction between neurons.

Based on the 1D periodic regular ring, we construct delayed Newman-Watts SWNNs [38] by introducing LRCs such that each neuron receives an unidirectional time delayed LRD from a randomly chosen cell with probability P [39,40]. We thus add an additional coupling term to Eq. (1) if neuron i receives an unidirectionally time delayed LRD from cell j. Now the delayed Newman-Watts SWNN is governed by the following equations:

$$\frac{du_i(t)}{dt} = -\frac{1}{\epsilon} u_i(t)[u_i(t)-1]\left[u_i(t)-\frac{v_i(t)+b}{a}\right] + D[u_{i-1}(t)+u_{i+1}(t)-2u_i(t)] + D[u_j(t-\tau)-u_i(t)], \tag{3}$$

$$\frac{dv_i(t)}{dt} = f[u_i(t)] - v_i(t). \tag{4}$$

In Eq. (3) cell j is randomly chosen in the 1D periodic regular ring and τ is the time delay in information transmission. By manipulating LRC probability P, we can obtain different kinds of time delayed Newman-Watts SWNNs. The schematic diagram of the considered networks for different LRC probability with 10 neurons is illustrated in Fig. 1. Here we should mention that for a given LRC probability there are a lot of network realizations. For a specific network structure, the interactions between neighboring neurons are bidirectional (shown by bidirectional arrowed lines), while the LRDs are unidirectional (shown by unidirectional arrowed lines). Time delays are only considered in these unidirectional LRDs, which will cause inhomogeneity in information transmission between neighboring and long-range interactions. As we know that the interactions from neighboring neurons are usually instantaneous in actual biological systems. And the LRDs from distant cells will have time delays due to the finite propagation velocities. Therefore, the model considered in present paper may be more realistic, and the results obtained may be more practical.

In this paper, the delayed Newman-Watts SWNNs are integrated by forward Euler integration scheme with time step $\Delta t = 0.001$. The initial variables $(u_i(t=0), v_i(t=0))$ are randomly given between 0 and 1 for each simulation. To investigate the synchronization transitions in delayed Newman-Watts SWNNs quantitatively, the synchronization parameter R will be used, which has been introduced in the previous study [41]. It is numerically calculated as:

$$R = \frac{<\bar{u}(t)^2> - <\bar{u}(t)>^2}{\frac{1}{N}\sum_{i=1}^{N}[<u_i(t)^2> - <u_i(t)>^2]}, \tag{5}$$

where

$$\bar{u}(t) = \frac{1}{N}\sum_{i=1}^{N} u_i(t). \tag{6}$$

The angular brackets denote the average over time. In present paper the synchronization parameters are calculated over last 30 time units. From Eq. (5) it is evident that the larger the synchronization parameter R is, the more synchronization is realized in neuronal network. Accordingly, the value of R close to unity indicates all neurons in the network are in complete synchronization. Therefore, the synchronization parameter R is an excellent indicator to reveal the spatiotemporal synchronization in delayed Newman-Watts SWNNs and the related transitions.

To guarantee the statistical accuracy with respect to the network structure and initial condition, 10 independent samples are executed for each set of parameter values in the simulation. And we will use

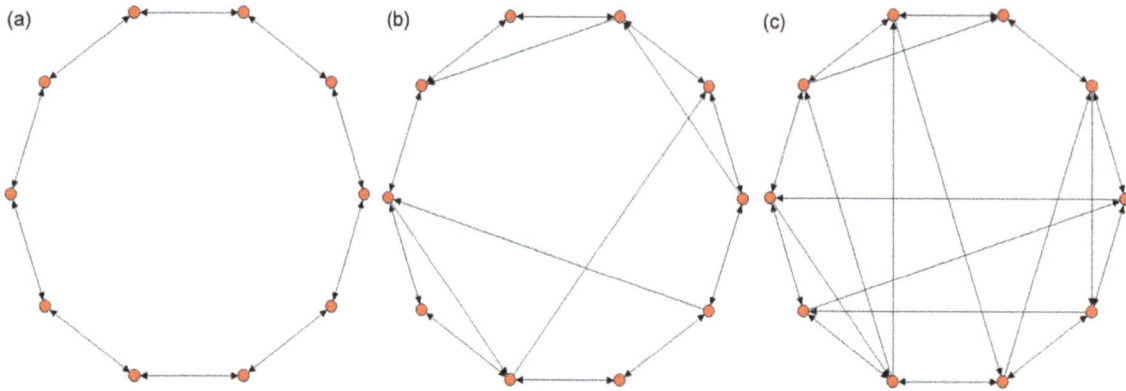

Figure 1. Schematic diagram of the considered Newman-Watts small-world neuronal networks for different long-range connection (LRC) probability P with 10 neurons. (a) $P=0.0$ (one-dimensional regular ring with periodic boundary condition); (b) $P=0.5$; (c) $P=1.0$. Here we should mention that the interactions between neighboring neurons are bidirectional (shown by bidirectional arrowed lines), while the long-range drivings (LRDs) are unidirectional (shown by unidirectional arrowed lines). Time delays are only considered in these unidirectional LRDs.

$$\bar{R} = \frac{1}{10} \sum_{i=1}^{10} R_i \qquad (7)$$

as an order parameter to measure the degree of synchronization and the related transitions induced by time delay and long-range connection in Newman-Watts SWNNs.

Results

Time Delay Induced Synchronization Transitions

In this part, we firstly investigate time delay induced synchronization transitions in Newman-Watts SWNNs at certain LRC probability. Figure 2 displays the dependence of synchronization parameters R (10 samples for each τ, depicted by black dots) and $\bar{R}$ (the average of Rs for 10 samples, depicted by red dots) on time delay τ at $P=1.0$. Four distinct parameter regions have been revealed by synchronization parameters as time delay is increased. When time delay is small ($\tau \leq 2.6$), synchronization parameters are all close to zero. It indicates that the states of individual neurons are significantly different and the whole network oscillates asynchronously at all (domain I in Fig. 2, called as asynchronous region). It means that small time delay has no effect on synchronization in delayed Newman-Watts SWNNs. A typical asynchronous spatiotemporal pattern is shown in Fig. 3(a) for $\tau = 1.0$. In the white regions, the nodes fire, while in the black ones they are quiescent. Time passes from left to right. Most of neurons in the network oscillate asynchronously and irregular spatiotemporal dynamics is observed. As τ is in the narrow region of [2.8,3.0], some synchronization parameters increase abruptly. It indicates that synchronous performance of neuronal network improves remarkably in some samples. A weak synchronization state for $\tau = 2.8$ is revealed in Fig. 3(b). The excitatory fronts are more ordered both in time and space. Time delay induced synchronization transition has been detected in Newman-Watts SWNNs. And we call this narrow parameter region as the transition region (domain II in Fig. 2, indicated by grey rectangle).

When time delay is moderate ($3.2 \leq \tau \leq 5.4$, domain III in Fig. 2), synchronization parameters R and $\bar{R}$ jump to unity simultaneously. It implies that moderate time delay in information transmission can induce complete synchronization in Newman-Watts SWNNs. Therefore, synchronous region is defined in this

parameter region. Fig. 3(c) exhibits a completely synchronous

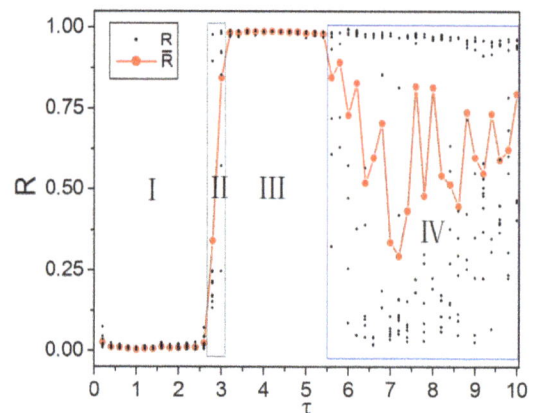

Figure 2. Time delay induced synchronization transitions. Dependence of synchronization parameters R (10 samples for each τ, depicted by black dots) and $\bar{R}$ (the average of Rs for 10 samples, depicted by red dots) on time delay τ at $P=1.0$. Four distinct parameter regions, i.e., asynchronous region (domain I for small τ), transition region (domain II for narrow region of time delay τ, indicated by grey rectangle), synchronous region (domain III for moderate τ) and oscillatory region (domain IV for large τ, indicated by blue rectangle) are revealed.

spatiotemporal pattern for $\tau = 4.0$. All neurons in the network fire simultaneously and damp to their rest state together. As time delay is further increased ($\tau \geq 5.6$), to our surprise, desynchronization occurs in Newman-Watts SWNNs. A distinct new parameter region, composed by asynchronous state, weak synchronization and complete synchronization, has been discovered. And oscillating behaviour of the order parameter is detected. Accordingly, we call this parameter region as the oscillatory region (domain IV in Fig. 2, indicated by blue rectangle). Fig. 3(d) displays a typical desynchronized spatiotemporal dynamics in oscillatory region at $\tau = 7.0$. Large time delay can effectively improve synchronization in the beginning (can be indicated by the second excitatory front in Fig. 3(d)). However, the ordered excitatory front degenerates and desynchronization occurs as the system evolves. Finally, asynchro-

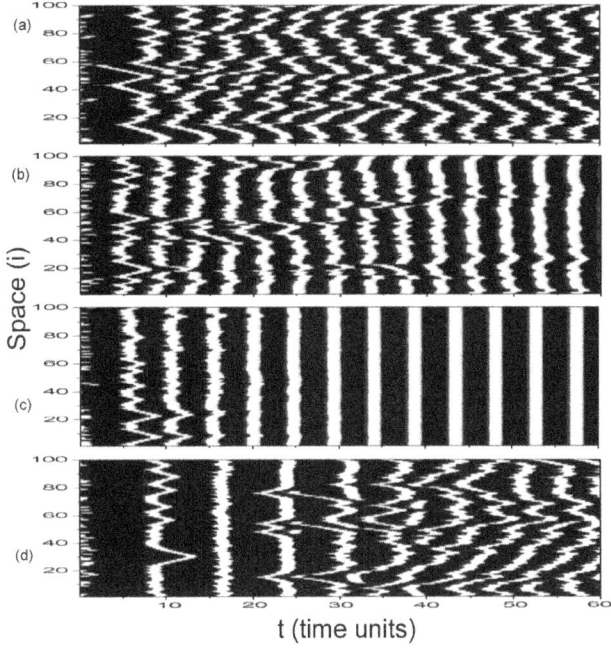

Figure 3. Space-time plots of u **for different time delay** τ **at** $P = 1.0$.
(a) $\tau = 1.0$ (asynchronous state), (b) $\tau = 2.8$ (weak synchronization), (c) $\tau = 4.0$ (complete synchronization), (d) $\tau = 7.0$ (desynchronized state). The figures are plotted in greyscale from black (lowest value at 0.0) to white (highest value at 1.0). And this greyscale will be used throughout this paper.

nous state is obtained in oscillatory region. According to the results shown in Fig. 2, we can conclude that moderate time delay is needed for synchronization in delayed Newman-Watts SWNNs.

For further investigating the synchronous oscillations, the dependence of oscillation period T on time delay τ in synchronous region is shown in Fig. 4(a). It is seen that synchronization oscillation period is monotonously increased with time delay. And approximate linear relationship is revealed. However, a time difference between T and τ can be detected. To explain the above phenomenon, time series u of neurons 79 (shown by black curve), 78 and 80 (two neighboring neurons of 79, shown by green and yellow curves) and 42 (the LRD neuron of 79, shown by red curve) of Fig. 3(c) are shown in Fig. 4(b). The blue dashed curve denotes time series u of neuron 42 with time delay translation. The pink line indicates excitation threshold. From Fig. 4(b) we can find that synchronization oscillation period T is composed by time delay τ and excitation time t_E. That's why there exists a time difference between synchronization oscillation period and time delay.

The mechanism of synchronous oscillations can also be explained by Fig. 4(b). As complete synchronization is achieved in delayed Newman-Watts SWNNs, all neurons can excite simultaneously and damp to their rest state together, oscillate just as a single cell (can be indicated by the overlap of the four solid curves). Since time delays exist in LRCs, neurons can be excited synchronously again by their corresponding delayed LRDs (can be indicated by the black solid and blue dashed curves). Synchronous oscillations can self-sustain in delayed Newman-Watts SWNNs in this manner (such as the two excitation periods shown in Fig. 4(b)). However, due to the existence of refractory period for excitable neuron, a minimal time delay τ_{min} is needed for LRDs sustaining synchronous oscillations. Accordingly, complete synchronization can emerge in delayed Newman-Watts SWNNs as $\tau \geq \tau_{min}$. Based

on the results shown in Fig. 2, we can find $\tau_{min} \approx 2.8$ under current parameter settings. Now the transition from non-synchronization to complete synchronization can be explained as follow: For small time delays (i.e., $\tau < \tau_{min}$), LRDs can not occupy the whole network entirely and simultaneously due to the existence of refractory period for excitable dynamics. Neurons in the network are mostly driven by their neighbors. As a result, zigzag excitation fronts (i.e., asynchronous spatiotemporal patterns) are obtained. As τ_{min} is reached, LRDs can dominate the neuronal network absolutely, and complete synchronization can emerge in delayed Newman-Watts SWNNs.

From the above discussion, we can find that LRDs play a key role in synchronization transition. To qualitatively investigate the effects of LRDs on the spatiotemporal dynamics obtained in delayed Newman-Watts SWNNs, the LRD proportion p is used, which can be calculated as:

$$p = \frac{N_{LRD}}{N}, \tag{8}$$

where N_{LRD} is the total number of neurons driven by LRDs. The evolvement of LRD proportion p between adjacent intervals for different time delay τ (corresponding to Figs. 3(a)–d)) is shown in Fig. 4(c). As time delay is small ($\tau = 1.0$, below τ_{min}, shown by black squares), p increases slightly at first and then tends to 0.5. It indicates that the neuronal network is governed by local and long-range drivings together. Accordingly, irregular asynchronous spatiotemporal dynamics of Fig. 3(a) is obtained. When τ is in the transition region ($\tau = 2.8$, close to τ_{min}, shown by green triangles), LRD proportion p increases abruptly, but can never reach 1.0. It means that most of neurons in the network are sustained by LRDs, and can fire simultaneously. However, few neurons are still excited by their corresponding neighbors. Therefore, weak synchronization can be observed. As synchronous region is reached ($\tau = 4.0$, beyond τ_{min}, shown by red dots), LRD proportion p jumps to unity rapidly. With the help of moderate time delay, LRDs can suppress neighboring interactions to dominate the system entirely. All neurons in the network can be excited by their corresponding LRDs simultaneously, and complete synchronization can emerge in delayed Newman-Watts SWNNs. When time delay is large ($\tau = 7.0$, also beyond τ_{min}, shown by blue diamonds), p increases abruptly at first and goes through a peak, then deceases monotonously, and finally tends to 0.5. It means that LRDs can take effect so long as τ_{min} is reached. And LRDs can dominate the neuronal network in the beginning and weak synchronization such as the second excitatory front of Fig. 3(d) can be achieved. However, LRD loses its predominance as the system evolves. It may be caused by the too long resting time which can increase the chance for neighboring interactions. As a result, the ordered excitatory front degenerates and desynchronization occurs in the oscillatory region. So we consider that too large time delay may be harmful for synchronization to a certain degree.

Based on the above discussion, we can infer that the mechanism behind spatiotemporal dynamics obtained in delayed Newman-Watts SWNNs is the competition between LRDs and neighboring interactions. This kind of competition is caused by inhomogeneity in information transmission between neighboring and long-range interactions of the present model. More importantly, the competition results, which will decide the spatiotemporal dynamics in the network, are largely dependent on time delays. Therefore, we can expect that the LRD proportion is also a good indicator to study the synchronization transitions in delayed Newman-Watts SWNNs. The dependence of LRD proportion p (10 samples for

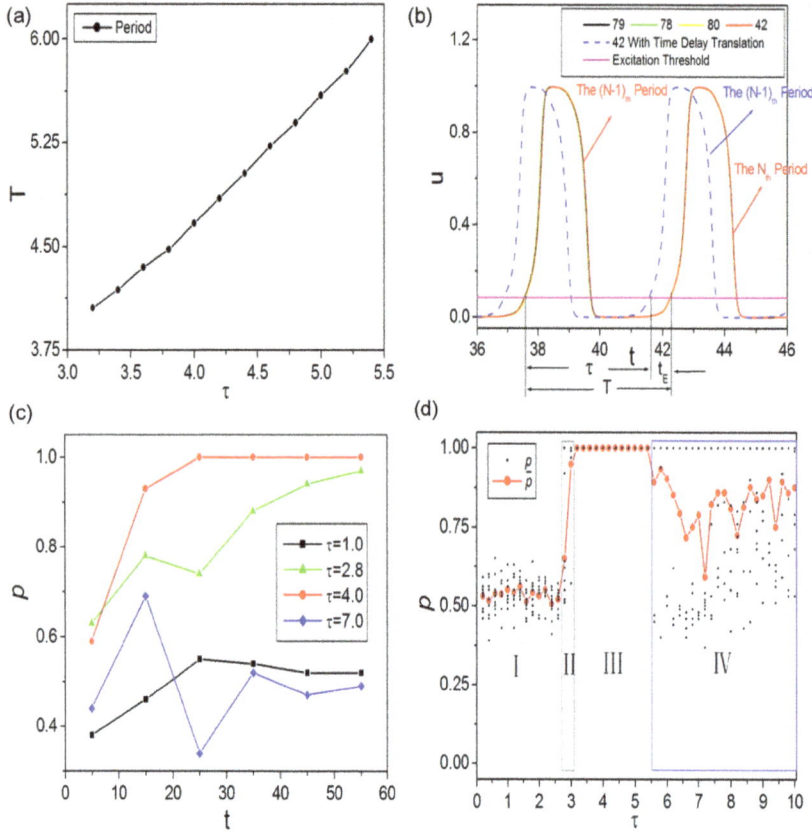

Figure 4. Dynamical analysis of synchronous oscillations and time delay induced synchronization transitions. (a) Dependence of oscillation period T on time delay τ in synchronous region. (b) Time series u of neurons 79 (shown by black curve), 78 and 80 (two neighboring neurons of 79, shown by green and yellow curves) and 42 (the LRD neuron of 79, shown by red curve) of Fig. 3(c). The blue dashed curve denotes time series u of neuron 42 with time delay translation. The pink line indicates excitation threshold. The oscillation period T is composed by time delay τ and excitation time t_E. (c) The LRD proportion p between adjacent intervals for different time delay τ (corresponding to Figs. 3(a)–(d)). (d) Dependence of LRD proportion p (10 samples for each τ, depicted by black dots) and $\bar{p}$ (the average of p_s for 10 samples, depicted by red dots) on time delay τ. The four distinct parameter regions can also be revealed by LRD proportion clearly.

each τ, depicted by black dots) and $\bar{p}$ (the average of p_s for 10 samples, depicted by red dots) on time delay τ is shown in Fig. 4(d). The four distinct parameter regions are revealed by LRD proportion clearly. Moreover, we can also find that moderate time delay can help LRDs to beat neighboring interactions to dominate the network absolutely. The conclusion that moderate time delay is needed for synchronization in delayed Newman-Watts SWNNs is further verified.

LRC Induced Synchronization Transitions

From the above understanding we can find that LRDs play an important role in deciding the spatiotemporal dynamics. Therefore, a detailed study on LRC induced synchronization transitions needs to be taken in delayed Newman-Watts SWNNs. Fig. 5(a) displays the dependence of synchronization parameter $\bar{R}$ on LRC probability P for different time delay τ. For small time delay ($\tau = 1.0$, below τ_{min}, shown by black triangles), LRDs can not occupy the system due to the existence of refractory period. As a result, LRCs have no effect on synchronization transitions in asynchronous region. When time delay is in transition region ($\tau = 2.8$, close to τ_{min}, shown by pink squares), few LRDs can occupy the neuronal network under this circumstance. Therefore, lots of LRCs are needed to slightly improve the synchronization. For moderate time delay ($\tau = 4.0$, beyond τ_{min}, shown by red dots),

LRDs can suppress neighboring interactions to dominate the system entirely. Consequentially, synchronization in delayed Newman-Watts SWNNs can be enhanced remarkably by increasing LRC probability P. For large time delay ($\tau = 7.0$, also beyond τ_{min}, shown by blue diamonds), synchronization of delayed Newman-Watts SWNN improves as LRC probability increases. However, as we have identified, too large time delay can increase the chance for neighboring interactions and is harmful for synchronization to a certain degree, oscillating behaviour of the order parameter can be observed. Fig. 5(b) displays the dependence of synchronization parameter $\bar{R}$ on time delay τ for different LRC probability P. An optimal time delay interval is needed to enhance the synchronization for Newman-Watts SWNNs. The centers of optimal time delay interval are all around 4.5 and are largely independent of LRC probability. The width of optimal time delay interval broadens as LRC probability increases.

To give more intuitive understanding on LRC induced synchronization transitions in delayed Newman-Watts SWNNs, space-time plots of u for different LRC probability P at $\tau = 4.0$ is given in Fig. 6. Remarkable enhancement of synchronization induced by LRCs in delayed Newman-Watts SWNNs is revealed obviously. Besides the asynchronous state ($P = 0.30$ for Fig. 6(a)), weak synchronization ($P = 0.70$ for Fig. 6(b)) and complete synchronization ($P = 1.00$ for Fig. 6(d)), another new synchroni-

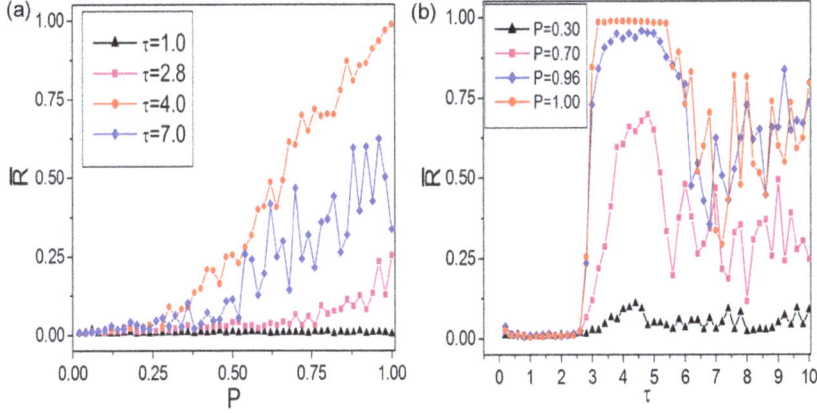

Figure 5. LRC induced synchronization transitions. (a) Dependence of synchronization parameter $\bar{R}$ on LRC probability P for different time delay τ. (b) Dependence of synchronization parameter $\bar{R}$ on time delay τ for different LRC probability P.

zation mode has been found at $P=0.96$ and is shown in Fig. 6(c). From visual assessment, we guess this kind of new synchronization mode is the lag synchronization. To test our idea, the similarity function is introduced, which was proposed to detect lag synchronization [5]. It is numerically calculated as:

$$S^2 = \frac{<[v_{78}(t+\tau_S) - v_{79}(t)]^2>}{[<v_{79}(t)^2> <v_{78}(t)^2>]^{1/2}}. \qquad (9)$$

Here v_{79} and v_{78} are the time series v of neurons 79 and 78 of Fig. 6(c). And τ_S is the time shift. Fig. 7(a) displays the dependence of similarity function S on time shift τ_S. The minimal value of S

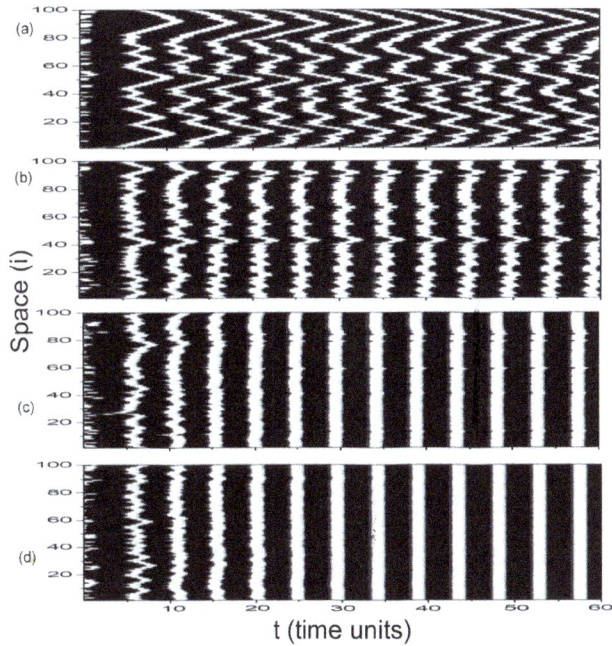

Figure 6. Space-time plots of u for different LRC probability P at $\tau=4.0$. (a) $P=0.30$ (asynchronous state), (b) $P=0.70$ (weak synchronization), (c) $P=0.96$ (lag synchronization), (d) $P=1.00$ (complete synchronization).

appears at $\tau_{S0}=0.363$, which indicates the lag synchronization between neurons 79 and 78. Fig. 7(b) shows the projection of the attractor on the time shifted plane $(v_{78}(t+\tau_{S0}), v_{79}(t))$. It demonstrates that the state of neuron 79 is delayed in time with respect to neuron 78. Accordingly, lag synchronization has been confirmed in delayed Newman-Watts SWNN. To explain the mechanism of lag synchronization, time series u of neurons 79 (without LRC, shown by black curve), 78 and 80 (two neighboring neurons of 79, shown by red and blue curves) of Fig. 6(c) are shown in Fig. 7(c). And the red dotted and blue dashed curves denote time series u of neurons 65 and 93 (the two LRD neurons of 78 and 80) with time delay translation, respectively. As LRC probability P is a little less than 1.0, some neurons in network will have no LRCs due to finite connection probability. All neurons without LRCs must be driven by their neighbors. And these neighboring neurons are excited by their corresponding delayed LRDs. The successive driving relationship is revealed in Fig. 7(c). And lag synchronization between neurons without LRCs and their corresponding neighbors is identified. Therefore, we can observe lag synchronization in delayed Newman-Watts SWNNs as LRC probability P is a little less than 1.0 at moderate time delay. Fig. 7(d) exhibits the LRD proportion p between adjacent intervals for different LRC probability P at $\tau=4.0$ (corresponding to Figs. 6(a)–(d)). Anticipated LRD proportions can be quickly approached so long as time delay is moderate. And large numbers of LRCs are needed to dominate the network for synchronization under this circumstance.

According to the results obtained in this part, the conclusion that moderate time delay can help LRDs to dominate the network has been verified again. And large numbers of LRCs are needed for synchronization under this circumstance. Therefore, the two necessary conditions, moderate time delay and large numbers of LRCs, are exposed explicitly for synchronization in delayed Newman-Watts SWNNs.

The Combined Effects on Synchronization Transitions

To have a overall inspection of time delay and LRC induced synchronization transitions in Newman-Watts SWNNs, the contour plot of synchronization parameter $\bar{R}$ in the plane (τ, P) is revealed in Fig 8. The color intensity denotes the synchronization degree in delayed Newman-Watts SWNNs. Specifically, lighter color representing larger synchronization parameter, which indicates higher degree of synchronization. The four distinct

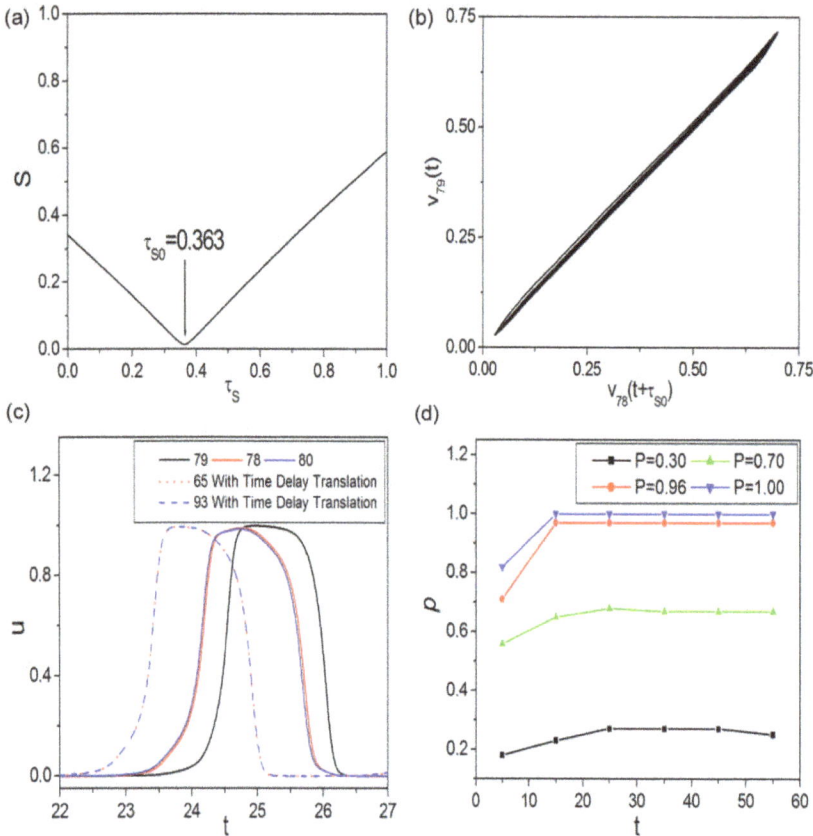

Figure 7. Dynamical analysis of lag synchronization and LRC induced synchronization transitions. (a) Dependence of similarity function S on time shift τ_S. The minimal value of S appears at $\tau_{S0}=0.363$, which indicates the lag synchronization between neurons 79 and 78 of Fig. 6(c). (b) Projection of the attractor on the time shifted plane $(v_{78}(t+\tau_{S0}), v_{79}(t))$. It demonstrates that the state of neuron 79 is delayed in time with respect to neuron 78. (c) Time series u of neurons 79 (without LRC, shown by black curve), 78 and 80 (two neighboring neurons of 79, shown by red and blue curves). The red dotted and blue dashed curves denote time series u of neurons 65 and 93 (the two LRD neurons of 78 and 80) with time delay translation, respectively. Lag synchronization is discovered in delayed Newman-Watts SWNN and the mechanism is also revealed. (d) The LRD proportion p between adjacent intervals for different LRC probability P (corresponding to Figs 6(a)–(d)).

parameter regions, i.e., asynchronous region, transition region, synchronous region and oscillatory region at certain LRC probability $P=1.0$ are exposed clearly. And the remarkable enhancement of synchronization transitions induced by LRCs under moderate time delay is also indicated explicitly. From Fig 8 the optimal combinations of time delay and LRC probability on synchronization transitions in delayed Newman-Watts SWNNs are revealed intuitively, which may has a useful impact for actual biological systems.

The Universality of Time Delay Induced Synchronization Transitions

In order to test the universality of time delay induced synchronization transitions, heterogeneous Newman-Watts SWNNs are considered. Diversity is introduced to system parameter b, i.e., the values of b_i are different in the network. And it satisfies the following Gaussian distribution:

$$<b_i> = b, <(b_i-b)(b_j-b)> = \sigma^2\delta(i-j). \quad (10)$$

The value of b is fixed at 0.07. Here σ is the standard deviation of the Gaussian probability distribution of system parameter b. It indicates the strength of the diversity in delayed Newman-Watts

SWNNs. Fig. 9(a) shows the dependence of synchronization parameter $\bar{R}$ on time delay τ for different diversity σ at LRC probability $P=1.0$. Although synchronization transition becomes

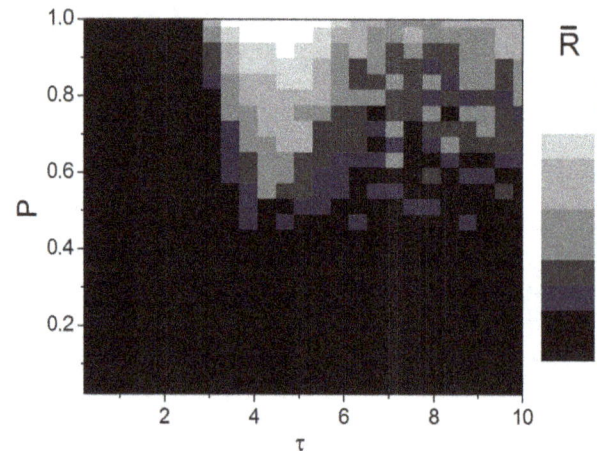

Figure 8. The combined effects on synchronization transitions. Dependence of synchronization parameter $\bar{R}$ on time delay τ and LRC probability P.

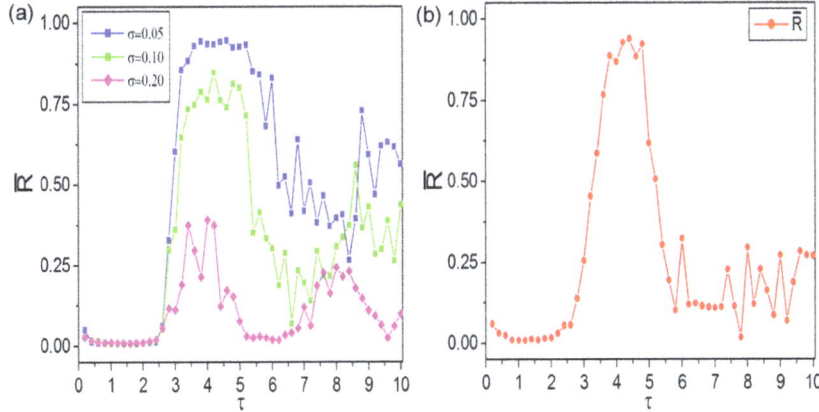

Figure 9. The universality of time delay induced synchronization transitions. (a) Dependence of synchronization parameter $\bar{R}$ on time delay τ for different diversity σ. (b) Dependence of synchronization parameter $\bar{R}$ on time delay τ for the new coupling.

less profound as diversity increases, similar time delay induced synchronization transitions can be observed in heterogeneous Newman-Watts SWNNs. More importantly, all these synchronization transitions appear at approximatively same τ. It indicates that time delay plays a significant role in synchronization transitions in Newman-Watts SWNNs. Moreover, to further test the generality of our findings, the following new coupling form is used:

$$\frac{du_i(t)}{dt} = -\frac{1}{\epsilon} u_i(t)[u_i(t)-1]\left[u_i(t)-\frac{v_i(t)+b_i}{a}\right] + D\left(\frac{W_{i,j}}{W_{i,j}+C_K}-u_i(t)\right), \qquad (11)$$

where

$$W_{i,j} = [u_{i-1}(t)+u_{i+1}(t)-2u_i(t)]+[u_j(t-\tau)-u_i(t)]. \qquad (12)$$

This type of coupling has been widely used in neural models and excitable complex networks. In simulations, we set $C_K = 0.5$. Fig. 9(b) displays the dependence of synchronization parameter $\bar{R}$ on time delay τ. Similar time delay induced synchronization transitions can also be observed for the new coupling form. Now we can conclude that time delay induced synchronization transitions in Newman-Watts SWNNs are a robust phenomenon. The results revealed in present paper are universal.

Conclusions

In conclusion, time delay and long-range connection induced synchronization transitions in Newman-Watts small-world neuronal networks are systematically investigated by synchronization parameter and space-time plots. We have found four distinct parameter regions, i.e., asynchronous region, transition region,

synchronous region and oscillatory region, at certain LRC probability $P = 1.0$ as time delay is increased. Interestingly, desynchronization and oscillating behaviour of the order parameter are observed in oscillatory region. More importantly, the mechanisms of synchronous oscillations and the transition from non-synchronization to complete synchronization are discussed. We consider the spatiotemporal patterns obtained in delayed Newman-Watts SWNNs are the competition results between long-range drivings and neighboring interactions. And our point of view has been verified by LRD proportion, which can also reveal the four distinct parameter regions clearly. In addition, for moderate time delay, the synchronization of neuronal network can be enhanced remarkably by increasing LRC probability. Furthermore, lag synchronization has been found between weak synchronization and complete synchronization as LRC probability P is a little less than 1.0. Finally, the two necessary conditions, moderate time delay and large numbers of LRCs, are exposed explicitly for synchronization in delayed Newman-Watts SWNNs.

As we know that synchronization transitions in neuronal networks are very important issues in related research fields and are associated with some specific physiological functions. A systematical investigation of synchronization transitions induced by time delay and long-range connection is expected to be useful both for theoretical understandings and practical applications. The results obtained in the present paper are universal. Similar time delay induced synchronization transitions can also be observed for heterogeneous Newman-Watts SWNNs and the new coupling form. We do hope that our work will be a useful supplement to the previous contributions and will have a useful impact in related fields.

Author Contributions

Conceived and designed the experiments: YQ. Performed the experiments: YQ. Analyzed the data: YQ. Contributed reagents/materials/analysis tools: YQ. Wrote the paper: YQ.

References

1. West BJ, Geneston EL, Grigolini P (2008) Maximizing information exchange between complex networks. Phys Rep 468: 1–99.
2. Arenas A, Díaz-Guilera A, Kurths J, Moreno Y, Zhou C (2008) Synchronization in complex networks. Phys Rep 469: 93–153.
3. Pecora LM, Carroll TL (1990) Synchronization in chaotic systems. Phys Rev Lett 64: 821–824.
4. Pyragas K (1996) Weak and strong synchronization of chaos. Phys Rev E 54: R4508–R4511.
5. Rosenblum MG, Pikovsky AS, Kurths J (1997) From phase to lag synchronization in coupled chaotic oscillators. Phys Rev Lett 78: 4193–4196.

6. Liu Z, Lai YC, Hoppensteadt FC (2001) Phase clustering and transition to phase synchronization in a large number of coupled nonlinear oscillators. Phys Rev E 63: R055201.

7. Yu HT, Wang J, Deng B, Wei XL, Wong YK, et al. (2011) Chaotic phase synchronization in small-world networks of bursting neurons. Chaos 21: 013127.

8. Gray CM, Singer W (1989) Stimulus-specific neuronal oscillations in orientation columns of cat visual cortex. Proc Natl Acad Sci 86: 1698–1702.

9. Bazhenov M, Stopfer M, Rabinovich M, Huerta R, Abarbanel HDI, et al. (2001) Model of transient oscillatory synchronization in the locust antennal lobe. Neuron 30: 553–567.

10. Mehta MR, Lee AK, Wilson MA (2002) Role of experience and oscillations in transforming a rate code into a temporal code. Nature 417: 741–746.

11. Stopfer M, Bhagavan S, Smith BH, Laurent G (1997) Impaired odour discrimination on desynchronization of odour-encoding neural assemblies. Nature 390: 70–74.

12. Usrey WM, Reid RC (1999) Synchronous activity in the visual system. Annu Rev Physiol 61: 435–456.

13. Ward LM (2003) Synchronous neural oscillations and cognitive processes. Trends in Cognitive Sciences 7: 553–559.

14. Fries P, Nikolić D, Singer W (2007) The gamma cycle. Trends in Neurosciences 30: 309–316.

15. Watts DJ, Strogatz SH (1998) Collective dynamics of 'small-world' networks. Nature 393: 440–442.

16. He D, Hu G, Zhan M, Ren W, Gao Z (2002) Pattern formation of spiral waves in an inhomogeneous medium with small-world connections. Phys Rev E 65: 055204(R).

17. Qi F, Hou Z, Xin H (2003) Ordering chaos by random shortcuts. Phys Rev Lett 91: 064102.

18. Zumdieck A, Timme M, Geisel T, Wolf F (2004) Long chaotic transients in complex networks. Phys Rev Lett 93: 244103.

19. Qian Y, Huang X, Hu G, Liao X (2010) Structure and control of self-sustained target waves in excitable small-world networks. Phys Rev E 81: 036101.

20. Kandel ER, Schwartz JH, Jessell TM (1991) Principles of Neural Science. (Elsevier, Amsterdam).

21. Dhamala M, Jirsa VK, Ding M (2004) Enhancement of neural synchrony by time delay. Phys Rev Lett 92: 074104.

22. Roxin A, Brunel N, Hansel D (2005) Role of delays in shaping spatiotemporal dynamics of neuronal activity in large networks. Phys Rev Lett 94: 238103.

23. Ko TW, Ermentrout GB (2007) Effects of axonal time delay on synchronization and wave formation in sparsely coupled neuronal oscillators. Phys Rev E 76: 056206.

24. Burić N, Todorović K, Vasović N (2008) Synchronization of bursting neurons with delayed chemical synapses. Phys Rev E 78: 036211.

25. Liang X, Tang M, Dhamala M, Liu Z (2009) Phase synchronization of inhibitory bursting neurons induced by distributed time delays in chemical coupling. Phys Rev E 80: 066202.

26. Tang J, Ma J, Yi M, Xia H, Yang X (2011) Delay and diversity-induced synchronization transitions in a small-world neuronal network. Phys Rev E 83: 046207.

27. Wang Q, Perc M, Duan Z, Chen G (2008) Delay-enhanced coherence of spiral waves in noisy hodgkin-huxley neuronal networks. Phys Lett A 372: 5681–5687.

28. Wang Q, Murks A, Perc M, Lu Q (2011) Taming desynchronized bursting with delays in the macaque cortical network. Chin Phys B 20: 040504.

29. Wang Q, Perc M, Duan Z, Chen G (2009) Delay-induced multiple stochastic resonances on scale-free neuronal networks. Chaos 19: 023112.

30. Wang Q, Duan Z, Perc M, Chen G (2008) Synchronization transitions on small-world neuronal networks: effects of information transmission delay and rewiring probability. Europhys Lett 83: 50008.

31. Wang Q, Perc M, Duan Z, Chen G (2009) Synchronization transitions on scale-free neuronal networks due to finite information transmission delays. Phys Rev E 80: 026206.

32. Wang Q, Perc M, Duan Z, Chen G (2010) Impact of delays and rewiring on the dynamics of small-world neuronal networks with two types of coupling. Physica A 389: 3299–3306.

33. Wang Q, Chen G, Perc M (2011) Synchronous bursts on scale-free neuronal networks with attractive and repulsive coupling. Plos One 6: e15851.

34. Guo D, Wang Q, Perc M (2012) Complex synchronous behavior in interneuronal networks with delayed inhibitory and fast electrical synapses. Phys Rev E 85: 061905.

35. Yu HT, Wang J, Liu C, Deng B, Wei XL (2013) Delay-induced synchronization transitions in small-world neuronal networks with hybrid electrical and chemical synapses. Physica A 392: 5473–5480.

36. Yu HT, Wang J, Liu QX, Sun JB, Yu HF (2013) Delay-induced synchronization transitions in small-world neuronal networks with hybrid synapses. Chaos, Solitons & Fractals 48: 68–74.

37. Bär M, Eiswirth M (1993) Turbulence due to spiral breakup in a continuous excitable medium. Phys Rev E 48: R1635–R1637.

38. Newmam MEJ, Watts DJ (1999) Renormalization group analysis of the small-world network model. Phys Lett A 263: 341–346.

39. Sinha S, Saramäki J, Kaski K (2007) Emergence of self-sustained patterns in small-world excitable media. Phys Rev E 76: R015101.

40. Qian Y, Liao X, Huang X, Mi Y, Zhang L, et al. (2010) Diverse self-sustained oscillatory patterns and their mechanisms in excitable small-world networks. Phys Rev E 82: 026107.

41. Gonze D, Bernard S, Waltermann C, Kramer A, Herzel H (2005) Spontaneous synchronization of coupled circadian oscillators. Biophys J 89: 120–129.

5

Motor Network Plasticity and Low-Frequency Oscillations Abnormalities in Patients with Brain Gliomas: A Functional MRI Study

Chen Niu[1], Ming Zhang[1]*, Zhigang Min[1], Netra Rana[1], Qiuli Zhang[1], Xin Liu[2], Min Li[1], Pan Lin[2]*

1 Department of Medical Imaging, First Affiliated Hospital of Xi'an Jiaotong University, Xi'an, Shaanxi-Province, P. R. China, **2** Institute of Biomedical Engineering, Xi'an Jiaotong University, Xi'an, Shaanxi-Province, P.R. China

Abstract

Brain plasticity is often associated with the process of slow-growing tumor formation, which remodels neural organization and optimizes brain network function. In this study, we aimed to investigate whether motor function plasticity would display deficits in patients with slow-growing brain tumors located in or near motor areas, but who were without motor neurological deficits. We used resting-state functional magnetic resonance imaging to probe motor networks in 15 patients with histopathologically confirmed brain gliomas and 15 age-matched healthy controls. All subjects performed a motor task to help identify individual motor activity in the bilateral primary motor cortex (PMC) and supplementary motor area (SMA). Frequency-based analysis at three different frequencies was then used to investigate possible alterations in the power spectral density (PSD) of low-frequency oscillations. For each group, the average PSD was determined for each brain region and a nonparametric test was performed to determine the difference in power between the two groups. Significantly reduced inter-hemispheric functional connectivity between the left and right PMC was observed in patients compared with controls ($P<0.05$). We also found significantly decreased PSD in patients compared to that in controls, in all three frequency bands (low: 0.01–0.02 Hz; middle: 0.02–0.06 Hz; and high: 0.06–0.1 Hz), at three key motor regions. These findings suggest that in asymptomatic patients with brain tumors located in eloquent regions, inter-hemispheric connection may be more vulnerable. A comparison of the two approaches indicated that power spectral analysis is more sensitive than functional connectivity analysis for identifying the neurological abnormalities underlying motor function plasticity induced by slow-growing tumors.

Editor: Emmanuel Andreas Stamatakis, University Of Cambridge, United Kingdom

Funding: This study was supported by the National Natural Science Foundation of China (Projects No. 81171318 and No. 31271061), the Doctoral Fund of Ministry of Education of China (20120201120071), and the Fundamental Research Funds for the Central Universities of China. The funders had no role in study design, data collection and analysis, decision to publish, or preparation of the manuscript.

Competing Interests: The authors have declared that no competing interests exist.

* E-mail: profzmmri@gmail.com (MZ); linpan@mail.xjtu.edu.cn (PL)

Introduction

Brain plasticity is the reshaping of the nervous system during routine activities (e.g., learning or memory) or following pathological conditions (e.g., neoplasms or traumatic brain injury). This continuous remodeling process aims to optimize the functioning of brain networks [1–3]. Progressive lesions, such as slow-growing tumors, may induce a larger functional reshaping. Many believe that this is the explanation for why neurological deficits do not appear earlier, even though the lesion lies within the so-called eloquent areas [4]. Additionally, the reorganization of functional areas may take place during tumor growth. Therefore, understanding such functional reorganization is not only important for mapping the resection margin, but is also helpful for to predict the functional outcomes of surgery and to prepare for rehabilitation. Yet, the exact neurobiological mechanisms underlying functional plasticity caused by brain tumors remain elusive.

In the last two decades, resting-state functional magnetic resonance imaging (rs-fMRI) has been widely used in the study of both normal subjects [5–7] and patients with brain disorders for assessing functional connectivity (FC), which involves analysis of spatially distributed and temporally correlated signals between brain regions. Biswal et al. [5] first reported the presence of spontaneous low-frequency oscillations (LFOs) that were highly synchronous between the right and left primary motor cortex (PMC) at rest, using fMRI. In addition, abnormal FC was found in a wide range of brain disorders including autism [8,9], Alzheimer's disease [10], attention deficit hyperactivity disorder [11], mild cognitive impairment [12], and schizophrenia [13].

Recently, brain tumor induced network connectivity dysfunction has been proposed in several studies, involving language, sensorimotor, and default-mode network [14–18]. However, research on the regional properties of the brain's intrinsic functional dynamics is lacking. Some recent studies have indicated that power spectral density (PSD) analysis is a sensitive method for detecting and characterizing blood oxygen level-dependent (BOLD) signal oscillations. The advantage of this approach is that it can identify the oscillatory dynamics of the BOLD signal across a wider range of frequencies than FC [19,20]. Recent studies using PSD analysis demonstrated increased high-frequency oscillations within certain pain-related brain regions in several pain diseases [19,21]. Furthermore, in contrast to FC, PSD

Table 1. Demographic information and tumor classification for study subjects.

No.	Symptoms	Age (years)	Gender	Tumor location	Tumor type
1	Seizure	42	F	Left Frontal	Astrocytoma (Grade II)
2	Seizure	39	M	Left Parietal	Astrocytoma (Grade II)
3	Headache	45	F	Left Frontal/ Parietal	Astrocytoma (Grade II)
4	Persistent vomiting	27	M	Right Frontal/ Parietal	Oligodendroglioma (Grade II)
5	Seizure	38	M	Right Frontal/ Parietal	Oligodendroglioma (Grade II)
6	Seizure	47	M	Left Frontal	Oligodendroglioma (Grade II)
7	Headache	65	F	Right Parietal	Astrocytoma (Grade II)
8	Headache	61	M	Left Frontal	Astrocytoma (Grade III)
9	Headache	53	M	Left Frontal/ Parietal	Astrocytoma (Grade III)
10	Asymptomatic	41	M	Left Parietal	Oligodendroglioma (Grade II)
11	Headache	63	M	Right Parietal	Astrocytoma (Grade III)
12	Vomiting	56	M	Left Frontal	Astrocytoma glioma (Grade III)
13	Seizure	51	M	Left Frontal/ Temporal	Astrocytoma glioma (Grade II)
14	Headache	55	F	Right Frontal/ Parietal	Astrocytoma glioma (Grade II)
15	Headache	56	M	Left Frontal/ Parietal	Astrocytoma glioma (Grade III)

M = male; F = female.

analysis can provide valuable information on the regional characteristics of spontaneous changes in the low-frequency fluctuations, as well as of changes in BOLD signal dynamics associated with neural activity. [22–25]. A small number of studies show that independent frequency bands are associated with specific brain function [23,26,27]. Furthermore, it has been shown that patients with cognitive disorders exhibit frequency-dependent changes in abnormal LFO amplitudes [28,29]. However, it is still not clear whether any PSD abnormalities are related to specific frequency sub-bands of the LFOs.

Brain tumor infiltration and compression of the cortex and subcortical white matter are thought to result in cortical dysfunction [30,31]. Accordingly, the brain function and rhythmic oscillations may be altered in the brain regions which show functional connectivity disruption in patients with brain tumors [31]. Furthermore, individual differences in tumor location, histopathology, growth patterns, and brain functional plasticity may induce FC or PSD changes in tumor patients. Little is known about whether patients with brain gliomas show abnormal PSDs across the LFOs bands and whether any LFO sub-bands are especially informative scientifically and diagnostically in these patients.

To address the above issues, in the current study, we limited our patient selection to a single pathology (glioma) with a restricted location (within or close to the PMC) and measured the FC of the motor network using functional connectivity magnetic resonance imaging (fcMRI). We hypothesized that the brain tumor would infiltrate, compress, and destroy motor areas and induce abnormal PSD in motor cortical regions of patients with brain tumors even in those without motor weakness. Specifically, we used rs-fMRI to investigate the possible alteration of PSD in the oscillatory dynamics of the BOLD signal across different frequency bands in patients with brain gliomas, and compared them with those of age- and gender-matched healthy controls. Ultimately, using both fcMRI and power spectral analysis, we examined the relationship between alterations of LFOs and plastic changes in motor FC in patients with brain gliomas to achieve a better understanding of the underlying brain plasticity mechanisms.

Materials and Methods

Ethics statement

All subjects were fully informed of the nature of the study and all gave their written consent regarding participation. This study was approved by the local ethical committee of the Xi'an Jiaotong University Institutional Review Board for clinical research.

Patients and controls

We consecutively evaluated 143 patients with brain tumors using conventional MRI, based on a prospective study design. These patients were registered at the First Affiliated Hospital of Xi'an Jiaotong University between May 2011 and March 2013. After reviewing all conventional MRI scans obtained prior to surgery, as well as the post-surgical pathology results, 15 patients (11 male and 4 female; age range, 27–65 years; mean age, 49.27 ± 10.65 years, all right-handed) with a histopathologically confirmed brain glioma, were selected for the study (Table 1). All subjects had a space-occupying lesion located in the vicinity of the central sulcus (near or within the PMC) recognized based on a previous computed tomography (CT) or MRI examination (with or without contrast medium). Seven patients (46.7%) presented with headache, 5 (33.3%) with seizures, 2 (13.3%) with a history of vomiting, and 1 (6.7%) was asymptomatic and incidentally diagnosed during an imaging study performed for other reason. All patients had normal muscle strength and had no motor weakness according to both the manual muscle testing scale (MTT) and a clinical exam.

Additionally, 15 healthy volunteers, (11 male and 4 female; age range, 25–60 years; mean age, 46.07 ± 9.42 years, all right-handed), were recruited as a control group. The eligibility criteria for healthy volunteers consisted of the absence of any pre-existing or presenting abnormal neurological conditions, and the volunteers underwent structural MRI scanning without administration of contrast medium prior to undergoing fMRI.

Data acquisition

All images were acquired using a 3.0T whole-body scanner (GE Signa HDxt, Milwaukee, WI, USA) equipped with an 8-channel head receiver coil. Head movement was restricted using a pillow and foam, and earplugs were used to minimize scanner noise and maximize patient comfort.

Anatomical imaging. A three-dimensional T1-weighted fast spoiled gradient echo (FSPGR) sequence covering the whole brain was performed to coregister functional data and define regions of interest (ROI) (time of repetition [TR] /time of echo [TE] /flip angle [α] = 10.8 ms/4.8 ms/15°; field of view = 256 mm; matrix = 256×256; slice thickness = 1 mm; no gap; voxel size = 1×1×1 mm^3; 150 axial plane).

Functional imaging. BOLD functional images were acquired by means of a T2*-weighted single-shot gradient-echo-planar-imaging sequence with the following parameters: TR = 2500 ms; TE = 40 ms; α = 90°; field of view = 256 mm; acquired matrix = 64×64; slice thickness = 3 mm; voxel size = 3.75×3.75×3 mm^3; 47 slices; no gap. A total of 150 functional volumes were acquired.

fMRI motor task design

A "block" design sequence (ABAB) was used for the motor task, with six 30-s rest periods (A) alternated with five 30-s periods of visual cues for hand movement (B). All patients and healthy controls were instructed to repetitively open and close both hands in response to each flash used as a visual cue. All subjects were trained in the task and were observed before performing the experiment to ensure their understanding and ability to comply with the protocol. No cue was supplied during rest periods. The experimental stimuli were presented using E-Prime Version 2.0 (Psychology Software Tools, Pittsburgh, PA, USA), transmitted via a liquid crystal display projector, and viewed through a mirror placed above the subject's head.

We performed the resting-state scanning prior to the motor task scanning. For the task-free functional experiment, all participants were instructed to relax and remain calm with their eyes open. Subjects were instructed to not think of anything in particular without falling asleep.

Data analysis

Motor task fMRI data analysis. The motor task fMRI dataset was analyzed with FSL software (www.fmrib.ox.ac.uk/fsl/). The first four scans were discarded, and then motion correction was applied using FLIRT (MCFLIRT). Spatial smoothing was performed using a 6-mm full-width-half-maximum (FWHM) Gaussian kernel to reduce noise. The functional connectivity MRI images were filtered with a high-pass filter. The functional images were normalized to the MNI152 standard brain space through their structural images. General linear model (GLM) analysis was carried out using FSL FEAT. Z statistic images were thresholded using clusters determined by Z>2.3, a corrected cluster significance threshold of $P<0.05$. All 3 regions including the left PMC (LPMC), right PMC (RPMC), and supplementary motor area (SMA) could be detected via a task-evoked BOLD response. As a result, we extracted the maximum activation mapping to define the key motor regions for resting-state inter-regional functional analysis.

Inter- regional functional connectivity analysis. The rs-fMRI analysis was performed using AFNI (Cox, 1996) and FSL software (www.fmrib.ox.ac.uk/fsl/). Pre-processing consisted of motion correction, temporal band-pass filtering (0.008 Hz<f< 0.1 Hz), spatial normalization to standard Talairach space and spatial smoothing (Gaussian, FWHM 6 mm). Several sources of nuisance covariates (6 head motion parameters, signal from the white matter and the CSF) were eliminated using linear regression. The three key motor network regions (LPMC, RPMC, and SMA) were selected based on motor task functional mapping for each subject, and defined as a spherical region with a radius of 10 mm. Mean time series from three Regions of interest (ROIs) were estimated by averaging the time series of all voxels in a region. In the present study, Pearson's correlation coefficients were computed between each pair of brain regions for each subject. For further analysis, a Fisher's r-to-z transformation was applied to improve the normality of the correlation coefficients. In general, normal brain areas can be infiltrated and damaged by tumors. As a previous study indicated that functional zones could shift in the presence of neoplastic disease [4], we suspected the possibility that the spatial distribution of functional activation areas between patients and healthy subjects may be inconsistent. In order to test the reliability of our results, we further analyze our fMRI data based on different ROIs (6 mm and 8 mm).

Spectral power analysis. Spectral analysis was performed using home-made Matlab (The MathWorks, 2010) code. We derived the PSD estimation using a direct fast Fourier transform method for each subject's motor cortex region resting-state network (RSN) time series. Our specific interest was to compare the power spectral density within this frequency domain between patients and healthy controls, for measurements in the motor cortex. Previous studies have divided the full frequency band (0–0.25 Hz) into following sub-bands: slow-5 (0.01–0.027 Hz), slow-4 (0.027–0.073 Hz), slow-3 (0.073–0.198 Hz), and slow-2 (0.198–0.25 Hz) [23,26]. These can be further subdivided into additional sub-bands to better reflect the neural origins of the signal sources [23]. Cordes et al suggested that the respiratory and aliased cardiac signals fall into the range of slow 2–3 [7], while the oscillatory signals upon which resting-state FC is primarily fall within slow 4–5 [32,33]. To simplify this, we divided the low frequency (0.01–0.08 Hz) band into three sub-bands, including "low-band" (0.01–0.02 Hz), "middle-band" (0.02–0.06 Hz), and "high-band" (0.06–0.08 Hz). For each patient with tumor and normal subject, the predominant power spectral density of each motor cortical region (computed from the resting-state time-course) was estimated in each sub-band.

Statistical analysis. All statistical calculations were performed by using Statistical Package for the Social Sciences, Version 16.0 (SPSS, Chicago, Illinois). Shapiro-Wilks test was used to assess the normality of all data. Group differences in FC and PSD analysis were compared by using non-parametric Mann-Whitney U tests. For all group-level statistical significance threshold was set at $P<0.05$, two tailed.

Results

Functional Magnetic Resonance Imaging

Both healthy controls and patients with brain tumors underwent resting-state and task-based fMRI scans (Table 1). As shown in Figure 1, the BOLD fMRI activation map and BOLD signal time course of a single tumor patient differs dramatically from that of a control. The reorganization of functional areas could have been induced by the lesion in patients with gliomas. In order to avoid the possible shift of functional areas caused by the tumor, three key motor areas were selected based on the activation maps of the LPMC, RPMC, and SMA associated with motor task stimuli and identified by the GLM analysis. Full details of this analysis strategy are described in the Materials and Methods section. We present our data processing steps in the form of a flow chart in Figure S1.

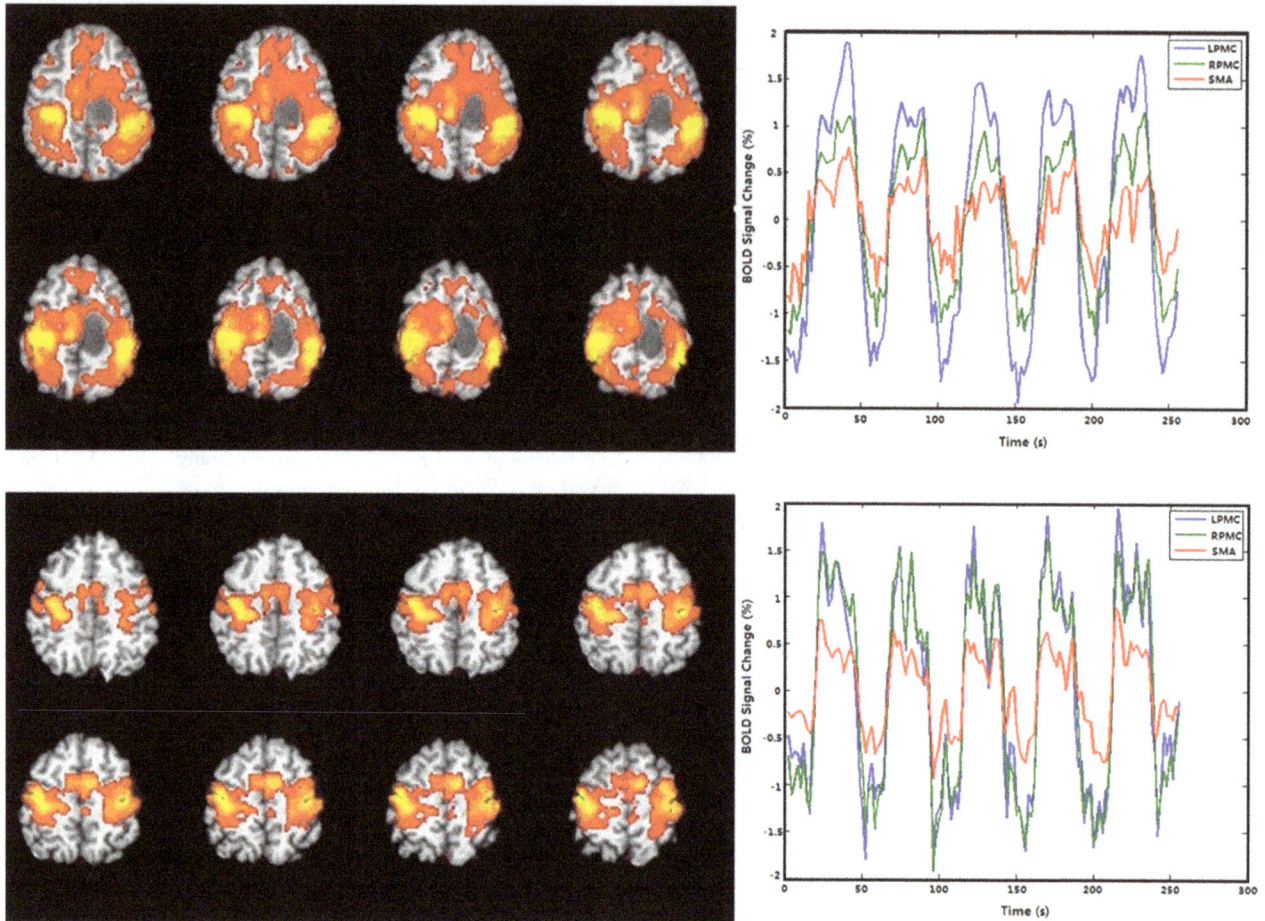

Figure 1. Example of BOLD functional magnetic resonance imaging activation maps and BOLD signal time courses in the LPMC, RPMC and SMA during a motor task in a single patient with glioma and a healthy control subject. BOLD, blood oxygen level dependent; LPMC, left primary motor cortex; RPMC, right primary motor cortex; SMA, supplementary motor area.

Functional connectivity within the motor network

The Pearson's correlation coefficients of inter-regional FC within the motor network were computed between each pair of brain regions (RPMC, LPMC, and SMA) for each subject. FC of control and patient groups are shown in Figure 2. We compared the averaged values of FC within ROIs of the 2 hemispheres, patients showed a statistically significant reduction in the connectivity of the LPMC-RPMC ($z = -3. 09$, $P = 0.002$, Mann-Whitney U test) compared to controls. In contrast, FC analysis of the LPMC-SMA and RPMC-SMA showed no significant differences between the two groups. (LPMC-SMA: $z = -0.892$, $P = 0.373$, Mann-Whitney U test; RPMC-SMA: $z = -0.145$, $P = 0.885$, Mann-Whitney U test; respectively). In order to test the consistency and reliability of the results, different size of ROIs (10 mm, 8 mm and 6 mm) were used in the analysis, all of which generated similar results (see Figure S2).

Changes in PSD

The PSDs of BOLD oscillations in the low-frequency band (0~0.1 Hz) within the LPMC, RPMC, and SMA of controls and patients are shown in Figure 3. Our results demonstrated a remarkable PSD decrease in patients compared to in controls in this range, as shown by the difference between the mean PSD of controls (red traces) and that of patients (blue traces) in the 0–

0.1 Hz frequency band within each key motor region. To further test the consistency and reliability of the results, PSD values in ROIs of different sizes (10 mm, 8 mm, and 6 mm) were also calculated and similar results were achieved (see Figure S3).

The PSDs of the BOLD oscillation in three frequency bands were estimated for controls and patients with gliomas in the three key motor regions (LPMC, RPMC, and SMA). For each of the frequency bands in the three key regions, we observed a significant decrease in PSD in patients compared to in controls ($P < 0.05$, Mann-Whitney U test), as shown in Figure 4 and Table 2. Again, when we used different ROI sizes (10 mm, 8 mm and 6 mm) in repeated analyses to test the consistency of our results, findings were consistent (see Figure S4).

Discussion

In this study, we employed FC and power spectral analyses to explore possible changes in the motor network of patients with gliomas. Our results showed a significant difference in the inter-regional FC of the LPMC-RPMC between patients and controls. In addition, patients with brain tumor exhibited abnormal amplitudes of low-frequency fluctuation activity during the resting state, and a significant decrease in PSD within three key motor cortical regions (LPMC, RPMC, and SMA) was found. These

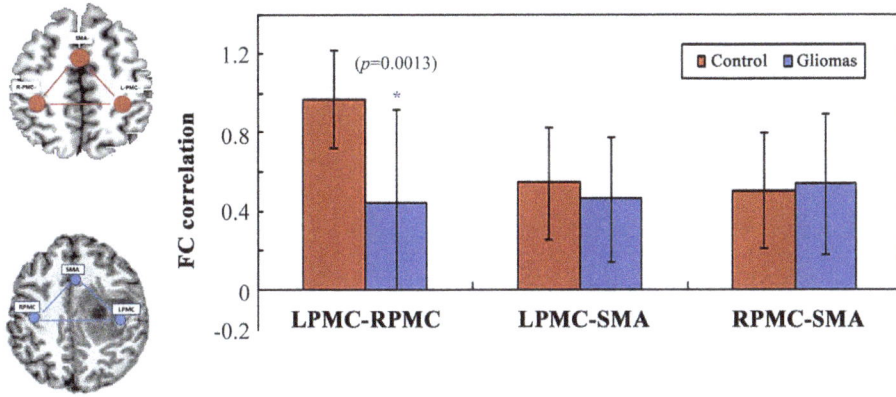

Figure 2. Group differences in the functional connectivity of the motor network between patients with brain gliomas and healthy controls. Error bars represent standard error of the mean. A blue asterisk indicates significant differences between groups ($z = -3.215$, $P = 0.001$, Mann-Whitney U test). LPMC, left primary motor cortex; RPMC, right primary motor cortex; SMA, supplementary motor area.

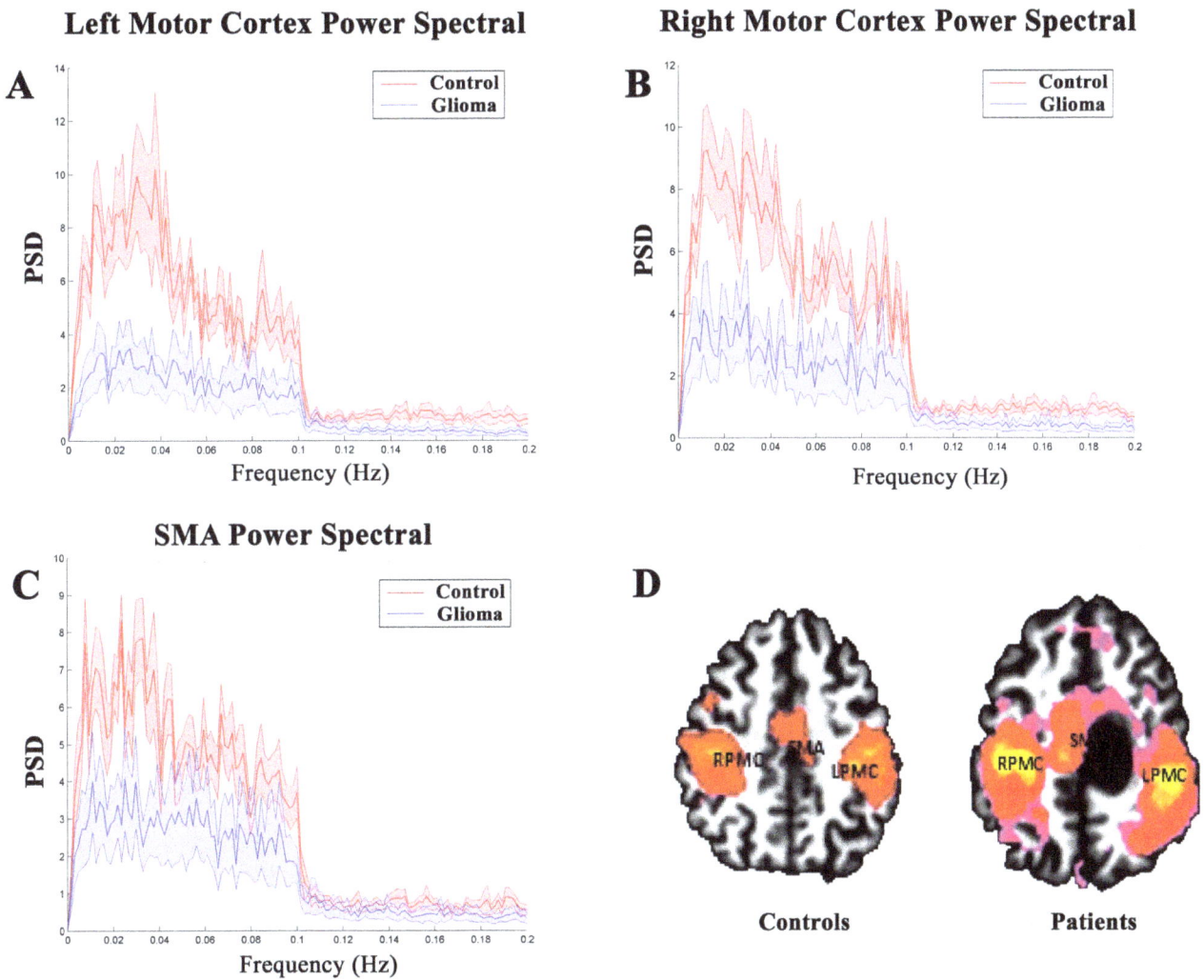

Figure 3. The power spectral density (PSD). A, B, and C show the group mean PSD in the LPMC, RPMC and SMA between healthy subjects (red traces) and patients with brain gliomas (blue traces). D, The localization of three key motor regions. In patients with brain gliomas, the PSDs in the LPMC, RPMC, and SMA are significantly lower than the PSDs of healthy controls ($P<0.05$). LPMC, left primary motor cortex; RPMC, right motor cortex; SMA, supplementary motor area.

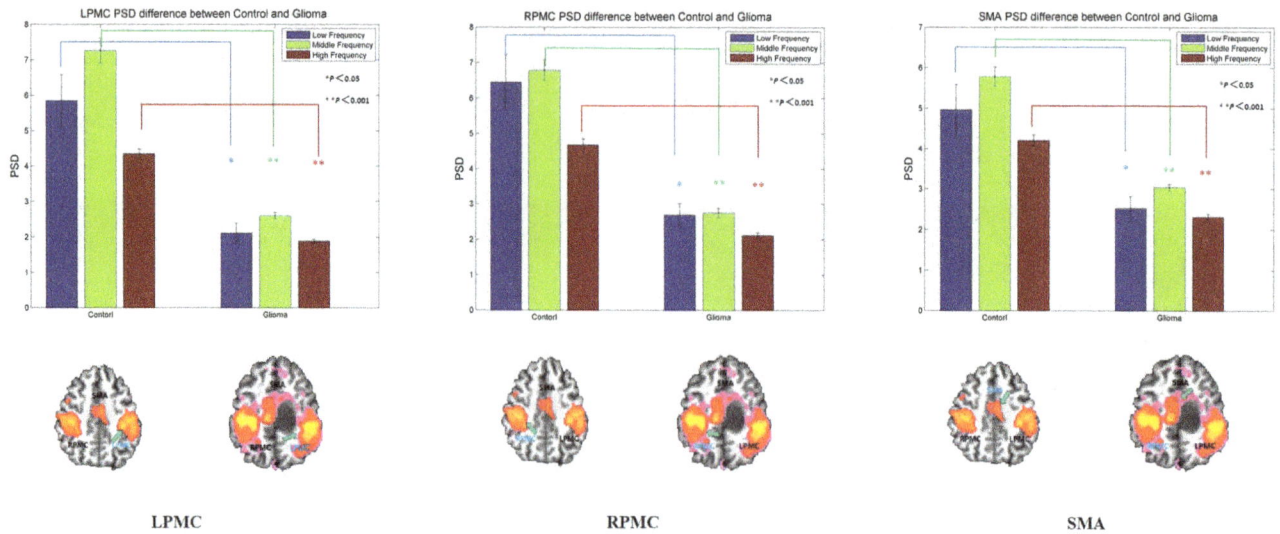

Figure 4. Bar graphs show the PSD in the three non-overlapping frequency bands for the three key regions of the motor network in healthy subjects and patients with brain gliomas. The sub-divisions of the low-frequency band were: low, 0.01–0.02 Hz; middle, 0.02–0.06 Hz; and high, 0.06–0.1 Hz. Patients with brain tumors show significant PSD decreases in all bands in all three key motor cortical regions (LPMC, RPMC, and SMA) (*$P<0.05$; ** $P<0.001$). PSD, power spectral density; LPMC, left primary motor cortex; RPMC, right motor cortex; SMA, supplementary motor area.

results suggest that the low-frequency brain oscillation changes in patients with brain tumors, even in the absence of motor deficits. This finding also indicates that power spectral analysis is more sensitive at detecting the underlying neural mechanism abnormalities during slow-growing tumor-induced brain motor plasticity, and provides a novel insight for explaining how abnormal oscillations might influence brain plasticity. Lastly, this study explores the underlying relationship linking brain plasticity to the LFOs.

Changes in resting-state functional connectivity within the motor cortex: relationship with motor function plasticity

For patients with brain tumors, brain plasticity plays an important role in motor and language areas. Moreover, brain reorganization is thought to explain why slow infiltrative low-grade gliomas near or in eloquent motor or language areas often do not induce detectable neurological deficits [34]. A number of studies have indicated that many brain diseases may produce a disruption of the normal architecture of the brain by inducing dysfunctional

Table 2. Statistical comparisons of power spectral density in different brain regions between groups.

PSD	Healthy Controls (N = 15)		Patients (N = 15)		Mann-Whitney U test
	Mean	SD	Mean	SD	P value
LPMC					
Low-frequency band*	5.85	2.61	2.11	1.00	$P=1.00\times10^{-3}$
Middle-frequency band**	7.26	1.81	2.60	0.46	$P=2.86\times10^{-10}$
High-frequency band**	4.34	0.69	1.88	0.28	$P=1.33\times10^{-9}$
RPMC					
Low-frequency band*	6.45	2.83	2.69	1.15	$P=1.00\times10^{-3}$
Middle-frequency band**	6.78	1.48	2.75	0.67	$P=2.87\times10^{-10}$
High-frequency band**	4.68	0.86	2.11	0.43	$P=1.50\times10^{-9}$
SMA					
Low-frequency band*	4.97	2.21	2.53	1.07	$P=2.00\times10^{-3}$
Middle-frequency band**	5.78	1.25	3.04	0.39	$P=4.47\times10^{-10}$
High-frequency band**	4.21	0.67	2.31	0.38	$P=1.33\times10^{-9}$

*implies significant group difference at $P<0.05$;
**implies significant group difference at $P<0.001$. PSD, power spectral density; SD, standard deviation; LPMC, left primary motor cortex; RPMC, right motor cortex; SMA, supplementary motor area. Group-differences were tested using SPSS software.

communication between neural networks [35,36]. According to this view, FC is useful for investigating communication within and between cortical networks. The current study reveals a remarkable difference in motor FC between the LPMC and RPMC in patients with brain tumors compared to in healthy controls, rather than a disruption in connectivity between the SMA and bilateral PMC. Consistent with a previous study [15], this finding confirms that long-distance connections, especially between hemispheres, are particularly vulnerable to damage. The presence of inter-hemispheric plasticity has been established in early brain lesions, while lesions occurring later in life show intra-hemispheric reorganization [37,38]. In addition, a hierarchically organized model, proposed by Duffau et al [34] explains the sensorimotor and language plasticity mechanisms in slow-growing low grade gliomas (LGG). Initially, intrinsic reorganization within injured areas occurs, and the perilesional structures play a major role in the functional compensation. However, if this reshaping is not sufficient, other regions are recruited to reorganize the functional network, starting with the ipsilateral hemisphere (remote to the damaged area) followed by the contralateral hemisphere [4,39]. Therefore, we speculate that the reduced inter-hemispheric FC observed in our patients was probably caused by the recruitment of compensating areas from the brain regions surrounding the slow-growing gliomas.

Interestingly, another recent study conducted by Otten et al. using rs-fMRI to investigate sixteen patients with brain neoplasms without motor weakness, reported no significant difference in the motor network connectivity of patients compared to that in controls [15]. However, the key differences include the large degree of heterogeneity in the pathological type and/or brain tumor location used in their study, as well as use of a different analytic method. Since it has been speculated that tumor type, growth pattern, and tumor locations can affect the FC of brain networks [14,16], the study design of Otten et al may have introduced confounding information via its relatively broad sample size whereas this study concerned a single population of slow-growing histopathologically confirmed gliomas. Therefore the discovery of the eloquent area induced specifically by the mass effect in the gliomas population remains a novel discovery [4]

Changes in PSD within the motor cortex: relationship with motor function plasticity

In addition to changes in FC within the motor network, our study has demonstrated that patients with gliomas exhibit a decreased PSD in low-frequency bands in each of the three key motor regions during the resting state. This observation provides direct evidence for the specificity of BOLD low-frequency changes in patients with brain tumors.

Previous studies have examined spontaneous LFO activities within the specific frequency band of 0.01–0.1 Hz, because this frequency band is hypothesized to be linked primarily to neural activity [28,40–42]. Additionally, several groups have suggested that a shift in LFOs is associated with some brain-related diseases [28,29,43]. These results suggest that changes in the brain's oscillatory dynamics may provide us with novel insights into the neural mechanisms underlying motor functional plasticity induced by brain gliomas. In addition to frequency-specific neural fluctuations, accumulating evidence suggests a possible relationship between PSD and regional spontaneous neural activity and cerebral metabolic rate [44,45]. Some recent studies have suggested that spontaneous fluctuations in brain activity are concentrated in specific frequency bands [28,46]. Although the physiological origin and specific functions of various frequency bands remain to be clarified, Zuo et al. [23] subdivided the power spectrum of spontaneous BOLD fluctuations into four different

slow-frequency ranges (slow-5, 0.01–0.027 Hz; slow-4, 0.027–0.073 Hz; slow-3, 0.073–0.198 Hz;, and slow-2, 0.198–0.25 Hz). The slow-4 oscillation was most prominent in the thalamus, basal ganglia, and sensorimotor regions, while slow-5 was more prominent in the ventromedial cortical areas. Slow-4 was the most reliable sub-band, with a more widespread spatial distribution of reliable voxels. Based on these observations, we further speculate that decreased PSD in low-frequency bands may indirectly reflect decreased local neural activity caused by tumor growth in the abovementioned motor regions.

Krings et al. [47] also observed a loss of signal intensity in lesions near the tumor, which may be related to tumor-induced hemodynamic changes or to a loss of active neurons. Furthermore, Hou et al. [48] suggested that physiological and biological changes caused by a tumor, such as neovascularization, mass effect, and edema, may alter the blood flow or induce a neurovascular uncoupling effect, thereby changing the hemodynamic responses to activations in functional areas. Ulmer et al. [49] have further suggested that lesion-induced neurovascular uncoupling could cause reduced fMRI signals in the perilesional eloquent cortex, in conjunction with normal or increased activity in homologous brain regions. This may stimulate hemispheric dominance and lesion-induced homotopic cortical reorganization. Taken together, these findings indicate that brain tumors may alter the brain microenvironment, possibly leading to hemodynamic changes and neurovascular uncoupling effects that ultimately result in a dysfunction of processes mediated by LFOs. Our findings provide further insight into the relationship between LFOs and brain function plasticity. It is possible that the dysfunction in LFOs within the motor network observed in this study could also be used in evaluating brain function for presurgical planning or postsurgical assessment.

Limitations and future perspectives

A few limitations need to be addressed in the interpretation of the results of our study.

Sample selection limitations. Although our results are encouraging, the current study is limited by the relatively small sample size; thus, statistical power is of potential concern. Future work should endeavor to increase the sample size so that brain network changes caused by different pathological types of brain tumors may be examined. In addition, in the present study, we only compared patients with gliomas and healthy controls. In our future studies, we intend to increase the sample size and select different histological types of tumor (such as meningioma or metastases) near or within the PMC to constitute an additional control group. This will help to determine whether the observed FC and PSD changes are glioma-specific or a consequence of brain tissue compression/edema.

Analysis method limitations. In our study, we observed a potential association between the PSD and functional reorganization in patients with brain gliomas. PSD analysis provides useful frequency information to characterize sensorimotor signal changes induced by brain gliomas. Recently, the frequency-based approach has been used to analyze sensorimotor function. These results indicated that brain low-frequency oscillation is associated with brain function [22,50]. Although the PSD differences between the patient and control groups were observed in the sensorimotor network, the small sample size means that our results must be treated with caution. Furthermore, only a small number of studies have employed the PSD method to analyze brain function, and its effectiveness needs to be further confirmed by future studies. In addition, other factors could contribute to the changes in PSD. Some studies suggest that the low-frequency fluctuation signal PSD is associated with neurovascular coupling. In particular, a recent cerebrovascular reactivity study showed that neurovascular uncoupling occurs in patients with low grade gliomas [51]. A potential explanation is that neurovascular uncoupling might be linked to brain motor function reorganization. Thus, these results could be helpful for understanding why a PSD shift occurs in patients with gliomas. Despite the interesting finding in our study, the neural basis of the low frequency fluctuation signal PSD deficit induced by brain tumors remains unclear and requires further investigation.

Furthermore, a study performed using only FC and frequency-based analytical approaches is not sufficient to understand the brain plasticity induced by brain tumors. The combination of diffusion tensor imaging and fMRI may provide valuable structure and function information for enhancing our understanding of this issue. Although our study subjects had normal muscle strength and no motor weakness, they were not scored using a behavioral testing method. Future studies should focus on investigating the relationship between LFO signal PSD and motor behavioral performance.

Conclusions

In summary, we used two different approaches to investigate the motor network plasticity in patients with brain gliomas. First, our results showed abnormal LFOs and dysfunction of inter-hemispheric FC in patients with gliomas without motor deficits. The clinical pre-symptomatic period could be the result of brain plasticity and the reorganization of the eloquent cortex induced by a slow-growing tumor. Secondly, according to our results, the frequency-based analysis may be more sensitive at detecting abnormal LFOs compared to traditional functional connectivity analysis. Emerging evidence suggests that frequency-based analysis is a good indicator of regional neural activity and cerebral metabolic rates in the resting state. Therefore, the frequency-based analysis may provides an important preoperative evaluation of the functionality of brain tissue surrounding the eloquent areas. This study further indicates that frequency-based analysis may have significant potential for addressing other clinical diseases related to abnormal LFOs.

Supporting Information

Figure S1 A flow chart of data processing steps. GLM, general linear model; FC, functional connectivity; ROI, region of interest; PSD, power spectral density.

Figure S2 Comparison of the functional connectivity of patients and healthy controls using different ROI size. Group differences in the functional connectivity of the motor network between patients with brain gliomas and healthy controls. Different ROIs (10 mm, 8 mm, and 6 mm) were used, which generate similar results. Error bars represent standard error of the mean. Asterisk indicates significant differences when compared to the control group (P<0.05, Mann-Whitney U test). LPMC, left primary motor cortex; RPMC, right motor cortex; SMA, supplementary motor area.

Figure S3 The power spectral density of patients and healthy controls using different ROI size. Power spectral density (PSD) computed using different sizes of ROI (10 mm, 8 mm, and 6 mm). The mean PSD of the left and right PMC between healthy subjects (red traces) and patients with brain gliomas (blue traces) and the group mean PSD of SMA are included. In patients with brain gliomas, the PSDs in the LPMC, RPMC, and SMA are significantly lower than the PSDs of healthy controls (P<0.05, Mann-Whitney U test). LPMC, left primary motor cortex; RPMC, right motor cortex; SMA, supplementary motor area.

Figure S4 Comparison of the power spectral density of patients and healthy controls in three frequency bands using different ROI size. Bar graphs show the PSD in the 3 non-overlapping frequency bands for the 3 key regions of motor network in healthy subjects and patients with brain gliomas. Different ROIs (10 mm, 8 mm, and 6 mm) were used, which generated similar results. The sub-divided low-frequency band (low, 0.01–0.02 Hz; middle, 0.02–0.06 Hz; and high, 0.06–0.1 Hz). Patients with brain tumors show a significant decrease in PSD in 3 key motor cortical regions (LPMC, RPMC, and SMA) (*, P<0.05; **, P<0.001).

Author Contributions

Conceived and designed the experiments: CN PL MZ. Performed the experiments: CN ZM QZ ML. Analyzed the data: PL XL. Contributed reagents/materials/analysis tools: PL MZ. Wrote the article: CN NR.

References

1. Duffau H (2008) Brain plasticity and tumors. In: Pickard JD, Akalan N, Rocco C, Dolenc VV, Antunes JL et al., editors.Advances and Technical Standards in Neurosurgery: Springer Vienna. pp. 3–33.
2. Duffau H (2007) Contribution of cortical and subcortical electrostimulation in brain glioma surgery: methodological and functional considerations. Neurophysiologie clinique = Clinical neurophysiology 37: 373–382.
3. Kadis DS, Iida K, Kerr EN, Logan WJ, McAndrews MP, et al. (2007) Intrahemispheric reorganization of language in children with medically intractable epilepsy of the left hemisphere. Journal of the International Neuropsychological Society 13: 505–516.
4. Duffau H, Capelle L, Denvil D, Sichez N, Gatignol P, et al. (2003) Functional recovery after surgical resection of low grade gliomas in eloquent brain: hypothesis of brain compensation. Journal of Neurology, Neurosurgery & Psychiatry 74: 901–907.
5. Biswal B, Zerrin Yetkin F, Haughton VM, Hyde JS (1995) Functional connectivity in the motor cortex of resting human brain using echo-planar mri. Magnetic Resonance in Medicine 34: 537–541.
6. Lowe MJ, Mock BJ, Sorenson JA (1998) Functional Connectivity in Single and Multislice Echoplanar Imaging Using Resting-State Fluctuations. Neuroimage 7: 119–132.
7. Cordes D, Haughton VM, Arfanakis K, Carew JD, Turski PA, et al. (2001) Frequencies Contributing to Functional Connectivity in the Cerebral Cortex in "Resting-state" Data. American Journal of Neuroradiology 22: 1326–1333.
8. Turner KC, Frost L, Linsenbardt D, McIlroy JR, Muller RA (2006) Atypically diffuse functional connectivity between caudate nuclei and cerebral cortex in autism. Behav Brain Funct 2: 34.
9. Villalobos ME, Mizuno A, Dahl BC, Kemmotsu N, Muller RA (2005) Reduced functional connectivity between V1 and inferior frontal cortex associated with visuomotor performance in autism. Neuroimage 25: 916–925.
10. Greicius MD, Srivastava G, Reiss AL, Menon V (2004) Default-mode network activity distinguishes Alzheimer's disease from healthy aging: Evidence from functional MRI. Proceedings of the National Academy of Sciences of the United States of America 101: 4637–4642.
11. Castellanos FX, Margulies DS, Kelly C, Uddin LQ, Ghaffari M, et al. (2008) Cingulate-precuneus interactions: a new locus of dysfunction in adult attention-deficit/hyperactivity disorder. Biol Psychiatry 63: 332–337.
12. Bokde ALW, Lopez-Bayo P, Meindl T, Pechler S, Born C, et al. (2006) Functional connectivity of the fusiform gyrus during a face-matching task in subjects with mild cognitive impairment. Brain 129: 1113–1124.
13. Jafri MJ, Pearlson GD, Stevens M, Calhoun VD (2008) A method for functional network connectivity among spatially independent resting-state components in schizophrenia. Neuroimage 39: 1666–1681.
14. Briganti C, Sestieri C, Mattei PA, Esposito R, Galzio RJ, et al. (2012) Reorganization of functional connectivity of the language network in patients with brain gliomas. AJNR Am J Neuroradiol 33: 1983–1990.

15. Otten ML, Mikell CB, Youngerman BE, Liston C, Sisti MB, et al. (2012) Motor deficits correlate with resting state motor network connectivity in patients with brain tumours. Brain 135: 1017–1026.

16. Esposito R, Mattei PA, Briganti C, Romani GL, Tartaro A, et al. (2012) Modifications of default-mode network connectivity in patients with cerebral glioma. PLoS One 7: e40231.

17. Lin P, Hasson U, Jovicich J, Robinson S (2011) A Neuronal Basis for Task-Negative Responses in the Human Brain. Cerebral Cortex 21: 821–830.

18. De Pisapia N, Turatto M, Lin P, Jovicich J, Caramazza A (2012) Unconscious Priming Instructions Modulate Activity in Default and Executive Networks of the Human Brain. Cerebral Cortex 22: 639–649.

19. Baliki MN, Baria AT, Apkarian AV (2011) The cortical rhythms of chronic back pain. J Neurosci 31: 13981–13990.

20. Robinson S, Basso G, Soldati N, Sailer U, Jovicich J, et al. (2009) A resting state network in the motor control circuit of the basal ganglia. BMC Neuroscience 10: 137.

21. Kim JY, Kim SH, Seo J, Kim SH, Han SW, et al. (2013) Increased power spectral density in resting-state pain-related brain networks in fibromyalgia. Pain.

22. Duff EP, Johnston LA, Xiong J, Fox PT, Mareels I, et al. (2008) The power of spectral density analysis for mapping endogenous BOLD signal fluctuations. Hum Brain Mapp 29: 778–790.

23. Zuo XN, Di Martino A, Kelly C, Shehzad ZE, Gee DG, et al. (2010) The oscillating brain: Complex and reliable. Neuroimage 49: 1432–1445.

24. Fransson P (2005) Spontaneous low-frequency BOLD signal fluctuations: an fMRI investigation of the resting-state default mode of brain function hypothesis. Hum Brain Mapp 26: 15–29.

25. Zou QH, Zhu CZ, Yang Y, Zuo XN, Long XY, et al. (2008) An improved approach to detection of amplitude of low-frequency fluctuation (ALFF) for resting-state fMRI: Fractional ALFF. Journal of Neuroscience Methods 172: 137–141.

26. Buzsáki G, Draguhn A (2004) Neuronal Oscillations in Cortical Networks. Science 304: 1926–1929.

27. Penttonen M, Buzsáki G (2003) Natural logarithmic relationship between brain oscillators. Thalamus & Related Systems 2: 145–152.

28. Hoptman MJ, Zuo XN, Butler PD, Javitt DC, D'Angelo D, et al. (2010) Amplitude of low-frequency oscillations in schizophrenia: a resting state fMRI study. Schizophr Res 117: 13–20.

29. Han Y, Wang J, Zhao Z, Min B, Lu J, et al. (2011) Frequency-dependent changes in the amplitude of low-frequency fluctuations in amnestic mild cognitive impairment: a resting-state fMRI study. Neuroimage 55: 287–295.

30. de Jongh A, de Munck JC, Baayen JC, Puligheddu M, Jonkman EJ, et al. (2003) Localization of Fast MEG Waves in Patients with Brain Tumors and Epilepsy. Brain Topography 15: 173–179.

31. Kamada K, Möller M, Saguer M, Ganslandt O, Kaltenhäuser M, et al. (2001) A combined study of tumor-related brain lesions using MEG and proton MR spectroscopic imaging. Journal of the Neurological Sciences 186: 13–21.

32. Salvador R, Martinez A, Pomarol-Clotet E, Gomar J, Vila F, et al. (2008) A simple view of the brain through a frequency-specific functional connectivity measure. Neuroimage 39: 279–289.

33. De Luca M, Beckmann CF, De Stefano N, Matthews PM, Smith SM (2006) fMRI resting state networks define distinct modes of long-distance interactions in the human brain. Neuroimage 29: 1359–1367.

34. Duffau H (2005) Lessons from brain mapping in surgery for low-grade glioma: insights into associations between tumour and brain plasticity. The Lancet Neurology 4: 476–486.

35. Oshino S, Kato A, Wakayama A, Taniguchi M, Hirata M, et al. (2007) Magnetoencephalographic analysis of cortical oscillatory activity in patients with brain tumors: Synthetic aperture magnetometry (SAM) functional imaging of delta band activity. Neuroimage 34: 957–964.

36. Guggisberg AG, Honma SM, Findlay AM, Dalal SS, Kirsch HE, et al. (2008) Mapping functional connectivity in patients with brain lesions. Ann Neurol 63: 193–203.

37. Hertz-Pannier L, Chiron C, Jambaqué I, Renaux-Kieffer V, Van de Moortele PF, et al. (2002) Late plasticity for language in a child's non-dominant hemisphere: A pre- and post-surgery fMRI study. Brain 125: 361–372.

38. Liégeois F, Connelly A, Cross JH, Boyd SG, Gadian DG, et al. (2004) Language reorganization in children with early-onset lesions of the left hemisphere: an fMRI study. Brain 127: 1229–1236.

39. Martino J, Taillandier L, Moritz-Gasser S, Gatignol P, Duffau H (2009) Re-operation is a safe and effective therapeutic strategy in recurrent WHO grade II gliomas within eloquent areas. Acta Neurochir (Wien) 151: 427–436.

40. Fox MD, Raichle ME (2007) Spontaneous fluctuations in brain activity observed with functional magnetic resonance imaging. Nat Rev Neurosci 8: 700–711.

41. Zhang D, Raichle ME (2010) Disease and the brain's dark energy. Nat Rev Neurol 6: 15–28.

42. Bianciardi M, Fukunaga M, van Gelderen P, Horovitz SG, de Zwart JA, et al. (2009) Sources of functional magnetic resonance imaging signal fluctuations in the human brain at rest: a 7 T study. Magn Reson Imaging 27: 1019–1029.

43. He Y, Wang L, Zang Y, Tian L, Zhang X, et al. (2007) Regional coherence changes in the early stages of Alzheimer's disease: A combined structural and resting-state functional MRI study. Neuroimage 35: 488–500.

44. Fukunaga M, Horovitz SG, de Zwart JA, van Gelderen P, Balkin TJ, et al. (2008) Metabolic origin of BOLD signal fluctuations in the absence of stimuli. J Cereb Blood Flow Metab 28: 1377–1387.

45. Wu CW, Gu H, Lu H, Stein EA, Chen JH, et al. (2009) Mapping functional connectivity based on synchronized CMRO2 fluctuations during the resting state. Neuroimage 45: 694–701.

46. Zhang J, Wei L, Hu X, Zhang Y, Zhou D, et al. (2013) Specific frequency band of amplitude low-frequency fluctuation predicts Parkinson's disease. Behavioural Brain Research 252: 18–23.

47. Krings T, Töpper R, Willmes K, Reinges MHT, Gilsbach JM, et al. (2002) Activation in primary and secondary motor areas in patients with CNS neoplasms and weakness. Neurology 58: 381–390.

48. Hou BL, Bradbury M, Peck KK, Petrovich NM, Gutin PH, et al. (2006) Effect of brain tumor neovasculature defined by rCBV on BOLD fMRI activation volume in the primary motor cortex. Neuroimage 32: 489–497.

49. Ulmer JL, Hacein-Bey L, Mathews VP, Mueller WM, DeYoe EA, et al. (2004) Lesion-induced Pseudo-dominance at Functional Magnetic Resonance Imaging: Implications for Preoperative Assessments. Neurosurgery 55: 569–581.

50. Bajaj S, Drake D, Butler AJ, Dhamala M (2014) Oscillatory motor network activity during rest and movement: an fNIRS study. Frontiers in Systems Neuroscience 8.

51. Zacà D, Jovicich J, Nadar SR, Voyvodic JT, Pillai JJ (2013) Cerebrovascular reactivity mapping in patients with low grade gliomas undergoing presurgical sensorimotor mapping with BOLD fMRI. Journal of magnetic resonance imaging : JMRI..

6

Observed Manipulation Enhances Left Fronto-Parietal Activations in the Processing of Unfamiliar Tools

Norma Naima Rüther[1,2]*, **Marco Tettamanti**[3,4], **Stefano F. Cappa**[4,5], **Christian Bellebaum**[6]

1 Institute of Cognitive Neuroscience, Dept. of Neuropsychology, Ruhr University Bochum, Bochum, Germany, 2 International Graduate School of Neuroscience, Ruhr University Bochum, Bochum, Germany, 3 Division Neuroscience, San Raffaele Scientific Institute, Milano, Italy, 4 Department of Nuclear Medicine, San Raffaele Scientific Institute, Milano, Italy, 5 Faculty of Psychology, Vita-Salute San Raffaele University, Milano, Italy, 6 Institute of Experimental Psychology, Heinrich Heine University Düsseldorf, Düsseldorf, Germany

Abstract

Tools represent a special class of objects, as functional details of tools can afford certain actions. In addition, information gained via prior experience with tools can be accessed on a semantic level, providing a basis for meaningful object interactions. Conceptual representations of tools also encompass knowledge about tool manipulation which can be acquired via direct (active manipulation) or indirect (observation of others manipulating objects) motor experience. The present study aimed to explore the impact of observation of manipulation on the neural processing of previously unfamiliar, manipulable objects. Brain activity was assessed by means of functional magnetic resonance imaging while participants accomplished a visual matching task involving pictures of the novel objects before and after they received object-related training. Three training session in which subjects observed an experimenter manipulating one set of objects and visually explored another set of objects were used to make subjects familiar with the tools and to allow the formation of new tool representations. A control object set was not part of the training. Training-related brain activation increases were found for observed manipulation objects compared to not trained objects in a left-hemispheric network consisting of inferior frontal gyrus (iFG) pars opercularis and triangularis and supramarginal/angular gyrus. This illustrates that direct manipulation experience is not required to elicit tool-associated activation changes in the action system. While the iFG activation might indicate a close relationship between the areas involved in tool representation and those involved in observational knowledge acquisition, the parietal activation is discussed in terms of non-semantic effects of object affordances and hand-tool spatial relationships.

Editor: Esteban Andres Fridman, Weill Cornell Medical College, United States of America

Funding: The authors thank the German Research Foundation for supporting this work (Deutsche Forschungsgemeinschaft, DFG; SFB 874/TP B6 to C.B.). The funders had no role in study design, data collection and analysis, decision to publish, or preparation of the manuscript.

Competing Interests: The authors have declared that no competing interests exist.

* E-mail: naima.ruether@rub.de

Introduction

To interact meaningfully with objects in the environment, individuals must be able to identify interaction sites that are part of the objects' appearances, an object-characteristic that is often related to the influential concept of "affordances" [1]. This concept states that the environment contains inherent cues offering possibilities to act upon, hence influencing perceptual processing. Tools are a special class of objects, because they have intrinsic manipulability. On the other hand, however, the exact function of a tool and the way in which it is manipulated must be learned. The neural organization of tool concepts in semantic memory is a central topic in cognitive neuroscience which is still unresolved. Many neuroimaging studies have shown activations in a fronto-parietal network during the processing of tool stimuli, suggesting that regions involved in tool-related actions are activated when pictures of tools are seen or tool sounds are heard. It appears that this activation reflects the automatic recruitment of underlying neural motor patterns related to hand movements and grasping as well as the access to object-associated goals, which are integrated into tool concepts (e.g., [2–6]; for review, see [7]). In support of this view, Grezes and Decety (2002) showed that the processing of

tool-stimuli leads to the activation of left inferior parietal lobule (iPL) and left inferior frontal gyrus (iFG; BA45), irrespective of a specific task [8].

Behavioral studies in healthy human subjects [2,9,10] provide only indirect evidence for an automatic motor cortex activation during the observation of tool stimuli, as shown by motor facilitation effects through tool picture presentations that can be attributable to the objects' inherent affordance cues. Studies using electroencephalography (EEG) show an early effect within 140–270 milliseconds (ms) that was interpreted as automatic affordance extraction [11,12].

Important insights on the neural underpinnings of tool use and tool representations can be gained by studying patients suffering from apraxia (for review see [13]). The use of tools and objects is affected in a large proportion of apraxic patients, and follows from damage to the left frontal and temporo-parietal cortex [14]. Some apraxic patients may misuse common tools, for example trying to cut a piece of paper with closed scissors [15–17]. These symptoms have been related by some researchers [15,16] to an impairment of stored conceptual knowledge ("action semantics"). Knowledge about object function has been suggested to contribute, together with general action knowledge and knowledge about action sequences, to a conceptual praxis system which, in turn, builds so-called action semantics along with a praxis production system [18–20]. The "sensory-motor theory" [21,22] proposes that object concepts are stored in the brain regions that were active during knowledge acquisition, thus ascribing a central role to individual object-related experience [21,23,24]. In accordance with this notion, models of praxis have postulated that prior experience leads to a "processing advantage" for each new experience, based on action semantics in memory, which entail not only concrete information on object function but possibly also on manipulation [19]. The recruitment of fronto-parietal brain regions in the processing of tool stimuli should thus not only reflect affordance related processes, but can also be related to previous sensory-motor experience with the objects, reflecting a reactivation of regions involved in acquisition of knowledge about the object. Several studies used training procedures with novel objects to control for individual object experience, aiming to elucidate the impact of modality-specific experience on conceptual representations of those objects [25–29]. Indeed, it was shown that after short periods of training, fronto-parietal brain regions were recruited during visual processing of the novel objects in an experience-dependent manner. Only when subjects learned to manipulate the objects, but not when they visually explored them, stronger post training activations were seen in the premotor and the posterior parietal cortex [27,29]. Experience effects are not specific for tools. A recent study in which participants were trained in either tying or naming knots showed recruitment of bilateral intraparietal sulcus (IPS) post training only when knots had been tied previously. In contrast, the left posterior IPS was active for knots that were learned to be named, showing that learning object-related information by linguistic or manipulation training leads to a recruitment of the parietal cortex independently of training experience [25].

Representations of tools, including information of associated action goals and manipulation sites, can be induced not only by active manipulation experience or, at least in part, by linguistic information, but also through indirect object experience, via observation of object manipulation, an important mechanism during the evolution of tool use behavior [30]. Models of praxis processing suggest that knowledge about tool use and function can be acquired via different routes [18,19], leaving open the issue whether direct object experience is necessary for tool representations to emerge. As outlined above, tools represent a class of objects that is mainly defined by their intrinsic properties that afford to interact and are associated with goal-relevant, conceptual information [31]. Changes in tool-associated brain activation elicited by active manipulation experience, as those described above, can be ascribed to a change in object affordances. Recently, it was shown that expectations about tool use behaviors can be modulated by an interaction of biomechanical affordance cues and experience-dependent probabilistic priors of observed goals coupled with observed action [32]. However, the impact of observation of manipulation on the neural representation of tool-like objects is still unclear and is addressed in the present study.

In the present study we hypothesized that indirect object related experience, similar to active experience, would influence the perception of object affordances and induce tool representations in a left fronto-parietal network related to tool-oriented actions. To this end, we investigated the impact of observed manipulation on the processing of previously unfamiliar, manipulable objects [27,29]. In three training sessions, participants observed one set of objects being actively manipulated by the experimenter (observation training objects, OTO), whereas a second set was visually explored (visually trained objects, VTO; see [27]). A third

object set served as a control condition (not trained objects, NTO). Processing of pictures of the manipulable objects was assessed by means of functional magnetic resonance imaging (fMRI). To control for potential affordance-related activations elicited by the objects pre training, processing of object pictures was compared before and after training. We hypothesized that regions involved in observation of hand-object interactions [33] and affordance processing [8] would be more strongly activated by OTO than by VTO pictures after training. After training, we found a specific training-related brain activation increase for OTO in left iFG pars opercularis/triangularis and parietal supramarginal/angular gyrus.

Materials and Methods

Ethics statement

Participants were informed about the testing procedure and gave written informed consent. The study complies with the Declaration of Helsinki and was approved by the ethics committee of the Medical Faculty at the Ruhr University Bochum, Germany.

Participants

19 healthy, right-handed students with a mean age of 23.21 years (SD = 3.36; range = 18–31) participated in the study (11 females). All participants had normal or corrected-to-normal vision.

Stimuli and experimental design

Object stimuli. Similar to the studies by [29] and [27], novel manipulable objects were used, constructed with K'nex (TM), a children's construction toy. Each object served one of six functions ("transport", "destroy", "push", "pull", "move" or "separate") that could be performed on other small everyday objects (e.g. plastic cups, tea boxes, or table tennis balls). All novel objects were photographed from four different perspectives for the visual matching task (see below). A separate group of volunteers (N = 33) rated the object pictures in terms of similarity to real objects, visual complexity, and singularity, that is, how outstanding each object was compared to the other objects. Based on these ratings, the total group of objects was divided into three matched sets of objects, each comprising 12 different objects, two of each function.

Training. Object-related training, which served to familiarize participants with the objects and to allow the formation of object representations, was divided into three training sessions of about 80 to 90 minutes that took place on three different days. On each training day, each participant received two qualitatively different types of object training with two different object sets during the course of one training session: "observation of manipulation training" with the first set of objects and "visual exploration training" with the second set (see Figure 1). The third, untrained object set served as a control and was only part of the visual matching task (see below). The allocation of object sets to "observation of manipulation training", "visual exploration training" and "no training" was counterbalanced and randomized across subjects.

In "observation of manipulation training", each object was first presented on a table in front of the participant before the concrete steps of manipulation were shown. The function of the object was named and subsequently the manipulation was demonstrated manually by the experimenter, simultaneously with a standardized verbal description of the discrete steps of manipulation. After demonstrating the use of the presented object, the participant was instructed to accurately observe the experimenter manipulating the object in the next 90 seconds and to furthermore count how

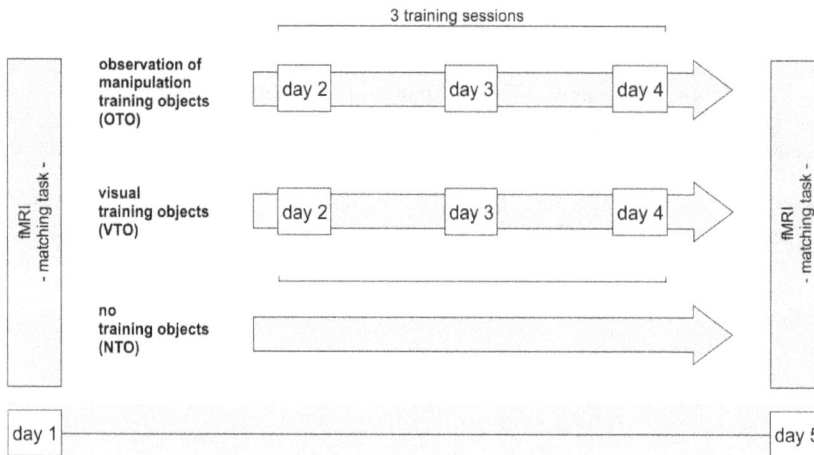

Figure 1. Experimental procedure.

often the experimenter performed the object-related action in this time period to ensure that the participant was paying attention.

In "visual exploration training", the object was also placed on a table in front of the participant and the function was named. However, neither a description of the discrete steps of manipulation was provided nor was the manipulation shown. Instead, participants were asked to verbally describe the visual form of the object for 90 seconds and to pay attention to its visual structure, with no reference to its function or ways of possible manipulation. If a participant took less than 90 seconds for the description, the experimenter prompted the visual exploration asking specific questions about the constituents of the object (e.g. "How many blue bars does the object have?"), ensuring that the procedures for observation of manipulation and visual exploration were comparable in terms of the time spent with each object. In both training conditions participants were not allowed to touch or grasp the object.

The visual matching task

To examine training-induced changes in the neural correlates of processing pictures of the novel objects, the participants underwent fMRI pre and post training with an identical visual matching task, similar to the tasks used in previous studies [27,29]. On each trial of the task, a fixation cross was first presented for 500 ms on a computer screen, which was projected on goggles worn by the subjects. Then a pair of pictures of the novel objects or a pair of scrambled images (SCI) of the objects, which served as a baseline condition, were shown for 3000 ms. Participants had to indicate whether the picture displayed the same object or not or, in case of the baseline condition, whether the SCI were identical or not. To respond, participants pressed either the index (for "identical") or middle finger (for "not identical") of the left hand during both tasks. Maximum response time was 3000 ms (see Figure 2). For the SCI, one picture per object was fragmented into 18 * 18 mosaic pieces which were then rearranged to yield a scrambled image of the object. To guarantee a comparable color distribution and distribution of the relevant information between center and periphery between SCI and unscrambled object pictures, the position of the 15×15 central mosaics was scrambled independently from the position of the peripheral mosaics.

The experiment was organized in a block design with four scan sessions, each comprising 16 blocks. Of the 16 blocks per session, four blocks contained trials exclusively showing OTO, VTO,

NTO or SCI, respectively, with each block containing six trials. One block lasted 27.7 seconds. Half of the trials per block were matches showing the same object or the same SCI on both pictures and half were non-matches. Importantly, the pictures presented during a particular trial showed objects from different perspectives. For each object there were four different perspectives. During the experiment, each individual object was shown 16 times. Thus, each individual picture showing an object from a specific perspective appeared four times. Each SCI was presented five or six times. Stimulus timing, response and scanner pulse recording were controlled with Presentation software (Neurobehavioral Systems, Inc., Albany, California, USA).

After the second fMRI acquisition, subjects were successively shown pictures of all 36 objects outside of the scanner and participants were asked to specify by means of a printed questionnaire if the object had been part of the training or not. If yes, they were asked to indicate whether they had observed the manipulation of the object or visually explored the object (assignment of objects to the training condition). The interval between the last training session and the second fMRI acquisition was on average 3.21 days (SD = 2.90) and the mean time for accomplishment of the whole experiment including all five sessions was 11.26 days (SD = 5.36).

Behavioral data analysis

Mean accuracy and reaction times in the matching task were analyzed with a repeated-measures ANOVA (Analysis of Variance) with the factors TIME (pre, post) and OBJECT SET (NTO, VTO, OTO). Correct assignment of object to training type after the second fMRI acquisition was analyzed by means of repeated-measures ANOVA with the factor OBJECT SET (NTO, VTO, OTO). In case of significant violation of sphericity, Greenhouse-Geisser corrected results and degrees of freedom are reported [34].

Imaging parameters and analysis

Participants were scanned with a 3 Tesla Philips Achieva Scanner equipped with a 32-channel head coil. A high-resolution, three-dimensional anatomical T1-weighted MR image was acquired with a spoiled-gradient-recalled sequence during the first fMRI acquisition (pre training) with 220 slices, slice thickness 1 mm, TE = 3.74 ms, TR = 8.19 ms, flip angle = 8° and an in-plane resolution of 1×1 mm. The T2*-weighted MR images during the functional sessions were acquired parallel to the

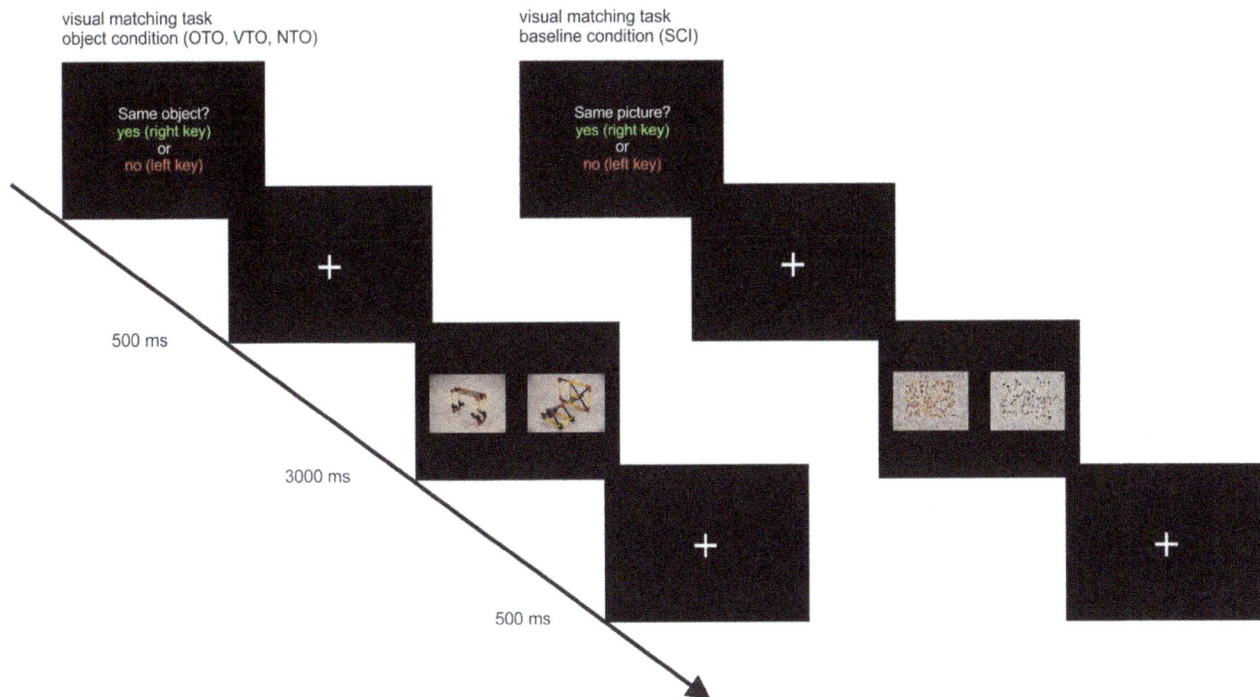

Figure 2. Example trials for object and scrambled image matching.

anterior-commissure-posterior-commissural plane using an echo-planar (EPI) pulse sequence with 30 ascending slices of 4 mm thickness, TR = 2000 ms, TE = 30 ms, flip angle = 90°, field of view of 224×240×120 mm and 2×2 mm pixel size. Each of the four functional imaging sequences started with 6 dummy scans that did not enter data analysis, and comprised 230 sequential volumes in total.

For preprocessing and statistical analysis, SPM8 (Statistical Parametric Mapping, Wellcome Department of Imaging Neuro-science, London, UK) was used in Matlab (Mathworks, Natick, Massachusetts, USA). Before preprocessing, all images were manually reoriented to the anterior commissure. Images were then corrected for slice timing, were realigned and unwarped [35], coregistered to the structural T1-weighted image and segmented and normalized to the Montreal Neurological Institute (MNI) standard space. Finally, an 8 mm FWHM Gaussian smoothing kernel was applied.

General linear model

Data were temporally filtered with a non-linear high-pass filter with a 128 s cutoff. A global normalization was not performed.

First-level GLM. FMRI responses of each subject were modeled with a canonical hemodynamic response function, aligned to the onsets of blocks of trials belonging to one experimental condition. In a 4×2 factorial design with the factors TIME (pre, post) and CONDITION (NTO, VTO, OTO, SCI), t-Student contrasts were specified, each contrasting the different object sets (NTO, VTO, OTO) with the SCI baseline, separately for the pre and post training assessment. This procedure yielded six contrasts (NTO pre and post, VTO pre and post, OTO pre and post) for each subject, representing the activation for the respective object set relative to the baseline condition pre and post training.

Second-level GLM. On the second level, a full factorial design was specified with the within-subjects factors TIME (pre, post) and OBJECT SET (NTO, VTO, OTO), based on the first-level contrast images of the object sets relative to SCI baseline for each subject. Dependency and equal variance were determined for the factors. To control for between-condition differences in object memory, as reflected in the performance differences in assigning object photographs to the correct training condition after the second fMRI acquisition, (see Results section for details), a masking procedure was used on the second level. More specifically, individual subjects' performance scores for OTO, VTO and NTO, reflecting a measure of post training object familiarity, were entered as a regressor in a separate second level analysis comprising only the post training contrast images (see above). The brain activation pattern correlating with object familiarity was then used as an explicit mask for the second level analysis on object training effects to make sure that these effects were not related to object familiarity. Note that data of three participants were missing. For those, the mean scores of the remaining subjects were entered.

In our analysis, we aimed to identify brain regions that showed activation differences in response to pictures of specific object sets after, but not before training. We thus expected a specific activation increase for those objects the participants had experience with during training and were not interested in general activation increases across all conditions from pre to post training. Thus, activations of interest had to fulfill two criteria. First, the interaction contrast of the factors OBJECT SET and TIME had to be significant. Second, within the brain regions showing a significant interaction there had to be significant post training activation differences between object sets, examined by means of T-contrasts (e.g. OTO post >NTO post). At the same time, the respective contrasts between object sets before training were expected to not yield significant activations.

Statistics referring to whole brain analyses are reported. To keep type I (false alarms) and at the same time type II (missing true results) errors low during multiple comparisons, Monte Carlo simulation [36] was used to correct whole brain analyses for a threshold of p<.05, corrected. The threshold for single voxels was set at p<.001 and Monte Carlo simulation with 10.000 iterations was run, resulting in an extent threshold of 22 resampled voxels, defining a volume of 176 mm^3. The SPM Anatomy Toolbox Version 1.8 was used to localize the activation peaks in MNI space [37].

As a further confirmation of the results, we applied small volume correction (SVC; [38]) both for the interaction F-contrast and the post training T-contrasts, focusing on relevant regions of interest. As already stated in the introduction, activation of a fronto-parietal network consisting of iFG (pars opercularis and triangularis) and iPL was expected for OTO stimuli. We hypothesized that regions involved in action observation of meaningful gestures, particularly in the left iFG [33], and potentially regions playing a role in affordance processing in the left parietal cortex [8] would be activated by OTO pictures after but not before training, indicating that action observation specifically modulated object processing in these areas. Hence, peak coordinates for SVC in the left inferior frontal cortex were derived from [33] (pars opercularis: x = −38, y = 8, z = 18; pars triangularis: x = −48, y = 36, z = 12). With respect to left iPL, peak coordinates from [8] were used (x = −54, y = −46, z = 30). Coordinates from Talairach space were transformed into MNI space (http://imaging.mrc-cbu.cam.ac.uk/downloads/MNI2tal/mni2tal.m) before applying SVC. An 8 mm sphere around the mentioned peak activations was used. For SVC, results with a corrected statistical threshold of p<.05 (FWE-corrected for the ROI in question) are reported.

Results

Behavioral Data

Performance in the matching task. Figure 3 displays mean accuracy and mean reaction times in the visual matching task before and after training. Behavioral data of two participants were excluded as a result of technical problems during response recording. For accuracy data, ANOVA with the factors TIME (pre, post) and OBJECT SET (NTO, VTO, OTO) revealed a main effect of TIME, indicating that participants responded more accurately after training than before training (F(1,16) = 16.188; p = .001). No significant main effect of OBJECT SET and no significant interaction between the factors were found (all p>.179).

Analysis of reaction time data again revealed a significant main effect of TIME that indicated decreased response time post compared to pre training (F(1,16) = 6.732; p = .020). The main effect of OBJECT SET and the interaction did not reach significance (all p>.232).

Assignment of objects to the training condition. After the second fMRI session, participants were asked to assign photographs of all objects to the training conditions (NTO, VTO, OTO; questionnaires of two participants are missing; a further questionnaire by one subject was not considered due to incompleteness). On average, participants correctly assigned 11.00 objects to NTO (SD = 1.00), 10.88 to VTO (SD = 1.71) and 9.50 to OTO (SD = 1.79). A one-factorial ANOVA revealed a significant effect of OBJECT SET (F(2,30) = 7.26; p = .003) and post-hoc t-tests showed that the number of correct assignments of OTO was significantly reduced in comparison to VTO (t(15) = 2.961; p = .010) and NTO (t(15) = −4.240; p = .001), whereas no

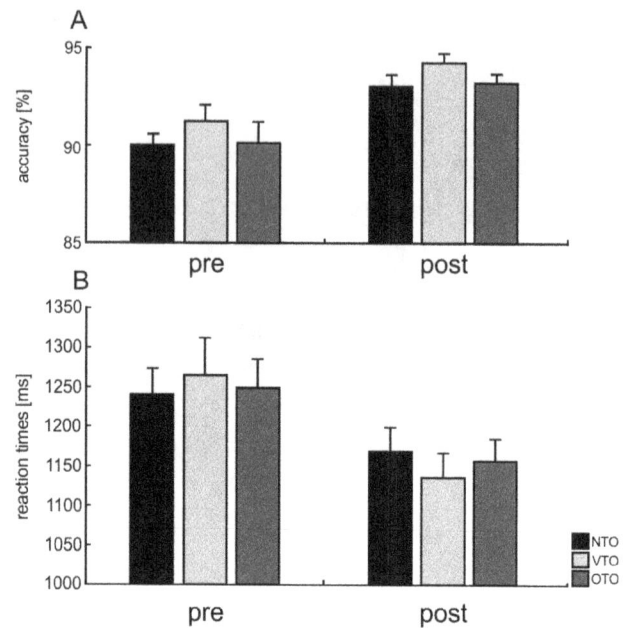

Figure 3. Mean accuracy and reaction times in the visual matching tasks before and after training. Error bars indicate standard error of mean.

significant difference was found comparing VTO and NTO assignments (p = .699).

Imaging data

As outlined in the Methods section, we identified brain regions on whole brain level for which brain activation during the visual matching task showed a) a significant interaction between the factors TIME and OBJECT SET and b) for which activation differences between object sets were seen after training, but not before training. Table 1 lists the brain activations fulfilling both these criteria at a corrected statistical significance threshold of p< .05 based on an extent threshold of 22 or more voxels defined by Monte Carlo simulations (see "Materials and Methods").

Brain regions with stronger post training activation for OTO relative to NTO were found in a left-lateralized fronto-parietal network consisting of two clusters in iFG (pars triangularis and pars opercularis, extending into rolandic operculum) and one cluster in the angular gyrus/supra marginal gyrus (see Figure 4 A).

Significant activations also emerged for the contrast OTO> VTO. Parts of the iFG (pars triangularis) cluster which was active for the contrast OTO>NTO were found to be active also in this contrast with comparable peak-coordinates, but reduced cluster size (see Table 1). Furthermore, an activation peak was found in precentral gyrus, with the cluster again overlapping in part the cluster found for OTO>NTO (see Figure 4 B).

To identify brain regions that were specifically activated by visual exploration training, VTO-related brain activation was contrasted with NTO- and OTO-related brain activation. Relative to OTO, VTO elicited higher activation in a large right hemispheric cluster extending from the precuneus to the calcarine gyrus and in a left hemispheric cluster including posterior cingulate cortex (extending into hippocampus) and calcarine gyrus (see Table 1). No significant activation was found for VTO in contrast to NTO. Moreover, no activations for NTO relative to VTO or OTO were found.

Table 1. Brain regions showing activation differences between object sets after training and an interaction between the factors TIME and OBJECT SET.

Brain region	Cluster size	Peak coordinates MNI (mm)			Peak Z-Score	Uncorrected P-value (peak-level)
		x	y	z		
OTO>NTO						
L inferior frontal gyrus (pars triangularis)	196	−48	36	8	4.78	<.001
		−46	36	−2	4.16	<.001
		−42	28	8	4.14	<.001
L inferior frontal gyrus (pars opercularis)	159	−42	12	16	4.68	<.001
		−54	14	22	4.58	<.001
L rolandic operculum		−48	4	16	4.48	<.001
L angular gyrus	44	−48	−50	32	4.40	<.001
L supramarginal gyrus		−56	−52	30	3.93	<.001
OTO > VTO						
L precentral gyrus	116	−50	4	18	4.50	<.001
		−40	4	20	3.83	<.001
L inferior frontal gyrus (pars triangularis)	25	−44	38	2	3.73	<.001
VTO>OTO						
R precuneus	101	18	−42	8	4.58	<.001
R calcarine gyrus		22	−50	12	3.20	.001
L posterior cingulate cortex	95	−16	−46	8	4.27	<.001
L calcarine gyrus	30	−16	−60	18	3.57	<.001
L hippocampus		−20	−38	6	3.45	<.001

Please note that only clusters surviving the extent threshold of 22 voxels are reported, as revealed by Monte Carlo simulation to correct for multiple comparisons at p< .05. L= left hemisphere, R = right hemisphere.

To confirm the specific involvement of a fronto-parietal network of brain regions by OTO after training, SVC was applied at brain regions hypothesized to be involved in action observation and action selection for interactions between hands and objects, as already pointed out in the methods section. SVC was applied for the interaction contrast as well as for the contrasts between OTO

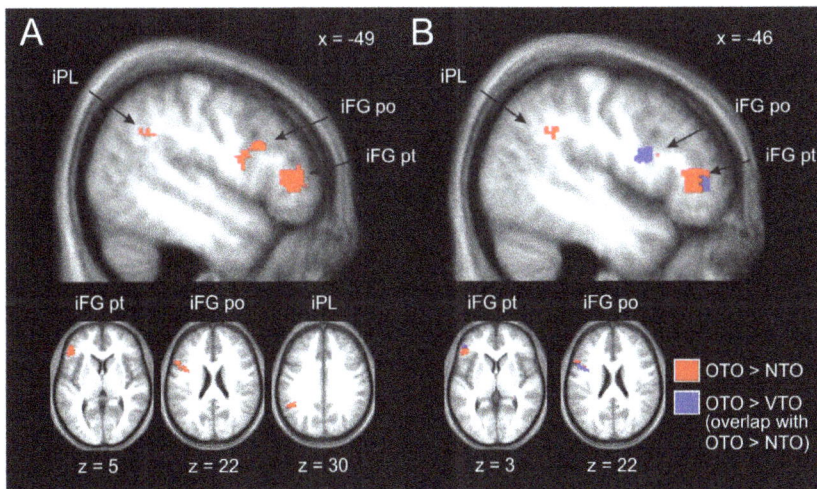

Figure 4. Significant post training activations projected on the mean T1 images of all study participants. Contrast A) displays OTO> NTO and B) displays OTO>VTO, overlapping completely with OTO>NTO (both p<.001, uncorrected). Note that all activations also had to show a significant interaction between the factors TIME and OBJECT SET. iFG =inferior frontal gyrus, pt = pars triangularis, po = pars opercularis, iPL = inferior parietal lobe.

on the one hand and VTO and NTO on the other hand after training. Both for the interaction contrast (pars triangularis, x = −50, y = 36, z = 8; 63 voxels; p = .002; pars opercularis, x = −40, y = 4, z = 18; 54 voxels; p = .003) and for OTO>NTO after training, activation within the left iFG was confirmed by SVC (pars triangularis: x = −48, y = 36, z = 8; 130 voxels; p<.001; pars opercularis: x = −42, y = 12, z = 16; 86 voxels; p<.001). Furthermore, we used coordinates from Grezes and Decety (2002) from an activation peak in parietal cortex. Again, a cluster of significant activation was found within this ROI for the interaction contrast (x = −48, y = −48, z = 30; 19 voxels; p = .018) and for OTO>NTO (x = −48, y = −50, z = 32; 159 voxels; p<.001).

Significant activations also emerged for the contrast OTO>VTO. SVC yielded significantly larger activations for OTO than VTO in the left inferior frontal cortex (pars triangularis: x = −48, y = 40, z = 6; 6 voxels; p = .012; pars opercularis: x = −44, y = 4, z = 18; 42 voxels; p = .005).

Discussion

The present study aimed to elucidate the impact of observed manipulation on the neural processing of previously unfamiliar tool-like objects. In three training sessions, participants observed one set of novel objects being manipulated by an experimenter and visually explored a second set of novel objects to induce qualitatively different histories of object-related experience (observation training objects and visually trained objects – OTO and VTO, respectively). A third (control) set of novel objects was not part of the training (not trained objects - NTO). Before and after training, participants accomplished a visual matching task comprising pictures of the objects during which brain activity was assessed by means of fMRI. In accordance with our expectations, training effects on neural activity were seen in a left fronto-parietal network of brain regions. More specifically, the processing of OTO in contrast to NTO after training significantly activated left-hemispheric regions comprising parts of the left iFG (pars triangularis and pars opercularis) and the angular/supramarginal gyrus within the left iPL. Activations in left iFG occurred as well, albeit with smaller cluster sizes, for OTO in contrast to VTO, whereas no activation in the left iPL was detected for this contrast. Moreover, for VTO, compared to OTO, stronger activity within a bilateral cluster in precuneus and calcarine gyrus was found. Additionally, VTO in contrast to OTO activated left posterior cingulate cortex, extending into left hippocampus. Finally, no specific recruitment of brain areas was found for VTO in contrast to NTO or for NTO relative to the other object sets after training.

To our knowledge, the present study is the first to examine neural correlates of the effect of observed manipulation on the processing of novel tools. Two previous fMRI studies have shown that direct experience with previously unfamiliar objects via active manipulation leads to a stronger recruitment of fronto-parietal brain regions during the processing of pictures of the objects [27,29]. This finding has been interpreted as support for sensory-motor theories of semantic object representations, proposing that conceptual knowledge is stored in or near brain regions associated with knowledge acquisition [21,39]. The sight of objects would thus reactivate brain regions that were involved in active object manipulation. Theories of embodied cognition, the broader framework in which sensory-motor theories of conceptual knowledge formation are proposed, suggest that object concepts in semantic memory are represented within modal systems of the brain-related to perception and action. Within this framework, however, direct manipulation experience is not considered to be

necessary for representations in motor regions to emerge (for review, see [24]). Similarly, models of praxis processing describe different access routes to action semantics, which provide a processing advantage when subjects are confronted with action-associated stimuli [18,19]. In this respect, the current study adds further evidence in favor of embodied cognition theories, showing that also indirect object experience can alter object processing, possibly, in part, due to the induction of new object representations in the fronto-parietal action system.

Considering the induced activations in detail, the strongest training effects were seen in the iFG. In general, ventral premotor cortex, including pars opercularis and precentral gyrus, has been suggested to represent a human homologue of monkey area F5, containing, among others, so-called canonical neurons that discharge in the presence of graspable objects [40] and visuo-motor neurons which fire when a monkey sees a goal-directed action of another individual acting with an object (also referred to as "mirror neurons"; [41–43]). Activation of iFG pars opercularis was reported by studies investigating the processing of tool stimuli [3,27] and when access to action concepts was required [44–46]. Furthermore, activation of pars opercularis and premotor cortex was reported in neuroimaging studies investigating neural correlates of action observation [47,48], with left-hemispheric activation of ventrolateral premotor cortex in tasks requiring access to object representations and right-hemispheric recruitment during tasks requiring analysis of movements [47]. Recruitment of iFG pars opercularis has also been interpreted to reflect the extraction of action goals during grasp observation [33]. The inferior frontal activations observed for OTO in the present study might thus, at first view, represent canonical neuron firing, since the OTO were "transformed" from meaningless objects into graspable tools via training. The pattern of activation does, however, support a different view: When objects had only been visually explored, no recruitment of pars opercularis was evident after training. Hence, pars opercularis is not activated by all kinds of graspable objects alike. Consequently, the stronger post training iFG activations for OTO might be interpreted as a re-enactment of regions relevant for action observation, possibly related to previous action goal coding associated with the object.

A similar explanation may hold for the activation within pars triangularis for OTO. IFG pars triangularis activation was reported in studies on perception and discrimination of objects [4,8] as well as during grasp observation [33,48,49]. With respect to the latter, Grafton et al. (1996) found activation at remarkably similar coordinates as the current study. Grasping as part of the observed object manipulation may thus have elicited activation in this region during the training procedure. After training, the object itself may then have been capable of eliciting an activation in or near this region.

It must be underlined that, both in the case of training studies involving active manipulation and of the present observational learning study, an interpretation in terms of a re-activation of brain regions that were active during knowledge acquisition while processing pictures of tool stimuli remains speculative, because brain activity during training was not assessed. Future studies will have to provide information on the degree of overlap of brain activations during acquisition of tool-related knowledge and tool processing. Another interesting topic for future research is whether the type of activation induced depends on the task subjects have to perform during active or observed manipulation.

Besides activation of frontal brain regions, parietal activation for OTO relative to NTO was found in the angular and supramarginal gyri (BA 40). Some previous studies investigating processing of tool-like stimuli reported activation of the parietal lobule

[8,27,29]. Using transcranial magnetic stimulation, Tunik et al. (2008) showed the importance of the left supramarginal gyrus within the parietal lobule in goal-oriented object-directed action, and proposed that it plays a crucial role in the construction of action plans and in action selection for purposeful hand-object interactions. Corroborating this interpretation, Grafton et al. (1996), investigating neural correlates of grasp imagination, reported activation in BA 40 close to the activation seen in the current study, suggesting that the role of BA40 in action plan construction is independent of actual grasp execution. In further support of this view, Culham et al. (2006) proposed that the activation of the parietal cortex during tool observation is related to the strong affordances of tools for the various hand actions with the objects.

Patient studies also suggest that the parietal lobe plays an important role in tool use and manipulation [50,51]. Randerath et al. (2010), for example, reported that patients suffering from apraxia characterized by deficits in tool use show a large lesion overlap in left supramarginal gyrus, whereas in patients mostly showing grasping errors the maximal overlap was seen in left iFG and angular gyrus. The authors propose that the angular gyrus provides information for grasping, while the supramarginal gyrus serves the integration of online and stored tool-related action knowledge. While this interpretation would be in line with the assumption that the parietal cortex stores tool representations along with information on manipulation, there are also theories claiming that the parietal lobe contribution is mostly inferring possible object uses on the basis the visual and tactile object properties affording certain actions (mechanical knowledge: [52–54]). An interesting double dissociation between object identification and object in patients suffering from semantic dementia or corticobasal degeneration does not support the notion of a separate action semantic system in the dorsal stream. Tool use in semantic dementia patients was characterized by a mechanical problem solving approach rather than by intact knowledge about proper tool use, probably guided by the intact parietal cortex. The corticobasal degeneration patient, with a prominent parietal involvement, on the other hand, showed chance level performance on mechanical problem solving. This observation suggests that viewing objects triggers a mechanical knowledge system, possibly located in parietal cortex, which extracts affordance cues to infer potential object use (e.g. [52]). With respect to the results of the present study, these findings might mean that the parietal activations do not reflect the induction of new semantic tool representations. Instead, a more general affordance-related process may be the trigger of this activation, in line with the finding that no activation of parietal cortex is found in the contrast of OTO compared to VTO. The latter result may be due to the fact that affordance-related activations were also triggered by VTO to some extent. At the same time, the parietal activations were clearly experience-dependent, as they occurred only after training and in contrast to the NTO. Thus, both observed manipulation and, to a lesser extent, visual exploration led to a strengthening of affordance-related processes during visual processing of tool-like stimuli. Learning about object function, which was provided to the subjects also in visual exploration training, may have played a key role for this process. Roy & Square (1985) and also Rothi, Ochipa & Heilman (1991, 1997) proposed that the action and the linguistic system are interconnected and that information about tool function as part of the conceptual praxis system can be acquired in different ways.

An alternative view on the role of the parietal cortex in motor performance has been put forward by Goldenberg (2009) in a recent review on the typical deficits associated with parietal brain damage in apraxia. Based on the observation that parietal lesions affect the imitation of meaningless gestures and the actual use of tools, but not the pantomime of tool use, he concludes that the parietal cortex does not store mental representations of movements. Rather, the degree of parietal recruitment depends on the "demands on categorical apprehension of spatial relationships between multiple objects" (p.1455), with the latter referring to objects, parts of objects or body parts [55]. This view was corroborated by the observation that parietal lesions affect the use of novel tools more than the use of common tools [14]. It is conceivable that increased object familiarity and/or the acquisition of object-function or object-action associations in the present study led to higher parietal involvement in the processing of object pictures, because an associated imagination of tool use required the apprehension of spatial relationships between the hands and the different object parts.

In the same study, Goldenberg and Spatt (2009) addressed also the differential role of the frontal and parietal cortex for apractic symptoms. Frontal lesions extending from the precentral gyrus to the middle and inferior frontal gyrus affected all functions assessed, from mechanical problem solving to functional knowledge and common tool selection and use. Accordingly, the authors concluded that the premotor cortex does not underlie the automatic planning of motor actions in response to the sight of tools, as suggested on the basis of imaging studies (e.g. [5]), but abstract aspects of movement planning [14].

The contrast VTO>OTO activated two large clusters in the medial parietal cortex, encompassing the calcarine gyrus bilaterally, in the left hemisphere protruding into the posterior hippocampus, and right precuneus. Additionally, VTO (in contrast to OTO) activated the left posterior cingulate cortex. Precuneus and hippocampus have been associated with episodic retrieval (e.g. [56,57]). It cannot be excluded that VTO images elicited retrieval of training episodes, whereas OTO primarily activated non-episodic memory contents. This interpretation would also explain why participants showed better assignment of VTO than OTO pictures to the correct training condition. It must be underlined, however, that we accounted for this difference in performance in our fMRI analysis.

In summary, results from the current study show that a short history of observation of object manipulation can induce activation changes in the processing of previously unfamiliar tools in fronto-parietal brain regions associated with motor actions. These activations were elicited by the mere sight of the objects and may in part constitute a reactivation of regions active during the observation of manipulation itself, especially in the case of the iFG. Alternatively, the activations, especially those involving the parietal cortex, may be related to induced object affordances, possibly triggering the activation of a mechanical problem solving system, and/or a system processing spatial relationships. With the current study design we cannot distinguish which of these processes is responsible for the fronto-parietal activation changes following training, and future research is needed to clarify if these activation changes reflect the formation of new object representations or more general action-related processes.

Author Contributions

Conceived and designed the experiments: NNR MT SFC CB. Performed the experiments: NNR. Analyzed the data: NNR MT CB. Wrote the paper: NNR MT SFC CB.

References

1. Gibson JJ (1977) The theory of affordances. In: Shaw R, Bransford J, editors.Perceiving, acting and knowing: Toward an ecological psychology. Hillsdale, NJ: Erlbaum. pp. 67–82.
2. Tucker M, Ellis R (1998) On the relations between seen objects and components of potential actions. J Exp Psychol Hum Percept Perform 24: 830–846.
3. Martin A, Wiggs CL, Ungerleider LG, Haxby JV (1996) Neural correlates of category-specific knowledge. Nature 379: 649–652.
4. Perani D, Schnur T, Tettamanti M, Gorno-Tempini M, Cappa SF, et al. (1999) Word and picture matching: a PET study of semantic category effects. Neuropsychologia 37: 293–306.
5. Chao LL, Martin A (2000) Representation of manipulable man-made objects in the dorsal stream. Neuroimage 12: 478–484.
6. Creem-Regehr SH, Lee JN (2005) Neural representations of graspable objects: are tools special? Brain Res Cogn Brain Res 22: 457–469.
7. Lewis JW (2006) Cortical networks related to human use of tools. Neuroscientist 12: 211–231.
8. Grezes J, Decety J (2002) Does visual perception of object afford action? Evidence from a neuroimaging study. Neuropsychologia 40: 212–222.
9. Symes E, Ellis R, Tucker M (2007) Visual object affordances: object orientation. Acta Psychol (Amst) 124: 238–255.
10. Tucker M, Ellis R (2001) The potentiation of grasp types during visual object categorization. Visual Cognition 8: 769–800.
11. Proverbio AM (2012) Tool perception suppresses 10-12 Hz mu rhythm of EEG over the somatosensory area. Biological Psychology 91: 1–7.
12. Proverbio AM, Adorni R, D'Aniello GE (2011) 250 ms to code for action affordance during observation of manipulable objects. Neuropsychologia 49: 2711–2717.
13. Goldenberg G (2013) Apraxia. Wiley Interdisciplinary Reviews: Cognitive Science 4: 453–462.
14. Goldenberg G, Spatt J (2009) The neural basis of tool use. Brain 132: 1645–1655. awp080 [pii];10.1093/brain/awp080 [doi].
15. De Renzi, Lucchelli F (1988) Ideational apraxia. Brain 111 (Pt 5): 1173–1185.
16. Lehmkuhl G, Poeck K (1981) A disturbance in the conceptual organization of actions in patients with ideational apraxia. Cortex 17: 153–158.
17. Heilman KM, Rothi LJG (2003) Apraxia. In: Heilman KM, Valenstein E, editors.Clinical Neuropsychology. New York: Oxford University Press. pp. 215–235.
18. Roy EA, Square PA (1985) Common considerations in the study of limb, verbal and oral apraxia. 23: 111–161.
19. Rothi LJG, Ochipa C, Heilman KM (1991) A Cognitive Neuropsychological Model of Limb Praxis. Cognitive Neuropsychology 8: 443–458.
20. Rothi LJG, Ochipa C, Heilman KM (1997) A cognitive neuropsychological model of limb praxis and apraxia. In: Rothi LJG, Heilman KM, editors.Apraxia: The Neuropsychology of Action. Psychology Press. pp. 29–49.
21. Martin A (1998) The organization of semantic knowledge and the origins of words in the brain. In: Jablonski N, Aiello L, editors.The origins and diversification of language.San Francisco: Californian Academy of Science. pp. 69–98.
22. Martin A, Chao LL (2001) Semantic memory and the brain: structure and processes. Curr Opin Neurobiol 11: 194–201.
23. Martin A (2001) Functional Neuroimaging of Semantic Memory. In: Cabeza R, Kingstone A, editors.Handbook of Functional Neuroimaging of Cognition.MA: MIT Press. pp. 153–186.
24. Barsalou LW, Kyle SW, Barbey AK, Wilson CD (2003) Grounding conceptual knowledge in modality-specific systems. Trends Cogn Sci 7: 84–91.
25. Cross ES, Cohen NR, Hamilton AFD, Ramsey R, Wolford G, et al. (2012) Physical experience leads to enhanced object perception in parietal cortex: Insights from knot tying. Neuropsychologia 50: 3207–3217.
26. Creem-Regehr SH, Dilda V, Vicchrilli AE, Federer F, Lee JN (2007) The influence of complex action knowledge on representations of novel graspable objects: evidence from functional magnetic resonance imaging. J Int Neuropsychol Soc 13: 1009–1020.
27. Bellebaum C, Tettamanti M, Marchetta E, Della Rosa P, Rizzo G, et al. (2013) Neural representations of unfamiliar objects are modulated by sensorimotor experience. Cortex 49: 1110–1125.
28. Kiefer M, Sim EJ, Liebich S, Hauk O, Tanaka J (2007) Experience-dependent plasticity of conceptual representations in human sensory-motor areas. J Cogn Neurosci 19: 525–542.
29. Weisberg J, Turennout M, Martin A (2007) A neural system for learning about object function. Cereb Cortex 17: 513–521.
30. van Schaik CP, Deaner RO, Merrill MY (1999) The conditions for tool use in primates: implications for the evolution of material culture. 36: 719–741.

31. Buxbaum LJ, Kalenine S (2010) Action knowledge, visuomotor activation, and embodiment in the two action systems. Ann N Y Acad Sci 1191: 201–218.
32. Jacquet PO, Chambon V, Borghi AM, Tessari A (2012) Object Affordances Tune Observers' Prior Expectations about Tool-Use Behaviors. Plos One 7.
33. Johnson-Frey SH, Maloof FR, Newman-Norlund R, Farrer C, Inati S, et al. (2003) Actions or hand-object interactions? Human inferior frontal cortex and action observation. Neuron 39: 1053–1058.
34. Greenhouse SW, Geisser S (1959) On Methods in the Analysis of Profile Data. Psychometrika 24: 95–112.
35. Andersson JLR, Hutton C, Ashburner J, Turner R, Friston K (2001) Modeling geometric deformations in EPI time series. Neuroimage 13: 903–919.
36. Slotnick SD, Moo LR, Segal JB, Hart J Jr (2003) Distinct prefrontal cortex activity associated with item memory and source memory for visual shapes. Brain Res Cogn Brain Res 17: 75–82.
37. Eickhoff SB, Stephan KE, Mohlberg H, Grefkes C, Fink GR, et al. (2005) A new SPM toolbox for combining probabilistic cytoarchitectonic maps and functional imaging data. Neuroimage 25: 1325–1335.
38. Worsley KJ, Marrett S, Neelin P, Vandal AC, Friston KJ, et al. (1996) A unified statistical approach for determining significant signals in images of cerebral activation. Human Brain Mapping 4: 58–73.
39. Martin A, Ungerleider LG, Haxby JV (2000) Category specificity and the brain: The sensory-motor model of semantic representations of objects. In: Gazzaniga MS, editors.The new cognitive neurosciences.Cambridge, M.A.: MIT Press. pp. 1023–1036.
40. Rizzolatti G, Fadiga L (1998) Grasping objects and grasping action meanings: the dual role of monkey rostroventral premotor cortex (area F5). Novartis Found Symp 218: 81–95.
41. Dipellegrino G, Fadiga L, Fogassi L, Gallese V, Rizzolatti G (1992) Understanding Motor Events - A Neurophysiological Study. Experimental Brain Research 91: 176–180.
42. Gallese V, Fadiga L, Fogassi L, Rizzolatti G (1996) Action recognition in the premotor cortex. Brain 119: 593–609.
43. Rizzolatti G, Fadiga L, Gallese V, Fogassi L (1996) Premotor cortex and the recognition of motor actions. Cognitive Brain Research 3: 131–141.
44. Martin A, Haxby JV, Lalonde FM, Wiggs CL, Ungerleider LG (1995) Discrete cortical regions associated with knowledge of color and knowledge of action. Science 270: 102–105.
45. Grafton ST, Fadiga L, Arbib MA, Rizzolatti G (1997) Premotor cortex activation during observation and naming of familiar tools. Neuroimage 6: 231–236.
46. Tettamanti M, Buccino G, Saccuman MC, Gallese V, Danna M, et al. (2005) Listening to action-related sentences activates fronto-parietal motor circuits. J Cogn Neurosci 17: 273–281.
47. Manthey S, Schubotz RI, von Cramon DY (2003) Premotor cortex in observing erroneous action: an fMRI study. Brain Res Cogn Brain Res 15: 296–307.
48. Molnar-Szakacs I, Iacoboni M, Koski L, Mazziotta JC (2005) Functional segregation within pars opercularis of the inferior frontal gyrus: evidence from fMRI studies of imitation and action observation. Cereb Cortex 15: 986–994.
49. Grafton ST, Arbib MA, Fadiga L, Rizzolatti G (1996) Localization of grasp representations in humans by positron emission tomography. 2. Observation compared with imagination. Exp Brain Res 112: 103–111.
50. Buxbaum LJ, Sirigu A, Schwartz MF, Klatzky R (2003) Cognitive representations of hand posture in ideomotor apraxia. Neuropsychologia 41: 1091–1113.
51. Buxbaum LJ, Saffran EM (2002) Knowledge of object manipulation and object function: dissociations in apraxic and nonapraxic subjects. Brain and Language 82: 179–199.
52. Hodges JR, Spatt J, Patterson K (1999) "What" and "how": evidence for the dissociation of object knowledge and mechanical problem-solving skills in the human brain. Proc Natl Acad Sci U S A 96: 9444–9448.
53. Goldenberg G, Hagmann S (1998) Tool use and mechanical problem solving in apraxia. Neuropsychologia 36: 581–589. S0028-3932(97)00165-6 [pii].
54. Sirigu A, Duhamel JR, Poncet M (1991) The role of sensorimotor experience in object recognition. A case of multimodal agnosia. Brain 114 (Pt 6): 2555–2573.
55. Goldenberg G (2009) Apraxia and the parietal lobes. Neuropsychologia 47: 1449–1459. S0028-3932(08)00298-4 [pii];10.1016/j.neuropsychologia. 2008.07.014 [doi].
56. Shallice T, Fletcher P, Frith CD, Grasby P, Frackowiak RSJ, et al. (1994) Brain-Regions Associated with Acquisition and Retrieval of Verbal Episodic Memory. Nature 368: 633–635.
57. Eldridge LL, Knowlton BJ, Furmanski CS, Bookheimer SY, Engel SA (2000) Remembering episodes: a selective role for the hippocampus during retrieval. Nat Neurosci 3: 1149–1152.

7

A Neural Network Approach to fMRI Binocular Visual Rivalry Task Analysis

Nicola Bertolino[1]*, Stefania Ferraro[2], Anna Nigri[2], Maria Grazia Bruzzone[2], Francesco Ghielmetti[1], and on behalf of the Coma Research Centre (CRC) – Besta Institute

1 Health Department, Carlo Besta Neurological Institute, Milan, Italy, **2** Neuro-Radiology Department, Carlo Besta Neurological Institute, Milan, Italy

Abstract

The purpose of this study was to investigate whether artificial neural networks (ANN) are able to decode participants' conscious experience perception from brain activity alone, using complex and ecological stimuli. To reach the aim we conducted pattern recognition data analysis on fMRI data acquired during the execution of a binocular visual rivalry paradigm (BR). Twelve healthy participants were submitted to fMRI during the execution of a binocular non-rivalry (BNR) and a BR paradigm in which two classes of stimuli (faces and houses) were presented. During the binocular rivalry paradigm, behavioral responses related to the switching between consciously perceived stimuli were also collected. First, we used the BNR paradigm as a functional localizer to identify the brain areas involved the processing of the stimuli. Second, we trained the ANN on the BNR fMRI data restricted to these regions of interest. Third, we applied the trained ANN to the BR data as a 'brain reading' tool to discriminate the pattern of neural activity between the two stimuli. Fourth, we verified the consistency of the ANN outputs with the collected behavioral indicators of which stimulus was consciously perceived by the participants. Our main results showed that the trained ANN was able to generalize across the two different tasks (i.e. BNR and BR) and to identify with high accuracy the cognitive state of the participants (i.e. which stimulus was consciously perceived) during the BR condition. The behavioral response, employed as control parameter, was compared with the network output and a statistically significant percentage of correspondences (p-value <0.05) were obtained for all subjects. In conclusion the present study provides a method based on multivariate pattern analysis to investigate the neural basis of visual consciousness during the BR phenomenon when behavioral indicators lack or are inconsistent, like in disorders of consciousness or sedated patients.

Editor: Emmanuel Andreas Stamatakis, University Of Cambridge, United Kingdom

Funding: The start-up Coma Research Centre (CRC) project was funded by a healthcare grant (N° IX/000407 - 05/08/2010) awarded by Regione Lombardia. The funders had no role in study design, data collection and analysis, decision to publish, or preparation of the manuscript.

Competing Interests: The authors have declared that no competing interests exist.

* Email: nicola.bertolino@istituto-besta.it

Introduction

Multivariate pattern analysis (MVPA) is able to process information coming from differently located clusters of voxels and makes it possible to detect particular patterns of neural activity that may remain hidden to conventional analyses (e.g., univariate statistical methods) [1]. Indeed, in these last years, MVPA has been extensively applied as a "mind reading" tool to decode mental states from functional magnetic resonance imaging (fMRI) data, such as to assess perceptual states [2] or to evaluate deception and differentiate lying from truth-telling [3], [4], [5]. A great interest arose around fMRI studies using MVPA that allowed the investigation of how the contents of conscious experience are encoded in the brain [6].

Most of the work on this topic examined only the prediction of static and unchanging perceptual states during extended periods of stimulation [7], [8], [9].

A dynamic perceptual phenomenon particularly suitable to be studied with MVPA is the binocular visual rivalry (BR): two different visual stimuli are presented, one to each eye, and the two conflicting monocular images compete for access to consciousness and the subject usually experiences an alternate perception of the two images. The perceptual dominance of one image can endure for a few seconds before switching to the other, fluctuating stochastically over time [10], [11]. Thus, the visual input is the same, but the perceptual interpretation changes. Due to this characteristic, the BR paradigm was shown to be an important tool to explore the neural correlates of visual conscious experience [11], [12].

In this framework, Haynes et al. (2005) investigated BR using MVPA on fMRI signals [13]. They showed that linear discriminant analysis was able to predict in healthy subjects from brain activity alone the stream of visual consciousness by means of the fluctuation between two classes of simple stimuli (blue and red orthogonal rotating gratings). This study also demonstrated that accurate prediction of the perception during BR could be established with signals recorded during stable monocular viewing, suggesting the possibility to use this approach in the absence of behavioral indicators, such as in animals or patients with locked-in syndrome.

A seminal study by Tong et al. (1998) demonstrated that during BR in which houses and faces were presented, the fusiform face area (FFA) and the parahippocampal place area (PPA) reflected the perceived stimulus, showing that changes from house to face led to an increase in blood oxygen level dependent (BOLD) signal in FFA and a decrease in PPA, while changes from face to house led to the opposite pattern. Moreover they showed a striking resemblance of BOLD signal changes during non-rivalry and rivalry paradigms, not only in the qualitative pattern but also in the amplitude of FFA and PPA responses [14]. However, they did not test for generalization between training with non-rivalry, and testing with rivalry in absence of behavior.

The brain regions involved in the processing of these stimuli are the bilateral occipital area, collateral sulcus, PPA, occipital face area (OFA), and FFA. In particular FFA and OFA were identified as areas responding more to face stimuli, whereas bilateral PPA as more reactive to houses and objects [15], [16].

These results allowed us to investigate whether multivariate classification methods are able to decode a dynamic perception phenomenon of complex and ecological stimuli using rivalry and non-rivalry paradigms.

The aim of our study was to provide a method based on artificial neural networks (ANN) [17] able to identify the different neural pattern of activity related to the processing of two classes of visual stimuli (houses and faces) during a visual rivalry paradigm, applicable in the absence of behavioral indicators, indicating which stimulus is perceived by participant.

We studied 12 healthy subjects with fMRI as they viewed binocular non-rivalry (BNR) and BR tasks. First we used the BNR to identify brain areas involved in face and house decoding, then we trained the ANN on these data, and finally we employed the trained ANN in order to discriminate the pattern of activity in BR task analysis and verified the consistency of these results with the behavioral response.

A major challenge of this study was the signal decoding due to a low signal to noise ratio (SNR). Many system imperfections and physical phenomena (eddy currents, asymmetric anti-aliasing filter response, concomitant magnetic field, mismatched gradient group delays, and hysteresis) affected echo planar imaging (EPI), and especially sequences with short TR, by artifacts and signal loss [18]. Hence, a processing protocol for signal optimization was implemented in order to increase the network performance.

Materials and Methods

Participants

We recruited 12 healthy volunteers for this study (mean age 32.5 years, range 18–47 years) with no history of neurological disease, 5 of whom were female. The experimental protocol was approved by the ethics committee (Comitato Etico) of IRCCS Carlo Besta Neurological Institute and all the participants gave written informed consent. All clinical investigation has been conducted according to the principles expressed in the Declaration of Helsinki.

MRI acquisitions

Anatomical and functional data were collected using a 3.0 Tesla MRI scanner (Achieva TX, Philips Medical Systems BV, Best, NL) equipped with a 32 channel phase-array head coil. Each participant underwent to an imaging protocol including anatomical 3D T1 (TFE with FOV = 240×240 mm^2 and voxel = $1 \times 1 \times 1$ mm^3, TR/TE = 9.8/4.6 ms) and two EPI sequences, one for the BNR (200 volumes) and the other for the BR fMRI paradigm (600 volumes). Both fMRI sequences had a FOV = 240×240 mm^2, an isotropic voxel ($3 \times 3 \times 3$ mm^3), a 90° flip angle and a TE = 40 ms. The TR of the BNR-localizer sequence was 3000 ms, while for the rivalry sequence TR was 1000 ms. We chose a short TR of 1000 ms for the BR sequence in order to be sure to capture the rapid alternate perception between

the two images. The perception dominance of one image was shown to be in the range between 2.5 to 5.5 s [14]. Because of the different TR, slices number of the package was set to 30 for the first EPI sequence and 16 for the second.

fMRI paradigms

All participants performed two fMRI block design tasks (Fig. 1): the BNR-localizer and the BR paradigm. During the BNR-localizer task participants were presented with 5 blocks showing a set of faces alternating with 5 blocks showing a set of houses, spaced out by 10 rest blocks. Each block duration was 30 seconds and included 10 stimuli, each shown for 3 seconds.

During the BR task participants were presented with 15 picture blocks broken up by 15 rest blocks. For the picture blocks, a house was shown to one eye and a face was shown to the other simultaneously. These two pictures were chosen from those used for the BNR-localizer task. Each block duration was 20 seconds. The house and face images were presented to the right and left eye, respectively, for half of the participants, and vice versa for the other half. For both tasks a white fixation cross on a black background was presented during rest blocks. Additionally the house pictures were red-filtered while the face pictures were blue-filtered in order to employ stimuli similar to the ones used in the previous literature [13], [14] and to increase the perceptual differences between the two classes of stimuli.

All the participants were provided with a pair of stereo LCD goggles for visual stimulation, a pair of headphones, and two keypads (VisuaStim, Resonance Technology Inc., Northridge CA, USA). During the BR task participants were asked to indicate which picture they perceived by pressing a button on the keypad at transition points from one stimulus perception to the other, and behavioral data were collected.

Data Analysis

In order to illustrate the multiple steps of the method employed, a flow chart is provided in Fig. 2.

For all the data analyses we used SPM 8 (Statistical Parametric Mapping, http://www.fil.ion.ucl.ac.uk), MatLab 7.13 (The Math-Works Inc., Natick, MA, 2012), and SPSS 17.0 (SPSS Inc., Chicago, 2008).

Behavioral data analysis

During the BR task, the mean value of the duration of the perceptual dominance for each image (house or face) and its standard deviation were calculated for each participant and for the whole group.

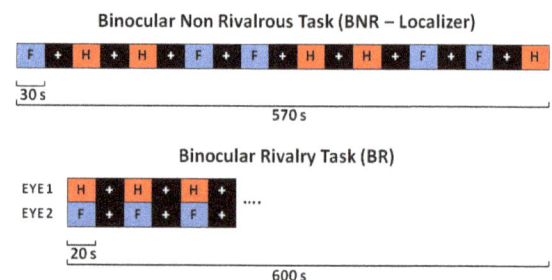

Binocular Non Rivalrous Task (BNR – Localizer)

Binocular Rivalry Task (BR)

Figure 1. Diagrams showing the fMRI block tasks design. The letter H in the red box represents the house block, the letter F in the blue box represents the face block, and the white cross in the black box represents the rest block. The BNR task is shown on the top, while the BR task is shown on the bottom.

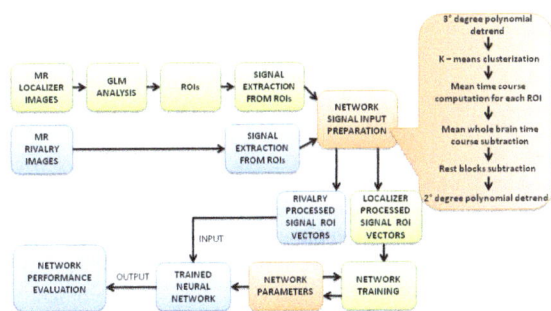

Figure 2. Diagram illustrating signal processing steps. In the green boxes the steps concerning the BNR ROI signals are described, in the blue boxes the steps concerning BR ROI signals are described, and in the orange boxes the steps in common for both signals are described.

Data preprocessing

Both fMRI acquisitions (i.e., BNR and BR scans) were co-registered to the T1 and pre-processed to correct 3D motion artifacts, linear drifts, and low-frequency non linear drifts. Spatial smoothing was applied using a Gaussian kernel with a 5 mm full width at half maximum isotropic. For the BR scan, a slice timing correction was also performed.

Single-subject analysis and ROIs identification

In order to identify the functional regions of interest (ROIs) (i.e., FFA, PPA, and OFA) necessary to extract the time course signals to train and to run the ANN we performed standard single-subject analyses [19] on the BNR-localizer data in the framework of the general linear model (GLM). In the design matrix we modeled the presentations of faces and houses as predictors. We performed two t-contrasts: faces>houses and houses>faces [14]. The package volume of the sequence, employed in the BR task, was applied as an inclusive mask to the obtained con-images in order to verify that the identified areas were included in the BR acquisition package and to control for I type error [20]. For every single subject the activations clusters, resulting from the analysis, were selected as ROIs with a voxel-level threshold of $P<0.05$ FWE-corrected and a minimum cluster size of 5 voxels. If using these threshold at least N = 3 ROIs (1 ROI for the first t-contrast and 2 ROIs for the second) were not identified, the voxel-level threshold was moved to $p<0.05$ FDR corrected. A maximum of 3 ROIs for contrast was extracted based on higher T-score. The peak MNI coordinates of every activation cluster, selected as ROI for each subject, is provided in Table 1.

Network input signal preparation

For both BNR and BR datasets, we extracted the fMRI signal time-courses from each voxel in the identified N ROIs and the mean fMRI signal time-course from the whole brain. The ROIs and the mean whole brain signal time-courses obtained from both fMRI task scans were detrended with a third degree polynomial function to eliminate the signal drift. Afterwards, the k-means clusterization algorithm [21] was employed to split the BR detrended ROI signal time-courses in two clusters. Considering that the ROIs were selected by the analysis on BNR data, we employed the clusterization algorithm in order to discriminate the voxels participating in BR phenomenon and remove the voxels not involved in the activation pattern and also affected by higher noise. Then, the mean fMRI signal time-course of the remaining voxels of each ROI was calculated.

Table 1. Selected ROIs coordinates.

Subject #	Faces-houses t-contrast												Houses-Faces t-contrast					
	FFA right			FFA left			OFA right			OFA left			PPA right			PPA left		
	x	y	z	x	y	z	x	y	z	x	y	z	x	y	z	x	y	z
1	40	-46	-22	-42	-60	-20	42	-68	-10	-	-	-	28	-46	-10	-28	-54	-8
2	40	-54	-16	-	-	-	-	-	-	-	-	-	30	-50	-8	-26	-50	-10
3	58	-28	16	-	-	-	-	-	-	-	-	-	36	-26	-12	-28	-36	-4
4	46	-48	-18	-42	-48	-20	-	-	-	-	-	-	32	-48	-10	-28	-50	-8
5	38	-44	-20	-	-	-	50	-68	-2	-	-	-	24	-42	-10	-26	-46	-12
6	44	-52	-22	-	-	-	40	-70	-10	-	-	-	32	-48	-10	-28	-56	-10
7	-	-	-	-44	-50	-24	38	-72	-20	-38	-78	-10	26	-50	-14	-24	-52	-14
8	40	-60	-18	-	-	-	-	-	-	-	-	-	30	-52	-8	-26	-44	-10
9	-	-	-	-38	-56	-18	44	-80	-18	-	-	-	28	-60	-6	-26	-52	-10
10	40	-40	-16	-36	-48	-14	-	-	-	-	-	-	28	-40	-8	-26	-44	-6

The table shows the peak MNI coordinates of every activation cluster, selected as ROI for each subject for PPAs, FFAs and OFAs.

These signals and the mean fMRI time-course from the whole brain were converted in percent signal changes relative to their mean values over time. In order to minimize most of the non-task-related signal fluctuations, the percent signal changes of the whole brain fMRI signal time-course was subtracted from the percent signal changes of each single ROI [22]; the resulting signal was shifted to account for the BOLD response delay. Finally, we removed the rest block time points and detrended the signals with a second degree polynomial, obtaining the ultimate neural network input signal. In order to assess the reliability of the network output we used the removed rest block time points of the BR dataset as a control signal.

Training and Running the network

We implemented a one-layer Feed-Forward Neural Network with a Log-Sigmoid Transfer Function [17]. We chose an hidden layer size of 65 neurons and, as performance function, the Mean Square Error (MSE) relative to the difference between the target outputs (presented stimuli) and the values predicted by the model (network outputs).

The network was trained and run separately for each subject. As a training dataset, we used a matrix in which the columns were the processed BNR ROIs time courses, divided randomly in train set (75%) and valuation set (25%). The training set was used for computing the gradient descent and updating the network weights and biases in the direction in which the performance function decreases more rapidly, while the evaluation set was used for the MSE value computation. At the end of the training, the network weights and biases were saved at the minimum of the MSE. If the training process performance did not achieve a selected threshold (MSE <0.02), chosen to have a good and homogeneous training between subjects [23], the algorithm repeated the process using new initialization seeds (weights and biases).

Next, we ran the trained network using the matrix in which the columns were the processed ROIs BR time courses as input data. The ANN produced an output matrix **X**, in which the rows were the time points and the two columns were the outputs of classification for the presented stimuli in a range between zero and one. The ideal output matrix row (1 0) represented the face, while (0 1) represented the house. In order to assign time points to one of the two conditions, we set up a threshold $|X_{t,1} - X_{t,2}| > 0.9$, where $t = 1,...,N$, with N number of time points. If a time point did not reach the threshold, it was labeled as not assigned and discarded; the whole process, including training and run, was reiterated until the number of unassigned time points was smaller than 16.7%.

To evaluate the accuracy of the network to discriminate between perception status, we computed (1) the percentage of successes, obtained comparing the network output with the behavioral response vector, and (2) the p-value, obtained by using a binomial distribution, considering two conditions with a probability of 50% to be equal or different from behavioral responses.

Assessment of reliability of the network output

As the network weights and biases change during initialization and optimization, the resulting output is affected by a certain variability, reflecting the stochastic nature of ANN training [23]. Hence, to evaluate the consistency of the results, for each subject we repeated the whole process described in the previous section 1000 times. In order to have a negative control set of data we applied the 1000 repetition again substituting the BR with the rest block time-course. For each repetition we collected the number of time points assigned to houses or faces. Based on the hypothesis

that the rest block signal is unrelated to BR phenomenon, in order to highlight differences between the distribution of predicted stimuli (houses and faces), we analyzed the different outputs. Frequency histograms of houses and faces were produced and normality tests [24] were performed on the distribution of percentage value of the two stimuli over the total time points allocated along with mean, variance, kurtosis, and asymmetry computation. We expect that for participants who experienced the phenomenon, the event distribution in the BR-task signal ANN output is balanced between the two stimuli (i.e. ratio between the percentage of number of houses and faces >1/4) and leptokurtic or at the most normally distributed over the 1000 reiterations. We also collected evaluative information performing a comparison between the task and the rest block signal ANN output (control). This signal is expected to be characterized by a more asymmetric and/or platykurtic events distribution and/or an unbalanced distribution between stimuli, with a larger variance, because of the unpredictable random effects involved in the ANN time points attribution of a non-task-related signal.

Results

We discarded two of the subjects from our analysis: the first because we did not find the expected activations (FFAs, OFAs, PPAs) during the GLM analysis of BNR paradigm, and the second because the subject declared that he did not experience the perception alternation phenomenon.

During the BR paradigm, the participants reported alternations between face-dominant and house-dominant percepts. The mean phase duration was 3.37 s (range: 1.78 to 4.47 s; standard deviation = 0.93 s).

Consistent with the literature [15], [16], the single-subject analysis of BNR data revealed that the participants showed activity for the contrast faces>houses in the posterior fusiform gyrus (i.e., FFA) and in the inferior occipital gyrus (i.e., OFA) (Fig. 3A), while for the contrast houses>faces in the parahippocampal gyrus (Fig. 3B). We identified a maximum of 5 ROIs for 2 participants, 4 ROIs for 5 participants, and 3 ROIs for 3 participants (Table 1).

The mean number of signal time points not assigned to each of the two conditions was 10.7±3.7%.

For 9 of the 10 participants, combined information of 3 ROIs was sufficient to allow the neural network to predict which

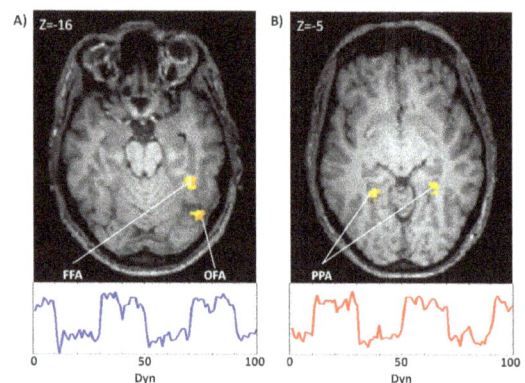

Figure 3. Example of resulting BOLD activity from GLM single-subject analysis of BNR-localizer task. Picture A shows t-contrast activations of face-house (FWE<0.05) in BNR time-course of PPA on top and FFA ROI on the bottom. Picture B shows t-contrast activations of house-face (FWE<0.05) in BNR-localizer time-course of FFA on top and PPA ROI on the bottom.

stimulus the subject was experiencing with up to 75% accuracy ($p<0.05$). When the signals from 4 ROIs were combined the classification accuracy improved slightly for all but 1 participant, and the ANN predicted the perceived stimulus in all the participants (up to 78% accuracy; $p<0.05$). The only 2 participants in which 5 ROIs were detected showed a further slight increase of the accuracy of the neural network (up to 80%; $p<0.05$) combining the information coming from all of them (Table 2; Fig. 4).

We tested the reliability of ANN output for all 10 participants, as described in the previous section. Analyzing the BR task signal, we found that in all cases the events distributions were leptokurtic (kurtosis coefficient >0) or normal (Shapiro-Wilk, $p>0.05$) and the mean number of predicted stimuli was balanced, with a percentage of houses and faces in the range between 25% and 75% for all the participants, except one. Moreover for the rest block signal output the events distribution was unbalanced and/or platykurtic (Kurtosis coefficient <0), with a larger variance and asymmetry than for task signal in all cases (Fig. 5A).

We also performed the reliability assessment for the discarded participant who declared that he did not experience the rivalry phenomenon. In this case the events distribution was unbalanced, platykurtic for both task and rest signal ANN output; moreover, asymmetry was larger for task than for rest ANN output (Fig. 5B).

Discussion and Conclusions

The present study provides a method based on MVPA to investigate the neural basis of visual consciousness during the BR phenomenon when behavioral indicators, of what the participant is experiencing, are lacking or inconsistent.

Our main results showed that the trained ANN was able to generalize across two different fMRI paradigms (i.e. BNR and BR) and to identify with high accuracy the cognitive state of the participant (i.e. which stimulus was consciously perceived) during the BR condition. These results were obtained combining information from 3 ROIs in all the participants, except one, although the best performances were obtained by combining information from 4 or 5 ROIs. The possibility to apply this procedure using a limited number of ROIs makes it applicable to a wide variety of patients with cerebral insult.

Based on the literature, we decided to use faces and houses as stimuli because they induce very different patterns of neural activity supporting an optimal training of ANN and because faces, due to their ecological relevance, are easily discriminated than other stimuli [25].

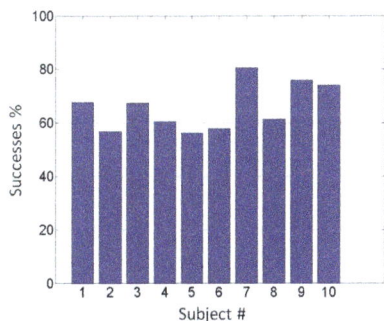

Figure 4. Bar plot of ANN percentage of successes for each subject. The plot shows in ordinate the percentage of time points correctly allocate to conditions (house or face) and in abscissa the number associated to the participants.

Table 2. Results summary.

#	sex	age	3 ROI Successes %	3 ROI p	3 ROI Descarded trials (%)	4 ROI Successes %	4 ROI p	4 ROI Descarded trials (%)	5 ROI Successes %	5 ROI p	5 ROI Descarded trials (%)	Behavioral mean (s)	Behavioral SD (s)
1	M	32	58,1	0,004	6,7	61,7	0,000	8,7	67,6	0,000	12,6	3,13	1,28
2	M	47	56,8	0,016	10	–	–	–	–	–	–	2,89	1,28
3	F	24	67,3	0,000	13,3	–	–	–	–	–	–	2,97	1,08
4	M	35	59,2	0,000	10	60,5	0,000	8	–	–	–	4,47	1,6
5	M	40	49,4	0,603	16,7	56,3	0,026	10,3	–	–	–	2,57	1,58
6	M	17	58,2	0,005	9,7	57,8	0,009	14,3	–	–	–	1,78	0,76
7	F	40	75,5	0,000	1,1	78,3	0,000	13,7	80,6	0,000	12,6	4,35	2,03
8	M	37	61,3	0,000	9,7	–	–	–	–	–	–	3,97	2,4
9	F	23	65,3	0,000	15,3	75,9	0,000	14,3	–	–	–	2,94	2,5
10	M	32	69,2	0,000	2,6	74,0	0,000	6,3	–	–	–	4,6	3,15

Neural Network results obtained from all participants, making use of 3, 4, or 5 ROIs as input data for the algorithm. The rate of success increases with the number of ROIs employed.

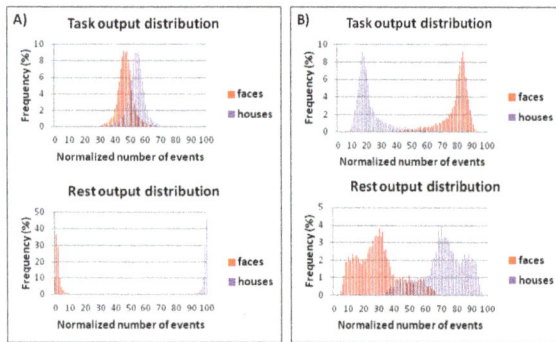

Figure 5. Examples of stimuli distributions after 1000 output repetitions. In panel A on top the bar histogram shows for subject 7 the results of the 1000 reiterations using the BR task time course signal. In y axis is represented the percentage number (frequency) of house and face over all time points in a reiteration, and in the x axis the percentage number of reiterations (events) in which we obtained a determined frequency of houses and faces over all 1000 reiterations. In the plot on the bottom of panel A the BR time course signal has been replaced with Rest time course signal. In panel B the same bar histograms, for BR and rest time courses, are shown for the subject excluded because he did not experience the BR phenomenon.

The ability to identify a common pattern of neural activity during two different paradigms is extremely important in a context where behavioral indicators lack or are difficult to detect. As in the study by Haynes et al. [13], we trained the neural network with data obtained in a controlled condition (i.e., BNR condition) that allowed us to know what the participant was perceiving, and tested it on data obtained in a condition where there was no external control (except for the behavioral response, used only to assess the prediction accuracy of the algorithm) of what the individual was perceiving (i.e., the BR condition). This clearly supports the use of our ANN in conditions where the conscious perception of an individual is not accessible to an external observer. Unlike Haynes [13], who trained the neural network on data obtained from a monocular non-rivalry condition, we trained it on data obtained from a binocular non-rivalry condition. The ability of the ANN to predict the conscious perception during BR using a training on BNR fMRI signal indicates that the BOLD signal changes in the ROIs were strictly modulated by the conscious percept and not by the eye of origin of the stimuli.

The behavioral data showed that the mean perception dominance duration was variable between subjects and consistent with the previous studies using similar stimuli [14], although an EEG study reported a shorter perception dominance duration using rotating gratings as stimuli [26]. Interestingly, we noticed that the worst performance of our brain states classifier was obtained from subjects 5 and 6, who experienced shorter mean perception durations (respectively 2.57 s and 1.78 s); we speculate that it may be harder to decode a signal when perception changes are too quick.

The single-subject GLM analysis of the BNR task did not activate the same number of areas in all participants. Thus, it was not feasible to identify 4 or 5 ROIs for each subject, because OFA and FFA are functional areas and they do not correspond to an easily recognizable and circumscribed anatomical location [15]. For this reason we trained and tested the ANN using information extracted from 3, 4 and 5 ROIs, based on the available identified regions for each participant.

In order to create a non-user dependent standard procedure, two thresholds were fixed, one related to the network training

performance (MSE <0.02) and the other to the time points assignment ($|X_{t,1}-X_{t,2}| >0.9$), based on the best results obtained for our group of healthy volunteers.

In the last decade there has been a great ongoing debate about the neural processes underlying BR, with some studies describing this phenomenon as a high-level and representation-based process [14], [27], [28], [29] and others describing it as a low-level and eye-based process [13], [30], [31]. In our study, we decided to use a paradigm based on the hypothesis of high-level and representation based processes during BR.

The future development of this study lies in the application of the described method to investigate BR phenomenon in patients with different levels of sedation, disorder of consciousness or patients with profound physical disabilities, where it is difficult even for experienced clinicians to diagnose cognitive ability [32]. The neuroscience community used fMRI paradigms extensively to detect willful behavior in these patients [33], [34].

The absence of any feedback from these patients creates the tricky problem of the ANN output truthfulness assessment.

We addressed this criticism by outlining some criteria that were derived from the described training method and reliability assessment. The conditions that should be fulfilled to consider the ANN output reliable and infer that the subject experienced the perception of BR, even in absence of any feedback, are as follows:

i. activation clusters present in BNR task single-subject analysis necessary to identify at least 3 ROIs;

ii. high network training performance: MSE <0.02;

iii. after 1000 runs the BR-task signal ANN outputs must be balanced between stimuli and presenting a leptokurtic, or at most normal, events distribution;

iv. the BR-task signal ANN output events distribution must have a smaller variance and symmetry than the rest events distribution.

Despite the significance of the results obtained, we underline that the classification performances of the ANN could have been more accurate in consideration of some limits of our study. The main issues that cannot be easily resolved lies in the behavioral responses registration method and more specifically we identified three critical aspects: first we did not ask to the participants to inform us when the two percepts were overlapping, second subject reaction times and errors in button-pressing may alter our recorded data and bias our final estimation on ANN output and third during BNR task registration the motor behavioral responses were absent.

Another limit of this study may be linked to pulse sequences parameters used for BNR and BR scans: it would likely be possible to achieve a better performance of the network using the same EPI sequence parameters for both tasks, though differences between the two sequences are slight.

In conclusion, the present study provides a method based on multivariate pattern analysis to investigate the neural basis of visual consciousness during the BR phenomenon when behavioral indicators lack or are inconsistent.

Acknowledgments

The authors are grateful to Domenico Aquino for excellent support during data processing and insightful advice.

The Coma Research Centre (CRC) multidisciplinary team, on behalf of which the present publication was submitted, acknowledges the following members: Matilde Leonardi (Scientific Director CRC), Eugenio Agostino Parati, Maria Grazia Bruzzone, Silvana Franceschetti, Dario Caldiroli, Davide Sattin, Ambra Giovannetti, Marco Pagani, Venusia Covelli,

Francesca Ciaraffa, Jesus Vela Gomez, Barbara Reggiori, Stefania Ferraro, Anna Nigri, Ludovico D'Incerti, Ludovico Minati, Adrian Andronache, Cristina Rosazza, Patrik Fazio, Davide Rossi, Giulia Varotto, Ferruccio Panzica, Riccardo Benti, Giorgio Marotta, Franco Molteni.

Study realized also in collaboration with FERB- European Federation Biomedical Research.

The authors are grateful to two anonymous reviewers for insightful feedback on an earlier draft of this paper.

Author Contributions

Conceived and designed the experiments: NB SF AN MGB FG. Performed the experiments: NB FS AN. Analyzed the data: NB SF AN FG. Contributed reagents/materials/analysis tools: MGB. Wrote the paper: NB SF AN MGB FG.

References

1. Norman KA, Polyn SM, Detre GJ, Haxby JV (2006) Beyond mind-reading: multi-voxel pattern analysis of fMRI data. Trends Cogn Sci, 10(9), 424–430.
2. Pereira F, Mitchell T, Botvinick M (2009) Machine learning classifiers and fMRI: A tutorial overview. NeuroImage, 45(1 Suppl), S199–209.
3. Gao J, Wang Z, Yang Y, Zhang W, Tao C, et al. (2013) A novel approach for lie detection based on F-score and extreme learning machine. PloS One, 8(6), e64704.
4. Langleben DD, Moriarty JC (2013) Using brain imaging for lie detection: Where science, law and research policy collide. Psychol Public Policy Law, 19(2), 222–234.
5. Davatzikos C, Ruparel K, Fan Y, Shen DG, Acharyya M, et al. (2005) Classifying spatial patterns of brain activity with machine learning methods: application to lie detection. NeuroImage, 28(3), 663–668.
6. Weil RS, Rees G (2010) Decoding the neural correlates of consciousness. Curr Opin Neurol, 23(6), 649–655.
7. Minati L, Nigri A, Rosazza C, Bruzzone MG (2012) Thoughts turned into high-level commands: Proof-of-concept study of a vision-guided robot arm driven by functional MRI (fMRI) signals. Med Eng Phys, 34(5), 650–658.
8. Mourao-Miranda J, Almeida JR, Hassel S, De Oliveira L, Versace A, et al. (2012) Pattern recognition analyses of brain activation elicited by happy and neutral faces in unipolar and bipolar depression. Bipolar Disord, 14(4), 451–460.
9. Yamamura H, Sawahata Y, Yamamoto M, Kamitani Y (2009) Neural art appraisal of painter: Dali or picasso? Neuroreport, 20(18), 1630–1633.
10. Blake R, Wilson H (2011) Binocular vision. Vision Res, 51(7), 754–770.
11. Blake R, Logothetis NK (2002) Visual competition. Nat Rev Neurosci, 3(1), 13–21.
12. Zhang P, Jiang Y, He S (2012) Voluntary attention modulates processing of eye-specific visual information. Psychol Sci, 23(3), 254–260.
13. Haynes JD, Rees G (2005) Predicting the stream of consciousness from activity in human visual cortex. Curr Biol : CB, 15(14), 1301–1307.
14. Tong F, Nakayama K, Vaughan JT, Kanwisher N (1998) Binocular rivalry and visual awareness in human extrastriate cortex. Neuron, 21(4), 753–759.
15. Rossion B, Hanseeuw B, Dricot L (2012) Defining face perception areas in the human brain: A large-scale factorial fMRI face localizer analysis. Brain Cogn, 79(2), 138–157.
16. Cant JS, Goodale MA (2011) Scratching beneath the surface: New insights into the functional properties of the lateral occipital area and parahippocampal place area. J Neurosci, 31(22), 8248–8258.
17. Picton P (2000) Neural networks. Basingstoke, UK: Palgrave Macmillan. 195 p.
18. Bernstein MA, King KF, Zhou XJ (2004) Handbook of MRI pulse sequences. ELSEVIER ACADEMIC PRESS. 1017 p.
19. Turner R, Howseman A, Rees GE, Josephs O, Friston K (1998) Functional magnetic resonance imaging of the human brain: Data acquisition and analysis. Exp Brain Res, 123(1–2), 5–12.
20. Poldrack RA (2007) Region of interest analysis for fMRI. Soc Cogn Affect Neurosci, 2(1), 67–70.
21. Goutte C, Toft P, Rostrup E, Nielsen F, Hansen LK (1999) On clustering fMRI time series. NeuroImage, 9(3), 298–310.
22. Desjardins AE, Kiehl KA, Liddle PF (2001) Removal of confounding effects of global signal in functional MRI analyses. NeuroImage, 13(4), 751–8.
23. Jiang Y (2003) Uncertainty in the output of artificial neural networks. IEEE Trans Med Imaging, 22(7), 913–21.
24. Shapiro S, Wilk MB (1965) An analysis of variance test for normality. Biometrika, 52(3), 591.
25. Hoshiyama M, Kakigi R, Takeshima Y, Miki K, Watanabe S (2006) Priority of face perception during subliminal stimulation using a new color-opponent flicker stimulation. Neurosci Lett, 402(1–2), 57–61.
26. Roeber U, Veser S, Schroger E, O'Shea RP (2011) On the role of attention in binocular rivalry: Electrophysiological evidence PloS One, 6(7), e22612.
27. Hsieh PJ, Colas JT, Kanwisher NG (2012) Pre-stimulus pattern of activity in the fusiform face area predicts face percepts during binocular rivalry. Neuropsychologia, 50(4), 522–9.
28. Logothetis NK (1998) Single units and conscious vision. Philos Trans R Soc Lond B Biol Sci, 353(1377), 1801–18.
29. Lumer ED, Friston KJ, Rees G (1998) Neural correlates of perceptual rivalry in the human brain. Science, 280(5371), 1930–4.
30. Wunderlich K, Schneider KA, Kastner S (2005) Neural correlates of binocular rivalry in the human lateral geniculate nucleus. Nat Neurosci, 8(11), 1595–602.
31. Tong F, Engel SA (2001) Interocular rivalry revealed in the human cortical blind-spot representation. Nature, 411(6834), 195–9.
32. Andrews K, Murphy L, Munday R, Littlewood C (1996) Misdiagnosis of the vegetative state: Retrospective study in a rehabilitation unit. BMJ, 313(7048), 13–16.
33. Laureys S, Giacino JT, Schiff ND, Schabus M, Owen AM (2006) How should functional imaging of patients with disorders of consciousness contribute to their clinical rehabilitation needs? Curr Opin Neurol, 19(6), 520–7.
34. Monti MM, Coleman MR, Owen AM (2009) Neuroimaging and the vegetative state: Resolving the behavioral assessment dilemma? Ann N Y Acad Sci, 1157, 81–9.

8

Alterations in Low-Level Perceptual Networks Related to Clinical Severity in PTSD after an Earthquake: A Resting-State fMRI Study

Jing Shang[1], Su Lui[2,3]*[9], Yajing Meng[1], Hongru Zhu[1], Changjian Qiu[1], Qiyong Gong[2], Wei Liao[4], Wei Zhang[1]*[9]

1 Mental Health Center, Department of Psychiatry, West China Hospital of Sichuan University, Chengdu, Sichuan, People's Republic of China, 2 Huaxi MR Research Center (HMRRC), Department of Radiology, West China Hospital of Sichuan University, Chengdu, Sichuan, People's Republic of China, 3 Radiology Department of the Second Affiliated Hospital, Wenzhou Medical University, Wenzhou, Zhejiang, People's Republic of China, 4 Center for Cognition and Brain Disorders (CCBD), Hangzhou Normal University, Hangzhou, Zhejiang, People's Republic of China

Abstract

Background: Several task-based functional MRI (fMRI) studies have highlighted abnormal activation in specific regions involving the low-level perceptual (auditory, visual, and somato-motor) network in posttraumatic stress disorder (PTSD) patients. However, little is known about whether the functional connectivity of the low-level perceptual and higher-order cognitive (attention, central-execution, and default-mode) networks change in medication-naïve PTSD patients during the resting state.

Methods: We investigated the resting state networks (RSNs) using independent component analysis (ICA) in 18 chronic Wenchuan earthquake-related PTSD patients versus 20 healthy survivors (HSs).

Results: Compared to the HSs, PTSD patients displayed both increased and decreased functional connectivity within the salience network (SN), central executive network (CEN), default mode network (DMN), somato-motor network (SMN), auditory network (AN), and visual network (VN). Furthermore, strengthened connectivity involving the inferior temporal gyrus (ITG) and supplementary motor area (SMA) was negatively correlated with clinical severity in PTSD patients.

Limitations: Given the absence of a healthy control group that never experienced the earthquake, our results cannot be used to compare alterations between the PTSD patients, physically healthy trauma survivors, and healthy controls. In addition, the breathing and heart rates were not monitored in our small sample size of subjects. In future studies, specific task paradigms should be used to reveal perceptual impairments.

Conclusions: These findings suggest that PTSD patients have widespread deficits in both the low-level perceptual and higher-order cognitive networks. Decreased connectivity within the low-level perceptual networks was related to clinical symptoms, which may be associated with traumatic reminders causing attentional bias to negative emotion in response to threatening stimuli and resulting in emotional dysregulation.

Editor: Huafu Chen, University of Electronic Science and Technology of China, China

Funding: Funding of the research was provided by the National High-tech R&D Program of China (863 Programme 2008AA022601 for Wei Zhang) and National Natural Science Foundation (Grant Nos. 81222018, 81371527 for Su Lui). The funders had no role in study design, data collection and analysis, decision to publish, or preparation of the manuscript.

Competing Interests: The authors have declared that no competing interests exist.

* E-mail: weizhang27@163.com (WZ); lusuwcums@tom.com (SL)

[9] These authors contributed equally to this work.

Introduction

Posttraumatic stress disorder (PTSD) is one of the most common psychiatric disorders [1]. The core feature of PTSD is the development of characteristic symptoms following a traumatic event, including a lack of emotional equilibrium [2] and the persistent re-experience of stressors, which is accompanied by continuous physiological hyperarousal [3], sustained avoidance of event reminders and a "numbing" of general responsiveness [4]. Although PTSD has a growing and serious impact on the population, little is known about the mechanisms by which this disorder develops. One hypothesis regarding the development of PTSD is the aberrant organization or dysfunction of distributed neural networks involving a triple network model correlation with cognition, including the salience network (SN), central executive network (CEN), and default mode network (DMN) [5]; this hypothesis is supported by previous studies [6,7]. However, the findings were inconsistent due to confounding factors, including medication, different sources of trauma, and various analysis methods. Furthermore, several recent task-based functional MRI

Table 1. Psychological or behavioral data.

| | PTSD (n = 18) | HS (n = 20) | PTSD vs. HS | |
	M± SD	M± SD	T value	p value
Gender(n: male/female)	4M/14W	11M/9W	–	0.052[a]
Age (yrs)	43.33±8.04	40.30±9.32	1.07	0.293
Education (yrs)	7.11±3.68	8.65±3.39	−1.34	0.188
CAPS	63.94±13.53	11.35±8.32	14.60	<0.0001
HAMD	13.83±5.39	4.00±3.49	6.59	<0.0001
HAMA	13.94±4.53	3.95±4.12	7.06	<0.0001

Data from questionnaires are presented in terms of mean score (M) and standard deviation (SD) in PTSD and HS groups. Statistical comparisons between the two groups are also provided.
PTSD, posttraumatic stress disorder; HS, healthy survivors; CAPS, Clinician-Administered Posttraumatic Stress Disorder Scale; HAMA, Hamilton Anxiety Rating Scale; HAMD, Hamilton Depression Rating Scale.
[a]The p value was Fisher's Exact test. The other p values were obtained by two-sample two-tailed t -test.

(fMRI) studies have highlighted an abnormal activation in specific regions involving the low-level perceptual (auditory, visual, somato-motor) network in PTSD patients [8,9]. However, whether the functional connectivity of low-level perceptual and higher-order cognitive (attention, central-execution, and default-mode) networks changes in medication-naïve PTSD patients during the resting state remains unclear. This issue is important for elucidating the pathogenesis of PTSD because the identification of different levels of brain networks and the reorganization of networks may provide evidence that validates the network impairment hypothesis. This modified model involves regions in the circuits that mediate the "contextualization" of stimuli and supplies a novel way to examine the neuro-pathophysiological mechanisms in PTSD patients.

In recent years, the resting-state fMRI has been identified as a marker of neural connectivity to explore the alterations of coherent intrinsic neuronal activity of blood oxygen level-dependent (BOLD) fluctuations in the brain. ICA is a data-driven analysis that separates a set of signals into independent, uncorrelated, and non-Gaussian spatiotemporal components without requiring a priori specification of a seed region [10]. ICA is particularly valuable for the investigation of brain networks modulated by task performance [11] and at rest [12,13]. Among them, the auditory network (AN), the visual network (VN), and the sensory-motor network (SMN) are composed of elementary networks that would be of considerable interest because they have connections with the situationally accessible memory system (SAMs). This system is triggered involuntarily by environmental or internal cues that are reminiscent of the original trauma for individuals and form the basis for flashbacks that are re-experienced by the individuals [14].

The primary aims of the present work were to use the task-free resting-state fMRI to investigate the two-level network effects on the pathogenesis of PTSD. Two hypotheses were considered. First, whether the functional connectivity of RSNs related to perceptual and higher cognitive processes may be aberrant in traumatized participants with PTSD. Second, whether any of the changes identified would be related to the measured clinical severity.

Methods

2.1 Subjects

The study was approved by the Medical Research Ethics Committee of West China Hospital, Sichuan University and all the subjects' written informed consents were obtained before the study. We acquired whole-brain resting-state fMRI for 18 patients (43.33±8.04 years, all right-handed) and 20 non-PTSD individuals with a history of trauma exposure (40.62±9.20 years, all right-handed). All participants were recruited two years after the Wenchuan earthquake through the Mental Health Center of the Huaxi Hospital, Chengdu, China (Table 1). Population age, gender and education characteristics were matched between patient and control groups. All participants were less than 60 years of age and were interviewed to confirm that there was no history of psychiatric illness among their first-degree relatives, no history of head injury or neurologic disorders, and no history of drug or alcohol abuse in the six months preceding the scan. Participants were evaluated with the Clinician-Administered Posttraumatic Stress Disorder Scale (CAPS) [15], which had excellent test-retest reliability across all clients and displayed moderate convergent validity for PTSD [16]; the Hamilton Anxiety Rating Scale (HAMA) and the Hamilton Depression Rating Scale (HAMD) were also used. The diagnosis of PTSD was determined by a consensus between the two attending psychiatrists and a trained interviewer using the Structured Clinical Interview DSM-IV (SCID)–Patients Version. PTSD patients receiving psychotherapy or psychiatric medications and participants with a total CAPS score of less than 40 points were excluded.

2.2 Image Acquisition

Experiments were performed on a 3.0-T GE-Signa MRI scanner (EXCITE, General Electric, Milwaukee, WI, USA) with an eight-channel phased array head coil at the Huaxi MR Research Center. We immobilized the participants' heads with foam padding. Functional images were acquired using a single-shot, gradient-recalled echo-planar imaging sequence (TR = 2,000 ms, TE = 30 ms, and flip angle = 90°). Thirty transverse slices (FOV = 240×240 mm), which had a matrix size of 64×64 and a slice thickness of 5 mm without a gap, yielded a voxel size of 3.75×3.75×5. A total of 200 volumes were acquired and images were aligned along the anterior commissure–posterior commissure (AC–PC) line. Subjects were instructed to relax, let their minds wander, keep their eyes closed, and not fall asleep.

2.3 Data Preprocessing

The data were preprocessed using SPM8 software (http://www.fil.ion.ucl.ac.uk/spm). All data were corrected for slice timing, and head motion correction of the functional scans was performed.

Next, the functional images were coregistered to the mean functional image and normalized to the echo-planar imaging template in SPM8. The data from 1 of the 19 subjects in the PTSD group were excluded because the translation and rotation of the head motion exceeded ±1.5 mm and ±1.5°, respectively. Images were then spatially smoothed by convolution with a half-maximum isotropic Gaussian filter (FWHM = 8 mm).

2.4 ICA and Identification of RSNs

Briefly, ICA is a mathematical procedure to decompose, for example, a spatiotemporal signal into independent, uncorrelated, and non-Gaussian components. We performed a spatial ICA using the GIFT software (http://icatb.sourceforge.net/,version 1.3e) [17]. To determine the number of independent components (ICs), we estimated the dimensions of the datasets from the two groups using the minimum description length (MDL) criterion to account for spatial correlation [18]. FMRI data from all subjects in each group were then concatenated, and the temporal dimension of the aggregate dataset was reduced via principal component analysis (PCA), decomposed by IC estimation (with time courses and spatial maps) using the Informax algorithm [17,18]. Two separate analyses based on the spatial ICA were conducted on the PTSD and healthy survivor (HS) groups, with 44 and 46 ICs, respectively. The intensity values in each map were scaled to z scores because ICA of fMRI data intrinsically extracts patterns of coherent neuronal responses (i.e., networks) [11,19–21].

2.5 Component Identification

Our RSNs were chosen according to the available knowledge on the psychopathology of PTSD and its neuronal correlates. Similar to other anxiety disorders, PTSD is related to difficulty in managing emotions, but particularly with an attentional bias for threatening stimuli [22], and intrusive memories [23]; these factors rely on the SN, CEN, and DMN. Because neurobiological studies of episodic memory retrieval have also shown that the visual cortex and auditory cortex are preferentially activated during reminder exposure tasks [8,9], we also chose the VN, AN, and SMN. To date, there is no consensus on how to select the optimal number of components, although methods to do so are in development [17]. We used RSN templates provided by previous studies [24], ensuring that the RSNs had a similar spatial pattern in the two groups [18]. The components were selected based on the largest spatial correlation [25], extracted from all subjects, and corresponded to six RSNs in the current work: the SN, DMN, CEN, SMN, VN, and AN.

2.6 Second-level Analysis of the RSNs

The spatial maps of each RSN were then gathered in each group for a random-effect analysis using one-sample t-tests (Fig. 1); data were corrected using a false discovery rate (FDR) with a threshold of $p<0.05$ in SPM8. The spatial distribution of the RSNs was the same as in previous studies [24,26]. To qualitatively and quantitatively compare the RSNs between the PTSD patients and HSs, the resulting maps of two-sample t-tests were thresholded at $p<0.05$ and corrected for multiple comparisons using a FDR correction [27] with an extent threshold of 10 voxels using the toolbox of REST (http://www.restfmri.net/forum/). The group comparisons were restricted to the voxels within the corresponding RSNs.

2.7 Post hoc Correlation Analysis

Pearson correlation analysis was performed between the connectivity strength (mean z-values) and the CAPS, HAMD, and HAMA scores to investigate the relationship between the z-values in the network maps and clinical severity. We extracted the z-values emerging from significant clusters of interest between the PTSD and HS groups as a mask consisting of several regions of interest (ROIs), which were applied to all subjects. The mean z-values of each individual within these ROIs were correlated to the clinical scales and then thresholded at a significance level of $p<0.05$.

Results

3.1 Psychological and Behavioral Data

Group demographic characteristics and psychological and behavioral scores are shown in Table 1. Compared with the HSs, PTSD patients displayed significantly impaired performance of CAPS, HAMD, and HAMA with higher scores.

3.2 Spatial Pattern of RSNs in Each Group

Our analysis indicated that the six RSNs were spatially consistent across patients and controls; the findings were consistent with previous fMRI studies on RSNs [12,21,26,28]. According to the one-sample t-tests, these six RSNs in both the PTSD and HS groups were the SN, CEN, DMN, SMN, AN, and VN (Fig. 1 shows the ICs of the PTSD and HS groups corrected using FDR with a threshold of $p<0.05$). The SN primarily contains the superior and middle prefrontal cortices, the anterior cingulate and paracingulate gyri, and the ventrolateral prefrontal cortex. The CEN connects the dorsolateral frontal cortex with the parietal cortex. The DMN is composed of the posterior cingulate cortex (PCC), the anterior cingulate cortex (ACC), the middle temporal gyrus, and the medial prefrontal cortex (mPFC). The SMN includes the pre- and post-central gyrus, the primary sensory-motor cortices, and the supplementary motor area (SMA). The AN primarily encompasses the bilateral middle and superior temporal gyrus, the Heschl gyrus, and the temporal pole. The VN is anchored in the inferior, middle, and superior occipital gyrus, the temporal–occipital regions, and along with the superior parietal gyrus.

3.3 Aberrant RSNs in Patients with PTSD

The two-sample t-tests revealed differences in the functional connectivity between the two groups (Fig. 2; Table 2). Direct group contrasts confirmed that both increased and decreased ($p<0.05$, FDR corrected) functional connectivity were illustrated in the SN, CEN, DMN, AN, VN, and SMN of PTSD patients. Moreover, supplementary HAMA values in the PTSD patients exhibited a significant ($p<0.05$) negative correlation with the mean z-values of the inferior temporal gyrus (IFG) in the AN. The negative connection strengthened between the mean z-values of the SMA in the SMN and the HAMA values, as well as the mean z-values of the SMA in the SMN and the HAMD values.

Discussion

Consistent with our hypothesis, the current study reveals the different functional connectivities in both low-level perceptual and higher-order cognitive networks in earthquake survivors with and without PTSD. Furthermore, both decreased and increased functional connectivity were found in all six networks in PTSD patients relative to HSs, whereas only changes of low-level perceptual networks were related to clinical severity, as assessed by the HAMA and HAMD scores. We also noticed that PTSD patients displayed significantly higher scores of HAMD, and HAMA when compared with the HSs, because most of PTSD

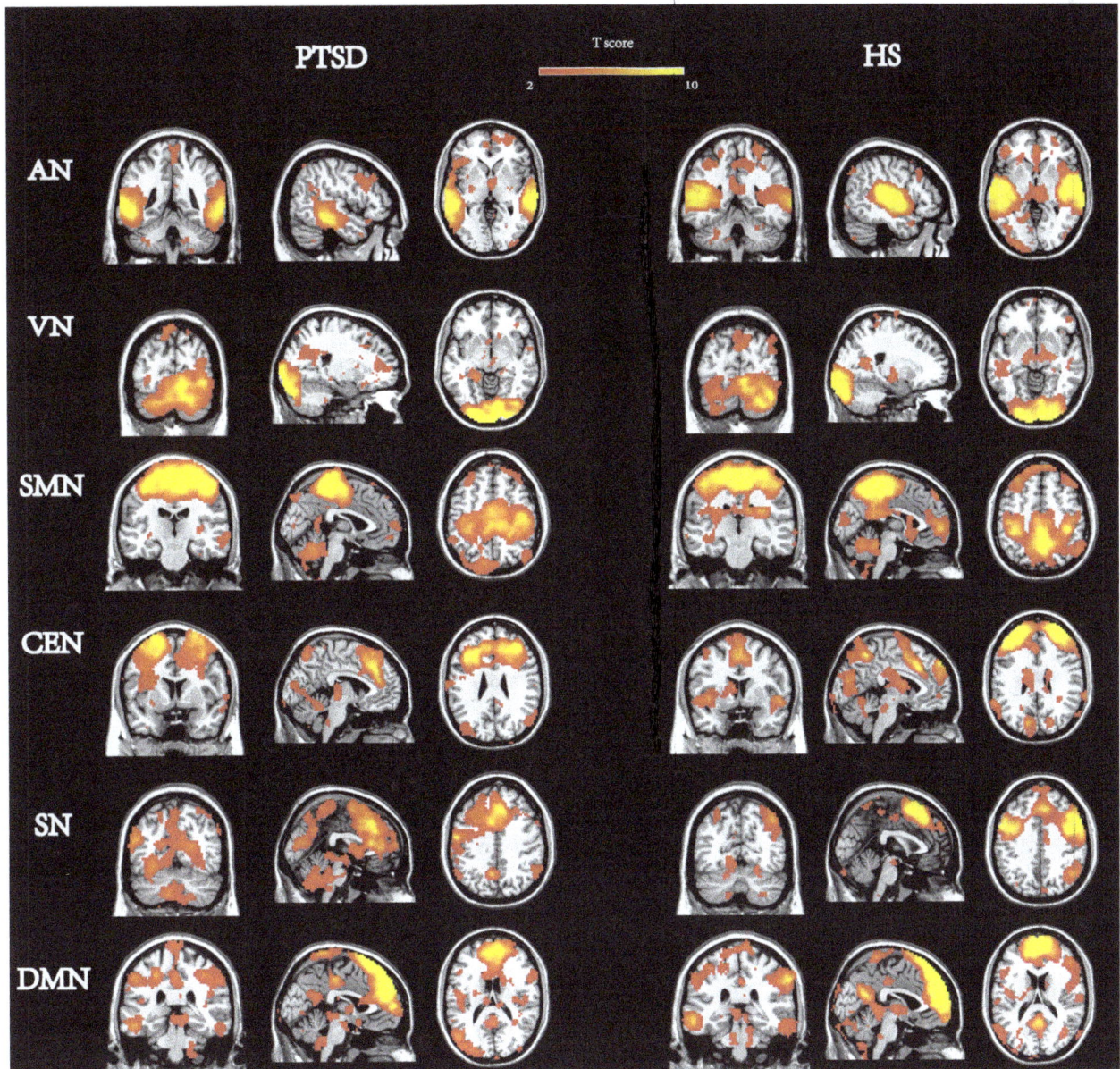

Figure 1. Six networks between PTSD and Healthy survivors (HS). (p<0.05, FDR corrected).

patients are accompanied by physiological anxiety symptoms and negative apprehension. These findings provide further evidence that widespread changes occur in the cognitive networks of PTSD patients; these alterations may be related to stress-related impairments, possible functional reorganization, and/or a compensatory mechanism [29]. Changes to low-level perceptual networks may play a critical role in the pathogenesis of PTSD symptoms.

4.1 Low-level Perceptual Networks in PTSD

The most interesting findings of the current study were those of the deficits of the AN and SMN, which were related to clinical severity in these earthquake-related PTSD patients. The AN and SMN are the most important components of the low-level perceptual network; this network can be accessed involuntarily and forms the basis for the flashbacks and nightmares that relate to

the traumatic moments in PTSD [30]. These findings support the dual representation theory of the development of PTSD, which was developed by Brewin [31] and in which the SAMs contains detailed sensory and perceptual images and holds low-level representations that are tightly bound to their sensory and affective qualities. In PTSD, extremely stressful events are stored as SAMs that are linked with sensory systems, including the AN, VN, and SMN.

4.1.1 The AN in PTSD. Lesions of the AN are influential for tinnitus, which was one of the most frequently reported problems among veterans returning from two recent armed conflicts, often co-occurring with PTSD [32]. The current study extended the previous findings by indicating complex changes of strengthened interconnection within the AN in PTSD patients relative to HSs, i.e., PTSD patients had both higher connectivity involving the inferior temporal gyrus (IFG)/fusiform and lower connectivity

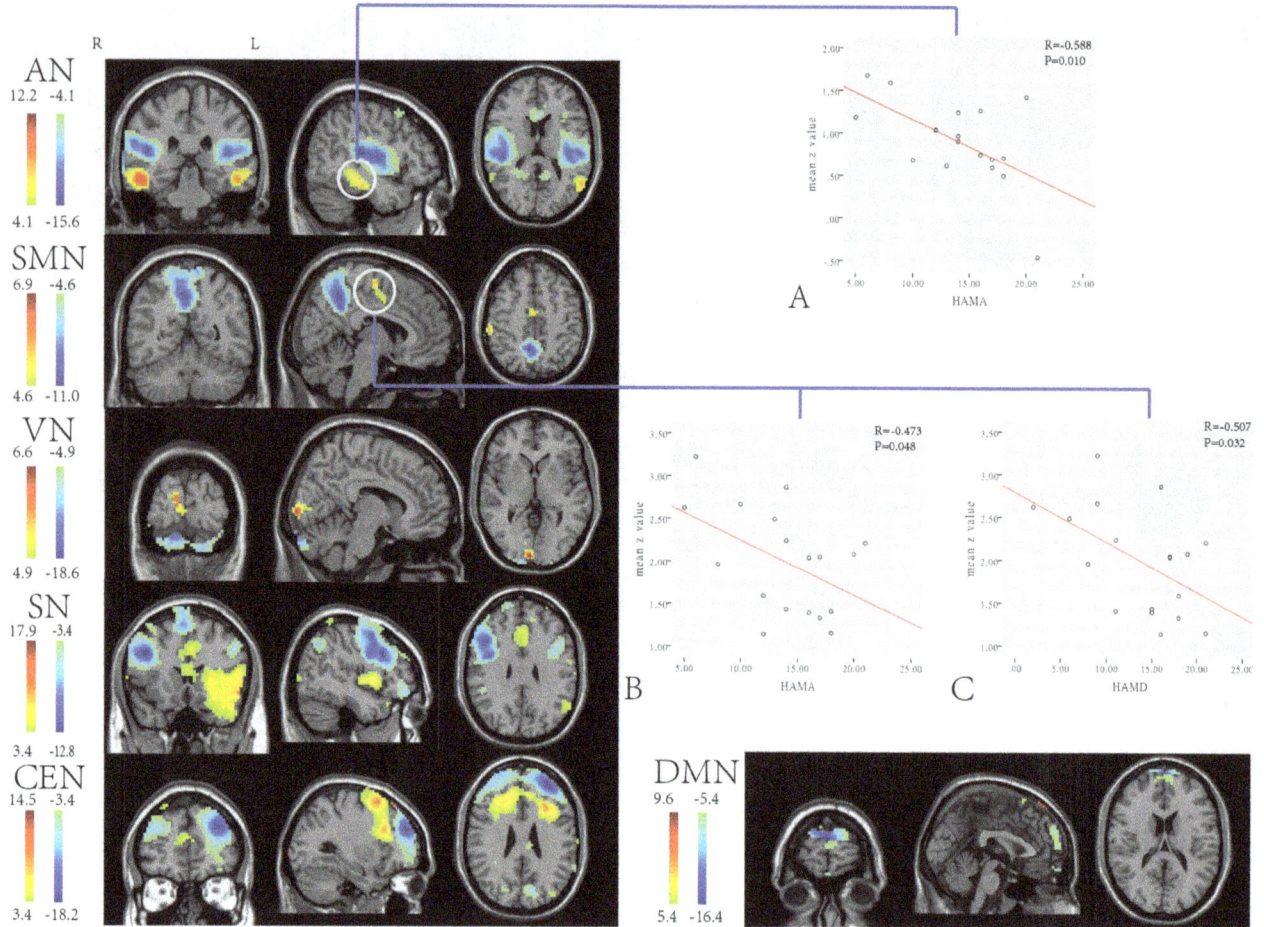

Figure 2. Anatomic templates implement of a two-sample t -test each RSNs in the PTSD vs. HS (p<0.05, FDR corrected). The warm and cold colors indicate the brain regions with significantly increased and decreased functional connectivity in PTSD, respectively. Correlation plots (p<0.05) between functional connectivity and psychometric measures, between mean Z values of ROIs(regionals of interest)and the clinical severity scores in PTSD patients. (A) Correlation between inferior temporal gyrus and HAMA score. (B) Correlation between supplementary motor area(SMA) and HAMA score. (C) Correlation between supplementary motor area(SMA) and HAMD score.

involving the superior temporal gyrus. Downar et al. [33] used event-related fMRI to identify IFG responses to oddball or otherwise salient stimuli and inferred that IFG may play a broad role in evaluating the potential relevance of sensory stimuli and in inhibiting prepotent responses to stimuli. Because PTSD is typically associated with traumatic reminders, elevated functional connectivity of the visual association cortex, such as the IFG reported in previous studies, can be interpreted as representing vivid intrusive memories that occur spontaneously and are accompanied by dissociative distortions to the perception of time, place, and self from even relatively mild stimuli [34,35]. In addition, the negative correlation between functional connectivity in the IFG and HAMA score provides further evidence for anticipatory anxiety, the discontinuity of conscious experience, and impaired memory retrieval in PTSD patients in the resting state.

The superior temporal gyrus (STG) is involved in nonverbal auditory and language processing and has been found to be activated in dissociated PTSD subjects during recall of the traumatic memory [36]. The disrupted function of the STG observed in patients with PTSD suggests that temporal or limbic structures may contribute to the patients' dissociative responses, which involve the fragmentation of the typically integrated

function of consciousness, memory, identity, or perception of the environment [37]. Alternatively, our findings may be due to the critical role of the STG in social cognition [38], which is connected with the avoidance of necessary cognition and affective processing of trauma [39] that is typical in PTSD. The above data are attributed to the anatomy of the STG, which is a vital structure in the pathway involving the amygdala and the prefrontal cortex that supports social cognition processes and encodes memory involvement [38,40].

4.1.2 The SMN in PTSD. Another network showing correlations with the severity of clinical symptoms in PTSD was the SMN. The SMN is operationally defined as the region that has significant functional connectivity with the primary somato-motor cortex (pre- and post- central gyrus) [41]. The SMN contributes to motor skill learning, as evidenced in animal models and human motor controls, which is accompanied by changes in the strength of connections within the primary motor cortex [42–44]. The current investigation demonstrates that regional connectivity in the SMA is a key part of the 'salience network' that processes autonomic, interoceptive, homeostatic, and cognitive information of personal relevance [33,45]. Thus, we propose here that increased functional connectivity of the motor cortex may represent the neural correlate of preparation for coping with a

Table 2. Difference of functional connectivity of the brain regions (PTSD- HS) in each RSN, along with the MNI coordinates of the peak foci and the associated Brodmann areas (BA).

RSN	ROI	BA	cluster	t-value(peak)	MNI x	MNI y	MNI z
SN	Middle frontal gyrus (L)	8	797	−12.82	45	18	30
CEN	Medial frontal gyrus (L)	9	439	−18.23	−30	48	27
DMN	Orbital frontal gyrus (L)	10	64	−16.43	0	66	18
AN	Superior temporal gyrus(R)	22	492	−15.65	45	−30	15
	Inferior temporal gyrus (R)	20	69	8.17	60	−54	30
SMN	Precuneus (R)	31	473	−11.00	6	−54	48
	Supplementary motor area(R)	6	37	5.62	9	−15	60
VN	Cuneus(R)	18	60	6.55	6	−96	0
	Cerebelum(R)	–	159	−18.63	15	−87	−27

BA, Brodmann area; MNI, Montreal Neurological Institute; ROI, region of interest; threshold was set at P<0.05 (FDR corrected).

physical threat [46], in line with the psychobiological mechanisms underlying PTSD. Cunnington et al. [47] have found that the SMA plays a common role in encoding or representing actions prior to voluntary self-initiated movements; the early component of premovement activity is strongly influenced by higher cognitive factors, such as attention. Our findings of a significant negative correlation between the SMA and the HAMA and HAMD factors further indicate that patients with PTSD tend to focus their attention upon and are hypervigilant for information related to 'emotional alarms' and associated stimuli. Furthermore, this attentional bias to negative emotion has been evidenced with the Stroop task [48].

The precuneus has been proposed to be involved in cognitive function, such as memory processing and spatial location encoding [49,50]. A reduced-strength connectivity of the precuneus correlated with other regions typically involved in the default mode network has been observed in PTSD patients during the resting state in previous fMRI studies [51]. This finding suggests the possible involvement of the region in the cognitive deficits seen in PTSD [52,53]. Given that the process of mental image generation requires reactivation of a stored percept, the precuneus may therefore be important in the retrieval of spatial information [54], which is associated with the core PTSD symptoms related to intrusive thoughts and memories.

4.1.3 The VN in PTSD. Excessive vigilance as a hallmark of PTSD may be associated with increased demands on the brain areas that are involved in the visual association cortex in pathological memories and planning a response to potentially threatening stimuli [46]. Our findings indicate an increased functional connectivity of the cuneus in the VN, which is consistent with previous studies [36]. This increased functional connectivity of the region is likely associated with an ongoing vigilance response [55] and with spontaneous dissociative experiences, including modulations of mental imagery [56]. Patients with cerebellar damage have been found to have reduced cognition and motor capacity in the verbal-visual span-matching task. Therefore, the breakdown in the functional connectivity of the cerebellum seen in our research provide further evidence for the impairment of verbal working memory (VWM) that is typical in PTSD [57].

4.2 High-level Cognitive Networks in PTSD

The present findings indicate that the Brodmann 8, 9 and 10 which are the constituents of the SN, CEN, and DMN, respectively, have decreased functional connectivity in PTSD patients when compared to HSs (Fig. 2 and Table 2). These regions belong to an extension of the medial prefrontal cortex (mPFC) [58] and involve the most replicated findings in PTSD, including diminished activation in the mPFC in PTSD patients relative to healthy controls regardless of a history of trauma exposure [5]. Further, these findings are in harmony with the anatomy and function of the mPFC, which was noted through the inhibition of excessive cortico-limbic activity [59]. Given that the mPFC has been shown to activate during self-referential and emotional-processing tasks [60,61], we speculate that the reduced activation of the mPFC in PTSD may be a reflection of the self-relevant nature of the traumatic stimuli and signify a deficiency in emotional self-awareness during traumatic memory recall [62]. In addition, the above findings support the prominent cognitive behavioral models of PTSD, which include an excess of fear memory of the traumatic event, a failure of expression, derealization states, and dissociative amnesia [63]. Interestingly, we did not identify any activation of the amygdala, which has been a focal point in the high-level cognitive networks; from this, we inferred that there may only be a consistent site of greater activation of the amygdala in comparison to individuals from a non-trauma-exposed group rather than the traumatic exposure control group. These data are in line with the notion that diminished medial prefrontal function is a reliable neural marker of PTSD and makes contribution to trauma-related resilience whereas amygdala may be connected more with arousal experience [5].

Limitations

Our results have several limitations. First, the absence of a healthy group that never experienced the earthquake limited the investigation of the discrepancy among the three groups. Alterations in cerebral function may be driven by trauma exposure rather than being unique in PTSD [64]. A second limitation is the small sample size considered in this study. Furthermore, we did not use physiological monitoring of the breathing and heart rates, which may interfere with the detection of spontaneously occurring low-frequency ranges of brain activity during the scan. For slow sampling rates (as in this study where one brain volume was scanned every 2 s), structured noise from these two physiological mechanisms can interfere with the low-frequency oscillations at which the resting-state connectivity is detected [65,66]. The majority of the PTSD patients were women, which is attributed to patient recruitment bias. The sex difference between subjects did not affect the within-study results because the patient and control groups were matched on all variables.

Future research should also use specific task paradigms that may reveal perceptual impairments. Ideally, such an optimized network metric may prove efficacious in making the critical clinical distinction regarding which at-risk subjects will develop PTSD or remain healthy.

Conclusions

In summary, the results of our baseline study provide a comprehensive examination of the relationship between the elementary and higher cognitive networks in PTSD patients exposed to a single trauma. The lower order of the cognitive processing hierarchy is directly related to symptom severity and contributes to our understanding of the mechanisms involved in emotion regulation and memory recall from trauma in patients with PTSD. Diminished medial prefrontal function as a reliable biomarker of PTSD provides evidence for contextualization impairments, including emotion regulation, social cognition, and self-referential processing [5]. Future studies that are combined with more sophisticated techniques, such as genetics, pupillometry, heart rate variability, and electroencephalographs (EEG), or integrated with task-related activities may yield more refined results about the neurophysiological processes of PTSD.

Acknowledgments

We thank Ph.D. Wei Liao for helpful discussion and providing us the RSNs image which was used as the template in the present study.

Author Contributions

Conceived and designed the experiments: WZ QG SL. Performed the experiments: YM HZ CQ. Analyzed the data: JS SL. Contributed reagents/materials/analysis tools: WL. Wrote the paper: JS SL.

References

1. Yehuda R (2002) Post-Traumatic Stress Disorder. New England Journal of Medicine 346: 108–114.
2. Dolan RJ (2002) Emotion, cognition, and behavior. Science 298: 1191–1194.
3. Bremner JD (1999) Alterations in brain structure and function associated with post-traumatic stress disorder. Seminars in clinical neuropsychiatry 4: 249–255.
4. Bremner JD, Southwick S, Brett E, Fontana A, Rosenheck R, et al. (1992) Dissociation and posttraumatic stress disorder in Vietnam combat veterans. American Journal of Psychiatry 149: 328–332.
5. Patel R, Spreng RN, Shin LM, Girard TA (2012) Neurocircuitry models of posttraumatic stress disorder and beyond: a meta-analysis of functional neuroimaging studies. Neurosci Biobehav Rev 36: 2130–2142.
6. Daniels JK, McFarlane AC, Bluhm RL, Moores KA, Clark CR, et al. (2010) Switching between executive and default mode networks in posttraumatic stress disorder: alterations in functional connectivity. Journal of psychiatry & neuroscience: JPN 35: 258.
7. Sripada RK, King AP, Welsh RC, Garfinkel SN, Wang X, et al. (2012) Neural dysregulation in posttraumatic stress disorder: evidence for disrupted equilibrium between salience and default mode brain networks. Psychosom Med 74: 904–911.
8. Nyberg L, Habib R, McIntosh AR, Tulving E (2000) Reactivation of encoding-related brain activity during memory retrieval. Proceedings of the National Academy of Sciences 97: 11120–11124.
9. Wheeler ME, Petersen SE, Buckner RL (2000) Memory's echo: Vivid remembering reactivates sensory-specific cortex. Proceedings of the National Academy of Sciences 97: 11125–11129.
10. Beckmann CF, Smith SM (2004) Probabilistic independent component analysis for functional magnetic resonance imaging. Medical Imaging, IEEE Transactions on 23: 137–152.
11. Bartels A, Zeki S (2005) Brain dynamics during natural viewing conditions–a new guide for mapping connectivity in vivo. Neuroimage 24: 339–349.
12. Damoiseaux JS, Rombouts SA, Barkhof F, Scheltens P, Stam CJ, et al. (2006) Consistent resting-state networks across healthy subjects. Proc Natl Acad Sci U S A 103: 13848–13853.
13. De Luca M, Beckmann CF, De Stefano N, Matthews PM, Smith SM (2006) fMRI resting state networks define distinct modes of long-distance interactions in the human brain. NeuroImage 29: 1359–1367.
14. Brewin CR, Gregory JD, Lipton M, Burgess N (2010) Intrusive images in psychological disorders: characteristics, neural mechanisms, and treatment implications. Psychol Rev 117: 210–232.
15. Blake DD, Weathers FW, Nagy LM, Kaloupek DG, Gusman FD, et al. (1995) The development of a clinician-administered PTSD scale. Journal of traumatic stress 8: 75–90.
16. Mueser KT, Rosenberg SD, Fox L, Salyers MP, Ford JD, et al. (2001) Psychometric evaluation of trauma and posttraumatic stress disorder assessments in persons with severe mental illness. Psychological Assessment 13: 110.
17. Calhoun V, Adali T, Pearlson G, Pekar J (2001) A method for making group inferences using independent component analysis of functional MRI data: Exploring the visual system. NeuroImage 13: 88–88.
18. Jafri MJ, Pearlson GD, Stevens M, Calhoun VD (2008) A method for functional network connectivity among spatially independent resting-state components in schizophrenia. NeuroImage 39: 1666–1681.
19. D'Argembeau A, Collette F, Van der Linden M, Laureys S, Del Fiore G, et al. (2005) Self-referential reflective activity and its relationship with rest: a PET study. NeuroImage 25: 616–624.
20. Calhoun VD, Liu J, Adali T (2009) A review of group ICA for fMRI data and ICA for joint inference of imaging, genetic, and ERP data. NeuroImage 45: S163–172.
21. Beckmann CF, DeLuca M, Devlin JT, Smith SM (2005) Investigations into resting-state connectivity using independent component analysis. Philos Trans R Soc Lond B Biol Sci 360: 1001–1013.
22. Pine DS, Mogg K, Bradley BP, Montgomery L, Monk CS, et al. (2005) Attention bias to threat in maltreated children: implications for vulnerability to stress-related psychopathology. American Journal of Psychiatry 162: 291–296.
23. Brewin CR (2001) Memory processes in post-traumatic stress disorder. International Review of Psychiatry 13: 159–163.
24. Ding JR, Liao W, Zhang Z, Mantini D, Xu Q, et al. (2011) Topological fractionation of resting-state networks. PLoS One 6: e26596.
25. Greicius MD, Flores BH, Menon V, Glover GH, Solvason HB, et al. (2007) Resting-state functional connectivity in major depression: abnormally increased contributions from subgenual cingulate cortex and thalamus. Biol Psychiatry 62: 429–437.
26. Liao W, Chen H, Feng Y, Mantini D, Gentili C, et al. (2010) Selective aberrant functional connectivity of resting state networks in social anxiety disorder. NeuroImage 52: 1549–1558.
27. Genovese CR, Lazar NA, Nichols T (2002) Thresholding of statistical maps in functional neuroimaging using the false discovery rate. Neuroimage 15: 870–878.
28. Damoiseaux JS, Beckmann CF, Arigita EJ, Barkhof F, Scheltens P, et al. (2008) Reduced resting-state brain activity in the "default network" in normal aging. Cereb Cortex 18: 1856–1864.
29. Wang Z, Lu G, Zhang Z, Zhong Y, Jiao Q, et al. (2011) Altered resting state networks in epileptic patients with generalized tonic-clonic seizures. Brain Res 1374: 134–141.

30. Whalley MG, Kroes MC, Huntley Z, Rugg MD, Davis SW, et al. (2013) An fMRI investigation of posttraumatic flashbacks. Brain Cogn 81: 151–159.

31. Brewin CR, Dalgleish T, Joseph S (1996) A dual representation theory of posttraumatic stress disorder. Psychol Rev 103: 670–686.

32. Rauschecker JP, Leaver AM, Muhlau M (2010) Tuning out the noise: limbic-auditory interactions in tinnitus. Neuron 66: 819–826.

33. Downar J, Crawley AP, Mikulis DJ, Davis KD (2002) A cortical network sensitive to stimulus salience in a neutral behavioral context across multiple sensory modalities. J Neurophysiol 87: 615–620.

34. Flatten G, Perlitz V, Pestinger M, Arin T, Kohl B, et al. (2004) Neural processing of traumatic events in subjects suffering PTSD-a case study of two surgical patients with severe accident trauma. GMS Psycho-social Medicine 1.

35. Lanius RA, Bluhm R, Lanius U, Pain C (2006) A review of neuroimaging studies in PTSD: heterogeneity of response to symptom provocation. J Psychiatr Res 40: 709–729.

36. Lanius RA, Williamson PC, Bluhm RL, Densmore M, Boksman K, et al. (2005) Functional connectivity of dissociative responses in posttraumatic stress disorder: a functional magnetic resonance imaging investigation. Biol Psychiatry 57: 873–884.

37. Lanius RA, Williamson PC, Boksman K, Densmore M, Gupta M, et al. (2002) Brain activation during script-driven imagery induced dissociative responses in PTSD: a functional magnetic resonance imaging investigation. Biological psychiatry 52: 305–311.

38. Bigler ED, Mortensen S, Neeley ES, Ozonoff S, Krasny L, et al. (2007) Superior temporal gyrus, language function, and autism. Dev Neuropsychol 31: 217–238.

39. Hopper JW, Frewen PA, van der Kolk BA, Lanius RA (2007) Neural correlates of reexperiencing, avoidance, and dissociation in PTSD: symptom dimensions and emotion dysregulation in responses to script-driven trauma imagery. J Trauma Stress 20: 713–725.

40. Adolphs R (2003) Cognitive neuroscience of human social behaviour. Nat Rev Neurosci 4: 165–178.

41. Biswal B, Yetkin FZ, Haughton VM, Hyde JS (1995) Functional connectivity in the motor cortex of resting human brain using echo-planar MRI. Magn Reson Med 34: 537–541.

42. Rioult-Pedotti MS, Friedman D, Hess G, Donoghue JP (1998) Strengthening of horizontal cortical connections following skill learning. Nat Neurosci 1: 230–234.

43. Butefisch CM, Davis BC, Wise SP, Sawaki L, Kopylev L, et al. (2000) Mechanisms of use-dependent plasticity in the human motor cortex. Proc Natl Acad Sci U S A 97: 3661–3665.

44. Ziemann U, Ilic TV, Pauli C, Meintzschel F, Ruge D (2004) Learning modifies subsequent induction of long-term potentiation-like and long-term depression-like plasticity in human motor cortex. J Neurosci 24: 1666–1672.

45. Seeley WW, Menon V, Schatzberg AF, Keller J, Glover GH, et al. (2007) Dissociable intrinsic connectivity networks for salience processing and executive control. J Neurosci 27: 2349–2356.

46. Bremner JD, Narayan M, Staib LH, Southwick SM, McGlashan T, et al. (1999) Neural correlates of memories of childhood sexual abuse in women with and without posttraumatic stress disorder. The American journal of psychiatry 156: 1787.

47. Cunnington R, Windischberger C, Moser E (2005) Premovement activity of the pre-supplementary motor area and the readiness for action: studies of time-resolved event-related functional MRI. Hum Mov Sci 24: 644–656.

48. Vythilingam M, Blair KS, McCaffrey D, Scaramozza M, Jones M, et al. (2007) Biased emotional attention in post-traumatic stress disorder: a help as well as a hindrance? Psychol Med 37: 1445–1455.

49. Lundstrom BN, Ingvar M, Petersson KM (2005) The role of precuneus and left inferior frontal cortex during source memory episodic retrieval. Neuroimage 27: 824–834.

50. Frings L, Wagner K, Quiske A, Schwarzwald R, Spreer J, et al. (2006) Precuneus is involved in allocentric spatial location encoding and recognition. Exp Brain Res 173: 661–672.

51. Lanius RA, Bluhm RL, Coupland NJ, Hegadoren KM, Rowe B, et al. (2010) Default mode network connectivity as a predictor of post-traumatic stress disorder symptom severity in acutely traumatized subjects. Acta Psychiatr Scand 121: 33–40.

52. Bluhm RL, Williamson PC, Osuch EA, Frewen PA, Stevens TK, et al. (2009) Alterations in default network connectivity in posttraumatic stress disorder related to early-life trauma. Journal of psychiatry & neuroscience: JPN 34: 187.

53. Molina ME, Isoardi R, Prado MN, Bentolila S (2010) Basal cerebral glucose distribution in long-term post-traumatic stress disorder. The World Journal of Biological Psychiatry 11: 493–501.

54. Fujii T, Suzuki M, Okuda J, Ohtake H, Tanji K, et al. (2004) Neural correlates of context memory with real-world events. Neuroimage 21: 1596–1603.

55. Sander D, Grandjean D, Pourtois G, Schwartz S, Seghier ML, et al. (2005) Emotion and attention interactions in social cognition: brain regions involved in processing anger prosody. Neuroimage 28: 848–858.

56. Gardini S, Cornoldi C, De Beni R, Venneri A (2006) Left mediotemporal structures mediate the retrieval of episodic autobiographical mental images. Neuroimage 30: 645–655.

57. Schmahmann JD, Caplan D (2006) Cognition, emotion and the cerebellum. Brain 129: 290–292.

58. Gusnard DA, Akbudak E, Shulman GL, Raichle ME (2001) Medial prefrontal cortex and self-referential mental activity: relation to a default mode of brain function. Proc Natl Acad Sci U S A 98: 4259–4264.

59. Rosenkranz JA, Grace AA (2002) Cellular mechanisms of infralimbic and prelimbic prefrontal cortical inhibition and dopaminergic modulation of basolateral amygdala neurons in vivo. The Journal of neuroscience 22: 324–337.

60. Northoff G, Heinzel A, de Greck M, Bermpohl F, Dobrowolny H, et al. (2006) Self-referential processing in our brain–a meta-analysis of imaging studies on the self. Neuroimage 31: 440–457.

61. Ochsner KN, Ray RD, Cooper JC, Robertson ER, Chopra S, et al. (2004) For better or for worse: neural systems supporting the cognitive down- and up-regulation of negative emotion. Neuroimage 23: 483–499.

62. Frewen PA, Lanius RA (2006) Toward a psychobiology of posttraumatic self-dysregulation: reexperiencing, hyperarousal, dissociation, and emotional numbing. Ann N Y Acad Sci 1071: 110–124.

63. Elzinga BM, Ardon AM, Heijnis MK, De Ruiter MB, Van Dyck R, et al. (2007) Neural correlates of enhanced working-memory performance in dissociative disorder: a functional MRI study. Psychol Med 37: 235–245.

64. Lui S, Huang X, Chen L, Tang H, Zhang T, et al. (2009) High-field MRI reveals an acute impact on brain function in survivors of the magnitude 8.0 earthquake in China. Proc Natl Acad Sci U S A 106: 15412–15417.

65. Lowe M, Mock B, Sorenson J (1998) Functional connectivity in single and multislice echoplanar imaging using resting-state fluctuations. Neuroimage 7: 119–132.

66. Birn RM, Diamond JB, Smith MA, Bandettini PA (2006) Separating respiratory-variation-related fluctuations from neuronal-activity-related fluctuations in fMRI. NeuroImage 31: 1536–1548.

9

Are All Beliefs Equal? Implicit Belief Attributions Recruiting Core Brain Regions of Theory of Mind

Ágnes Melinda Kovács[1]*[9], Simone Kühn[2][9], György Gergely[1], Gergely Csibra[1], Marcel Brass[3,4]

1 Cognitive Development Centre, Central European University, Budapest, Hungary, 2 Max Planck Institute for Human Development, Center for Lifespan Psychology, Berlin, Germany, 3 Department of Experimental Psychology and Ghent Institute of Functional and Metabolic Imaging, Ghent University, Ghent, Belgium, 4 Behavioural Science Institute, Radboud University, Nijmegen, The Netherlands

Abstract

Humans possess efficient mechanisms to behave adaptively in social contexts. They ascribe goals and beliefs to others and use these for behavioural predictions. Researchers argued for two separate mental attribution systems: an implicit and automatic one involved in online interactions, and an explicit one mainly used in offline deliberations. However, the underlying mechanisms of these systems and the types of beliefs represented in the implicit system are still unclear. Using neuroimaging methods, we show that the right temporo-parietal junction and the medial prefrontal cortex, brain regions consistently found to be involved in explicit mental state reasoning, are also recruited by spontaneous belief tracking. While the medial prefrontal cortex was more active when both the participant and another agent believed an object to be at a specific location, the right temporo-parietal junction was selectively activated during tracking the false beliefs of another agent about the presence, but not the absence of objects. While humans can explicitly attribute to a conspecific any possible belief they themselves can entertain, implicit belief tracking seems to be restricted to beliefs with specific contents, a content selectivity that may reflect a crucial functional characteristic and signature property of implicit belief attribution.

Editor: Sam Gilbert, University College London, United Kingdom

Funding: MB was supported by a grant of the Special Research Fund of Ghent University (BOF06/24JZAP). Further support came from the European Research Council under the European Union's Seventh Framework Programme (FP7/2007–2013)/ERC Advanced Investigator Grant to GC (249519-OSTREFCOM), by an ERC Starting Grant to AMK (284236-REPCOLLAB) and by a grant from the Hungarian Science Foundation (OTKA NK 83997) to GG. The funders had no role in study design, data collection and analysis, decision to publish, or preparation of the manuscript.

Competing Interests: The authors have declared that no competing interests exist.

* Email: kovacsag@ceu.hu

9 These authors contributed equally to this work.

Introduction

To successfully participate in social interactions, one must take into account that people are guided by mental states, such as desires and beliefs. Such "theory of mind" (ToM) abilities allow us to predict and interpret others' behavior based on attributed mental states. Remarkably, human adults can attribute to another person any possible mental state that they themselves can hold, ranging from a belief about the location of an object, to more complex ones that, for instance, a juror may have when inferring criminal intent. ToM sometimes involves explicit and verbally expressed reasoning about mental states, but it could also operate implicitly and automatically without much deliberation.

According to a recent proposal the implicit ToM system employs different representations than does the explicit system [1]. Such 'two-system' approaches assume that automatic ToM relies on cognitive processes that are distinct from those employed by explicit mechanisms that are manifested in judgments of veridicality of others' beliefs. In this view, only the latter can be considered proper ToM, while the implicit system is considered as a precursor. Alternatively, it was argued that implicit mental attributions reflect proper ToM, and their fast and efficient mechanisms may be crucial for real-life interactions from early on

[2–4]. However, while there is extensive behavioral and neuro-imaging research on explicit ToM, the functional properties and the underlying neural mechanisms of implicit ToM are less clear.

Neuroimaging research targeting explicit ToM reasoning has provided extensive evidence suggesting that a consistent set of brain regions is recruited when participants are required to reason about other people. This brain network (also termed social brain network or mentalizing network) includes the medial prefrontal cortex (MPFC), the bilateral temporo-parietal junction (TPJ), the superior temporal sulcus (STS), precuneus (PC) and the temporal poles [5–11]. In particular, two brain areas within the social brain network have been claimed to be crucial for ToM, namely the TPJ and MPFC. These brain areas are assumed to have well defined roles in reasoning about other people's mental states. Specifically, Frith & Frith [7] have argued that the MPFC is involved in decoupling mental states from physical state representations and according to Saxe [12] the right TPJ is selectively involved in reasoning about other's representational mental states.

However, most neuroimaging studies investigating ToM have employed paradigms following the standard false belief tasks, which require off-line deliberate reasoning and explicit and often verbal predictions based on mental states. A few investigations have used online or implicit tasks that elicited attributing goals to other agents, perspective taking or involved moral judgments, and reported the involvement of the social brain network in these tasks, such as the MPFC, or the TPJ, PC and STS regions [13–16]. Studies have also implemented methods where participants had an apparently unrelated task, but the situation could implicitly elicit thinking about other people. For instance, presentations of static natural scenes containing people while making simple category judgments (e.g., animal/vegetable) activated parts of the mentalizing network, specifically, the dorsomedial PFC and temporal poles [17]. Other studies, using online virtual reality tasks such as driving a taxi, found an increased activity in the right posterior STS, MPFC and right temporal pole for the events participants reported offline that they were engaged in thinking about other people [18]. Further investigations have addressed the question whether spontaneous trait inferences recruit the same brain networks as intentional inferences, revealing the involvement of the MPFC for both [19]. While most of these paradigms targeting implicit social cognition required attributing goals, traits or intentionality, rather than attributing representational mental states (i.e., beliefs) to other agents, in the present study we use a paradigm that directly taps on spontaneous computations concerning an agent's false beliefs.

In a recent behavioral study investigating automatic ToM mechanisms, Kovács et al. [4] found that adults spontaneously tracked an agent's belief about a location of an object, even when the agent and his beliefs were completely irrelevant for their task. The participants' task was to detect the presence of an object, and their own belief that the object was present at a target location facilitated their performance. Importantly, object detection was also speeded when an additional observer, based on the perceptual input that was accessible for him, could have entertained the belief that the object was present, even though participants later observed the object having left the scene.

Two aspects of these results deserve closer attention. First, facilitation occurred without the instruction to encode the observer's belief. This suggests that tracking the epistemic states of others, just like tracking others' behavior in joint action [20] may be automatic [21]. Second, the above study of Kovács et al. [4] found asymmetric effects: While the detection of the object was facilitated by the false belief of the other observer that the object was present, the observer's belief about the opposite state of affairs (i.e., that the ball was absent) did not interfere with object detection. Such an asymmetry might have been due to task demands, which required participants to respond only to the presence of the target, but not to its absence. However, it is also possible that this asymmetry is a functional characteristic of the implicit belief tracking system, which leads to preferential encoding of certain types of belief contents, while ignoring others in specific situations. The implicit ToM system may be specialized to track false beliefs about the presence, but not about the absence of objects.

In the current study we investigate implicit ToM by using functional MRI and a literature-based region of interest (ROI) approach. If automatic belief tracking recruits the same representational systems as explicit judgments, we expect that core brain regions previously reported to be active for explicit ToM tasks (i.e. MPFC and TPJ) to be also active in an implicit ToM task. Furthermore, by measuring brain activation during implicit belief tracking we can investigate whether the asymmetric sensitivity to false beliefs about the presence, but not the absence of objects reflects a genuine content-selectivity of the implicit system. We reasoned that if brain regions that are known to reflect belief attribution are active when an observer should think that an object is at a location (though it is not), and are not active when the observer should think that the object is not at a location (though it is), it would be evidence for the claim that automatic ToM tracks only specific kinds of beliefs (that is, beliefs with positive content, e.g., object at location, but not with negative content, e.g., object not at location).

Materials and Methods

We recorded BOLD signal while participants were lying in the MRI scanner watching short movies, in which the movements of an agent, an occluder, and a ball were arranged to give rise to various potential belief contents to the agent. Like in the original study by Kovács et al. [4], participants were not required to monitor the agent's beliefs. However, unlike in the original study, they had to respond to both the presence and the absence of the ball (eliminating the asymmetry of task demands).

Participants

Fifteen healthy students (6 male; age: mean = 21.6, ranging from 18 to 27) participated on the basis of written informed consent. The study was conducted according to the Declaration of Helsinki, with approval of the local ethics committee of the University Hospital Gent. All subjects had normal or corrected-to-normal vision. No subject had a history of neurological, major medical, or psychiatric disorder. All participants were right-handed as assessed by the Edinburgh handedness questionnaire (mean score = 92).

Design and stimuli

Participants were lying in the MRI scanner while watching short videos via a mirror. We have adapted the design and stimuli from Experiment 1 of Kovács et al. [4] with the modifications described below. We have used the same movies, except that they were 25% faster in this study, and we introduced a variable jitter between the two phases. All movies consisted of two phases: the belief formation phase and the outcome phase. Since we were specifically interested in the neural correlates of implicit belief formation, we introduced a variable jitter interval of 2, 3.5, 5, 6.5, 8, or 9.5 seconds between the two phases.

The movies in the belief formation phase differed along two aspects of the belief attributable to the agent: Content (Positive: ball present vs. Negative: ball absent) and Veridicality (True: matching reality vs. False: mismatching reality). Combined with the two versions of the outcome phase (ball does or does not appear from behind the occluder), there were 8 different trials, 6 jitter intervals, and movies were repeated twice during the study in a random order resulting in a total of 96 experimental trials. In addition, we inserted 12 null events consisting of a blank screen presented for the entire trial length.

Belief formation phase. As shown in Figure 1, all movies started with an agent placing a ball on a table in front of an occluder. Then the ball rolled behind the occluder. Following this, the movies could continue in four ways depending on the experimental conditions:

1. In the True Belief-Positive Content condition, the ball rolled out of the scene from behind the occluder, and then rolled back behind the occluder (ball last seen by the participant at 10 s; time information is given relative to the beginning of the movie) in the agent's presence. The agent left the scene at 11 s. Thus, the agent could rightly believe the ball to be behind the occluder.

2. In the True Belief-Negative Content condition, the ball emerged from behind the occluder without leaving the scene,

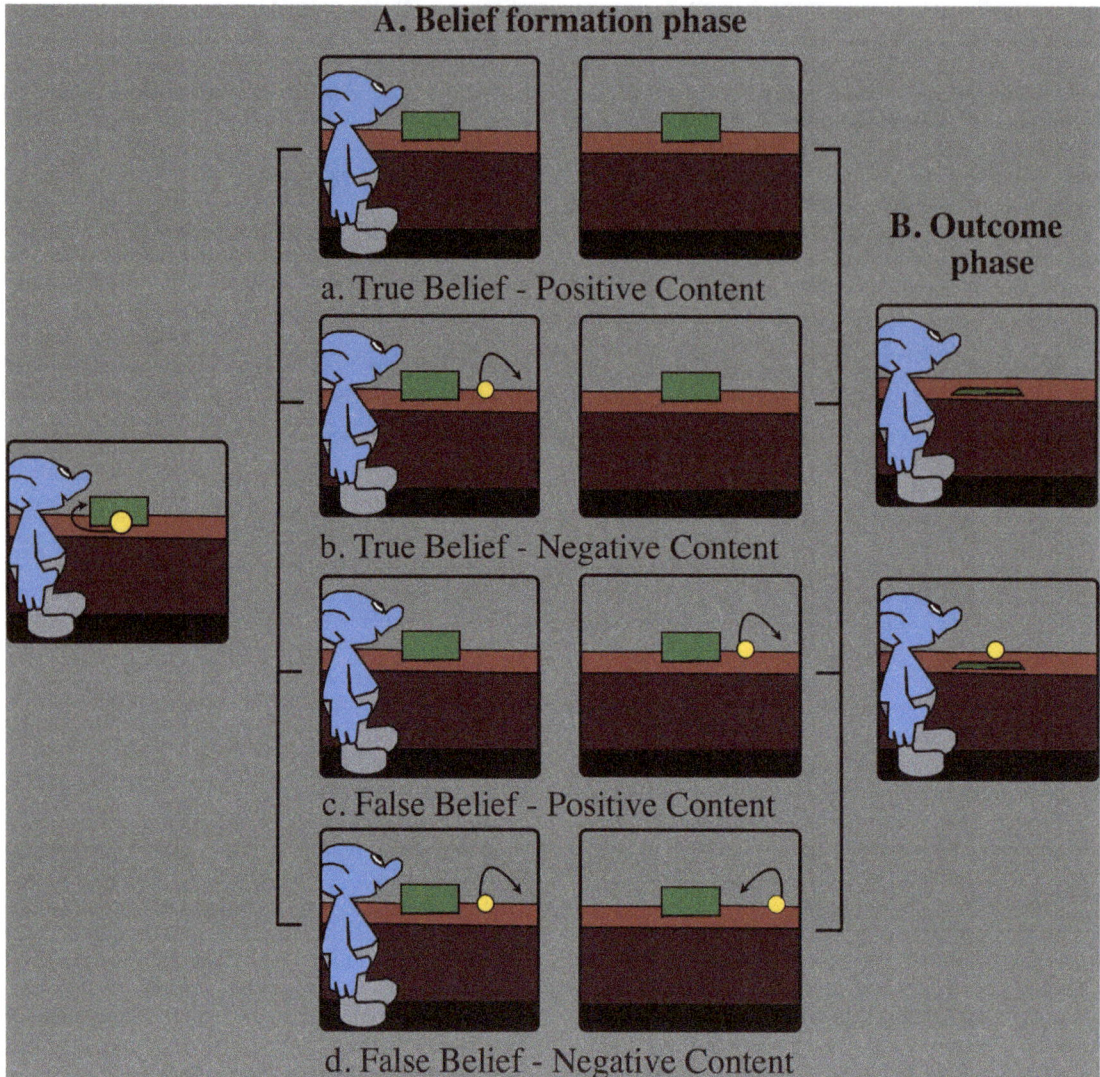

Figure 1. The logical structure of events in the experimental conditions. In the figure only the critical events are depicted, specifically, the final location of the ball and whether the agent was present or not when the event leading the outcome occurred (for the exact events and the timing see Methods).

then rolled back behind the occluder, and finally left the scene (ball last seen at 10 s), all in the agent's presence. The agent left the scene at 11 s. Thus, the agent could rightly believe the ball not to be behind the occluder.

3. In False Belief -Positive Content condition, we reversed the order of when the ball and the agent left the scene, respectively, relative to the True Belief –Negative Content condition. Thus, the agent left the scene at 6 s. Then, the ball emerged from behind the occluder without leaving the scene, rolled back behind the occluder, and finally left the scene (ball last seen at 11 s), all in the agent's absence. Thus, the agent could wrongly believe the ball to be behind the occluder.

4. In the False Belief-Negative Content condition, the ball rolled out of the scene from behind the occluder in the agent's presence. Then, the agent left the scene at 9 s. In his absence, the ball rolled back behind the occluder at 11 s. Thus, the agent could wrongly believe the ball not to be behind the occluder.

Outcome phase. At the end of each movie, the agent re-entered the scene and the occluder was lowered. The four conditions were paired with two outcomes, in which the ball was either present or absent behind the occluder. Participants were instructed to press one key when they detected the ball, and another key when they detected that the ball was not there (see Supporting Information, Additional analysis S1). Unlike in the Kovács et al. study [4], participants did not press a button when the agent left the scene, as we aimed to measure BOLD signal in the belief formation phase without possible movement artifacts. It is important to note that the required two alternative choice response (ball present/ball absent) in the outcome phase differed from that of Kovács et al. [4], where a detection (go-nogo) task was used rather than a choice response task. We changed the response in order to equate manual responses for ball presence and absence, and to make each outcome equally relevant. The ball was present in 50% of the trials in all conditions. Importantly, the agent's beliefs were never mentioned and were irrelevant to the task. As we were interested in belief attribution processes, we restricted our analyses to the four conditions defined by the belief formation phase, independently of the outcome.

MRI-Scanning Procedure

Images were collected with a 3T Magnetom Trio MRI scanner system (Siemens Medical Systems, Erlangen, Germany) using an 8-channel radiofrequency head coil. First, high-resolution anatomical images were acquired using a T1-weighted 3D MPRAGE sequence (TR = 2530 ms, TE = 2.58 ms, TI = 1100 ms, acquisition matrix = 256×256×176, sagittal FOV = 220 mm, flip angle = 7°, voxel size = 0.86×0.86×0.9 mm^3). Whole brain functional images were collected using a T2*-weighted EPI sequence sensitive to BOLD contrast (TR = 2000 ms, TE = 35 ms, image matrix = 64×64, FOV = 224 mm, flip angle = 80°, slice thickness = 3.0 mm, distance factor = 17%, voxel size 3.5×3.5×3 mm^3, 30 axial slices). Volumes aligned to AC-PC.

FMRI analysis

The fMRI data were analysed with statistical parametric mapping using SPM5 software (Wellcome Department of Cognitive Neurology, London, UK). The first 4 volumes of all EPI series were excluded from the analysis to allow the magnetisation to approach a dynamic equilibrium. Data processing started with slice time correction and realignment of the EPI datasets. A mean image for all EPI volumes was created, to which individual volumes were spatially realigned by rigid body transformations. The high-resolution structural image was co-registered with the mean image of the EPI series. Then the structural image was normalised to the Montreal Neurological Institute (MNI) template, and the normalisation parameters were applied to the EPI images to ensure an anatomically informed normalisation. During normalisation the anatomy image volumes were resampled to 1×1×1 mm^3. A filter of 8 mm FWHM (full-width at half maximum) was used. Low-frequency drifts in the time domain were removed by modelling the time series for each voxel by a set of discrete cosine functions to which a cut-off of 128 s was applied.

The subject-level statistical analyses were performed using the general linear model (GLM). The model contained separate regressors for all possible combinations of Veridicality (True vs. False), Content (Positive vs. Negative), phase (belief vs. outcome) and actual presence of the ball (present/absent) (duration of 0 seconds) resulting in 16 regressors in total. The percent signal change was extracted for the whole duration of the events of interest. Movement parameters were included to account for variance associated with head motion. All resulting vectors were convolved with the canonical haemodynamic response function (HRF) and its temporal derivative to form the main regressors in the design matrix (the regression model). The statistical parameter estimates were computed separately for each voxel for all columns in the design matrix.

The coordinates reported correspond to the MNI coordinate system.

Literature based ROIs in TPJ and MPFC. In order to obtain a ROI of TPJ and MPFC we conducted an activation-likelihood estimation (ALE) [22] meta-analysis on 26 studies on mentalizing that reported 31 peaks of activation in the proximity of TPJ and 31 in MPFC [23]. We used a threshold of FDR $p <$ 0.01 and a cluster size above 200 mm^3. The cluster identified in TPJ was centred around the coordinate 56–47 33 (cluster size: 4448 mm^3) and we used the mirrored ROI for the localization of left TPJ whereas the literature-based MPFC ROI was located at 2 53 13 (cluster size: 3368 mm^3). Separately for each subject, each literature-based ROI, and each condition, the mean percent signal change over a time window of 4–13 s after stimulus onset was

extracted (http://marsbar.sourceforge.net/) [24] and used for further analysis.

Results

We carried out signal-change analyses in the a-priori defined ROIs based on a meta-analysis of peaks reported in 26 studies on mentalizing. In right TPJ we found a main effect of belief (F(1,14) = 6.34, p = .025). Participants showed higher activation values for false than for true beliefs. Furthermore, there was a statistical trend for a main effect of content (F(1,14) = 4.37, p = .055). Importantly, a significant interaction effect of belief and content was found (F(1,14) = 5.35, p = .036) (Fig. 2A). Post-hoc t-tests revealed significant differences between the False Belief, Positive Content condition and all other conditions (True Belief, Negative Content: t(14) = −3.65, p<0.01; True Belief, Positive Content: t(14) = −2.64, p<0.05; False Belief, Negative Content: t(14) = −3.0, p<0.01).

In the left TPJ we did not observe any significant activation differences (Belief: F(1,14) = 0.22, p = .645, Content: F(1,14) = .784, p = .391, Belief*Content: F(1,14) = 1.09, p = .313). Furthermore, the signal-change analyses in the literature based MPFC ROI did not reveal any significant main effects (Belief: F(1,14) = 2.20, p = .160, Content: F(1,14) = 3.30, p = .091). Interestingly, however, it also showed a significant interaction of belief and content (Belief*Content: F(1,14) = 4.79, p = .046) (Fig. 2B). Post-hoc t-tests revealed significant differences between True Belief, Positive Content and True Belief, Negative Content (t(14) = −2.0, p<0.01) as well as False Belief, Positive Content (t(14) = −2.58, p<0.05), the difference to False Belief, Negative Content only revealed a tendency (t(14) = −1.98, p = 0.068).

Discussion

The aim of the current study was to investigate two questions regarding the mechanisms and the underlying neural substrates of implicit belief tracking. One question was related to the neural mechanism of implicit ToM, and the other concerned the potential content selectivity of the implicit system. Regarding the first question, we found that implicit belief tracking, similarly to what is repeatedly found in studies targeting explicit ToM reasoning, recruits right TPJ and MPFC regions.

The finding that the right TPJ is only active when a false belief attributed to another person has a positive content reveals a crucial functional characteristic of the automatic belief tracking system, more specifically, a genuine content selectivity. This implies that spontaneous belief tracking may be initiated only for certain types of belief contents. When this content is about the occurrence of an object at a certain location, a positive content is attributed, while potential beliefs with negative content are ignored. One possible explanation for such pattern could be that this system may represent only false beliefs about the presence of an object (e.g., 'he believes the ball is there') because only these yield definite transitive action predictions related to the represented object, while false beliefs about the absence of an object (e.g., 'he believes the ball is not there') do not allow such predictions. Although we are certainly able to explicitly attribute to others any possible belief that we ourselves can entertain, including beliefs about the absence of objects (negative content), we conjecture that these might pose representational demands that the implicit system is not prepared to tackle.

Alternatively, such a limitation of the spontaneous belief tracking system may stem from the conflicting relation between the content of one's own reality representation and that of an attributed belief. According to this possibility, one would

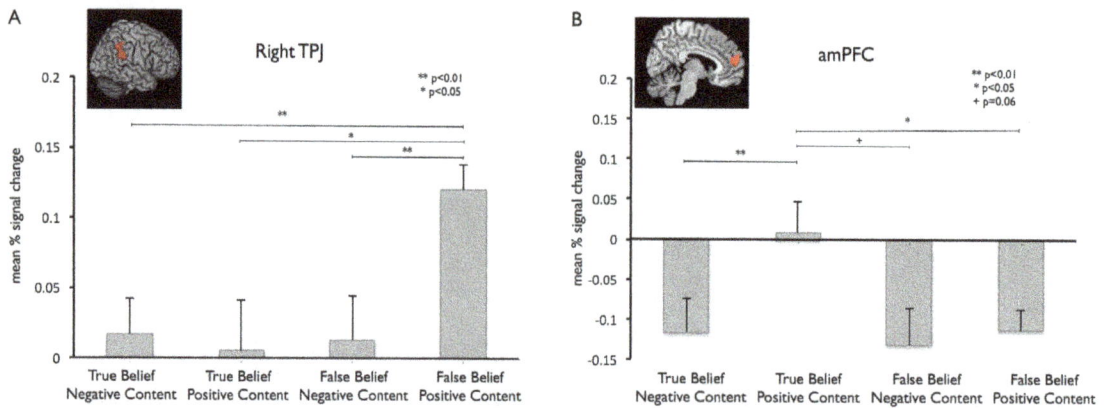

Figure 2. ROI mean percent signal change analysis for the right TPJ (A) and the amPFC (B).

spontaneously track someone else's belief only when one does not have a strong competing own belief. Thus, in our case one would compute the belief of the agent in the condition where one believes nothing to be present behind the occluder, but not when one believes the ball to be behind the occluder. While it is difficult to separate the two alternatives with the current design, data from other studies with infants and adults seem to support the interpretation that the limitation may be related to the negative belief content. Indeed, both infants and adults seem to spontaneously track others' beliefs and perspective even if these are strongly competing with their own representations [25,10].

On the other hand, the MPFC was more active in the condition where both the participant and the agent believed that the ball was behind the occluder (true belief with a positive content). Recent studies have found that the MPFC is recruited in situations where an actor searches in a location where an object is present compared to an empty location [26]. While there was no explicit object search induced in the present task, we have also found a higher activation pattern in the condition where both the participant and the agent believed that the object was behind the occluder, thus allowing for a possible search. Furthermore, this higher MPFC activation pattern in the true belief- object present condition is also in line with proposals suggesting that the MPFC is involved in reasoning about triadic relations between Me, You and an object [12], but might not be selectively recruited for attributing representational mental states [27,28]. Indeed, in the present study, using an implicit belief attribution task that is analogous to earlier used explicit ToM task, we found an activation of the MPFC in the true belief - object present condition, but not in the false belief conditions. Earlier studies have found that the MPFC is involved in representing various characteristics of other agents besides their beliefs, such as their appearance and emotions [27,28] or a viewpoint-independent perspective selection [15].

While in the last years there seems to be more consensus on the selective role of the right TPJ in processing mental states with representational content [12,27,29], researchers have also proposed that right TPJ activity may not be selective for social cognition, as both ToM and attentional reorienting tasks were found recruit this area [30]. Additionally, research has shown that the TPJ and the MPFC are also associated with self-other distinction [23]. Our finding that implicit ToM seems to recruit the right TPJ is consistent with what is usually found using explicit ToM tasks, although the left TPJ might also play a role in ToM reasoning, as lesion studies have reported that damage to left TPJ is associated to deficits on explicit ToM tasks [31–33].

One might wonder whether the implicit vs. explicit distinction is warranted in ToM research, as it is unclear whether it refers to the nature of the task or to the underlying cognitive processes, and we concur with such worries. After all, one could argue that even in our study participants could have spontaneously engaged in explicit, besides implicit, mentalizing, even if they were not instructed to do so. However, if our participants recruited similar computations as the participants in the Kovács et al. [4] study, where equivalent belief tracking effects were found in adults and infants, than given that young infants are thought to lack an explicit belief tracking system, one could argue that our participants most likely have relied on their implicit ToM system as well. Additionally, according to standard views, explicit ToM, in contrast to implicit ToM, should be effortful, highly dependent on cognitive resources and occur offline [1]. However, since we measured the BOLD signal online as the belief scenario unfolded, we find it unlikely that participants could have engaged in explicit and effortful ToM processes. While we did not systematically debrief the participants in the present study, in the earlier Kovács et al. study participants reported that they had believed the agent to be irrelevant or that it was a mere distractor [4] (Supplementary Material, Additional analysis S1, p. 5).

Furthermore, regarding the issue of automaticity in mental state reasoning, earlier studies have found a modulation of the dorsomedial prefrontal cortex by cognitive load when participants were instructed to think of the reasons why a character might perform specific actions [34]. In a framework where automaticity is not seen a unitary construct but instead as comprising a set of relatively independent dimensions, such as efficiency, awareness, intention, and control [35], our study seems to speak mostly to the intention and awareness dimensions, as participants were not instructed to intentionally track the agent's beliefs (and were likely not aware of doing so).

In summary, our findings suggest that the mechanisms underlying the automatic tracking of others' beliefs exploit partly similar representational systems as explicit ToM judgments do. Furthermore, we have found evidence for a content-dependent representational constraint on implicit ToM, which restricts the system to tracking false beliefs that may allow fast and efficient predictions about others' actions. Such a content-selectivity favoring potential behaviorally relevant beliefs may represent the signature limit of the implicit ToM system and may signal a functional difference between implicit and explicit ToM attributions.

Supporting Information

Additional analysis S1

Author Contributions

Conceived and designed the experiments: AMK SK GG GC MB. Performed the experiments: SK. Analyzed the data: SK. Contributed to the writing of the manuscript: AMK SK GG GC MB.

References

1. Apperly IA, Butterfill SA (2009) Do humans have two systems to track beliefs and belief-like states? Psychological Review 116: 953–70.
2. Fodor JA (1992) A theory of the child's theory of mind. Cognition 44: 283–296.
3. Friedman O, Leslie AM (2004) Mechanisms of belief-desire reasoning: inhibition and bias. Psychological Science 15: 547–552.
4. Kovács ÁM, Téglás E, Endress AD (2010) The social sense: susceptibly to others' beliefs in human infants and adults. Science 330: 1830–1834.
5. Gallagher HL, Happe F, Brunswick N, Fletcher PC, Frith U, et al. (2000) Reading the mind in cartoons and stories: An fmri study of 'theory of mind' in verbal and nonverbal tasks. Neuropsychologia 38: 11–21.
6. Fletcher PC, Happe F, Frith U, Baker SC, Dolan RJ, et al. (1995) Other minds in the brain: A functional imaging study of "theory of mind" in story comprehension. Cognition 57: 109–128.
7. Frith U, Frith CD (2003) Development and neurophysiology of mentalizing. Philos. Trans. R. Soc. Lond. B Biol. Sci. 358: 459–473.
8. Frith CD, Frith U (2006) The neural basis of mentalizing. Neuron 50: 531–4.
9. Ruby P, Decety J (2001) Effect of subjective perspective taking during simulation of action: a PET investigation of agency. Nat Neurosci 4: 546–550.
10. Saxe R, Kanwisher N (2003) People thinking about thinking people. The role of the temporo-parietal junction in "theory of mind". Neuroimage 19: 1835–1842.
11. Vogeley K, Bussfeld P, Newen A, Herrmann S, Happé F, et al. (2001) Mind reading: Neural mechanisms of theory of mind and self-perspective. NeuroImage 14: 170–181.
12. Saxe R (2006) Uniquely human social cognition. Curr Opin Neurobiol 16: 235–239.
13. Castelli F, Frith C, Happe F, Frith U (2002) Autism, Asperger syndrome and brain mechanisms for the attribution of mental states to animated shapes. Brain 125: 1839–1849.
14. Schilbach L, Wohlschlager AM, Newen A, Kramer N, Shah NJ, et al. (2006) Being with virtual others: neural correlates of social interaction. Neuropsychologia 44: 718–730. (doi:10.1016/j.neuropsychologia.2005.07.017)
15. Ramsey R, Hansen P, Apperly I, Samson D (2013) Seeing it my way or your way: frontoparietal brain areas sustain viewpoint-independent perspective selection processes. Journal of Cognitive Neuroscience 25: 670–684.
16. Young L, Saxe R (2009) An fMRI Investigation of Spontaneous Mental State Inference for Moral Judgment. Journal of Cognitive Neuroscience 21: 1396–1405.
17. Wagner DD, Kelley WM, Heatherton TF (2011) Individual Differences in the Spontaneous Recruitment of Brain Regions Supporting Mental State Understanding When Viewing Natural Social Scenes. Cerebral Cortex 21: 2788–2796.
18. Spiers HJ, Maguire EA (2006) Spontaneous mentalizing during an interactive real world task: An fMRI study. Neuropsychologia 44: 1674–1682.
19. Ma N, Vandekerckhove M, Baetens K, Van Overwalle F, Seurinck R, et al. (2012) Inconsistencies in spontaneous and intentional trait inferences. Social Cognitive and Affective Neuroscience 7: 937–950.
20. Sebanz N, Knoblich G, Prinz W (2005) How two share a task: Corepresenting stimulus–response mappings. J Exp Psychol Hum 31: 1234–1246.
21. Samson D, Apperly IA, Braithwaite J, Andrews B (2010) Seeing it their way: Evidence for rapid and involuntary computation of what other people see. J Exp Psychol Hum 36: 1255–1266.
22. Eickhoff SB, et al. (2009) Coordinate-based activation likelihood estimation meta-analysis of neuroimaging data: A random effects approach based on empirical estimates of spatial uncertainty. Hum Brain Mapp 30: 2907–2926.
23. Brass M, Ruby P, Spengler S (2009) Inhibition of imitative behaviour and social cognition. Philos Trans R So. Lond B 364: 2359–2367.
24. Brett M, Anton JC, Valabregue R, Poline JB (2002) Region of interest analysis using an SPM toolbox. 8th International Conference on Functional Mapping of the Human Brain, June 2–6.
25. Onishi KH, Baillargeon R (2005) Do 15-month-old infants understand false beliefs? Science 308: 255–258.
26. Ramsey R, Hamilton AF de C (2012) How does your own knowledge influence the perception of other people's actions in the human brain? Social Cognitive and Affective Neuroscience 7: 242–251.
27. Saxe R, Powell LJ (2006) It's the thought that counts: specific brain regions for one component of theory of mind. Psychological Science 17: 692–699.
28. Saxe R, Wexler A (2005) Making sense of another mind: the role of the right temporo-parietal junction. Neuropsychologia 43: 1391–1399.
29. Aichhorn M, Perner J, Weiss B, Kronbichler M, Staffen W, et al. (2008) Temporo-parietal junction activity in Theory-of-Mind tasks: Falseness, beliefs, or attention. J Cognit Neurosci 21: 1179–1192.
30. Mitchell JP (2008) Activity in right temporo-parietal junction is not selective for theory-of-mind. Cerebral Cortex 18: 262–271.
31. Apperly IA, Samson D, Chiavarino C, Humphreys GW (2004) Frontal and temporo-parietal lobe contributions to theory of mind: neuropsychological evidence from a false-belief task with reduced language and executive demands. J Cogn Neurosci 16: 1773–1784.
32. Apperly IA, Samson D, Chiavarino C, Bickerton WL, Humphreys GW (2006) Testing the domain-specificity of a theory of mind deficit in brain-injured patients: evidence for consistent performance on nonverbal, "reality-unknown" false belief and false photograph tasks. Cognition 103: 300–321.
33. Samson D, Apperly IA, Chiavarino C, Humphreys GW (2004) Left temporoparietal junction is necessary for representing someone else's belief. Nat Neurosci 7: 499–500.
34. Spunt RP, Lieberman MD (2013) The Busy Social Brain: Evidence for Automaticity and Control in the Neural Systems Supporting Social Cognition and Action Understanding. Psychological Science 24: 80–86.
35. Bargh JA (1994) The four horsemen of automaticity: Awareness, intention, efficiency, and control in social cognition. In R. Wyer & T. Srull (Eds.), Handbook of social cognition (1–40). Hillsdale, NJ: Lawrence Erlbaum.

10

Autapse-Induced Spiral Wave in Network of Neurons under Noise

Huixin Qin[1], Jun Ma[1]*, Chunni Wang[1], Ying Wu[2]

1 Department of Physics, Lanzhou University of Technology, Lanzhou, China, **2** School of Aerospace, Xian Jiaotong University, Xian, China

Abstract

Autapse plays an important role in regulating the electric activity of neuron by feedbacking time-delayed current on the membrane of neuron. Autapses are considered in a local area of regular network of neurons to investigate the development of spatiotemporal pattern, and emergence of spiral wave is observed while it fails to grow up and occupy the network completely. It is found that spiral wave can be induced to occupy more area in the network under optimized noise on the network with periodical or no-flux boundary condition being used. The developed spiral wave with self-sustained property can regulate the collective behaviors of neurons as a pacemaker. To detect the collective behaviors, a statistical factor of synchronization is calculated to investigate the emergence of ordered state in the network. The network keeps ordered state when self-sustained spiral wave is formed under noise and autapse in local area of network, and it independent of the selection of periodical or no-flux boundary condition. The developed stable spiral wave could be helpful for memory due to the distinct self-sustained property.

Editor: Changsong Zhou, Hong Kong Baptist University, Hong Kong

Funding: This work is partially supported by the National Nature Science Foundation of China under the Grant No. 11265008, and is partially supported by the National Nature Science Foundation of China under the Grant No. 11372122, and it is also partially supported by the National Nature Science Foundation of China under the Grant No. 11365014. The funders had no role in study design, data collection and analysis, decision to publish, or preparation of the manuscript.

Competing Interests: The authors have declared that no competing interests exist.

* Email: hyperchaos@163.com

Introduction

Neuronal system consists of a large number of neurons, and the collective electric activities of neurons can emerge complex spatiotemporal patterns during the process of signals. It is believed that signals communication can be realized by synapse coupling, and the distribution of spatiotemporal pattern can present some useful clues to understand the information propagation between neurons [1−8]. In this way, some researchers show great interests in detecting the formation and transition of patterns in network of neurons [9−19]. It was reported that spiral wave can be found in the cortex of brain [20−22], and then some theoretical investigations [23,24] have been presented to explore the potential formation mechanism of spiral wave and multi-armed spiral wave in the network of neurons, indeed, these results [24] have confirmed that intermediate channels blocking in neurons in a local area of neuronal network can induce emergence of spiral wave, and the stability of multiarmed spiral wave was also discussed. It was also confirmed that artificial defects [25] can block travelling wave to induce perfect spiral wave under appropriate coupling intensity between neurons, and breakup of spiral wave occurs with strong noise or channel noise [26,27] being used.

Chemical and electric synapses bridge the neurons during signal transmission and the mutual connections can dominate the collective behaviors of neurons or oscillators. That is to say, an unusual kind of synapse is a specialized connection between neurons or between a neuron and a muscle, which is used for transmitting electrical signals. While an autapse is a self-synapse, which exists a connection between a neuron and itself [28−30].

Herrmann et al. [31] presented an experimental study to detect the functional significance that autapses offer for neural behavior, and they simulated a neural basket cell via the Hodgkin-Huxley equations and implemented an autapse which feeds back onto the soma of the neuron, interestingly, their results confirmed that neuron can become active due to the effect of autapse. Then the biophysical modeling for autapse [32] is achieved in terms of a stochastic Hodgkin-Huxley model containing such a built in delayed feedback, and the dynamics of electric activity of neurons was discussed. As a result, it is reasonable to model the effect of autapse on neuron by imposing a feedback term with time delay and feedback gain. In the case of dynamics of neuron and networks, the effect of autapse is often left out though time delay between neurons is considered in signal transmission [33,34]. As is well known, a negative feedback is often helpful to stabilize the system while a positive feedback can enhance the oscillating of the system. For example, Ao et al. [35] numerically investigated the influence of intrinsic channel noise on the dynamical response of delay-coupling in neuronal systems. Wang et al. [36] discussed the dynamics of electrical activity and the transition of firing patterns induced by three types of autapses in Hindmarsh-Rose neuron. Indeed, Refs. [37,38] gave a brief discussion about the potential biological function of autapse in neuron. The author of this paper ever investigated the effect of autapse on Hindmarsh-Rose neuron, and it was found that appropriate electric autapse can wake up quiescent neurons in ring network [39]. However, the effect of autapses on collective electric behaviors of neurons keeps open in the two-dimensional arrar network. In the case of ring network, stable and continuous pulses can regulate the collective behaviors of neurons? Is there any new 'pacemaker' in a two-dimensional array network induced by the distribution of electric autapses thus the collective behaviors of neurons can be regulated? If possible, how many neurons can be regulated by a target wave or spiral wave in the two-dimensional array network with electric autapses being considered? What is the difference if noise is also considered? It was confirmed that optimized noise on network can be active to develop a spiral wave [40] due to coherence resonance [41,42]. More often, target wave can also be induced in the media due to heterogeneity [43] and the emitting wave can be used to suppress the spiral wave and turbulence of the media [44], for example, the tip dynamics of spiral wave is changed by the fractal heterogeneity [43], and the heterogeneity by a rotating electric field [45] can emit ordered wave to regulate the behavior of excitable media.

Noise plays important role in regulating electric activities of neurons though breakup of spiral wave could be induced by noise beyond certain intensity. In this paper, a regular network of Hindmarsh-Rose neuron is designed in a two-dimensional array, some autapses are introduced into the neurons in a local area and noise is also considered on the whole network. A statistical function is defined to detect the transition of spiral wave under noise and autapses in a local area of the network. Breakup and development of spiral wave in the network induced by few autapses, and the effect of noise will be investigated, respectively. To discern the effect of boundary condition, no-flux boundary and periodical boundary condition is considered, respectively.

Model and Scheme

Hindmarsh-Rose(HR) neuron model is regarded as a simplified neuron model to describe the main properties of electric activities in neurons. A two-dimensional network of HR neurons with regular [46,47] or small-world connection type [48] can be used to study the pattern formation and selection of neurons. Then the network dynamics of HR neurons with autapses in local area under noise is described by

$$\begin{cases} \frac{dx_{ij}}{dt} = y_{ij} - ax_{ij}^3 + bx_{ij}^2 - z_{ij} + I_{ext} + \\ \quad I_{aut}\delta_{i\alpha}\delta_{j\beta} + \xi(t) + D(x_{i+1j} + \\ \quad x_{i-1j} + x_{ij+1} + x_{ij-1} - 4x_{ij}) \\ \frac{dy_{ij}}{dt} = c - dx_{ij}^2 - y_{ij} \\ \frac{dz_{ij}}{dt} = r[s(x_{ij} - x_0) - z_{ij}] \end{cases} \quad (1)$$

$$I_{aut} = g(x_{ij}(t-\tau) - x_{ij}(t)) \quad (2)$$

where x_{ij} represents the membrane potential of neuron in node (i, j), y_{ij}, z_{ij} denotes the recovery variable and slow adaption current in node (i, j), respectively. D is the intensity of coupling between adjacent neurons, I_{ext} is the external forcing current on each neuron. I_{aut} is the forcing current generated from a electric autapse, g, τ is the gain and time delay, respectively. Autapse current $I_{aut} \neq 0$ in a local area, and α, β are integers, for example, $\alpha = 100, 101, 102, \beta = 100, 101, 102$, it means that autapses are imposed on the neurons in a local area (3×3 nodes) as $100 \leq i, j \leq 102$, thus autapse currents are considered in these neurons. $\xi(t)$ is Gaussian white noise on each node, the statistical relation is described by $<\xi(t)> = 0, <\xi(t)\xi(t')> = 2D_0\delta(t-t')$, D_0 is the noise intensity. For a single neuron without autapse effect being considered, it can emerge chaotic state at $a = 1.0, b = 3.0, c = 1.0, d = 5.0, s = 4.0, r = 0.006, x_0 = -1.56$ by increasing the forcing current I_{ext} beyond certain threshold [46]. According to Eq. (2), negative feedback on membrane potential occurs for positive g values thus the neuron tends to be stable. While positive feedback on membrane potential emerges for negative g values so that the neuron can become active. In this paper, negative values will be selected for gain g to detect the development of spiral wave in the network induced by noise and a fraction of electric autapses in a local area of the network.

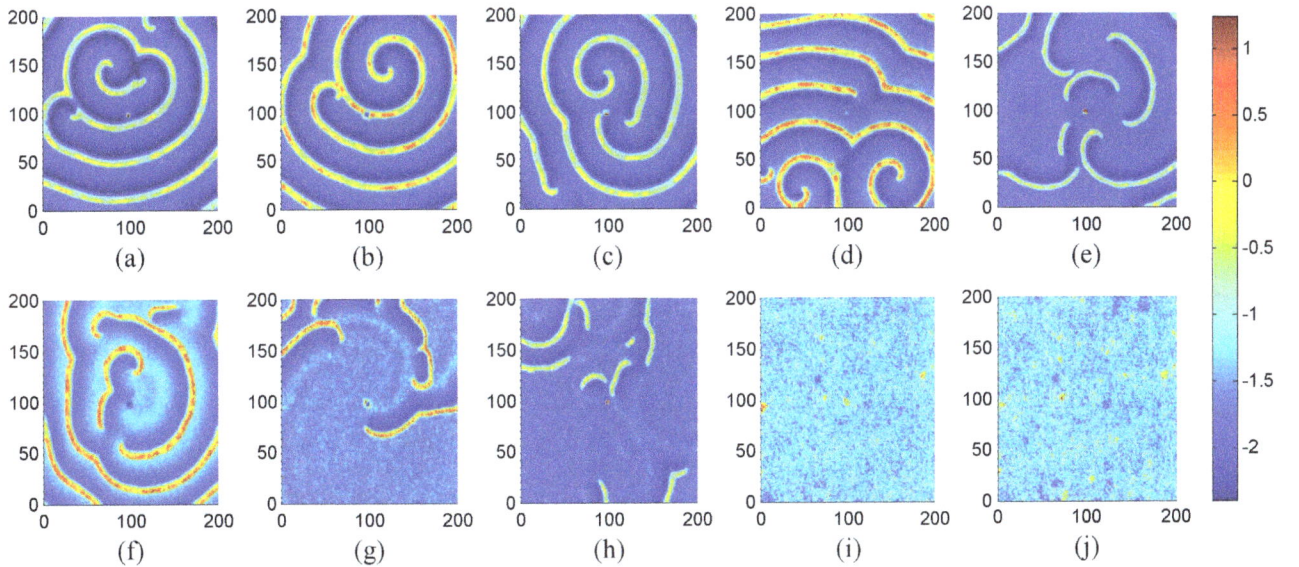

Figure 1. The developed states at $t = 16000$ time units in the network of neurons under different intensities of noise. For noise intensity (a) $D_0 = 0.005$, (b) $D_0 = 0.01$, (c) $D_0 = 0.02$, (d) $D_0 = 0.03$, (e) $D_0 = 0.04$, (f) $D_0 = 0.05$, (g) $D_0 = 0.08$, (h) $D_0 = 0.1$, (i) $D_0 = 0.5$, (j) $D_0 = 0.8$. Where $g = -1.5, \tau = 30, I_{ext} = 1.0, D = 1.0$ and no-flux boundary condition is used.

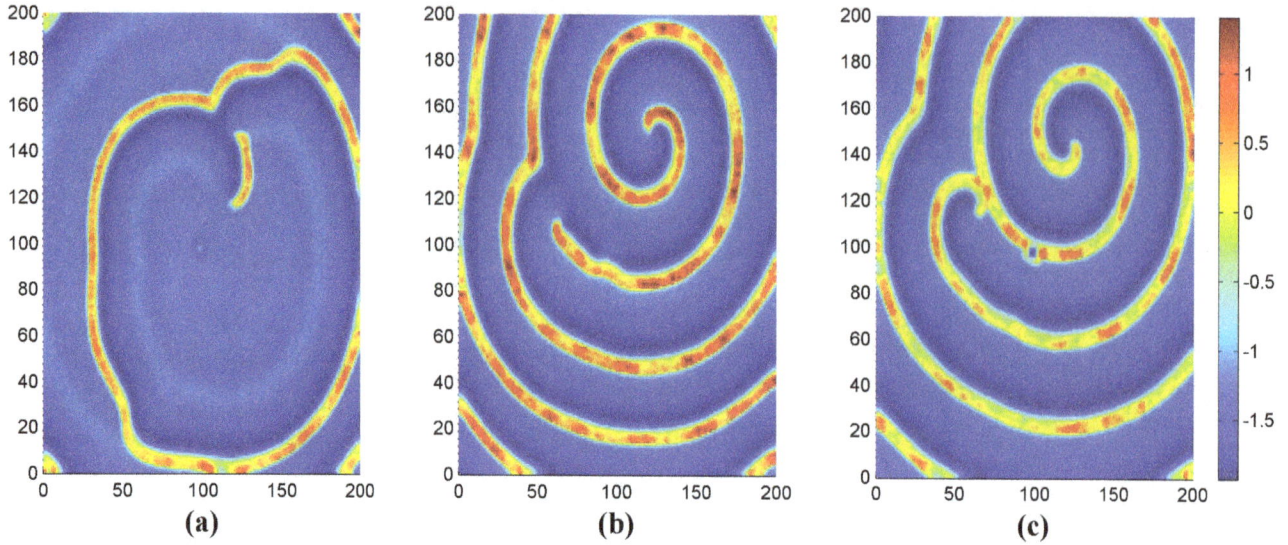

Figure 2. The development of spiral wave in the network. For (a) $t = 2000$, (b) $t = 4000$, (c) $t = 16000$ time units. Where $g = -1.5$, $\tau = 30$, $I_{ext} = 1.0$, $D = 1.0$, $D_0 = 0.01$ and no-flux boundary condition is used.

It is necessary to give some clarifications before further investigation in the following sections. For a single HR neuron without autapse, it is found that the neuron begins to emerge spiking at $I_{ext} > 1.1$, then bursting at $I_{ext} > 1.8$. To cares about the autapse effect, the external forcing current is selected as $I_{ext} = 1.0$ for a quiescent state without autapse. To detect the transition of collective behaviors of neurons in the network, a statistical factor of synchronization in a two-dimensional space is defined according to mean filed theory, and the factor of synchronization R is described by [18,27,47].

$$R = \frac{\langle F^2 \rangle - \langle F \rangle^2}{\frac{1}{N^2} \sum_{j=1}^{N} \sum_{i=1}^{N} \left(\langle V_{ij}^2 \rangle - \langle V_{ij} \rangle^2 \right)}, \quad F = \frac{1}{N^2} \sum_{j=1}^{N} \sum_{i=1}^{N} V_{ij}, \quad (3)$$

Where N^2 is the total number of neurons of the network, the symbol $\langle * \rangle$ represents an average over time, the V_{ij} is the observable variable in node (i, j) and it is replaced by the membrane potential x_{ij} in the following numerical studies. It predicates a perfect synchronization for $R \sim 1$, while it means non-perfect synchronization for $R \sim 0$. In realistic neuronal systems, the distribution of autapses connected to neurons in a local area of

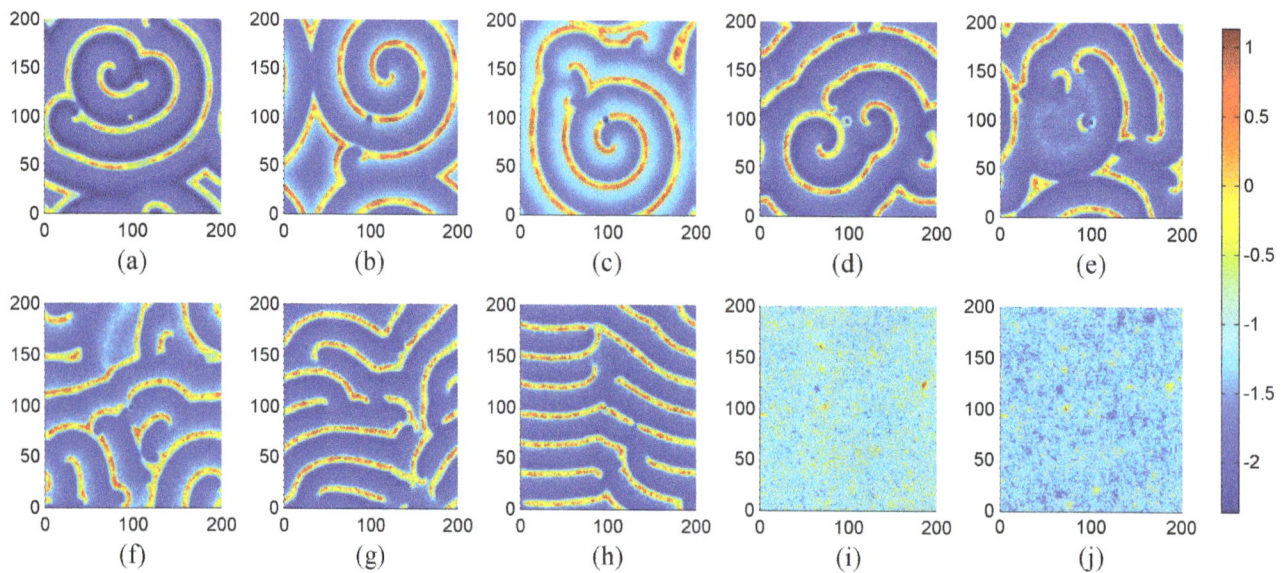

Figure 3. The developed states at $t = 16000$ time units in the network of neurons under different intensities of noise. For noise intensity (a) $D_0 = 0.005$, (b) $D_0 = 0.01$, (c) $D_0 = 0.02$, (d) $D_0 = 0.03$, (e) $D_0 = 0.04$, (f) $D_0 = 0.05$, (g) $D_0 = 0.08$, (h) $D_0 = 0.1$, (i) $D_0 = 0.5$, (j) $D_0 = 0.8$. Where $g = -1.5$, $\tau = 30$, $I_{ext} = 1.0$, $D = 1.0$ and periodical boundary condition is used.

network can be reliable and reasonable. In fact, the media becomes heterogeneous if autapses are considered on a few neurons in a local area of the network, thus target wave can be induced to occupy the network. Breakup of target waves occur under noise, thus spiral wave could be developed after collision between broken target waves. Extensive numerical results show that spiral wave can be observable easily when stronger gain g is used and the density of electric autapses (more autapses are included) is bigger. The potential cause is that powerful target wave occurs and spiral wave is induced via complex collision between broken target waves. For simplicity, $g=-1.5$, $\tau=30$ are used in the following numerical studies, the development of spiral wave is investigated by changing the coupling intensity D, noise intensity D_0, and this case is discussed under no-flux and periodical boundary condition, respectively.

Numerical Results and Discussion

In the numerical studies, the Euler forward difference algorithm is used with time step $h=0.01$, the initial values are selected as (3.0, 0.3, 0.1), all the neurons keep quiescent states, the transient period for calculation is about 16000 time units. The network size is 200×200. Autapses are imposed on neurons in a local area with 5×5 nodes ($96\leq i, j\leq100$). In mathematical models and computer simulations, periodic boundary conditions (PBC) are a set of boundary conditions that are often used to simulate a large system by modeling a small part that is far from its edge. The realistic neuronal system consists of a large number of neurons, the border effect from neurons outside but close to the system border should be considered, as a result, periodical boundary condition is often appreciated. Sometimes, no-flux boundary condition is also discussed for the case that the system keeps independent from cells outside the system (or an isolated system). In the following sections, A no-flux, and periodical boundary condition is used in the study of pattern formation and selection, respectively. It confirms that the development of spiral wave is much dependent on the distribution of electric autapses in the network, or the results are much independent of the selection of boundary condition. For a clear illustration, readers can refer to the two short movies in the supporting information, in the case of appropriate noise, the development of spiral wave induced by autapses can be observed under periodical and/or no-flux boundary conditions. In this way, it can give some clues to understand how the collective behaviors of neurons in network can

be regulated by a continuous 'pacemaker' like spiral wave induced by the electric autapses.

Subsection A: Noise on the formation of spiral wave

In this subsection, the coupling intensity is fixed at $D=1$, different intensities of noise are considered on the network. The gain intensity and time delay in autapse are selected as $g=-1.5$, $\tau=30$, and $I_{ext}=1.0$. Firstly, no-flux boundary condition is used for the network in numerical studies. As shown in Fig. 1, the developed states at $t=16000$ time units are illustrated under different intensities of noise.

The results in Fig. 1 show that spiral wave can be induced in the network under noise, breakup of spiral wave occurs and disordered state emerge with increasing the intensity of noise on the network. The developed spiral wave in Fig. 1(b) is much perfect than other snapshots, it means that the intensity of noise $D_0=0.01$ could be the most intermediate noise to develop a stable spiral wave. Then the development of spiral wave under $D_0=0.01$ is monitored, and snapshots under different time units are illustrated in Fig. 2.

The results in Fig. 2 confirm that stable spiral wave emerges with a transient period about 2000 time units, the potential mechanism is that autapses in a local area are critical to induce target wave, and the target wave begins to break up under noise, then spiral wave is formed under optimized noise. Surely, it is interesting to investigate this case under periodical boundary condition, and the results are plotted in Fig. 3.

The results in Fig. 3 confirm that spiral wave still emerges in the network under noise in the case of periodical boundary condition, breakup of target wave, spiral wave can still be observed with increasing the intensity of noise, and disordered state emerges in the network when the intensity of noise is beyond certain threshold. Clearly, the spiral wave seems perfect as shown in Fig. 3(b) but never covers the network completely as the emergence spiral wave in reaction-diffusion systems, and it is important to check its stability by monitoring its development under different time units, and the results are shown in Fig. 4.

The results in Fig. 4 show that the spiral wave becomes stable with a transient period about 4000 time units, and it grows up quickly to occupy most of the areas in the network. That is to say, the formation of spiral wave induced by noise and autapses in local area could be much independent of the selection of boundary condition. Extensive numerical results show that noise plays an important role in growing up the spiral wave and thus bigger area

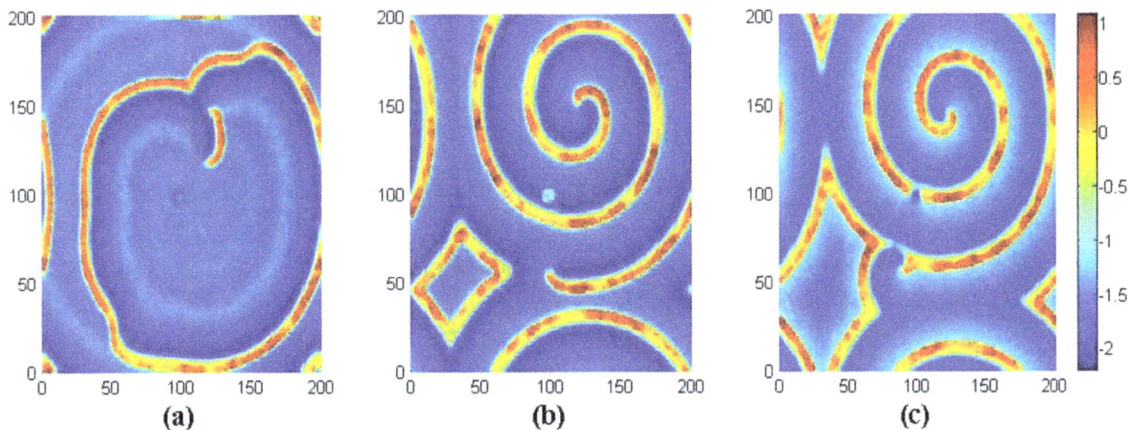

Figure 4. The development of spiral wave in the network. For (a) $t=2000$, (b) $t=4000$, (c) $t=16000$ time units. Where $g=-1.5$, $\tau=30$, $I_{ext}=1.0$, $D=1.0$, $D_0=0.01$ and periodical boundary condition is used.

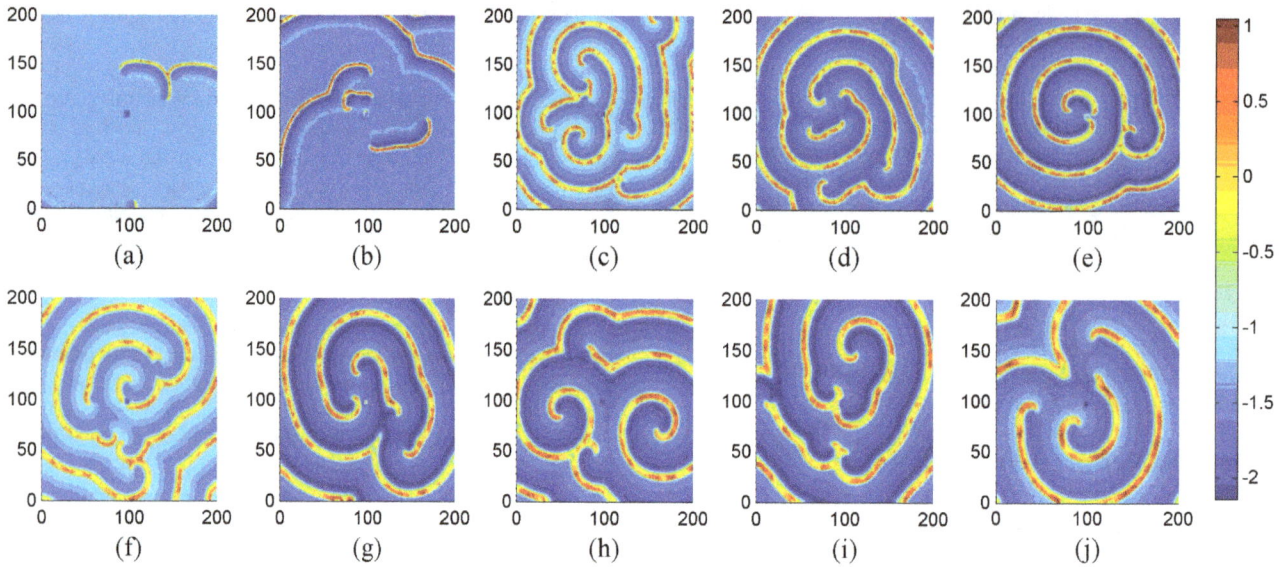

Figure 5. The developed states at $t=16000$ **time units in the network of neurons under different coupling intensities.** For coupling intensity (a) $D=0.4$, (b) $D=0.5$, (c) $D=0.6$, (d) $D=0.7$, (e) $D=0.8$, (f) $D=0.9$, (g) $D=1.1$, (h) $D=1.2$, (i) $D=1.3$, (j) $D=1.5$. Where $g=-1.5$, $\tau=30$, $I_{ext}=1.0$, $D_0=0.01$ and no-flux boundary condition is used.

of the network could be occupied by the spiral wave. The spiral wave shown in Fig. 4 is not as pefect as possible like the well-known spiral wave in reaction-diffusion system that spiral wave can cover the media completely. In fact, local distribution of electric autapse just induces spiral wave or segment in a local area but the spiral segment never grows up to occupy the network completely in the absence of noise, sometimes, broken spiral segments also emerges. Extensive numerical results seem to confirm that a developed spiral wave can cover more areas of the network by selecting noise intensity $D_0=0.01$, which can be regarded as a more optimized noise intensity to develop a spiral wave and thus more neuronal activities can be regulated by the spiral wave. It is also important to investigate the effect of coupling intensity on the development of spiral wave at $D_0=0.01$.

Subsection B: Coupling intensity on the formation of spiral wave

Spiral wave is self-sustained, the propagation of spiral wave is much dependent on the coupling intensity, appropriate coupling intensity is much helpful for those spiral seeds, thus stable spiral wave can be developed more quickly from the spiral seed (or segment) under appropriate noise, and then more area of the network can be occupied by the spiral wave completely. For simplicity, it selectes the noise intensity $D_0=0.01$, $I_{ext}=1.0$, $g=-1.5$, $\tau=30$, different coupling intensities are used to detect the development of spiral wave with a transient period about 16000 time units, and the results are shown in Fig. 5 when no-flux boundary condition is used for the network.

The results in Fig. 5 show that no spiral wave can be developed in the network under smaller intensity of coupling, and spiral wave begins to emerge with increasing the coupling intensity in the case

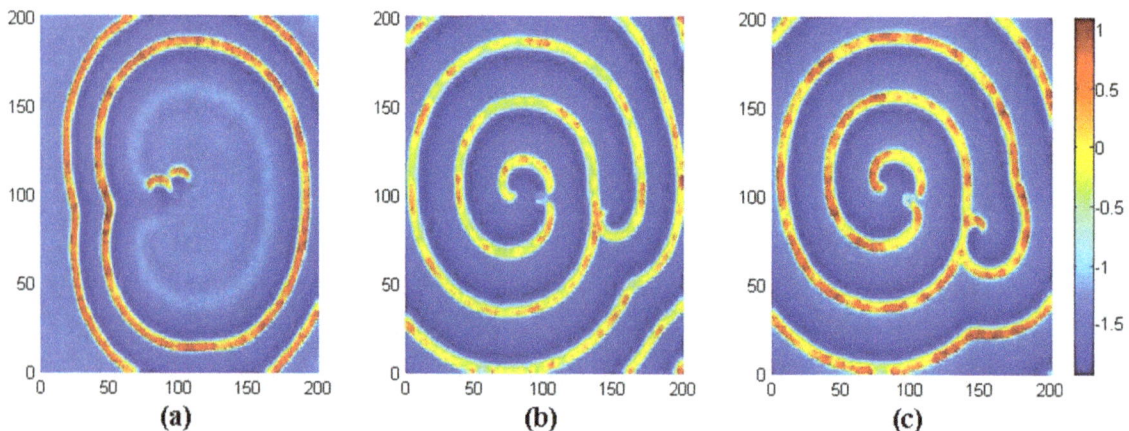

Figure 6. The development of spiral wave in the network. For (a) $t=2000$, (b) $t=4000$, (c) $t=16000$ time units. Where $g=-1.5$, $\tau=30$, $I_{ext}=1.0$, $D=0.8$, $D_0=0.01$ and no-flux boundary condition is used.

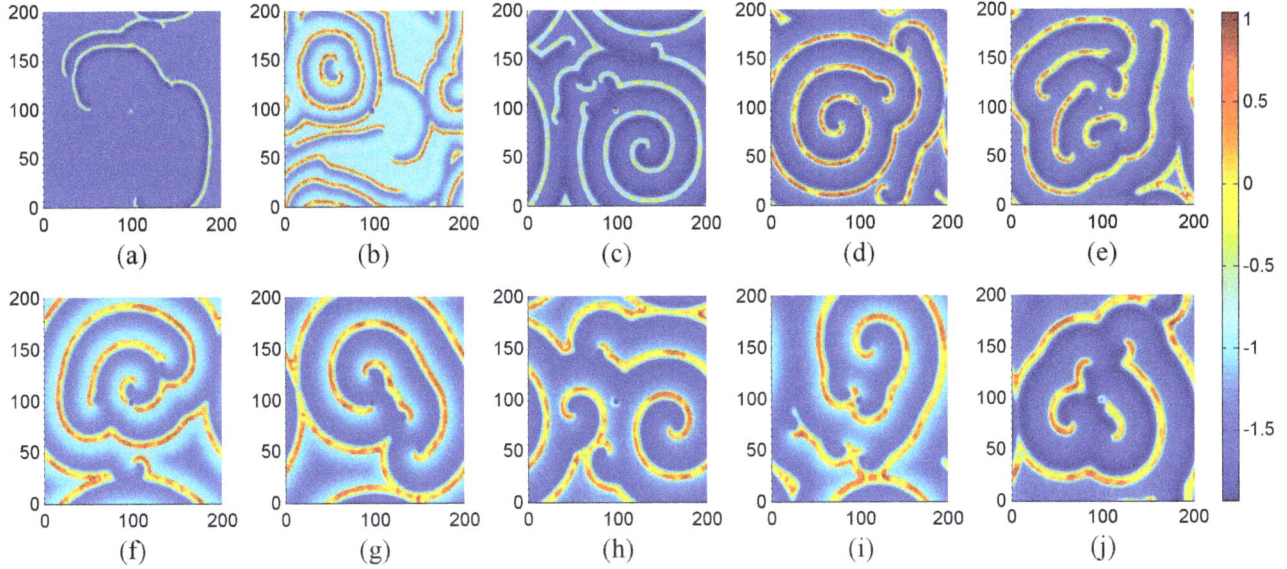

Figure 7. The developed states at $t=16000$ time units in the network of neurons under different coupling intensities. For coupling intensity (a) $D=0.4$, (b) $D=0.5$, (c) $D=0.6$, (d) $D=0.7$, (e) $D=0.8$, (f) $D=0.9$, (g) $D=1.1$, (h) $D=1.2$, (i) $D=1.3$, (j) $D=1.5$. Where $g=-1.5$, $\tau=30$, $I_{ext}=1.0$, $D_0=0.01$ and periodical boundary condition is used.

of no-flux boundary condition. To check the stability of spiral wave in Fig. 5(e), its development is monitored by illustrating the snapshots at different transient periods, and the results are shown in Fig. 6.

The results in Fig. 6 confirm that a spiral wave begins to emerge, and it occupies more and more nodes (size) vs. time, then it dominates most of the area in the network. It indicates that a perfect spiral wave induced by electric autapses in the network is also dependent on the selection of coupling intensity as the noise. It is also interesting to investigate this case under periodical boundary condition, and the results are shown in Fig. 7.

The results in Fig. 7 still show that spiral wave seldom emerges under smaller coupling intensity, and spiral wave begins to occur by using a stronger intensity of coupling. Then some perfect spiral wave is developed to occupy the network as shown in Fig. 7(d). However, more segments of spiral wave emerge in the network with increasing the intensity of coupling, and it shows some

difference from the case of no-flux boundary condition. That is to say, perfect spiral wave emerges at $D=0.8$ for no-flux boundary condition, while it emerges at $D=0.7$ for periodical boundary condition. The potential mechanism could be that noise enhances the boundary condition effect. To detect the stability of the developed spiral wave in Fig. 7(d), snapshots under different transient periods are illustrated in Fig. 8.

The results in Fig. 8 show that periodical boundary condition is also effective to support stable spiral wave, and the spiral wave occupies most of the area in the network with a transient period about 6000 time units. It is also confirmed that spiral wave emerges well by selecting appropriate coupling intensity at fixed intensity of noise, gain, time delay in the autapse.

Above all, the emergence of spiral wave in the network is just investigated by illustrating the snapshots under different autapse parameters (g, τ), coupling intensities and noise intensities. It is important to discern some statistical properties of the collective

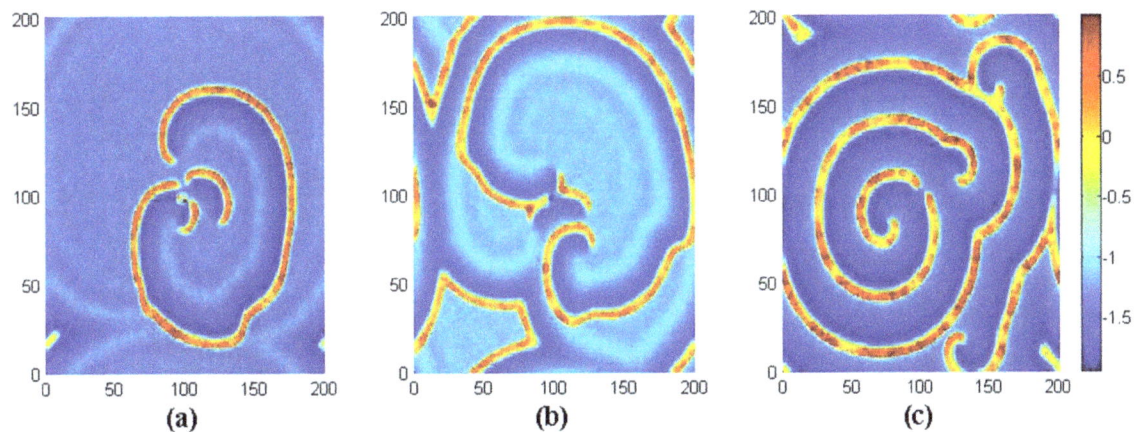

Figure 8. The development of spiral wave in the network. For (a) $t=2000$, (b) $t=4000$, (c) $t=16000$ time units. Where $g=-1.5$, $\tau=30$, $I_{ext}=1.0$, $D=0.7$, $D_0=0.01$ and periodical boundary condition is used.

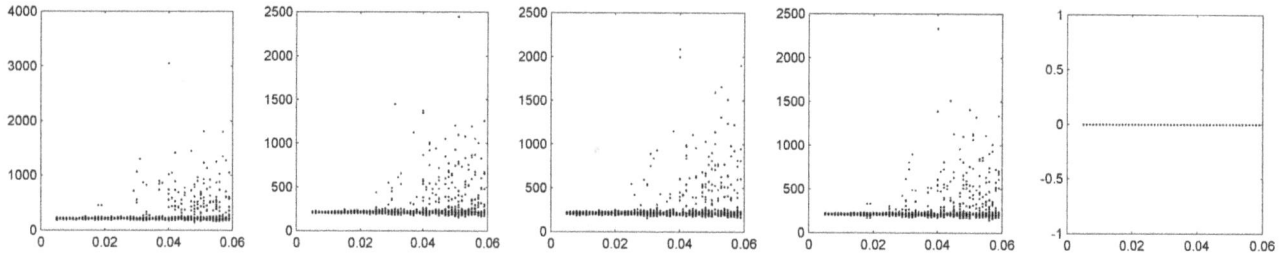

Figure 9. Bifurcation diagram for ISI vs. noise intensity. For (a) time series of membrane potentials in node ($i=90, j=100$), (b) time series of membrane potentials in node ($i=110, j=100$), (c) time series of membrane potentials in node ($i=100, j=90$), (d) time series of membrane potentials in node ($i=100, j=110$). No-flux boundary condition is used, and $D=1$, $I_{ext}=1.0$, $\tau=30$, $g=-1.5$.

behaviors in the network by calculating the factors of synchronization. For simplicity, it will discuss the case for $D=1$, $I_{ext}=1.0$, $\tau=30$, $g=-1.5$. The time series for four space symmetrical nodes ($i=90, j=100$), ($i=110, j=100$), ($i=100, j=90$), ($i=100, j=110$) are used for bifurcation analysis from the ISI (Inter-Spike Interval) vs. noise intensity $D_0 \sim [0.005 \sim 0.1]$. The bifurcation diagrams for the sampled time series vs., noise intensity are plotted in Fig. 9, and the distribution of factor of synchronization is plotted in Fig. 10.

The results in Fig. 9 show that the ISI values are much close to stable value about 250 when noise intensity is less than $D_0=0.03$, thus the network can generate periodic or quasi-periodic property, which is necessary to support a stable spiral wave with distinct periodicity that can be verified by using time series analysis. The time series often shows distinct periodicity when spiral wave regulates or dominates the network, while disordered state emerges when breakup of spiral wave occurs under noise. However, the ISI begins to fluctuate in random that means no dominant period can be sustained in the network with further increasing the intensity of noise, as a result, no spiral wave can be developed and disordered states emerge in the network of neurons. To discern the phase transition of spiral wave in the network with no-flux boundary condition being used, the distribution for factors

of synchronization is calculated by changing the intensity of noise carefully, and the results are shown in Fig. 10.

The results in Fig. 10 confirm that smaller factor of synchronization could be detected when the intensity of noise is low usually, and thus an ordered state could be reached, which is helpful to support a spiral wave in the network. The factor of synchronization tends to increase when stronger noise is used on the network, thus breakup of ordered wave occurs. Particularly, for the case $D_0=0.01$, the factor of synchronization is approached by a much smaller value for $D=0.8$ than $D=0.7, 1.0, 1.1$ as well, which means a perfect spiral wave is much easy to be induced in the network. In the case for $D=0.7$, the factor of synchronization fluctuates in the range from 0.02 to 0.04 when noise intensity is selected from $D_0=0.01$ to 0.04. In the case for $D=0.8, 1.0, 1.1$, slight deviation emerges for the factor of synchronization when noise intensity is changed below $D_0=0.06$. In fact, spiral segments emerge in a local area of the network when smaller factors of synchronization are approached within [0.02, 0.04] though different area sizes can be covered by the spiral wave under different noise intensities. Compared the results in Fig. 10(a) with Fig. 10(b, c, d), it is found that the maximal factor of synchronization is decreased from $0.3 \to 0.2 \to 0.1$ when the intensity is increased from $D=0.7 \to 0.8 \to 1.0 \to 1.1$ which makes the spiral segment propagate more quickly and regulate the

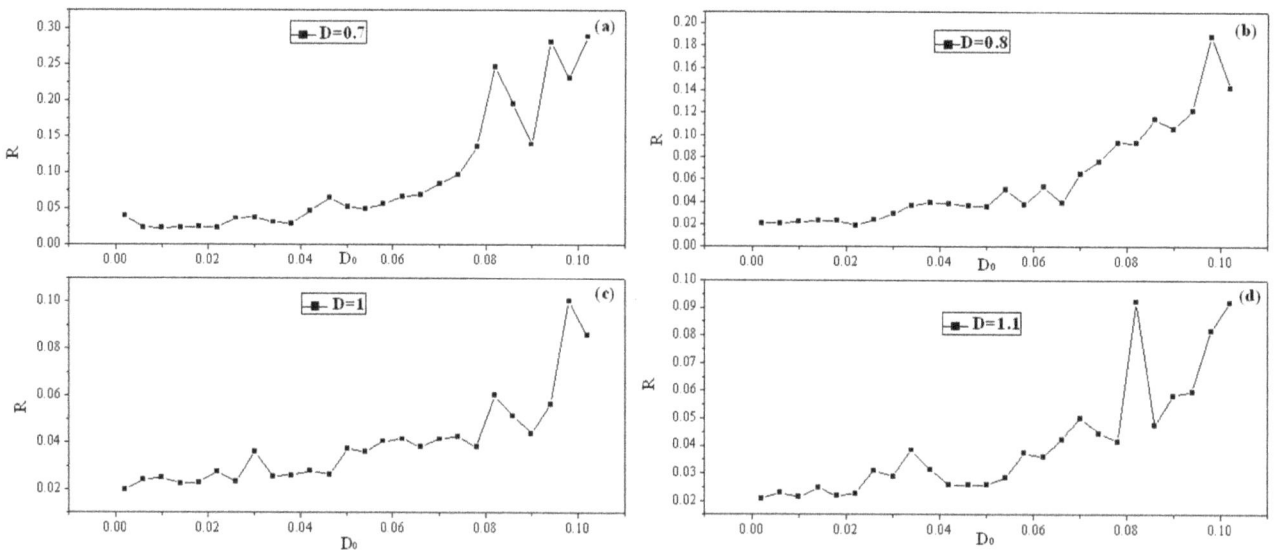

Figure 10. Distribution of factors of synchronization *vs.* noise intensity under no-flux boundary condition. For coupling intensity (a) $D=0.7$, (b) $D=0.8$, (c) $D=1$, (d) $D=1.1$. $I_{ext}=1.0$, $\tau=30$, $g=-1.5$, transient period t = 16000 time units, and the autapses are connected to neurons in the nodes ($96 \le i, j \le 100$).

collective behaviors of network more effectively. Extensive numerical results confirm that $D_0 = 0.01$ can be the most effective noise intensity to enhance the growth of spiral wave so that more large number of neurons can be regulated by the spiral wave. By further increasing the noise intensity, it finds distinct shift in the curve for factor of synchronization, which means that the previous ordered state is removed and the network becomes disorder due to breakup of spiral waves. The case for periodical boundary condition is also investigated, and similar distribution of factor of synchronization is observed, that means smaller factor of synchronization vs. noise is active to support stable spiral wave in the network.

In a summary, autapses connected to neuron in a local area of the network are helpful to induce target wave, spiral wave emerges resulting from the breakup and collision of target waves, and optimized noise, coupling intensity are much important in supporting a stable spiral wave in the network. It accounts for the emergence of spiral wave in the neuronal network with autapse being considered. Time delay in autapse of a single neuron used to record the previous information, and the network enhances the memory and information propagation. The spiral wave is often self-sustained and robust to certain noise, thus the formation of spiral wave induced by autapse under optimized noise is much helpful for information memory in the network of neurons. It plays like a pacemaker and thus the collective electric behaviors of neurons are regulated by the spiral wave, which can be induced by appropriate distribution of electric autapses in the network.

Conclusions

Autapses are observed in rat hippocampal neuron, and its functional roles are much attractive for study. The effect of autapse is often described by imposing self-feedback current with time delay on the membrane potential, and it is thought to be associated with memory and self-adjusting. In realistic neuronal system, a fraction of autapses can regulate the collective behaviors of neurons; therefore, it is interesting to study the transition and self-organization in neuronal network by detecting pattern dynamics. In this paper, the selection of spiral wave induced by autapses in a neuronal network is investigated, and the effect of noise on the network is also discussed. A statistical factor of synchronization is used to detect the transition of pattern induced by noise on the network, it is found that the emergence of spiral wave is often associated with a smaller factor of synchronization, which often represents an ordered state. Autapses connected to neurons in a local area can generate target wave in the network, breakup of target wave occurs due to noise, and optimized noise can enhance the ordered state by developing the broken target waves into a spiral wave, which regulates the collective electric behaviors of neurons like a pacemaker due to its intrinsic self-sustained dynamical property. Similar results are approached under no-flux and periodical boundary conditions.

Supporting Information

Movie S1 Supporting flash for spiral wave induced by autapses under periodical boundary condition.

Movie S2 Supporting flash for spiral wave induced by autapses under no-flux boundary condition. (SWF) The two short movies are supplied to observe the formation of autapse-induced spiral waves in the network under different boundary conditions. Coupling intensity $D = 1$, noise intensity $D_0 = 0.01$, $g = -1.5$, $\tau = 30$, transient period $t = 16000$ time units.

Author Contributions

Conceived and designed the experiments: HXQ JM CNW YW. Performed the experiments: HXQ JM CNW YW. Analyzed the data: HXQ JM CNW YW. Contributed reagents/materials/analysis tools: HXQ JM CNW YW. Wrote the paper: JM.

References

1. Hodgkin AL, Katz B (1949) The effect of temperature on the electrical activity of the giant axon of the squid, J Physiol (London) 109: 240–249.
2. Hodgkin AL, Huxley AF (1952) A quantitative description of membrane current and its application to conduction and excitation in nerve, J Physiol (London) 117(4): 500–544.
3. Morris C, Lecar H (1981) Voltage oscillations in the barnacle giant muscle fiber, Biophy J 35: 193–213.
4. Hindmarsh JL, Rose RM (1984) A model of neuronal bursting using three coupled first order differential equations, Proc R Soc Lond B 221(1222): 87–102.
5. Rinzel J, Ermentrout GB (1989) Analysis of neuronal excitability and oscillations, C Koch and I. Segev (Eds.), Methods in neuronal Modeling: from synapses to Networks, MIT press, London.
6. Izhikevich EM (2004) Which Model to Use for Cortical Spiking Neurons? IEEE Transactions on Neural Networks 15(5): 1063–1070.
7. Schmid G, Goychuk I, Hänggi P (2004) Effect of channel block on the spiking activity of excitable membranes in a stochastic Hodgkin-Huxley model, Phys Biol 1: 61–66.
8. Storace M, Linaro D, de Lange E (2008) The Hindmarsh-Rose neuron model: Bifurcation analysis and piecewise, linear approximations, Chaos 18: 033128.
9. He DH, Hu G, Zhan M, Ren W, Gao Z (2002) Pattern formation of spiral waves in an inhomogeneous medium with small-world connections, Phys Rev E 65: 055204.
10. Roxin A, Riecke H, Solla SA (2004) Self-sustained activity in a small-world network of excitable neurons, Phys Rev Lett 92: 198101.
11. Sinha S, Saramaki J, Kaski K (2007) Emergence of self-sustained patterns in small-world excitable media, Phys Rev E 76: 015101.
12. Perc M (2007) Effects of small-world connectivity on noise-induced temporal and spatial order in neural media, Chaos Solitons Fractals 31(2): 280–291.
13. Weber S, Hütt MT, Porto M (2008) Pattern formation and efficiency of reaction-diffusion processes on complex networks, Europhys Lett 83: 28003.
14. Jr Erichsen R, Brunnet LG (2008) Multistability in networks of Hindmarsh-Rose neurons, Phys Rev E 78: 061917.
15. Liao XH, Xia QZ, Qian Y, Zhang LS, Hu G, Mi YY (2011) Pattern formation in oscillatory complex networks consisting of excitable nodes, Phys Rev E 83: 056204.
16. Ma J, Wang CN, Ying H P, Chu RT (2013) Emergence of target waves in neuronal networks due to diverse forcing currents, Sci China Phys Mech Astro 56: 1126–1138.
17. Hou ZH, Xin HW (2002) Noise-sustained spiral waves: effect of spatial and temporal memory, Phys Rev Lett 89: 280601.
18. Ma J, Huang L, Ying HP, Pu ZS (2012) Detecting the breakup of spiral waves in small-world networks of neurons due to channel block, Chinese Sci Bull 57: 2094–2101.
19. Ma J, Hu BL, Wang CN, Jin WY (2013) Simulating the formation of spiral wave in the neuronal system, Nonlinear Dyn 73(1–2): 73–83.
20. Huang XY, Troy WC, Yang Q, Ma HT, Laing CR, et al. (2004) Spiral waves in disinhibited mammalian cortex, J Neurosci 24: 9897–9902.
21. Schiff SJ, Huang XY, Wu JY (2007) Dynamical evolution of spatiotemporal patterns in mammalian middle cortex, Phys Rev Lett 98: 178102.
22. Huang XY, Xu WF, Liang JM, Takagaki K, Gao X, et al. (2010) Spiral Wave Dynamics in Neocortex, Neuron 60: 978–990.
23. Wu XY, Ma J (2013) The formation mechanism of defects, spiral wave in the network of neurons, PLoS ONE 8(1): e55403.
24. Hu BL, Ma J, Tang J (2013) Selection of Multiarmed Spiral Waves in a Regular Network of Neurons, PLoS ONE 8(7): e69251.
25. Ma J, Liu Q R, Ying H P, Wu Y (2013) Emergence of spiral wave induced by defects block, Commun Nonlinear Sci Numer Simulat 18(7): 1665–1675.
26. Li F, Ma J (2013) Selection of spiral wave in the coupled network under Gaussian colored noise, Int J Mod Phys B 27(21): 1350115.
27. Ma J, Wu Y, Ying HP, Jia Y (2011) Channel noise-induced phase transition of spiral wave in networks of Hodgkin-Huxley neurons, Chinese Sci Bull 56: 151–157.
28. Bacci A, Huguenard JR (2006) Enhancement of spike-timing precision by autaptic transmission in neocortical inhibitory interneurons, Neuron 49: 119–130.

29. Bekkers JM (2003) Synaptic transmission: Functional autapses in the cortex, Curr Biol 13: R433–R435.
30. Tamás G, Buhl EH, Somogyi P (1997) Massive autaptic self-innervation of GABAergic neurons in cat visual cortex, J Neurosci 17: 6352–6364.
31. Herrmann CS, Klaus A (2004) Autapse turns neuron into oscillator, Int J Bifurcat Chaos 14(2): 623–633.
32. Li YY, Schmid G, Hänggi P, Schimansky-Geier L (2010) Spontaneous spiking in an autaptic Hodgkin- Huxley setup, Phys Rev E 82: 061907.
33. Wang QY, Perc M, Duan Z, Chen GR (2009) Synchronization transitions on scale- free neuronal networks due to finite information transmission delays, Phys Rev E 80: 026206.
34. Ao X, Hänggi P, Schmid G (2013) In-phase and anti-phase synchronization in noisy Hodgkin–Huxley neurons, Mathematical Biosciences 245(1): 49−55.
35. Wang HT, Ma J, Chen YL, Chen Y (2014) Effect of an Autapse on the Firing Pattern Transition in a Bursting Neuron, Commun Nonlinear Sci Numer Simulat 19: 3242–3254.
36. Bekkers JM (2002) Synaptic Transmission: A New Kind of Inhibition, Curr Biol 12 (19): R648−R650.
37. Bekkers JM(2009)Synaptic transmission: excitatory autapses find a function? Current Biology 19(7): R296−298.
38. Wang QY, Perc M, Duan ZS, Chen GR (2010) Impact of delays and rewiring on the dynamics of small-world neuronal networks with two types of coupling, Physica A 389: 3299−3306.
39. Qin HX, Ma J, Jin WY, Wang CN (2014) Dynamics of electric activities in neuron and neurons of networkinduced by autapses, Sci China Tech Sci 57: 936–946.
40. Perc M (2007) Effects of small-world connectivity on noise-induced temporal and spatial order in neural media, Chaos, Solitons & Fractals 31: 280–290.
41. Gu HG, Jia B, Li YY, Chen GR (2013) White noise-induced spiral waves and multiple spatial coherence resonances in a neuronal network with type I excitability, Physica A 392: 1361–1374.
42. Tang Z, Li YY, Xie L, Xi L, Gu HG (2012) Spiral Waves and Multiple Spatial Coherence Resonances Induced by Colored Noise in Neuronal Network, Commun Theor Phys 57(1): 61–67.
43. Tang J, Luo JM, Ma J, Yi M, Yang XQ (2013) Spiral waves in systems with fractal heterogeneity, Physica A 392(22): 5764–5771.
44. Lou Q, Chen JX, Zhao YH (2012) Control of turbulence in heterogeneous excitable media, Phys Rev E 85: 026213.
45. Zhao YH, Lou Q, Chen JX, Sun WG, Zhao YH (2013) Emitting waves from heterogeneity by a rotating electric field, Chaos 23: 033141.
46. Ma J, Ying HP, Liu Y, et al. (2009) Development and transition of spiral wave in the coupled Hindmarsh-Rose neurons in two-dimensional space, Chinese Phys B 18(1): 98–105.
47. Wang CN, Ma J, Tang J, Li YL (2010) Instability and Death of Spiral Wave in a Two-Dimensional Array of Hindmarsh-Rose Neurons, Commun Theor Phys 53(2): 382–388.
48. Ma J, Yang LJ, Wu Y, Zhang CR (2010) Spiral Wave in Small-World Networks of Hodgkin -Huxley Neurons, Commun Theor Phys 54(3): 583–588.

11

An Artificial Neural Network Estimation of Gait Balance Control in the Elderly Using Clinical Evaluations

Vipul Lugade[1], Victor Lin[2], Arthur Farley[3], Li-Shan Chou[1]*

1 Department of Human Physiology, University of Oregon, Eugene, Oregon, United States of America, 2 Rehabilitation Medicine Associates of Eugene-Springfield, P.C., Eugene, Oregon, United States of America, 3 Department of Computer and Information Sciences, University of Oregon, Eugene, Oregon, United States of America

Abstract

The use of motion analysis to assess balance is essential for determining the underlying mechanisms of falls during dynamic activities. Clinicians evaluate patients using clinical examinations of static balance control, gait performance, cognition, and neuromuscular ability. Mapping these data to measures of dynamic balance control, and the subsequent categorization and identification of community dwelling elderly fallers at risk of falls in a quick and inexpensive manner is needed. The purpose of this study was to demonstrate that given clinical measures, an artificial neural network (ANN) could determine dynamic balance control, as defined by the interaction of the center of mass (CoM) with the base of support (BoS), during gait. Fifty-six elderly adults were included in this study. Using a feed-forward neural network with back propagation, combinations of five functional domains, the number of hidden layers and error goals were evaluated to determine the best parameters to assess dynamic balance control. Functional domain input parameters included subject characteristics, clinical examinations, cognitive performance, muscle strength, and clinical balance performance. The use of these functional domains demonstrated the ability to quickly converge to a solution, with the network learning the mapping within 5 epochs, when using up to 30 hidden nodes and an error goal of 0.001. The ability to correctly identify the interaction of the CoM with BoS demonstrated correlation values up to 0.89 (P<.001). On average, using all clinical measures, the ANN was able to estimate the dynamic CoM to BoS distance to within 1 cm and BoS area to within 75 cm^2. Our results demonstrated that an ANN could be trained to map clinical variables to biomechanical measures of gait balance control. A neural network could provide physicians and patients with a cost effective means to identify dynamic balance issues and possible risk of falls from routinely collected clinical examinations.

Editor: Francisco J. Esteban, University of Jaén, Spain

Funding: This study was funded by the International Society of Biomechanics Student Dissertation Grant (to V. Lugade) and the University of Oregon. The funders had no role in study design, data collection and analysis, decision to publish, or preparation of the manuscript.

Competing Interests: The authors have declared that no competing interests exist.

* E-mail: chou@uoregon.edu

Introduction

Over one third of adults over the age of 65 will fall each year [1]. Falls are not only associated with injury and morbidity, but also reductions in physical, psychological, and social capacities [2,3]. The direct cost of falling exceeds $10 billion a year in the United States [1,2], with almost 9,500 deaths per year attributed to falling [2,3]. Epidemiological studies have shown that 30–70% of falls occur while level walking and thus understanding balance control during gait remains paramount.

Falls in the elderly are a complicated phenomenon comprising multifactoral risk factors, including both intrinsic and extrinsic issues [4]. Intrinsic factors, or those related to the individual, include a decreased performance in the balance control system, with loss of mobility being a strong indicator for increasing fall risk. In order to maintain stability, adequate levels of vision, vestibular function, musculoskeletal function, and proprioception are all required. Prior studies have also shown that decreased lower-extremity muscle strength and cognitive function are significant predictors of falls among older adults [4–6]. Extrinsic factors, or those pertaining to environmental hazards, contribute significantly to fall incidents and can include objects to trip over, poor lighting, slippery surfaces, or inappropriate furniture [3]. The ability to understand which of the multitude of neuromuscular, cognitive, and sensory factors most contribute to balance control ability during gait can provide further ability to diagnose and treat elderly at risk of falling.

While clinically valuable, gait analysis can be both expensive and time inefficient for laboratory technicians, with a data collection taking up to 2 hours and costing up to $2,000 [7]. Having a model that could predict the fall risk of elderly individuals based on calculated gait balance control parameters would be a clinically viable and inexpensive solution. In order to achieve this, models are needed which can find a mapping between clinical and laboratory biomechanical measures. Fall prediction models have previously used logistic regression as well as static posture variables and clinical measures to determine fall risk. These included predictions based on Berg balance scores, Timed Up and Go test, and self-reported history of imbalance and history of falls to determine the risk of falling among a group of elderly individuals [4,8]. Such models require that input predictors explain a high degree of variability and make the assumption that linear relationships exist between variables. Another approach which would allow for non-linear relationships and include a number of input variables is an artificial neural network (ANN) [9]. An advantage of ANN models is that they can be built to infer a function simply from observation or training. By exposing the model to set of elderly adult data, with known input and output values, the ANN can be trained to an appropriate level.

Neural networks have been previously trained to efficiently determine foot-strike and foot-off events [10], as well as identify temporal or amplitude asymmetry in bilateral vertical ground reaction forces [11]. The use of an ANN in gait analysis has additionally demonstrated greater accuracy in discriminating patient populations from healthy adults, when compared to using linear discriminant analysis [12]. Further applications include estimating joint kinetics and kinematics using electromyography [13], as well as mapping spatio-temporal gait and electromyographic measures to dynamic balance control measures and fall risk [9,14].

Since complete and accurate measurement of spatio-temporal gait variables is not possible in the clinical environment, the purpose of this study was to test the feasibility of a neural network model in mapping commonly used clinical measures to laboratory balance measures. Clinical measures included a history of falls, deficits in sensory motor function, visual and hearing impairment, presence of chronic disease or depression, number of medications, and clinical balance examinations. We hypothesized that an ANN model could determine the balance control of elderly individuals given easily assessable clinical measures such as static balance examinations, cognitive performance, and muscle strength.

Methods

Subjects

A total of 56 community living elderly subjects [age (SD) = 76.1 (6.5) years; 22 males] were recruited for this study. A phone screen was performed prior to recruitment. All subjects reported no history of head trauma, neurological disease, heart disease or visual impairment that was uncorrected by glasses. In addition, subjects confirmed that they were able to ambulate for up to 10 minutes without the use of an assistive device. A clinical and laboratory gait evaluation was then performed on all subjects by a physician and trained researchers, respectively. Each subject signed an informed consent statement, in accordance with ethics approval granted from the Institutional Review Board of University of Oregon, prior to participation in the study.

Clinical Evaluation

The body mass index (BMI) was computed for each subject along with a full medical history of prior fall history, the number of medications taken, and co-morbidities. In addition, physicians evaluated proprioceptive ability, vision, and hearing. The Geriatric Depression Scale (GDS) was used to evaluate depression [15]. The Activities Specific Balance Confidence Scale (ABC) provided information on a person's self-perception of balance ability [16]. Static balance was evaluated using the Berg Balance Scale (BBS) [17]. Dynamic gait performance was recorded through the Timed Up and Go test (TUG) [18]. Cognitive ability was estimated using the Trail Making Test (TMT) A and B, as well as the Saint Louis University Mental Status (SLUMS). The TMT test was evaluated based on the difference in scores on the B and A test [19]. This difference has been shown to demonstrate the task switching cost. The SLUMS was used to identify any dementia or mild neuro-cognitive disorder by conducting screening tests for orientation, memory, attention, and executive function [20].

Bilateral isometric muscle strength of the hip abductors, knee extensors, and ankle plantarflexors was tested using a Biodex System 3 dynamometer (Biodex Medical Systems, NY). For hip strength, the subject was instructed to abduct while standing in the neutral position. Knee extensor strength was evaluated in the seated position at 60 degrees of knee flexion. Ankle plantorflexor strength was tested while seated at 20 degrees of knee flexion and in a neutral ankle position. The peak torque value for each joint was recorded and normalized to a person's body mass.

Laboratory Gait Balance Evaluation

Subjects were asked to walk at a self-selected comfortable speed across a 10-meter walkway. During ambulation, 29 retro reflective markers were placed on bony landmarks of the body [21], with three dimensional marker trajectories captured with an 8-camera motion analysis system (Motion Analysis Corp, Santa Rosa, CA). Data were filtered using a fourth-order low pass Butterworth filter with an 8-Hz cutoff frequency. Ground reaction forces and

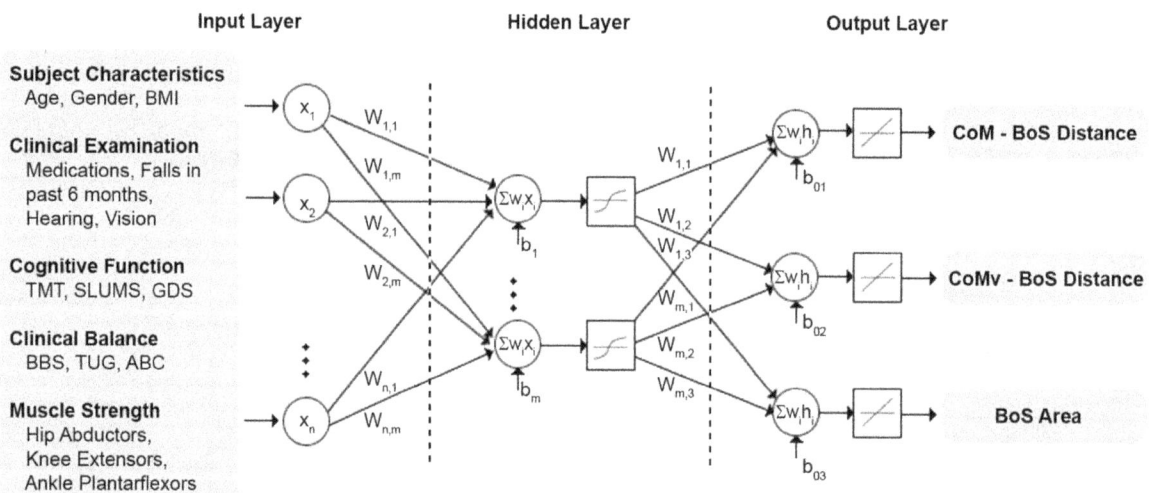

Figure 1. Neural network architecture representing the three layers as well as the tangential sigmoid and pure linear transfer functions in the hidden and output layers, respectively. All nodes are not represented in this diagram, though a weighted sum of all inputs and the bias is performed at each node in the hidden and output layers.

Table 1. Demographics of all 56 participants [mean (SD)].

Subject Characteristics	
Age (years)	76.1 (6.5)
Gender (Males/Females)	22/34
BMI	27.4 (6.1)
Clinical Examination	
Fall History (number in past year)	0.95 (1.35)
Number of Medications	3.8 (3.2)
Visual acuity (/20)	36.6 (11.7)
Hearing (number impaired)	14
Clinical Balance	
BBS (/56)	53.4 (3.8)
TUG (seconds)	9.0 (2.0)
ABC (%)	85.7 (13.6)
Cognitive Performance	
TMT B-A (seconds)	63.2 (63.0)
GDS (/15)	1.6 (1.9)
SLUMS (/30)	26.4 (3.3)
Muscle Strength [a]	
Ankle Plantarflexion	3.1 (2.3)
Knee Extension	3.8 (2.7)
Hip Abduction	1.9 (1.6)
Gait Balance Control [b]	
CoM-BoS distance (cm)	3.8 (1.1)
CoMv-BoS displacement (cm)	19.3 (3.5)
BoS Area (cm^2)	436 (88)

[a]Normalized to body weight and body height (Nm/BW*BH).
[b]Balance control measures evaluated at heel strike.

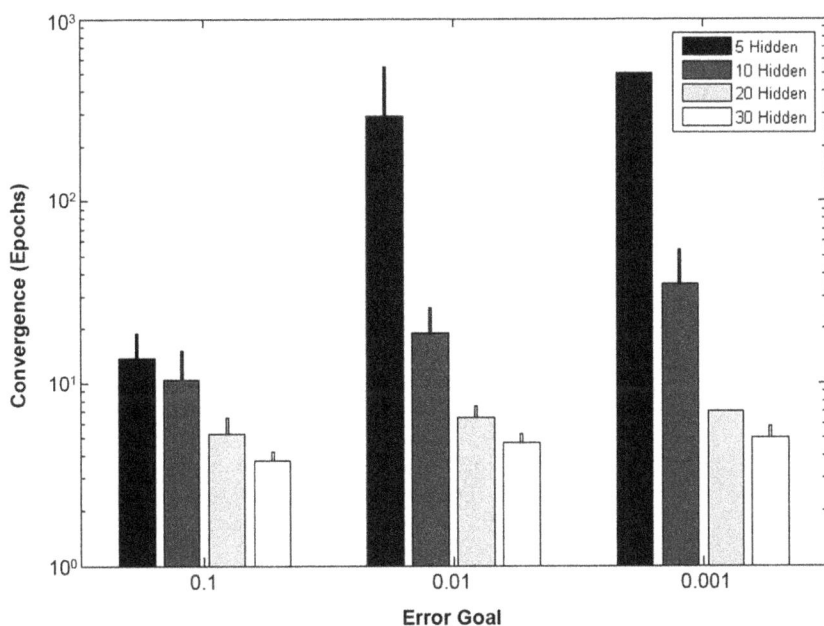

Figure 2. Number of epochs required for convergence to error goal given the number of hidden nodes during training of the neural network with all 16 input variables.

A

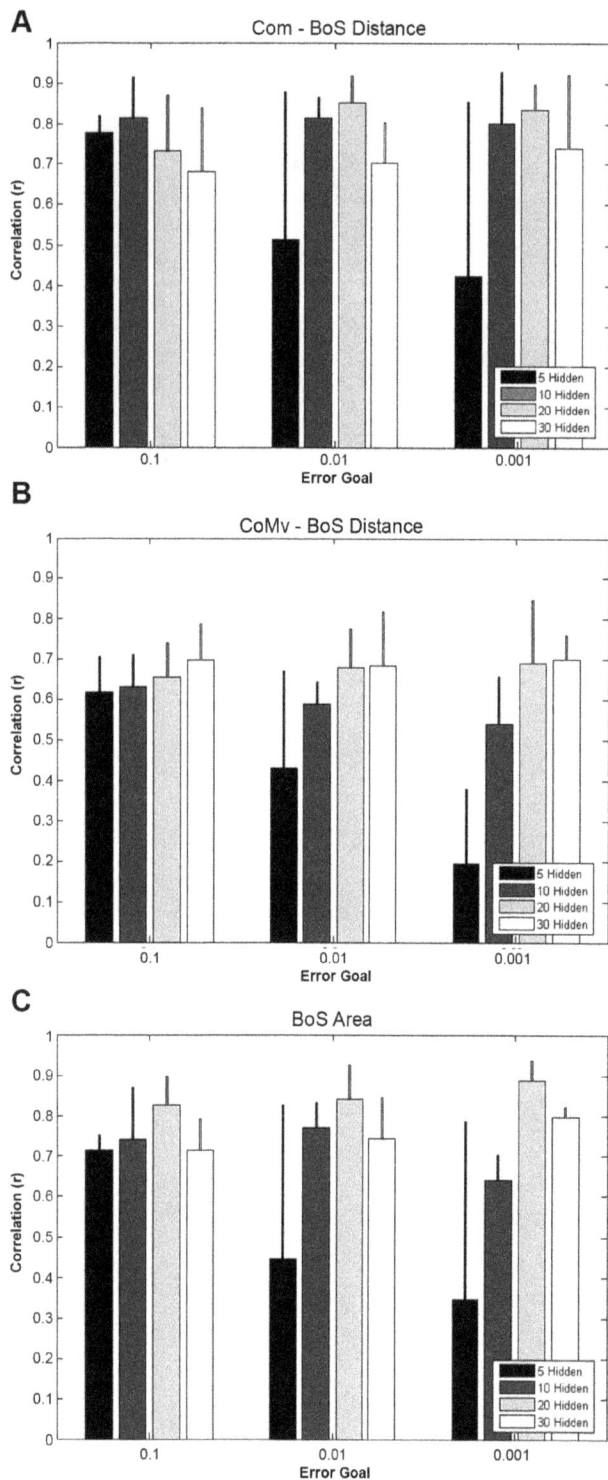

B

C

Figure 3. Performance of the neural network using all 16 input variables.

Balance control during gait included analysis of the position and velocity of the center of mass (CoM) in relation to the dynamically changing base of support (BoS) [22]. The distance from the CoM position to the closest border of the BoS (CoM-BoS) represented static balance control. The displacement of the CoM along the direction of the CoM velocity vector to the boundary of the BoS (CoMv-BoS) represented dynamic balance control. The BoS area was calculated based on the anthropometrics and configuration of the feet. These three measures were evaluated at heel strike of both limbs across all gait cycles.

ANN Development

An artificial neural network is a series of interconnected nodes (biological neurons) which approximates the relationships, or adaptive weightings, between input and output measures. Similar to biological nervous systems, connections (biological synapses) were established through a learned iterative process. Upon receiving one or more inputs (biological dendrites), a node was able to compute a weighted sum and pass a value through a non-linear transfer function to establish an output function. Training, or learning and the establishment of synapses, occurred by using the clinical (inputs) and balance control (outputs) data among a subset of individuals, then solving for the weights of the inter-connections in an optimal manner. Inferring the mapping implied by the data and finding the solution that has the smallest possible cost allows the ANN to arrive at a satisfactory weighting level. Once the ANN model was trained, it was then be used to predict outputs for the remaining subset of individuals.

The ANN used in this study was designed to calculate the gait balance control measures of each subject. Input data sets included subject characteristics (age, BMI, gender), clinical examination (fall history, medications, vision, hearing), clinical balance performance (BBS, TUG, ABC), cognitive evaluation (TMT, GDS, SLUMS), and muscle strength (bilateral ankles, knees and hips). The ANN program is provided as Program S1 in supplementary materials.

A three-layer, feed-forward back-propagation ANN was constructed using MATLAB (Mathworks Inc., Natick, MA; Figure 1; see Program S1). The first layer of the network consisted of different combinations of the normalized input data sets, with between three and 16 possible clinical measures included in each iteration of the analyses. The second layer included 5, 10, 20 or 30 hidden neurons. The third or output layer included the three laboratory gait balance control variables. Out of the 56 subjects, 42 were randomly selected for training, with testing performed on the other 14 subjects. This process was repeated 4 times in order to test the network on all 56 subjects, with training stopped when the mean squared error (MSE) error reached 0.1, 0.01 or 0.001. Error correction during training was conducted with the Levenberg-Marquardt algorithm [23]. Weighted incoming signals were summed at the hidden and output units, with a tangential sigmoid transfer function and pure linear transfer function used at each layer, respectively. Details of the network have been described previously by Hahn and colleagues [14].

After successful training, all balance control data was converted back to real world units of cm and cm^2, for the distance and area measures, respectively. The ability of the ANN model to accurately estimate CoM-BoS balance control measures in comparison to actual gait measurements was assessed via correlation analysis. Differences in accuracy in the correlation coefficient (R) between the number of hidden units (5, 10, 20 or 30), between the error goal (0.1, 0.01 and 0.001), and across grouping type were assessed with a 3 way ANOVA in SPSS 14.0 (IBM Inc., Armonk, NY).

moments were captured from three floor-embedded force plates (Advanced Mechanical Technologies Inc., Watertown, MA). Marker and force plate data were collected at 60 Hz and 960 Hz, respectively.

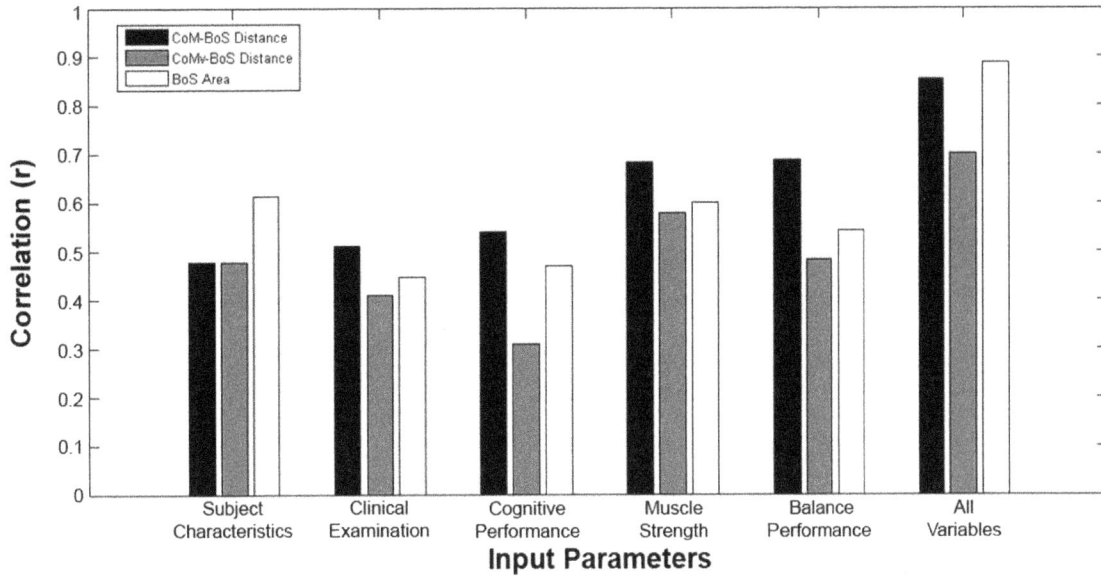

Figure 4. Maximum mapping performance of a three layer neural network in estimating the CoM-BoS distance, CoMv-Bos displacement and BoS area across the five different input variable categories as well as when using a combination of all input categories.

Results

The ability to calculate gait balance control using five functional domains as well as a combination of all variables were investigated (Table 1). In addition, 4 different hidden node sizes and 3 MSE error goals were assessed for a total of 72 network iterations. Minimal processing time was required for network training on all these combinations. When 5 hidden nodes were used, much greater time was needed for the solution to converge to an MSE error of less than 0.01 or 0.001, with much of the samples reaching the maximum limit of 500 epochs before failing to reach the goal (Figure 2). The use of 20 or 30 hidden nodes was much more efficient in training the data sets at all error goals.

The input type by error goal by hidden nodes interaction was not detected for the CoM-BoS (P = .849), CoMv-BoS (P = .877) or BoS Area (P = .477) correlations. Alternatively, an error goal main effect was demonstrated for all three balance control dependent variables (P<.001). Overall, as the error goal was decreased from 0.001 to 0.1 there was an increase in the correlation coefficient

(Figure 3), especially when utilizing 5 hidden nodes. Additionally, an increase in hidden nodes from 10 to 20 demonstrated on average a 0.10 greater correlation for the BoS area (P = 0.008) and a 0.08 greater correlation for the CoM-BoS distance (P = 0.057). Increasing to 30 hidden nodes demonstrated 0.08 and 0.11 greater correlation for the CoMv-BoS distance and BoS area, respectively (P = 0.016 and P = 0.004). No other hidden node or error goal differences were detected.

Input variable differences were also demonstrated, as greater correlations were demonstrated by using all variables, when compared to any single input type (Figure 4). The combination of all input variables, with 20 hidden nodes and a 0.001 error goal resulted in the best training across all three dependent variables (Table 2). The use of these parameters provided convergence within an average of 4 epochs to finish training the network and provided correlation values of R>0.80 for the CoM-BoS distance and BoS Area. On average, using all input variables, the ANN was able to calculate the CoMv-BoS distance to within 1 cm and the BoS Area to within 75 cm^2 for elderly adults (Figure 5).

Table 2. Average performance (SD) of selected combinations of inputs and the corresponding hidden nodes and error goal values that produced the highest accuracy.

Inputs	Hidden Nodes	Error goal	R[1]	R[2]	R[3]
All Input Variables	20	0.001	0.84 (0.06)	0.69 (0.16)	0.89 (0.05)
Clinical Balance and Clinical Exams	20	0.001	0.72 (0.22)	0.63 (0.12)	0.72 (0.10)
Clinical Balance and Cognitive Tests	20	0.01	0.67 (0.11)	0.54 (0.13)	0.63 (0.17)
Clinical Balance and Muscle Strength	20	0.01	0.74 (0.08)	0.73 (0.05)	0.63 (0.10)
Clinical Exams and Muscle Strength	20	0.01	0.71 (0.14)	0.57 (0.18)	0.72 (0.07)
Cognitive Tests and Muscle Strength	30	0.1	0.56 (0.08)	0.68 (0.04)	0.51 (0.05)

1 Correlations for the CoM-BoS distance.
2 Correlations for the CoMv-BoS displacement.
3 Correlations for the BoS Area.

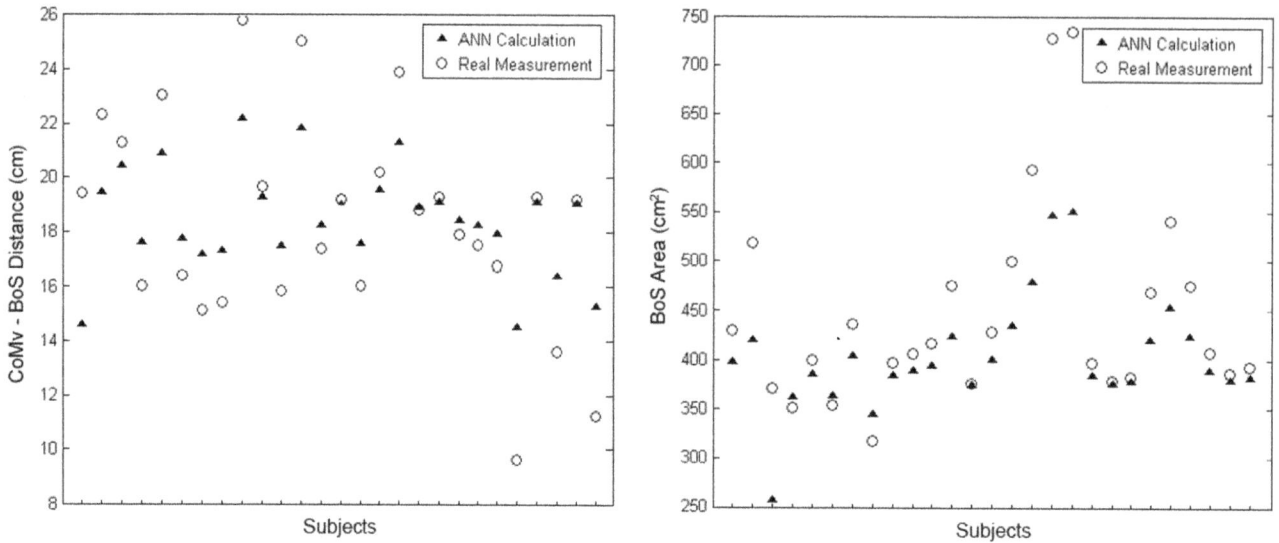

Figure 5. Representative data for the CoMv-BoS distance (A) and the BoS Area (B), as calculated by a neural network (triangles) with 20 hidden nodes and an error goal of 0.01. All input variables were included in this training set, with the actual values for these balance control measures represented by the open circles.

Utilizing all input variables, variability in input weights were demonstrated across all learning iterations of the neural network. While the predictive nature of the input weights is unknown, nonetheless, the largest weights in the input layer were found for the ABC test, vision performance, and hip abductor strength.

Discussion

The purpose of this study was to demonstrate that given clinical measures readily obtained by a physician, an artificial neural network can determine gait balance control among elderly adults ambulating in a laboratory. In support of our hypothesis, with the use of subject characteristics, clinical examinations, cognitive evaluations, and muscle strength, we were able to demonstrate that an ANN model could determine the balance control of elderly individuals during gait.

Utilizing a combination of all variables performed strongest in this study with correlation values for mapping clinical to balance control measures of up to 0.89. Among the various functional domains, muscle strength and clinical balance measures correlated to gait stability better than subject characteristics, clinical examinations, and cognitive performance. As the musculoskeletal system is the effector system which maintains posture and controls movement [24], it understandably plays an important role in predicting dynamic balance control. Among nursing home residents with a history of falls, the peak torque and power of knee extensors, knee flexors, ankle plantarflexors, and ankle dorsiflexors were significantly less than those of age-matched controls [25]. Similarly, clinical balance measures such as the BBS, though a measure of static balance ability, also maps strongly to dynamic CoM and BoS interactions during gait. Additionally, both muscle strength tests and clinical balance examinations are commonly used in the clinical setting to evaluate elderly adults at risk for falling.

As individual functional domains, subject characteristics, clinical examinations and cognitive performance did not map strongly to gait balance control performance. While age related differences have been reported for the BBS, TUG, and gait speed for male

and female older adults [26], these measures were not strongly correlated with gait balance control using the ANN mapping, as R values for these three domains ranged from 0.3 to 0.6. Interestingly, a combination of the TMT, SLUMS and GDS did not demonstrate strong mapping with gait balance control measures as well. Though depression has been associated with standing imbalance [27] and increased incidence of falls [28], similar relationships to gait balance control were weak. Similarly, medication use, prior falls and cognitive performance have all shown a relationship to falls, though they were not as strong when mapping to dynamic balance control [28]. Among our subject population though, most adults reported no depression, while being highly active and functional. Confirming the findings of the two strongly correlated functional domains, Rubenstein found that the important risk factors for falls are more often related to muscle weakness and gait or balance deficits [29].

Improvement in the ability to properly determine balance control measures were demonstrated with an increased number of hidden units. The use of additional hidden nodes has previously been hypothesized to be an indicator of enhanced generality, with greater plasticity and pathways to a solution [14]. Similar network architecture has been successful in gait research. The ability to characterize lower extremity joint kinematics and kinetics based on muscle electromyographic activity was shown to confirm with physiological expectations [13]. Prior studies have also utilized two hidden layer architectures and shown an ability to correctly identify gait conditions using fast Fourier transform of lower extremity kinematics as inputs, with up to 83% accuracy [30]. In the current study, single hidden layer architecture was utilized as this has been shown to be computationally faster and sufficient for learning functional relationships [31].

While neural network weights are variable and the predictive strengths unknown, the ABC score, vision, and hip abductor strength demonstrated the greatest weighting when all groupings were included as network inputs. The ABC, which is sometimes used as an indicator of fear of falling, has also been shown previously to be sensitive in discriminating fallers from non-fallers [32]. Similarly, the ability to maintain balance is a function of adequate visual information, with Nashner and Berthoz (1978) demonstrating that reduction in vision increased sway amplitude among older adults [33]. Furthermore, the hip abductor has been shown to be important in maintaining lateral stability, with changes in the base of support adapted by older adults in order to control the CoM and compensate for decreased hip abductor strength [34].

The use of biomechanics laboratory equipment to assess gait performance can be time consuming and expensive [7]. While biomechanical data are essential for determining the underlying mechanisms of balance impairment and possible fall incidents [35], the ability to categorize and identify community dwelling elderly fallers at risk of falls in a timely and inexpensive manner is needed. The strength of this study is the ability to map clinical measures routinely collected by physicians to dynamic gait measures which better characterize a person's balance control. The advantages of using an ANN is the ability to reveal the multifactorial factors that can lead to poor balance control during gait. By including a combination of five functional domains, it is possible to learn mappings from the clinical measures to dynamic balance control, and apply these connections to novel data sets.

A limitation of this study included the small sample size. Though only 56 adults have thus far been fully screened by a physician, the use of a neural network still demonstrated the ability to quickly be trained and showed high correlation values of up to 0.89. This provides further evidence that an ANN can successfully be used to assess a person's gait balance control, without the need for full assessment within a laboratory setting. Future research needs to investigate the generalizability of this algorithm to a larger sample of older adults. Additionally, utilization of a neural network to predict changes in balance control ability and fall risk in the elderly based on different interventions would be beneficial. The

ability for the network to provide predicted balance control outcomes based on improvements at the input layer, such as alterations in muscle strength, medications, or cognitive ability, will hopefully provide a quick and useful way to assess predicted changes in gait performance and possible fall risk. Similar assessments of fall risk are available for clinical examinations such as the BBS [4] or TUG [8], but a generalized form including all five domains would be a valuable tool for older adults and physicians.

In conclusion, results from this study demonstrated that an artificial neural network could be trained to map clinical variables to biomechanical measures of gait balance control. While further studies will investigate the generalizability of this network to a larger group of subjects, these initial findings suggest that an ANN can be used to assess balance impairment in the elderly.

Supporting Information

Program S1 MATLAB codes for the three-layer, feed-forward back-propagation ANN.

Acknowledgments

The authors would like to thank Drs. Tzurei Chen and Masahiro Fujimoto for their assistance during data collections.

Author Contributions

Conceived and designed the experiments: V. Lugade LCS. Performed the experiments: V. Lugade LSC V. Lin. Analyzed the data: V. Lugade LSC AF. Contributed reagents/materials/analysis tools: V. Lugade LSC AF. Wrote the paper: V. Lugade LSC AF V. Lin.

References

1. Sattin RW, Huber DAL, Devito CA, Rodriguez JG, Ros A, et al. (1990) The incidence of fall injury events among the elderly in a defined population. Am J Epidemiol 131: 1028–1037.
2. Lord SR, Sherrington C, Menz HB (2001) Falls in older people.
3. Tinetti ME, Speechley M (1989) Prevention of falls among the elderly. N Engl J Med 320: 1055–1059.
4. Shumway-Cook A, Baldwin M, Polissar NL, Gruber W (1997) Predicting the probability for falls in community-dwelling older adults. Phys Ther 77: 812–819.
5. Gabell A, Simons M, Nayak U (1985) Falls in the healthy elderly: predisposing causes. Ergonomics 28: 965–975.
6. Guralnik JM, Ferrucci L, Simonsick EM, Salive ME, Wallace RB (1995) Lower-extremity function in persons over the age of 70 years as a predictor of subsequent disability. N Engl J Med 332: 556–562.
7. Simon SR (2004) Quantification of human motion: gait analysis—benefits and limitations to its application to clinical problems. J Biomech 37: 1869–1880.
8. Shumway-Cook A, Brauer S, Woollacott M (2000) Predicting the probability for falls in community-dwelling older adults using the Timed Up & Go Test. Phys Ther 80: 896–903.
9. Hahn ME, Chou LS (2005) A model for detecting balance impairment and estimating falls risk in the elderly. Ann Biomed Eng 33: 811–820.
10. Miller A (2009) Gait event detection using a multilayer neural network. Gait & Posture 29: 542–545.
11. Michalski R, Wit A, Gajewski J (2011) Use of artificial neural networks for assessing parameters of gait symmetry. Acta of Bioengineering & Biomechanics 13.
12. Wu W-L, Su F-C (2000) Potential of the back propagation neural network in the assessment of gait patterns in ankle arthrodesis. Clinical Biomechanics 15: 143–145.
13. Sepulveda F, Wells DM, Vaughan CL (1993) A neural network representation of electromyography and joint dynamics in human gait. J Biomech 26: 101–109.
14. Hahn ME, Farley AM, Lin V, Chou LS (2005) Neural network estimation of balance control during locomotion. J Biomech 38: 717–724.
15. Sheikh JI, Yesavage JA (1986) Geriatric Depression Scale (GDS): Recent evidence and development of a shorter version. Clin Gerontol 5: 165–173.
16. Powell LE, Myers AM (1995) The activities-specific balance confidence (ABC) scale. J Gerontol A Biol Sci Med Sci 50: M28–M34.
17. Berg K (1989) Measuring balance in the elderly: preliminary development of an instrument. Physiother Can 41: 304–311.
18. Podsiadlo D, Richardson S (1991) The timed" Up & Go": a test of basic functional mobility for frail elderly persons. J Am Geriatr Soc 39: 142–148.
19. Corrigan JD, Hinkeldey NS (1987) Relationships between parts A and B of the Trail Making Test. J Clin Psychol 43: 402–409.
20. Tariq SH, Tumosa N, Chibnall JT, Perry III MH, Morley JE (2006) Comparison of the Saint Louis University mental status examination and the mini-mental state examination for detecting dementia and mild neurocognitive disorder—a pilot study. The American journal of geriatric psychiatry 14: 900–910.
21. Chou LS, Kaufman KR, Hahn ME, Brey RH (2003) Medio-lateral motion of the center of mass during obstacle crossing distinguishes elderly individuals with imbalance. Gait Posture 18: 125–133.
22. Lugade V, Lin V, Chou LS (2011) Center of mass and base of support interaction during gait. Gait Posture 33: 406–411.
23. Hagan MT, Menhaj MB (1994) Training feedforward networks with the Marquardt algorithm. Neural Networks, IEEE Transactions 5: 989–993.
24. Patla A, Frank J, Winter D (1992) Balance control in the elderly: implications for clinical assessment and rehabilitation. Can J Public Health 83: S29–33.
25. Whipple R, Wolfson L, Amerman P (1987) The relationship of knee and ankle weakness to falls in nursing home residents: an isokinetic study. J Am Geriatr Soc 35: 13–20.
26. Steffen TM, Hacker TA, Mollinger L (2002) Age-and gender-related test performance in community-dwelling elderly people: Six-Minute Walk Test, Berg Balance Scale, Timed Up & Go Test, and gait speeds. Phys Ther 82: 128–137.
27. Turcu A, Toubin S, Mourey F, D'Athis P, Manckoundia P, et al. (2004) Falls and depression in older people. Gerontology 50: 303–308.
28. Cesari M, Landi F, Torre S, Onder G, Lattanzio F, et al. (2002) Prevalence and risk factors for falls in an older community-dwelling population. J Gerontol A Biol Sci Med Sci 57: M722–M726.
29. Rubenstein LZ (2006) Falls in older people: epidemiology, risk factors and strategies for prevention. Age Ageing 35: ii37–ii41.
30. Barton JG, Lees A (1997) An application of neural networks for distinguishing gait patterns on the basis of hip-knee joint angle diagrams. Gait Posture 5: 28–33.
31. Chau T (2001) A review of analytical techniques for gait data. Part 2: neural network and wavelet methods. Gait Posture 13: 102–120.
32. Herman T, Mirelman A, Giladi N, Schweiger A, Hausdorff JM (2010) Executive control deficits as a prodrome to falls in healthy older adults: a prospective study

linking thinking, walking, and falling. J Gerontol A Biol Sci Med Sci 65: 1086–1092.

33. Nashner L, Berthoz A (1978) Visual contribution to rapid motor responses during postural control. Brain Res 150: 403–407.

34. Woollacott MH, Tang PF (1997) Balance control during walking in the older adult: research and its implications. Phys Ther 77: 646–660.

35. Bhatt T, Espy D, Yang F, Pai YC (2011) Dynamic gait stability, clinical correlates, and prognosis of falls among community-dwelling older adults. Arch Phys Med Rehabil 92: 799–805.

12

GABA Concentration in Posterior Cingulate Cortex Predicts Putamen Response during Resting State fMRI

Jorge Arrubla[1], Desmond H. Y. Tse[1], Christin Amkreutz[1,2], Irene Neuner[1,2,3], N. Jon Shah[1,3,4]*

1 Institute of Neuroscience and Medicine 4, INM 4, Forschungszentrum Jülich, Jülich, Germany, 2 Department of Psychiatry, Psychotherapy and Psychosomatics, RWTH Aachen University, Aachen, Germany, 3 JARA – BRAIN – Translational Medicine, RWTH Aachen University, Aachen, Germany, 4 Department of Neurology, RWTH Aachen University, Aachen, Germany

Abstract

The role of neurotransmitters in the activity of resting state networks has been gaining attention and has become a field of research with magnetic resonance spectroscopy (MRS) being one of the key techniques. MRS permits the measurement of γ-aminobutyric acid (GABA) and glutamate levels, the central biochemical constituents of the excitation-inhibition balance in vivo. The inhibitory effects of GABA in the brain have been largely investigated in relation to the activity of resting state networks in functional magnetic resonance imaging (fMRI). In this study GABA concentration in the posterior cingulate cortex (PCC) was measured using single voxel spectra acquired with standard point resolved spectroscopy (PRESS) from 20 healthy male volunteers at 3 T. Resting state fMRI was consecutively measured and the values of GABA/Creatine+ Phosphocreatine ratio (GABA ratio) were included in a general linear model matrix as a step of dual regression analysis in order to identify voxels whose neuroimaging metrics during rest were related to individual levels of the GABA ratio. Our data show that the connection strength of putamen to the default-mode network during resting state has a negative linear relationship with the GABA ratio measured in the PCC. These findings highlight the role of PCC and GABA in segregation of the motor input, which is an inherent condition that characterises resting state.

Editor: Yu-Feng Zang, Hangzhou Normal University, China

Funding: Jorge Arrubla and Desmond Tse are supported by the Marie Curie Initial Training Network Methods in Neuroimaging (MC-ITN-238593). N. Jon Shah is funded in part by the Helmholtz Alliance ICEMED - Imaging and Curing Environmental Metabolic Diseases, through the Initiative and Network Fund of the Helmholtz Association. Jorge Arrubla, Irene Neuner, and N. Jon Shah are also funded in part through the EU FP7 project TRIMAGE (Grant no. 602621). The funders had no role in study design, data collection and analysis, decision to publish, or preparation of the manuscript.

Competing Interests: The authors have declared that no competing interests exist.

* Email: n.j.shah@fz-juelich.de

Introduction

Resting state has become an emerging field of research the understanding of which has brought new insights into brain function. The concept of resting state arose from positron emission tomography (PET) and functional magnetic resonance imaging (fMRI) studies in which the focus moved from stimuli-related brain responses to the spontaneous fluctuations of activity when the brain is not engaged in any particular task [1–3]. It was thereby discovered that there exists a high correlation and temporal synchrony of the fMRI blood oxygen level-dependence (BOLD) series among relatively distant brain regions [3]. The analysis of resting state data is possible through independent component analysis (ICA) [4], where the low-frequency patterns of the resting state networks (RSN) are characterised and identified. The default-mode network (DMN) has gained particular interest due to its relationship with neurological and psychiatric conditions [5–13] as well as with normal aging [14].

The canonical DMN comprises precuneus, anterior cingulate cortex (ACC), posterior cingulate cortex (PCC), medial prefrontal cortex (MPfC) and lateral parietal inferior gyri (LPIG) [2,5,15]. The DMN is thought to characterise basal neural activity [16,17]

and has been linked to self-referential thought, introspection and integration of cognitive and emotional processing [18]. The DMN shows strong activity during rest, as well as rapid deactivation during externally directed tasks [19]. The DMN is also believed to represent an introspectively oriented mode of the mind which provides readiness and alertness to changes in the external and internal environment [15].

The posterior components of the DMN, precuneus and PCC, seem to act as an intrinsic mediatory node of this network [20,21]. Hagmann et al. [21] used diffusion imaging techniques to demonstrate the existence of a highly connected, complex brain network consisting of the posterior components of the DMN, and showed it to be highly activated at rest. Those regions showed a substantial correspondence between structural connectivity and resting-state functional connectivity.

The PCC has been extensively described as an 'evaluative region' [22], and includes Brodmann areas 29, 30, 23, and 31. This region is involved in spatial orientation and memory and it is likely that connections between posterior cingulate and parahippocampal cortices contribute to these processes [22]. Although PCC has been widely investigated, there is no consensus regarding its function [8]. The main functional characterisation of the PCC results from studies which investigate its role within the DMN [23]. PCC is implicated in awareness [24] and internally directed thoughts [13], which is supported by increased PCC activity during internally directed thoughts or during retrieval of autobiographical memories. Importantly, the PCC is one of the areas exhibiting significantly higher activity at rest, as it has been demonstrated by PET and arterial spin labelling [25]. Connectivity studies also demonstrate that the PCC is one of the regions with the highest local functional connectivity in resting conditions [26].

The role of neurotransmitter concentration in the activity of RSN is still not well understood and is an active field of research in magnetic resonance spectroscopy (MRS) [27]. MRS permits the measurement of γ-aminobutyric acid (GABA) and glutamate levels, the central biochemical constituents of the excitation-inhibition balance in vivo. In this sense, the presence of intra-regional and trans-regional neuro-biochemical modulation has been proposed [27]. The latter means that the concentration of a biochemical constituent, as measured by MRS, may predict activity in either the same region, i.e., intra-regionally, and/or another region, i.e., trans-regionally [27]. There is, for example, evidence which suggests the existence of complex interactions between neurotransmitters and the activity of the DMN [28]. Similarly, glutamate measured in the ACC was found to be related with the resting state activity in the same region [29]. The concentration of neurotransmitters has also been related to disease, such as depressive disorder, where abnormal levels of glutamate and GABA have been reported [30].

GABA is the most important inhibitory neurotransmitter in the brain; therefore, it has been linked to several neurological and psychiatric disorders such as epilepsy, panic disorder and depression [31]. Northoff et al. [32] found that the concentration of GABA in the ACC predicts negative BOLD responses of the same area during resting state. In a similar manner, Donahue et al. [33] reported that GABA concentration in the visual cortex is inversely correlated with BOLD signal variations and with cerebral blood flow, suggesting a link between neurochemical and MR-measured hemodynamic responses. In another study, BOLD magnitude was inversely correlated with GABA concentration in the visual cortex, suggesting that the excitation/inhibition cortical balance controls the functional neuroimaging measures [34]. Kapogiannis et al. [35] concluded that regional GABA and glutamate in the posteromedial cortex predict intrinsic functional connectivity of the DMN.

Based on evidence showing the importance of the PCC in the DMN and its importance during resting state [25], as well as the modulatory functions of GABA, we hypothesise that GABA concentration, explicitly the GABA/Cr+PCr ratio – hereafter referred to as the 'GABA ratio' – in the PCC measured by MRS has a direct relationship with the response of some areas in the DMN. Previous evidence shows the existence of linear correlations between neurochemicals and the BOLD contrast. Thus, we hypothesise that using a general linear model will reveal clusters exhibiting a linear relationship between the GABA ratio and the neuroimaging metrics measured during resting state, and therefore an assumption of 'predictability' could be made. 'Dual regression', an analysis tool proposed by Beckmann and co-workers [36], will be used in order to answer these questions. 'Dual regression' is a method which permits the identification of between-subject differences in resting functional connectivity [37] based on between-subject similarities using a dual regression approach within the framework of multi-subject-ICA analysis [38].

Materials and Methods

Subjects and data acquisition

Data were recorded from 20 healthy male volunteers (mean age = 25.4, SD = 3.7) in a 3 T Siemens Magnetom Trio scanner. Written, informed consent was obtained from all subjects and the study was approved by the Ethics Committee of the Medicine Faculty of the Rheinisch-Westfälischen Technischen Hochschule Aachen (RWTH Aachen University). The study was conducted in accordance with the Declaration of Helsinki. Subjects underwent medical interview and examination in order to exclude psychiatric and neurological conditions. Drug abuse, smoking status and medication intake were assessed using the DIA-X questionnaire (Diagnostisches Expertensystem für Psychische Störungen) [39]. All subjects were right-handed according to the Edinburgh handedness scale [40]. During the scanner procedure the subjects were requested to close their eyes and relax.

Functional images were acquired using a T2*-weighted EPI sequence (TR = 2.2 s, TE = 30 ms, field-of-view = 200 mm, slice thickness = 3 mm and number of slices = 36). The functional time series consisted of 165 volumes. Anatomical images were acquired for every subject by means of a Magnetization-Prepared, Rapid Acquisition Gradient-Echo (MP-RAGE) sequence (TR = 2250 ms, TE = 3.03 ms, field-of-view = 256 × 256 × 176 mm³, matrix size = 256 × 256, flip angle = 9°, 176 sagittal slices with 1 mm slice thickness and GRAPPA factor of 2 with 70 autocalibration signal lines).

To reliably resolve GABA resonance peaks at 1.9 ppm and 2.3 ppm, single voxel spectra were consecutively measured by standard point resolved spectroscopy (PRESS) with a set of optimised echo times reported by Napolitano et al. [41] (TE1 = 14 ms, TE = 105 ms, TR = 2.5 s, NA = 128, 25 mm × 25 mm × 25 mm voxel size, RF pulse centred at 2.4 ppm, 16 step phase cycling). The duration of the measurement was 5 minutes and 30 seconds. One extra complete phase cycle was measured without the water suppression RF pulse to record a water peak reference for eddy current correction and absolute metabolite concentration calibration. Before the spectroscopy measurements, the static magnetic field was homogenised by running FASTEST-MAP [42] iteratively to ensure that the full–width at half maximum (FWHM) of the reference water peak was below 0.05 ppm. The spectroscopy voxel was placed at the PCC by a trained operator (JA). See Figure 1.

MRS data analysis

The spectra were analysed with LCModel version 6.3-0I [43] using a GAMMA simulated basis set [44]. The simulation was 2D in the two directions where the slice selections were accomplished

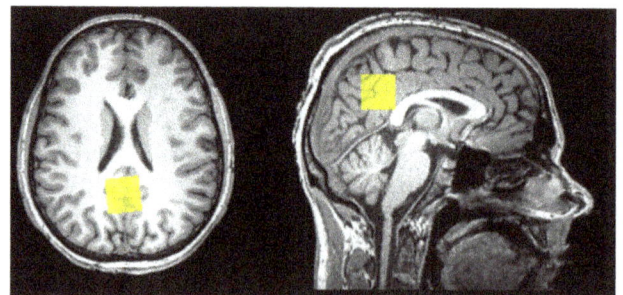

Figure 1. Depiction of voxel positioning for MRS on a background of a T1 individual structural image.

by 180-degree pulses [45]. The numerical waveforms of the 180-degree pulses were obtained directly from the scanner. The GABA ratio (GABA/Cr+PCr) was extracted and used as covariant in the fMRI resting state data analysis.

fMRI resting state data analysis

Analysis of functional data was carried out using Probabilistic Independent Component Analysis [38] as implemented in MELODIC (Multivariate Exploratory Linear Decomposition into Independent Components) Version 3.10, part of FSL (FMRIB's Software Library, www.fmrib.ox.ac.uk/fsl). Individual pre-processing consisted of motion correction using MCFLIRT [46], brain extraction using BET [47], spatial smoothing using a Gaussian kernel of FWHM of 5 mm, and high-pass temporal filtering of 100 s. Functional MRI volumes were registered to the structural scan of each individual and standard space (MNI152) images using FLIRT [46,48]. Temporal concatenation ICA was performed across all functional datasets from each subject using automatic dimensionality estimation [38]. The DMN was identified by visual inspection and comparison to previously published data [2,49] Finally, the dual regression algorithm [36] was applied to the ICs in order to identify the individual contribution of every subject to the RSNs using the GABA ratio in the PCC as a covariant in the second stage of dual regression analysis within the framework of the general linear model. Here, the subject-specific GABA ratio was tested for linear relationship with the subject-specific z–values of the IC representing the DMN. The different component maps were collected across subjects into single 4D files and tested voxel-wise for statistically significant correlation using nonparametric permutation testing (10000 permutations) [50] and 'threshold-free cluster enhancement' for improved sensitivity [51]. This resulted in spatial maps characterising the voxels with signal intensities that had a linear relationship (slope) with GABA ratio. The maps were thresholded and controlled for family-wise error rate at $p<0.05$ [52].

Additionally, a Pearson product-moment correlation was used to test whether the GABA ratio measured in the PCC had any relationship with the absolute and relative motion observed during the acquisition of the fMRI data.

Results

All the subjects reported full compliance with the instructions; no self-reports of having fallen asleep were given.

Twenty-three components were found after decomposition of the data by means of ICA. 'Meaningful' RSNs (i.e. representing neuronal signal as opposed to physiological and non-physiological noise such as vascular, respiratory and motion artefacts) were identified by matching them visually against a previously published set of data encompassing 20 'canonical' RSNs (http://fsl.fmrib.ox. ac.uk/analysis/brainmap+rsns) [49]. In accordance with the study by Smith et al. [49] the following 9 RSNs were identified in our data: right and left frontoparietal networks, medial visual network, occipital pole visual network, lateral visual network, DMN, auditory network, executive control network and sensorimotor network. The DMN was picked by visual inspection, comprising medial prefrontal cortex, anterior and posterior cingulate cortices, precuneus and lateral parietal inferior gyri [2,49]. See Figure 2.

The GABA ratio was successfully measured in the PCC using single voxel spectra (mean = 0.177, SD = 0.024).

The voxel-wise statistical maps, generated by the permutation test of dual regression, exhibited a cluster in the right putamen with significant values ($p<0.05$, corrected) where the connection strength within or to the DMN had a negative linear relationship

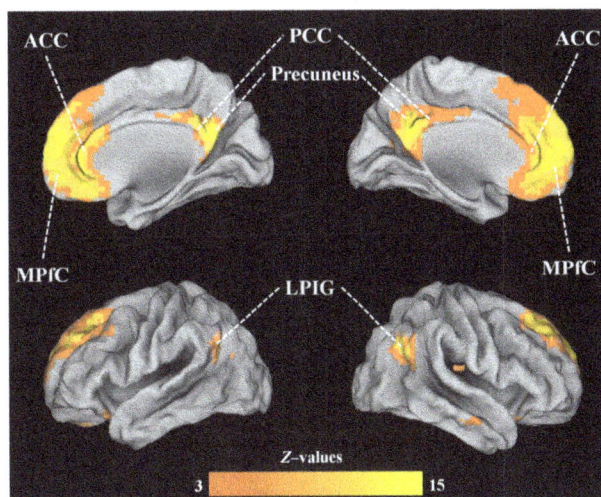

Figure 2. DMN identified in the group analysis of the 20 subjects; the DMN was picked by visual inspection, comprising medial prefrontal cortex (MPfC), anterior and posterior cingulate cortices (ACC and PCC), precuneus and lateral parietal inferior gyri (LPIG).

with GABA ratio measured in the PCC. See Table 1. The point of lowest p value (p = 0.0002) was located in the right putamen (MNI coordinates x = 26, y = 10, z = 4) according to the Harvard-Oxford Subcortical Structural Atlas (Figure 3).

The Pearson product-moment correlation between the GABA ratio and the absolute motion during the acquisition of the fMRI data was $r(18) = -0.321$, $p = 0.168$. In the case of the GABA ratio and the relative motion the correlation coefficient was $r(18) = -0.411$, $p = 0.072$.

Additionally, a region-of-interest analysis was performed in order to test whether a similar relationship between GABA ratio and signal intensity in the left putamen could be found. The mean z–values of the individual DMN maps were extracted from the left putamen according to the Harvard-Oxford Subcortical Structural Atlas and tested for correlation with the GABA ratio using the Pearson product-moment correlation. The correlation coefficient was $r(18) = -0.383$, $p = 0.095$ (Figure 4).

Discussion

Given the prior evidence of the modulatory role of GABA in the excitation/inhibition balance we investigated its role in the PCC, an important hub of the DMN. We conducted a study in healthy male volunteers in which the GABA ratio was measured in the PCC using MRS at 3 T. The measured values were included in the analysis of fMRI resting state data in order to identify the relationship between the GABA ratio values and the response of the DMN. Our results show that the activity of the right putamen in the DMN has a negative linear relationship with the GABA ratio measured in the PCC.

The results presented here confirm previous observations in which GABA concentration had an inverse relationship with the magnitude of BOLD signal [32,33], and suggest that the putamen is a structure whose activity during resting state is intrinsically modulated by the concentration of GABA. Previous investigations already showed how regional BOLD signal appears to be governed by local GABA concentration either in the same or other regions [27,32–34].

Table 1. MNI coordinates (2 mm template) of clusters with minimal P values of linear relationship between GABA ratio and z-values in the DMN.

Number of significant voxels in the cluster	Regions of minimum p value according to the Harvard-Oxford Cortical Structural Atlas	Min. corrected *P* value	MNI coordinates		
			x	*y*	*z*
65	96% Right Putamen, 4% Right Cerebral White Matter	0.0002	26	10	4

The negative relationship found between GABA ratio and the right putamen response seems to be also extended to the left putamen; although in our data it did not achieve statistical significance probably due to the number of participants and the strictness of the statistical model used for the voxel-wise analysis.

Noteworthy is the fact that the putamen is not part of the DMN, although it has been described as being part of a basal ganglia RSN, which corresponds to the motor control circuit [53,54]. The interactions among RSNs have been extensively described, particularly for the case of the DMN, which is the network holding hubs with the highest global functional connectivity [55]. A recent fMRI study suggests the presence of complex modulatory interactions among the DMN and the other networks in resting state. Such communications among networks seem to be modulated by critical brain structures such as the basal ganglia and the thalamus [56]. Moreover, there is evidence of negative interactions between the basal ganglia and the activity of the DMN [56]. In this regard, Tomasi et al. [53] described the existing segregation of the DMN from the other networks, which appears to be necessary for its deactivation during task performance. The results presented here suggest that GABA is a critical neurotransmitter for the interactions among RSNs, particularly for the case of the DMN and the basal ganglia RSN, where putamen is a relevant structure.

The importance of the putamen in the activity of the DMN has also been previously described. In a PET study Tomasi et al. [57] demonstrated that the availability of dopamine and dopamine transporters in the putamen had a negative linear correlation with deactivation in areas belonging to the DMN. Moreover, the putamen has been included as one of the regions with higher local functional connectivity density at rest [26], and there is evidence of segregation towards this structure to slow the access to cortical sources [55].

Functions of the putamen are majorly categorised as 'motor functions'. It has a well-known role in motor preparation, execution and control [58]. In an fMRI study it was established that putamen is a target area for proactive motor inhibition driven by the MPfC and the inferior parietal cortex [59]. Among the functions of putamen, learning and memory processes have also been described [60], particularly in studies where lesions of the putamen impair visual discrimination and learning in non-human primates [61]. Further evidence on the functions of the putamen is provided by the pathophysiology of Parkinson's and Huntington's disease, both exhibiting a variety of cognitive deficits as well as cell loss in the putamen. Nigrostriatal projection loss with dopamine deficiency in the putamen is the feature that characterises Parkinson's disease [62], while atrophy patterns in the putamen have been described at different stages of Huntington's disease [63].

Modulatory functions of neurotransmitters in relation to the putamen have also been described. In an animal study, Packard [64] demonstrated that rats which received an infusion of glutamate in the caudate-putamen exhibited increased place learning which influenced behaviour. This evidence suggests that the learning functions modulated by the putamen might depend on the concentration and/or balance of neurotransmitters. Our results extend the mutual modulatory role over the putamen also to GABA, although just in the sense of segregation of the motor input that occurs during resting state and that is driven by the activity of the DMN. Our results add to the existing evidence that GABA is an important neurotransmitter with diverse functions during resting state [32,33]. The results presented here highlight the role of GABA in the segregation of the motor engagement, which is an inherent condition that characterises resting state.

The inhibitory functions of GABA have also been well-described [65]. GABAergic systems mediate most fast synaptic inhibition in the mammalian brain, controlling activity at both the network and the cellular levels. There is evidence of the role of GABA in motor inhibition [66], and moreover, our results highlight its inhibitory functions during resting state. Based on the best evidence our study included only male volunteers. The effect of female gonadal steroids on GABAergic systems is well-known and has been described as a modulator factor [67]. In a MRS study, Epperson et al. [68] found a reduction in cortical GABA levels during the follicular phase of the human menstrual cycle, and therefore, this explorative study included only male volunteers.

Inhibitory functions direct multiple processes and networks in the central nervous system. In an fMRI study, Jaffard et al. [59] identified a network involved in motor inhibition which included the superior parietal lobule, PCC, precuneus, parahippocampal gyrus and thalamus. Some of these areas also belong to the DMN; hence they conclude that the resting state activity, which is not directly related to identifiable sensory or motor events, controls the balance between excitatory and inhibitory activations determining responsiveness to possible incoming events [59]. The PCC has been identified as a key structure in inhibition tasks with a possible role in alertness. Furthermore, activation of the putamen was identified when motor inhibition was expected to be 'on'. Additionally, Hu and Li [69] confirmed that the PCC and putamen were both identified as areas involved in preparatory motor execution during rest. Moreover, dense anatomical connections between the PCC and the striatum have been described [8], supporting the role of PCC in directing the segregation of the motor input.

The conclusion in the study by Jaffard et al. [59], according to which the activity at rest may be partly due to an active and sustained process consisting of locked movement initiation mechanism, is in line with our results and, moreover, we hypothesise that this mechanism is linked to the concentration of GABA. The fact that the concentration of GABA in the PCC, the 'core' of resting state, predicts the BOLD response of the putamen supports this hypothesis.

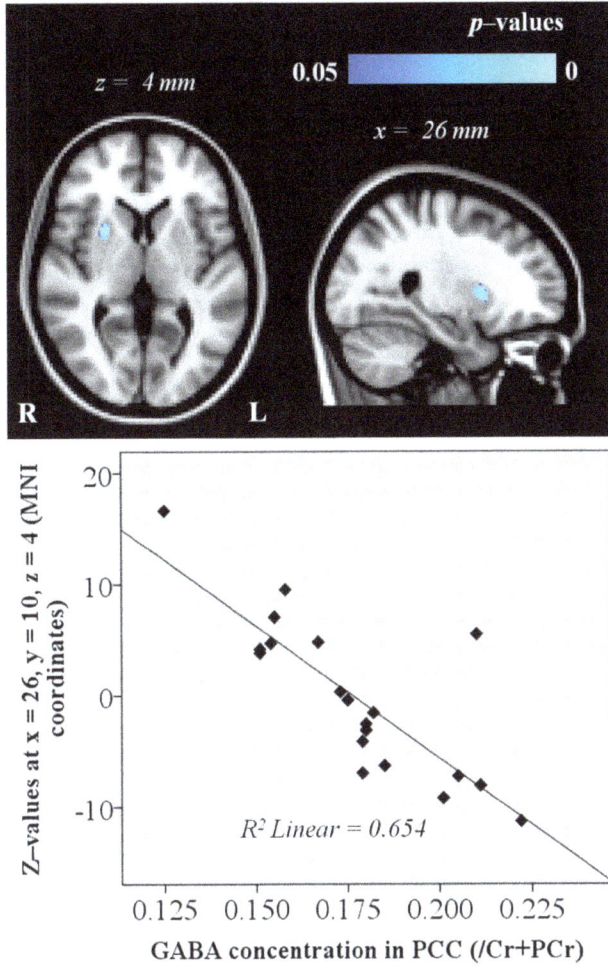

Figure 3. Voxel-wise statistical maps with the inclusion of the GABA ratio measured in the PCC and generated by the dual regression analysis of the DMN. Significant voxels thresholded at p<0.05 (corrected). The point of lowest p value (p = 0.0002) was located in MNI coordinates x = 26, y = 10, z = 4. The background image is the MNI152 T1 (2 mm) template.

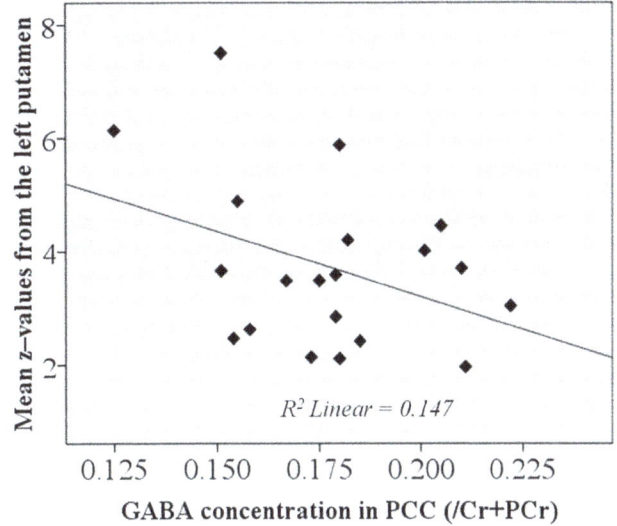

Figure 4. Mean z–values extracted from the left putamen in relation to GABA ratio in the PCC.

Even though our results appear plausible from a physiological point of view, some limitations must be mentioned. Unfortunately, the measures that each of the modalities provides are not necessarily complementary [27]. Furthermore, the concentrations of transmitters measured by MRS reflect also pools that are not used for neurotransmission, making it more difficult to understand the exact mechanisms of the neuro-biochemical relationships. Hence, the approach described here does not permit to answer questions of causality.

GABA has a concentration of about 1 mM in human brain. This is about an order of magnitude lower than that of some other metabolites and is about 40,000 times lower than the concentration of water [70]. At 3 T, resonance peaks of GABA at 1.9 ppm, 2.3 ppm and 3.0 ppm overlap with the large resonance peaks from n-acetyl aspartate (NAA), total glutamate and glutamine (Glx), and creatine (Cr), respectively. These overlaps make the detection of GABA error-prone. Currently, the most commonly applied MRS method to separate the GABA signal from the rest of the spectrum is Mescher-Garwood point resolved spectroscopy (MEGA-PRESS), in which the J-coupling between GABA-H3 at 1.9 ppm

and GABA-H4 at 3.0 ppm is exploited by an on/off frequency selective RF pulse applied at 1.9 ppm [71]. Due to the lack of J-coupling at 1.9 ppm for Cr, its signal at 3.0 ppm is removed by taking the difference from the two sets of measurements, leaving only the GABA-H4 peaks at 3.0 ppm. This method relies on the subtraction of two sets of spectra to remove any strong overlapping peaks; hence, it is vulnerable to any instability caused by the scanner, e.g., magnetic field drift, or by the subject, e.g., movement.

Another popular method to detect GABA is two-dimensional MRS [72] in which a series of spectra that differ by a single parameter, such as a delay duration or the timing of a refocusing pulse, are acquired. The second spectral dimension contains the coupling information which, in turn, allows overlapping multiplets to be resolved. However, these experiments usually require longer acquisition time due to the increased number of measurements. Recently, Napolitano et al. [41] demonstrated that using a standard PRESS sequence with a set of optimised echo time parameters, they could reliably detect GABA in the ACC and the precuneus region in a shorter measurement time and in a smaller voxel size than previous studies with MEGA-PRESS. Due to the time constrain of the multi-modality investigation in this study, the standard PRESS sequence with optimised echo time parameters was chosen to detect GABA.

The use of GABA ratio in the present study instead of absolute concentration is in agreement with previous publications [33,35], in which metabolite levels are commonly reported as their ratio to creatine. Creatine has been shown to be a stable metabolite in healthy individuals [73] and thus is commonly used as an internal reference in brain spectroscopy. Furthermore, in a study by Bogner et al. [74] GABA ratio exhibited the best reproducibility.

From a technical point of view, we must remark that the separation and quantification of metabolites are often ambiguous and difficult due to several factors. First, since 80% of brain tissue is endogenous water, the water resonance peaks is several orders of magnitude higher than that of the metabolites, which can potentially distorts nearby metabolite resonance signals. Second, large subcutaneous lipids signals can potentially ruin metabolite signals. Third, the spectral resolution as well as the signal-to-noise ratio are often reduced by the anatomical induced magnetic field spatial inhomogeneity. Despite these difficulties were overcome in this study, the process of separating metabolite signals is still challenging because of the large number of overlapping metabolite resonance peaks confined in a narrow chemical shift range of ~4 ppm.

Conclusions

The results presented here show that the connection strength of putamen to the DMN during resting state has a negative linear relationship with the GABA ratio measured in the PCC. These findings highlight the role of PCC and γ-aminobutyric acid in the segregation of the motor input that occurs during resting state.

Our data support the notion that the activity of the DMN implies deactivation of the motor control circuit, which corresponds to the basal ganglia RSN, where putamen is a relevant structure. This study confirms once more the possibility and utility of measuring local concentration of transmitters using MRS.

Author Contributions

Conceived and designed the experiments: JA IN. Performed the experiments: JA DT CA. Analyzed the data: JA DT. Contributed reagents/materials/analysis tools: IN NJS. Contributed to the writing of the manuscript: JA DT IN NJS.

References

1. Biswal B, Yetkin FZ, Haughton VM, Hyde JS (1995) Functional connectivity in the motor cortex of resting human brain using echo-planar MRI. Magn Reson Med 34: 537–541.
2. Raichle ME, MacLeod AM, Snyder AZ, Powers WJ, Gusnard DA, et al. (2001) A default mode of brain function. Proc Natl Acad Sci U S A 98: 676–682.
3. Biswal BB, Van Kylen J, Hyde JS (1997) Simultaneous assessment of flow and BOLD signals in resting-state functional connectivity maps. NMR Biomed 10: 165–170.
4. Beckmann CF, DeLuca M, Devlin JT, Smith SM (2005) Investigations into resting-state connectivity using independent component analysis. Philos Trans R Soc Lond B Biol Sci 360: 1001–1013.
5. Greicius MD, Srivastava G, Reiss AL, Menon V (2004) Default-mode network activity distinguishes Alzheimer's disease from healthy aging: evidence from functional MRI. Proc Natl Acad Sci U S A 101: 4637–4642.
6. Bluhm RL, Miller J, Lanius RA, Osuch EA, Boksman K, et al. (2007) Spontaneous low-frequency fluctuations in the BOLD signal in schizophrenic patients: anomalies in the default network. Schizophr Bull 33: 1004–1012.
7. Delaveau P, Salgado-Pineda P, Fossati P, Witjas T, Azulay J-P, et al. (2010) Dopaminergic modulation of the default mode network in Parkinson's disease. Eur Neuropsychopharmacol 20: 784–792.
8. Leech R, Sharp DJ (2014) The role of the posterior cingulate cortex in cognition and disease. Brain 137: 12–32.
9. Quarantelli M, Salvatore E, Giorgio SMDA, Filla A, Cervo A, et al. (2013) Default-mode network changes in Huntington's disease: an integrated MRI study of functional connectivity and morphometry. PLoS One 8: e72159.
10. Sorg C, Riedl V, Mühlau M, Calhoun VD, Eichele T, et al. (2007) Selective changes of resting-state networks in individuals at risk for Alzheimer's disease. Proc Natl Acad Sci U S A 104: 18760–18765.
11. Werner CJ, Dogan I, Saß C, Mirzazade S, Schiefer J, et al. (2014) Altered resting-state connectivity in Huntington's Disease. Hum Brain Mapp 35:2582–2593.
12. Whitfield-Gabrieli S, Thermenos HW, Milanovic S, Tsuang MT, Faraone S V, et al. (2009) Hyperactivity and hyperconnectivity of the default network in schizophrenia and in first-degree relatives of persons with schizophrenia. Proc Natl Acad Sci U S A 106: 1279–1284.
13. Buckner RL, Andrews-Hanna JR, Schacter DL (2008) The brain's default network: anatomy, function, and relevance to disease. Ann N Y Acad Sci 1124: 1–38.
14. Damoiseaux JS, Beckmann CF, Arigita EJS, Barkhof F, Scheltens P, et al. (2008) Reduced resting-state brain activity in the "default network" in normal aging. Cereb Cortex 18: 1856–1864.
15. Fransson P (2005) Spontaneous low-frequency BOLD signal fluctuations: an fMRI investigation of the resting-state default mode of brain function hypothesis. Hum Brain Mapp 26: 15–29.
16. Snyder AZ, Raichle ME (2012) A brief history of the resting state: The Washington University perspective. Neuroimage 62: 1–9.
17. Raichle ME, Snyder AZ (2007) A default mode of brain function: a brief history of an evolving idea. Neuroimage 37: 1083–90; discussion 1097–9.
18. Greicius MD, Krasnow B, Reiss AL, Menon V (2003) Functional connectivity in the resting brain: a network analysis of the default mode hypothesis. Proc Natl Acad Sci U S A 100: 253–258.
19. Fox MD, Snyder AZ, Vincent JL, Corbetta M, Van Essen DC, et al. (2005) The human brain is intrinsically organized into dynamic, anticorrelated functional networks. Proc Natl Acad Sci U S A 102: 9673–9678.
20. Cavanna AE, Trimble MR (2006) The precuneus: a review of its functional anatomy and behavioural correlates. Brain 129: 564–583.
21. Hagmann P, Cammoun L, Gigandet X, Meuli R, Honey CJ, et al. (2008) Mapping the structural core of human cerebral cortex. PLoS Biol 6: e159.
22. Vogt BA, Finch DM, Olson CR (1992) Functional heterogeneity in cingulate cortex: the anterior executive and posterior evaluative regions. Cereb Cortex 2: 435–443.
23. Greicius MD, Supekar K, Menon V, Dougherty RF (2009) Resting-state functional connectivity reflects structural connectivity in the default mode network. Cereb Cortex 19: 72–78.
24. Vogt BA, Laureys S (2005) Posterior cingulate, precuneal and retrosplenial cortices: cytology and components of the neural network correlates of consciousness. Prog Brain Res 150: 205–217.
25. Zou Q, Wu CW, Stein EA, Zang Y, Yang Y (2009) Static and dynamic characteristics of cerebral blood flow during the resting state. Neuroimage 48: 515–524.
26. Tomasi D, Volkow ND (2010) Functional connectivity density mapping. Proc Natl Acad Sci U S A 107: 9885–9890.
27. Duncan NW, Wiebking C, Muñoz-Torres Z, Northoff G (2014) How to investigate neuro-biochemical relationships on a regional level in humans? Methodological considerations for combining functional with biochemical imaging. J Neurosci Methods 221: 183–188.
28. Hahn A, Wadsak W, Windischberger C, Baldinger P, Höflich AS, et al. (2012) Differential modulation of the default mode network via serotonin-1A receptors. Proc Natl Acad Sci U S A 109: 2619–2624.
29. Enzi B, Duncan NW, Kaufmann J, Tempelmann C, Wiebking C, et al. (2012) Glutamate modulates resting state activity in the perigenual anterior cingulate cortex - a combined fMRI-MRS study. Neuroscience 227: 102–109.
30. Hasler G, van der Veen JW, Tumonis T, Meyers N, Shen J, et al. (2007) Reduced prefrontal glutamate/glutamine and gamma-aminobutyric acid levels in major depression determined using proton magnetic resonance spectroscopy. Arch Gen Psychiatry 64: 193–200.
31. Sanacora G, Gueorguieva R, Epperson CN, Wu Y-T, Appel M, et al. (2004) Subtype-specific alterations of gamma-aminobutyric acid and glutamate in patients with major depression. Arch Gen Psychiatry 61: 705–713.
32. Northoff G, Walter M, Schulte RF, Beck J, Dydak U, et al. (2007) GABA concentrations in the human anterior cingulate cortex predict negative BOLD responses in fMRI. Nat Neurosci 10: 1515–1517.
33. Donahue MJ, Near J, Blicher JU, Jezzard P (2010) Baseline GABA concentration and fMRI response. Neuroimage 53: 392–398.
34. Muthukumaraswamy SD, Edden RAE, Jones DK, Swettenham JB, Singh KD (2009) Resting GABA concentration predicts peak gamma frequency and fMRI amplitude in response to visual stimulation in humans. Proc Natl Acad Sci U S A 106: 8356–8361.
35. Kapogiannis D, Reiter DA, Willette AA, Mattson MP (2013) Posteromedial cortex glutamate and GABA predict intrinsic functional connectivity of the default mode network. Neuroimage 64: 112–119.
36. Filippini N, MacIntosh BJ, Hough MG, Goodwin GM, Frisoni GB, et al. (2009) Distinct patterns of brain activity in young carriers of the APOE-ε4 allele. Proc Natl Acad Sci 106: 7209–7214.
37. Zuo X-N, Kelly C, Adelstein JS, Klein DF, Castellanos FX, et al. (2010) Reliable intrinsic connectivity networks: test-retest evaluation using ICA and dual regression approach. Neuroimage 49: 2163–2177.
38. Beckmann CF, Smith SM (2004) Probabilistic independent component analysis for functional magnetic resonance imaging. IEEE Trans Med Imaging 23: 137–152.
39. Wittchen H-U, Pfister H (1997) DIA-X-Interviews: Manual für Screening-Verfahren und Interview; Interviewheft. Available: http://pubman.mpdl.mpg.de/pubman/faces/viewItemFullPage.jsp;jsessionid=7E7416C4873C2CE37AD0EAA806D6A319?itemId=escidoc:1646479:1&view=EXPORT.
40. Oldfield RC (1971) The assessment and analysis of handedness: the Edinburgh inventory. Neuropsychologia 9: 97–113.
41. Napolitano A, Kockenberger W, Auer DP (2013) Reliable gamma aminobutyric acid measurement using optimized PRESS at 3 T. Magn Reson Med 69: 1528–1533.
42. Gruetter R, Tkác I (2000) Field mapping without reference scan using asymmetric echo-planar techniques. Magn Reson Med 43: 319–323.
43. Provencher SW (2001) Automatic quantitation of localized in vivo 1H spectra with LCModel. NMR Biomed 14: 260–264.
44. Smith SA, Levante TO, Meier BH, Ernst RR (1994) Computer Simulations in Magnetic Resonance. An Object-Oriented Programming Approach. J Magn Reson Ser A 106: 75–105.

45. Maudsley AA, Govindaraju V, Young K, Aygula ZK, Pattany PM, et al. (2005) Numerical simulation of PRESS localized MR spectroscopy. J Magn Reson 173: 54–63.

46. Jenkinson M, Bannister P, Brady M, Smith S (2002) Improved optimization for the robust and accurate linear registration and motion correction of brain images. Neuroimage 17: 825–841.

47. Smith SM (2002) Fast robust automated brain extraction. Hum Brain Mapp 17: 143–155.

48. Jenkinson M, Smith S (2001) A global optimisation method for robust affine registration of brain images. Med Image Anal 5: 143–156.

49. Smith SM, Fox PT, Miller KL, Glahn DC, Fox PM, et al. (2009) Correspondence of the brain's functional architecture during activation and rest. Proc Natl Acad Sci U S A 106: 13040–13045.

50. Nichols TE, Holmes AP (2002) Nonparametric permutation tests for functional neuroimaging: a primer with examples. Hum Brain Mapp 15: 1–25.

51. Smith SM, Nichols TE (2009) Threshold-free cluster enhancement: addressing problems of smoothing, threshold dependence and localisation in cluster inference. Neuroimage 44: 83–98.

52. Nichols T, Hayasaka S (2003) Controlling the familywise error rate in functional neuroimaging: a comparative review. Stat Methods Med Res 12: 419–446.

53. Tomasi D, Volkow ND (2011) Association between functional connectivity hubs and brain networks. Cereb Cortex 21: 2003–2013.

54. Robinson S, Basso G, Soldati N, Sailer U, Jovicich J, et al. (2009) A resting state network in the motor control circuit of the basal ganglia. BMC Neurosci 10: 137.

55. Tomasi D, Volkow ND (2011) Functional connectivity hubs in the human brain. Neuroimage 57: 908–917.

56. Di X, Biswal BB (2014) Modulatory interactions between the default mode network and task positive networks in resting-state. PeerJ 2: e367.

57. Tomasi D, Volkow ND, Wang R, Telang F, Wang G-J, et al. (2009) Dopamine transporters in striatum correlate with deactivation in the default mode network during visuospatial attention. PLoS One 4: e6102.

58. DeLong MR, Alexander GE, Georgopoulos AP, Crutcher MD, Mitchell SJ, et al. (1984) Role of basal ganglia in limb movements. Hum Neurobiol 2: 235–244.

59. Jaffard M, Longcamp M, Velay J-L, Anton J-L, Roth M, et al. (2008) Proactive inhibitory control of movement assessed by event-related fMRI. Neuroimage 42: 1196–1206.

60. Packard MG, Knowlton BJ (2002) Learning and memory functions of the Basal Ganglia. Annu Rev Neurosci 25: 563–593.

61. Buerger AA, Gross CG, Rocha-Miranda CE (1974) Effects of ventral putamen lesions on discrimination learning by monkeys. J Comp Physiol Psychol 86: 440–446.

62. Brooks DJ (2010) Imaging approaches to Parkinson disease. J Nucl Med 51: 596–609.

63. Younes L, Ratnanather JT, Brown T, Aylward E, Nopoulos P, et al. (2012) Regionally selective atrophy of subcortical structures in prodromal HD as revealed by statistical shape analysis. Hum Brain Mapp 35:792–809.

64. Packard MG (1999) Glutamate infused posttraining into the hippocampus or caudate-putamen differentially strengthens place and response learning. Proc Natl Acad Sci U S A 96: 12881–12886.

65. Jacob TC, Moss SJ, Jurd R (2008) GABA(A) receptor trafficking and its role in the dynamic modulation of neuronal inhibition. Nat Rev Neurosci 9: 331–343.

66. Van den Wildenberg WPM, Burle B, Vidal F, van der Molen MW, Ridderinkhof KR, et al. (2010) Mechanisms and dynamics of cortical motor inhibition in the stop-signal paradigm: a TMS study. J Cogn Neurosci 22: 225–239.

67. Majewska MD, Harrison NL, Schwartz RD, Barker JL, Paul SM (1986) Steroid hormone metabolites are barbiturate-like modulators of the GABA receptor. Science 232: 1004–1007.

68. Epperson CN, Haga K, Mason GF, Sellers E, Gueorguieva R, et al. (2002) Cortical gamma-aminobutyric acid levels across the menstrual cycle in healthy women and those with premenstrual dysphoric disorder: a proton magnetic resonance spectroscopy study. Arch Gen Psychiatry 59: 851–858.

69. Hu S, Li C-SR (2012) Neural processes of preparatory control for stop signal inhibition. Hum Brain Mapp 33: 2785–2796.

70. Puts NAJ, Edden RAE (2012) In vivo magnetic resonance spectroscopy of GABA: a methodological review. Prog Nucl Magn Reson Spectrosc 60: 29–41.

71. Mescher M, Merkle H, Kirsch J, Garwood M, Gruetter R (1998) Simultaneous in vivo spectral editing and water suppression. NMR Biomed 11: 266–272.

72. Ke Y, Cohen BM, Bang JY, Yang M, Renshaw PF (2000) Assessment of GABA concentration in human brain using two-dimensional proton magnetic resonance spectroscopy. Psychiatry Res 100: 169–178.

73. Soher BJ, van Zijl PC, Duyn JH, Barker PB (1996) Quantitative proton MR spectroscopic imaging of the human brain. Magn Reson Med 35: 356–363.

74. Bogner W, Gruber S, Doelken M, Stadlbauer A, Ganslandt O, et al. (2010) In vivo quantification of intracerebral GABA by single-voxel (1)H-MRS-How reproducible are the results? Eur J Radiol 73: 526–531.

13

Influenza Virus Infection Induces the Nuclear Relocalization of the Hsp90 Co-Chaperone p23 and Inhibits the Glucocorticoid Receptor Response

Xingyi Ge[1,2,3◉], Marie-Anne Rameix-Welti[1,2,3,4◉], Elyanne Gault[1,2,3,4◉], Geoffrey Chase[5], Emmanuel dos Santos Afonso[1,2,3¤], Didier Picard[6], Martin Schwemmle[5], Nadia Naffakh[1,2,3*]

1 Institut Pasteur, Unité de Génétique Moléculaire des Virus à ARN, Département de Virologie, Paris, France, 2 CNRS, URA3015, Paris, France, 3 Université Paris Diderot, Sorbonne Paris Cité, Unité de Génétique Moléculaire des Virus à ARN, Paris, France, 4 Université Versailles Saint-Quentin-en-Yvelines, Guyancourt, France, 5 Department of Virology, Institute for Medical Microbiology and Hygiene, University of Freiburg, Germany, 6 Département de Biologie Cellulaire, Université de Genève, Genève, Switzerland

Abstract

The genomic RNAs of influenza A viruses are associated with the viral polymerase subunits (PB1, PB2, PA) and nucleoprotein (NP), forming ribonucleoprotein complexes (RNPs). Transcription/replication of the viral genome occurs in the nucleus of infected cells. A role for Hsp90 in nuclear import and assembly of newly synthetized RNA-polymerase subunits has been proposed. Here we report that the p23 cochaperone of Hsp90, which plays a major role in glucocorticoid receptor folding and function, associates with influenza virus polymerase. We show that p23 is not essential for viral multiplication in cultured cells but relocalizes to the nucleus in influenza virus-infected cells, which may alter some functions of p23 and Hsp90. Moreover, we show that influenza virus infection inhibits glucocorticoid receptor-mediated gene transactivation, and that this negative effect can occur through a p23-independent pathway. Viral-induced inhibition of the glucocorticoid receptor response might be of significant importance regarding the physiopathology of influenza infections in vivo.

Editor: Paul Digard, University of Cambridge, United Kingdom

Funding: Institut Pasteur (http://www.pasteur.fr), FLUINNATE SP5B-CT-2006-044161 EU program (http://www.fluinnate.org/), and FLUPHARM FP7-INFLUENZA-2010-259751 (http://flupharm.eu). X.G. was supported by a fellowship from the Chinese Academy of Sciences. The funders had no role in study design, data collection and analysis, decision to publish, or preparation of the manuscript.

Competing Interests: The authors have declared that no competing interests exist.

* E-mail: nadia.naffakh@pasteur.fr

¤ Current address: Promega France, Charbonnières-les-Bains, France

◉ These authors contributed equally to this work.

Introduction

The genome of influenza A viruses consists of eight molecules of single-stranded RNA of negative polarity. The viral RNAs (vRNAs) are associated with the nucleoprotein (NP) and with the three subunits of the polymerase complex (PB1, PB2 and PA) to form viral ribonucleoproteins (vRNPs) (reviewed in [1]). Once in the infected cells, the vRNPs are transported to the nucleus, where they undergo transcription and replication. Newly synthetised NP and polymerase subunits are imported from the cytoplasm into the nucleus to form new vRNPs. At late stages in infection, vRNPs are exported from the nucleus to the cytoplasm, and assembly with the other viral proteins occurs at the plasma membrane. There are evidence for physical and functional association between the vRNP components and the cellular machineries for transcription, nuclear import and nuclear export. A model for the import of newly synthetised polymerase has been proposed, based on the findings that the RanBP5 importin interacts with the PB1-PA dimer [2], and importins α interacts with PB2 [3,4]. The Hsp90 protein was found to interact with both PB1 and PB2 and to undergo nuclear relocalization in infected cells [5], suggesting that it could also be involved in nuclear import of newly synthetised

viral polymerase subunits. Nuclear proteins are clearly involved in the production of viral RNAs. In particular, the synthesis and processing of viral messenger RNAs (mRNAs) depends on cellular mRNAs transcription [1,6,7,8,9,10], splicing [11] and export [12,13] machineries. Nuclear export of the newly synthetized vRNPs is promoted by the M1 and NEP viral proteins and mediated by molecular interactions with the cellular CRM1 export pathway [14,15]. Further characterization of the interplay between vRNPs and host factors is needed for a better understanding of the molecular mechanisms of viral RNAs synthesis and trafficking in the host cell, and the role of the RNA polymerase as a determinant of influenza virus host range and pathogenicity. In the longer term, it could provide a rationale for the development of antivirals targeting essential interactions between vRNPs and host factors.

Here we used a recombinant influenza virus expressing a PB2 protein fused to a purification tag to identify vRNP-associated host factors. We report that the p23 cochaperone of Hsp90, which plays a major role in the folding and function of glucocorticoid receptors [16], associates with the viral polymerase and relocalizes to the nucleus in influenza virus-infected cells. We show that p23 is not essential for viral multiplication in cultured cells, and that glucocorticoid receptor-mediated signalling is impaired in influenza virus-infected cells.

Materials and Methods

Plasmids

The series of eight pPolI plasmids containing the sequences corresponding to the genomic segments of WSN virus, and the four recombinant pcDNA3.1 plasmids for the expression of WSN-PB1, -PB2, -PA and -NP proteins [17] were kindly provided by G. Brownlee (Sir William Dunn School of Pathology, Oxford, UK). In order to insert the Strep-tag sequence downstream the PB2-ORF into the pPolI-PB2 plasmid, two PCR reactions were performed in parallel, using pPolI-PB2 or pEXPR-IBA103 (IBA GmbH) as a template, and oligonucleotides designed so that the amplified products contained an overlapping sequence corresponding to the junction between the PB2 and Strep-tag coding sequences 5'-TGGATTATCAGAAACTGGGAAAC-3' and 5'GTCGTCA TCGTCTTTGTAGTCAGCTGCATTGATGGCCATCCGAA TTCTTTTGGTCG-3' on the one hand, 5'-CATCAATGCAGC TGACTACAAAGACGATGACGACAAATAGTGTCGAATA GTTTAAAAACGACCTTG-3' and 5'-CAGCTGGCGAAAG GGGGATGTGC-3' on the other hand). An equimolar mix of the amplified products was used as a template for a third PCR reaction, and the resulting amplicon was cloned between the NheI and BstXI sites of plasmid pPolI-PB2-Flag-143 [18]. The same protocol was used for insertion of the HA tag sequence downstream the PB2-ORF into the pPolI-PB2 plasmid. The pPR7-FluA-Luc plasmid was constructed by replacing the sequences encoding CAT by the sequences encoding the *Renilla* luciferase in the pPR7-FluA-CAT plasmid [19], using a standard PCR-based protocol.

The GR expression vector and GR luciferase reporter plasmid were described previously [20].

The p23 and EF1α coding sequences were amplified from a human spleen cDNA library (kindly provided by Y. Jacob, Institut Pasteur, Paris) with the oligonucleotides 5'-GGGGACAACTTTG TACAAAAAAGTTGGCATGCAGCCTGCTTCTGCAAAGT GGTACGATC-3' and 5'-GGGGACAACTTTGTACAAAAAA AGTTGGCAGTTACTCCAGATCTGGCATTTTTTCATCA TCAC-3' for p23, and 5'-GGGGACAACTTTGTACAAAAAAG TTGGCGGAAAGGAAAAGACTCATATCAACATTGTCG-3' and 5'-GGGACAACTTTGTACAAAAAAGTTGTTAGTTAT TTAGCCTTCTGAGCTTTCTGGGCAG-3' for EF1α). The resulting amplicons were subcloned using the Gateway technology downstream the GST coding sequences into a pCMV-GST plasmid (Y. Jacob, Institut Pasteur, Paris), for construction of the pCMV-GST-p23 and pCMV-GST-EF1α plasmids.

All constructs were verified by the sequencing of positive clones using a Big Dye terminator sequencing kit and an automated sequencer (Perkin Elmer). The sequences of the oligonucleotides used for amplification and sequencing can be obtained upon request.

Cell and viruses

Wild-type and p23$^{-/-}$ MEFs [21], 293T (ATCC, CRL-11268) and A549 (ATCC, CCL-185) cells were grown in complete Dulbecco's modified Eagle's medium (DMEM) supplemented with 10% fetal calf serum (FCS). MDCK cells were grown in modified Eagle's medium supplemented with 5% FCS.

The method used for the production of the WSN-PB2-Strep and P908-WSN-PB2-Strep recombinant influenza viruses by reverse genetics was adapted from previously described procedures [17,18]. Briefly, the eight pPolI and 4 pcDNA3.1 plasmids (0.5 μg of each) were co-transfected into a subclonfluent monolayer of

cocultivated 293T and MDCK cells (4×10^5 and 3×10^5 cells, respectively, in a 35-mm dish), using 10 μl of the Fugene 6 transfection reagent (Roche). After 24 hours of incubation at 35°C, the supernatant was removed and replaced with DMEM supplemented with 2% FCS, and the cells were incubated at 35°C for two more days. The efficiency of reverse genetics was evaluated by titrating the supernatant on MDCK cells, in a standard plaque assay using an agarose overlay in complete MEM with 2% FCS. Viral stocks were produced by infecting MDCK cells at a m.o.i. of 0.001 and collecting the supernatant after an incubation of 2 days at 35°C in DMEM supplemented with 2% FCS. Experimental infections were performed at 37°C, unless otherwise indicated.

PB2-strep complex purification on Strep-tactin colums

At 6 hours following infection of 293T cells (4×10^8 cells per 150 mm dishes) with the PB2-wt or PB2-Strep viruses at a m.o.i. of 5 pfu/cell, cells were washed twice with PBS, collected with a cell scraper and centrifuged at 450 g for 5 min. The packed cell volume (PCV) was estimated. Cells were resuspended in $5 \times$ PCV of a hypotonic lysis buffer (Hepes 100 mM, MgCl$_2$ 1.5 mM, KCl 100 mM, DTT 1 mM, Protease Inhibitor Cocktail-Sigma) and kept on ice for 15 mn. NP40 was added at a final concentration of 0.3%, and the lysate was centrifuged at 11,000 g for 2 mn at +4°C. The supernatant corresponding to the cytoplasmic fraction was transferred to a fresh tube, 1:20 of the volume was frozen at −80°C. The remaining volume was loaded on a 1 ml Strep-tactin column following the recommendations of the supplier (IBA GmbH). Following elution with 6×200 μl of a desthiobiotin solution (IBA GmbH), elution fractions n° 2 to 5 were pooled and concentrated approximately 15-fold using a 10,000 MWCO Vivaspin tube (Sartorius). One third of the resulting sample was subjected to electrophoresis on a 4–15% Tris-Glycine-SDS polyacrylamide gel (Biorad). Following overnight staining of the gel with SYPRO-Ruby (Invitrogen), or western-blotting as described below, the proteins were vizualized using the G-Box (Syngene).

Mass spectrometry analysis

Destaining of SYPRO-Ruby-stained gel slices, reduction, alkylation, trypsin digestion of the proteins followed by peptide extraction were carried out with the Progest Investigator (Genomic Solutions). Peptides were eluted directly using the ProMS Investigator, (Genomic Solutions) onto a 96-well stainless steel MALDI (Matrix Assisted Laser Desorption Ionisation) target plate (Applied Biosystems) with 0.5 μL of CHCA (alpha-cyano-4-hydroxy cinnamic acid) matrix (2,5 mg/ml in 70% Acetonitrile, 30% H$_2$O, 0.1% Trifluoroacetic acid).

Raw data for protein identification were obtained on the 4800 Proteomics Analyzer (Applied Biosystems) and analyzed by GPS Explorer 2.0 software (Applied Biosystems/MDS SCIEX). For positive-ion reflector mode spectra 3000 laser shots were averaged. For MS calibration, autolysis peaks of trypsin ([M+H]$^+$ = 842.5100 and 2211.1046) were used as internal calibrates. Monoisotopic peak masses were automatically determined within the mass range 800–4000 Da with a signal to noise ratio minimum set to 20. Up to 10 of the most intense ion signals were selected as precursors for Tandem Mass Spectrometry (MS/MS) acquisition excluding common trypsin autolysis peaks and matrix ion signals. In MS/MS positive ion mode, 4000 spectra were averaged, collision energy was 2 kV, collision gas was air and default calibration was set using the Glu^1-Fibrino-peptide B ([M+H]$^+$ = 1570.6696) spotted onto fourteen positions of the MALDI target. Combined Peptide Mass Fingerprinting (PMF) and MS/MS queries were performed using the MASCOT search engine 2.1 (Matrix Science

Ltd.) embedded into GPS-Explorer Software 3.5 (Applied Biosystems/MDS SCIEX,) on the NCBInr [20100119 (10348164 sequences; 3529470745 residues)] database with the following parameter settings: 50 ppm mass accuracy, trypsin cleavage, one missed cleavage allowed, carbamidomethylation set as fixed modification, oxidation of methionines was allowed as variable modification, MS/MS fragment tolerance was set to 0.3 Da. Protein hits with MASCOT Protein score $\geq$83 and a GPS Explorer Protein confidence index $\geq$95% were used for further manual validation.

Affinity purification of GST-fusion proteins

Plasmids pCMV-GST-p23, pCMV-GST-EF1α or pCMV-GST (1 µg) were transfected together with pcDNA3.1-PB1, -PB2, and/or -PA (1 µg) into a subconfluent monolayer of 293T cells (8×10^5 cells in a 35-mm dish) using 10 µl of the Fugene-6 transfection reagent (Roche). At 48 hours post-transfection, cells were lysed in 300 mL of Tris-HCl [pH 7.4] 50 mM, NaCl 120 mM, EDTA 1 mM, NP40 1% and Protease Inhibitor Cocktail 1X (Sigma). Gluthation Sepharose 4 Fast Flow beads (GE Healthcare) were added to the supernatant and incubated overnight under gentle rotation. Beads were washed three times in Tris-HCl [pH 7.4] 50 mM, NaCl 120 mM, EDTA 1 mM, NP40 1%, and bound proteins were eluted by incubation with 30 µl of Laemmli buffer.

siRNA transfection, viral-minigenome and GR-mediated gene transactivation assay

Subconfluent monolayers of 293T cells (2×10^5 cells per well in 24-well-plates) were transfected with anti-p23 or control siRNAs (ON-TARGET plus SMART pool L-004496-00 and ON-TARGET plus Non targeting pool, Dharmacon) at a final concentration of 25 nM using the DharmaFECT reagent (Dharmacon) according to the manufacturer's recommendations. For viral minigenome assays, plasmids pcDNA3.1-PB1, -PB2, -PA and -NP (0.25, 0.25, 0.25, 0.5 µg) were transfected together with the pPR7-FluA-Luc plasmid (0.1 µg) using 5 µl of the Fugene-HD transfection reagent (Roche). At 24 hours post-transfection, cell lysates were prepared and luciferase activity was measured, using the Lysis Buffer and substrate provided in the *Renilla* Luciferase Assay System kit (Promega) and a Tecan luminometer (Berthold).

For GR-mediated gene transactivation assays, subconfluent monolayers of 293T cells (4×10^5 cells per well in 12-well-plates) were pre-incubated for 16 hours in serum free medium prior to cotransfection with a GR expression vector, a GR-*Firefly* luciferase reporter plasmid and a pTK-*Renilla* luciferase expressing vector (0.5 µg of each plasmid) using 5 µL of the FuGENE HD reagent (Roche). At 24 hours post-transfection cells were infected at a m.o.i. of 5 pfu/cell with the A/WSN/33 virus. After one hour of adsorption, the viral suspension was replaced with medium supplemented with dexamethasone and cells were incubated at 35°C for 10 hours. Cell lysates were prepared and luciferase activities were measured using Luciferase Assay kits (Promega).

Indirect immunofluorescence assay

293T cells on coverslips were transfected using the FuGENE HD reagent (Roche) with a PB2-flag expression vector alone or in combination with PB1 and PA expression vectors. At 24 h post-transfection cells were fixed with PBS-4% paraformaldehyde for 20 min and permeabilized with PBS-0.1% Triton X100 for 15 min. They were incubated with a mixture of the mouse monoclonal anti-p23 (Abcam, diluted 1/250) and the rabbit polyclonal anti-Flag (Sigma, diluted 1/400) antibodies, and then with a mixture of AF555-coupled anti-mouse IgG and AF488

coupled anti-rabbit IgG secondary antibodies (Invitrogen, diluted 1/1000).

A549 or 293T cells on coverslips were infected with the PB2-HA recombinant virus at a m.o.i. of 5 pfu/cell or mock-infected, and incubated at 37°C. At 4–8 hours post-infection, cells were fixed and permeabilized as indicated above. They were incubated with a mixture of the mouse monoclonal anti-p23 and the rabbit polyclonal anti-Hsp90 (Santa Cruz Biotechnology, diluted 1/100) antibodies, and then with a mixture of AF640-coupled anti-mouse IgG secondary antibody (Invitrogen, diluted 1/500), AF555-coupled anti-rabbit IgG secondary antibody (Invitrogen, diluted 1/500), and AF488-coupled anti-HA antibody (Invitrogen, diluted 1/200). Alternatively, cells were incubated with dexamethasone 10 nM for 1 hour at 37°C prior to fixation and permeabilization. They were incubated with a mixture of the rat anti-HA (Roche, diluted 1/1,000) and mouse anti-glucocorticoid receptor (Affinity BioReagents, diluted 1/300) monoclonal antibodies, and then with a mixture of AF555-coupled anti-mouse IgG secondary antibody (Invitrogen, diluted 1/1,000) and AF488-coupled anti-rat IgG secondary antibody (Invitrogen, diluted 1/500). The samples were analyzed under a fluorescence microscope (Zeiss Axioplan 2 imaging- Zeiss ApoTome).

Western-blot assays

For western blot assays, cells in 35-mm dishes were resuspended directly in 300 µl of sample loading buffer. The cell lysates were centrifuged for 2 mn at 16,000 g on a QIAShredder column (QIAGEN), heated for 3 min at 95°C and analyzed by electrophoresis on a 4–12% Bis-Tris NuPAGE gel (Invitrogen) and western blotting using PVDF membranes. The membranes were incubated overnight at 4°C with primary antibodies directed against p23 (Abcam, diluted 1/1,000), GST (Upstate Cell Signalling Solutions, diluted 1/4,000), Hsp90 (Santa Cruz Biotechnology, diluted 1/1,000) or Histone3 (ab1791, Abcam, diluted 1/3,000), or with rabbit polyclonal serum directed against the PB1, PB2, or PA proteins (kindly provided by J. Ortin, Centro Nacional de Biotecnologia, Madrid, Spain, diluted 1/5,000) or against A/PR/8/34 virions ([22], diluted 1/10,000) in PBS with 1% BSA, 0.25% Tween20. Membranes were then incubated for 1 h at room temperature with peroxydase-conjugated secondary antibodies, with the ECL+ substrate (GE Healthcare), and scanned for chemiluminescence using a G-Box (Syngene).

Results

p23 associates with influenza virus polymerase

In order to identify cellular proteins associated to influenza virus RNPs, we produced a recombinant A/WSN/33 (WSN) influenza A virus expressing a PB2 protein fused to a Strep-tag epitope at the C-terminus (PB2-Strep virus). The Strep-tag is a short polypeptide which binds specifically to Strep-tactin, a derivative of streptavidin [23]. The packaging signal overlapping the coding and non-coding regions at the 5′ end of the PB2 segment was conserved by duplicating the 109 last nucleotides encoding PB2 between the Strep-tag sequence and the 5′NCR, as described previously [24]. The resulting PB2-Strep virus replicated efficiently, and showed no genetic instability upon sequential amplifications on MDCK cells (data not shown).

The PB2-Strep and wild-type (PB2-wt) viruses were used in parallel to infect 4×10^9 293T cells at a multiplicity of infection (m.o.i.) of 5 pfu/cell. Cytoplasmic extracts were prepared at 6 hours post-infection (hpi), and were loaded onto Strep-tactin columns. Native PB2-Strep complexes were eluted using desthio-biotin, and subjected to SDS-PAGE analysis. As shown in Figure 1,

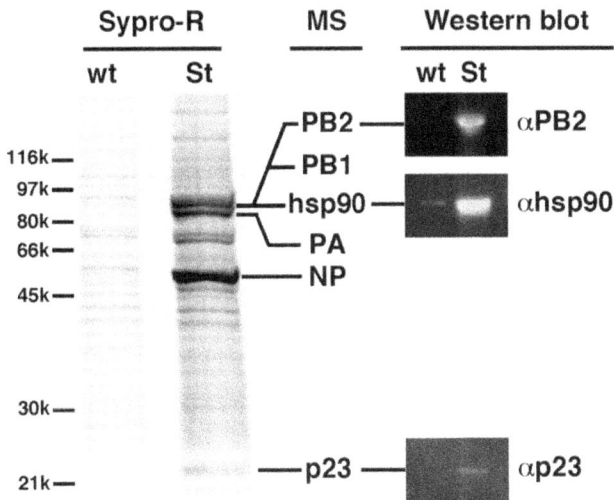

Figure 1. Co-purification of influenza virus polymerase and p23 upon infection of 293T cells with a PB2-Strep-WSN virus. 293T cells were infected with the WSN (WT) or WSN-PB2-Strep (Strep) virus at a m.o.i. of 5 for 6 hours. Cell lysates were loaded onto a Strep-tactin column, and bound proteins were eluted in desthiobiotine elution buffer. Eluted proteins were analysed on a 4–15% polyacrylamide gel and stained with Sypro-Ruby. Proteins from individual gel slices were analysed by mass spectrometry (MS). For confirmation, western blot analysis of eluted proteins was performed using antibodies specific for the PB2, Hsp90 and p23 proteins.

Sypro-Ruby staining of the gel revealed a number of bands which were present in the sample derived from cells infected with the PB2-Strep virus, but not from cells infected with the PB2-wt virus. Slices of the gel were sent to Institut Pasteur Proteomics Facility. As expected, slices corresponding to the major bands corresponded to the PB2, PB1, PA and NP viral proteins (Figure 1), which was in agreement with our previous observations using PB2-Strep viruses [24,25]. The slice containing PB2 and PB1 was also found

to contain the Hsp90 protein, whereas a band of lower molecular weight corresponded to the p23 co-chaperone of Hsp90. Western-blot analysis using anti-Hsp90 and anti-p23 antibodies confirmed that Hsp90 and p23 were specifically co-purified with PB2-Strep complexes (Figure 1).

Co-purification assays were then performed using a GST-p23 fusion protein transiently expressed in 293T cells. A pCMV-GST-p23 expression vector was transfected in 293T cells together with pcDNA3.1 expression vectors for the WSN-PB1, -PB2 or -PA proteins, separately or in combination. Similar to p23, EF1-α is an abundant, constitutively expressed, cytoplasmic protein, and therefore a GST-EF1α construct was used in parallel as a control. At 48 h post-transfection, total cell extracts were prepared and incubated with glutathion beads as described under the Materials and Methods section. The GST-p23 complexes were washed, eluted using Laemmli buffer and subjected to western-blot analysis. As expected the Hsp90 protein was co-purified with the GST-p23 protein, but not with the GST-EF1α protein (Figure 2). Each of the PB1, PB2 and PA subunits of the polymerase complex bound specifically to the GST-p23 protein, whether expressed alone, or in combination with one or both of the other subunits (Figure 2).

Viral replication is not impaired in p23-deficient cultured cells

To investigate the functional relevance of p23 interaction with the influenza polymerase complex in the replication cycle of influenza viruses, we compared viral growth on mouse embryonic fibroblasts either derived from p23-deficient mice (p23$^{-/-}$) or from control wild-type mice (wt) [21]. Following infection at a m.o.i. of 10^{-3} pfu/cell, viral titers in the culture supernatants were determined at different times post-infection by plaque assay on MDCK cells. The WSN virus replicated at a similar rate on p23$^{-/-}$ and wt cells, titers of 10^7–10^8 pfu/ml being observed at 48 hpi (Figure 3A). The same observations were made when the cells were incubated at 33°C or 39°C instead of 35°C upon infection, or when a recombinant virus expressing the PB1, PB2, PA and NP proteins derived from the A/Paris/908/97 (H3N2) human isolate was used instead of the A/WSN/33 virus (data not shown).

To further document the effect of p23 depletion on influenza virus replication, we performed single-cycle growth assays on

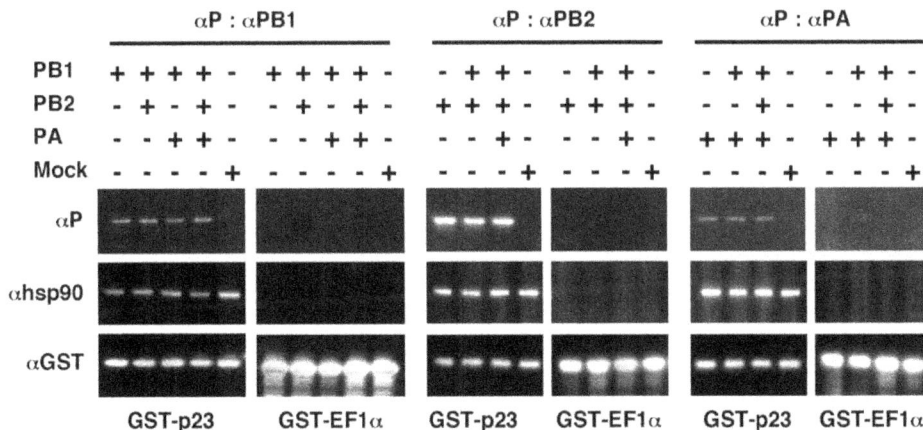

Figure 2. Co-purification of a GST-p23 fusion protein and the influenza virus polymerase subunits upon co-expression in 293T cells. 293T cells were co-transfected with expression plasmids for GST-p23 or GST-EF1α fusion proteins, together with expression plasmids for the WSN-PB1, WSN-PB2, and/or WSN-PA proteins. At 48 hours post-transfection, cell lysates were incubated with Glutathion Sepharose beads overnight, and bound proteins were eluted in Laemmli buffer. Eluted proteins were analysed by western blot using antibodies specific for the GST, Hsp90, p23, PB1, PB2 and PA proteins.

A

B

C

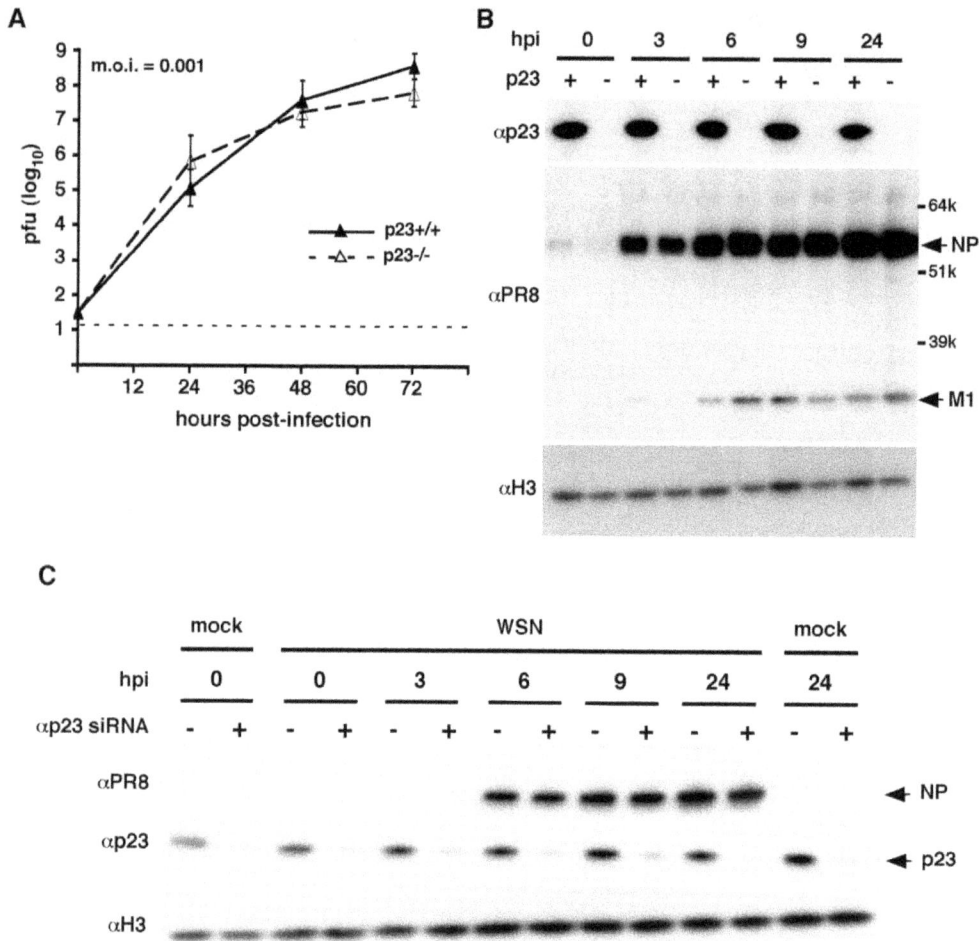

Figure 3. Influenza virus replication on p23$^{-/-}$ and wild-type mouse embryonic fibroblasts. A. Subconfluent monolayers of p23$^{-/-}$ and wild-type mouse embryonic fibroblasts (MEFs) were infected at a m.o.i. of 10^{-3} pfu/cell with the WSN virus and incubated for 72 h at 37°C. At the indicated time-points, supernatants were harvested and viral titers were determined by plaque assays on MDCK cells. The mean values ± SD from 3 independent experiments are shown. The horizontal dotted line represents the limit of detection in the plaque assays. **B.** Subconfluent monolayers of p23$^{-/-}$ and wild-type MEFs were infected at a m.o.i. of 10 pfu/cell with the WSN virus and incubated for 24 h at 37°C. Total cell lysates prepared at the indicated time-points were analysed by western blot, using an anti-p23 antibody, a polyclonal serum directed against the A/PR/8/34 virus which enables detection of the NP and M1 proteins of WSN, and a polyclonal anti-Histone3 antibody. Data are representative of two independent experiments. **C.** 293T cells were transfected with anti-p23 or control siRNAs. At 48 hours post-transfection, they were infected at a m.o.i. of 10 pfu/cell with the WSN virus and incubated for 24 h at 37°C. Total cell lysates prepared at the indicated time-points were analysed by western blot, as in **B**.

p23$^{-/-}$ and wt cells. Following infection with the WSN virus at a high m.o.i. of 10 pfu/cell, total cell extracts were prepared at various times post-infection and analyzed by western-blot using a polyclonal serum to detect the viral NP and M1 viral proteins, or cells were fixed and analyzed by immunofluorescence to detect the PB2 protein. As shown in Figure 3B the NP and M1 proteins steady-state levels were similar in p23$^{-/-}$ and wt cells. The nuclear accumulation of the PB2 viral polymerase subunit was not delayed in p23$^{-/-}$ cells (Figure S1). The viral titers in the supernatants of p23$^{-/-}$ and wt cells were in the same range, and reached 10^6–10^7 pfu/ml at 48 hpi (data not shown).

Single-cycle growth assays were also performed in 293T cells transiently transfected with anti-p23 siRNAs. The steady-state level of p23, as evaluated by western-blot analysis of serial dilutions of total cell extracts, showed a significant reduction in 293T transfected with the anti-p23 siRNAs as compared to the control siRNAs (Figure 3C, middle panel). Following infection with the WSN virus at a high m.o.i. of 10 pfu/cell, accumulation of the NP

and M1 proteins occurred at the same rate in anti-p23 and control siRNA-treated cells (Figure 3C, upper panel).

The viral polymerase activity was assayed in anti-p23 and control siRNA-treated 293T cells, by co-expressing transiently the PB1, PB2, PA and NP proteins of WSN together with an influenza-like RNA containing the luciferase reporter gene. The efficiency with which the influenza-like RNA underwent transcription/replication, as monitored by the levels of luciferase activity in transfected cell extracts, was similar in both types of cells (data not shown).

p23 relocalizes to the nucleus in influenza virus-infected cells

The subcellular localization of p23 in influenza virus- and mock-infected A549 and 293T cells was compared. A recombinant WSN virus expressing a PB2 protein fused with the HA tag at the C-terminus was used in these experiments, to allow simultaneous labeling of the viral PB2 and cellular p23 and

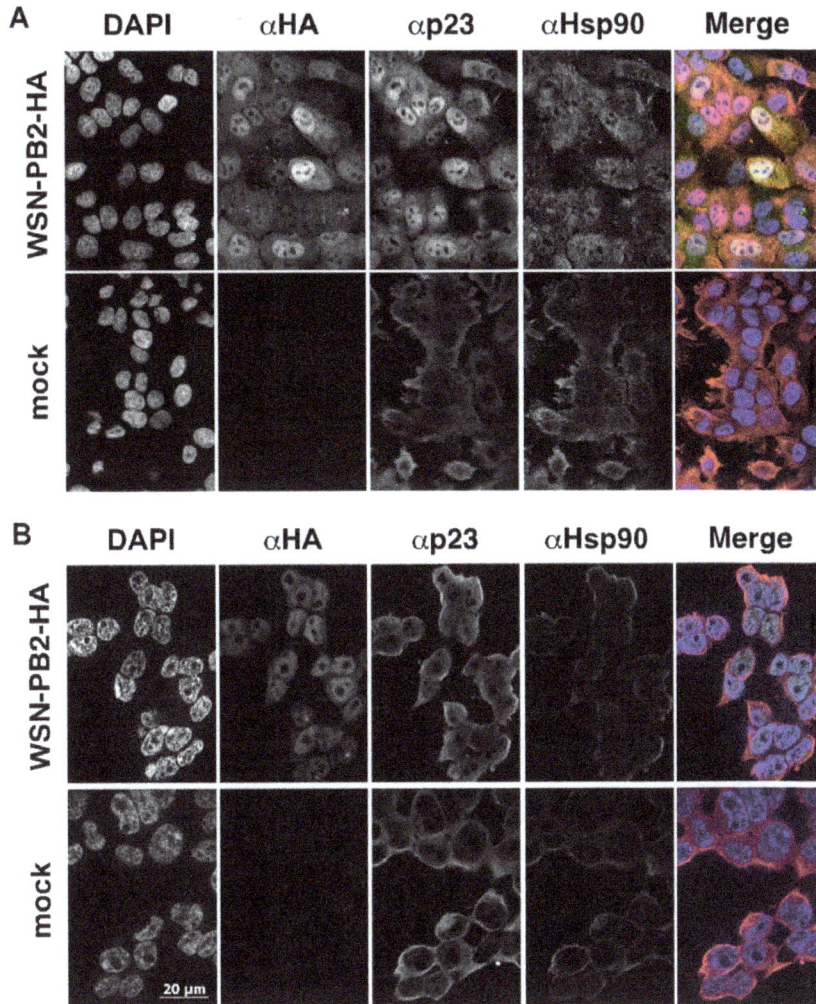

Figure 4. Relocalization of p23 to the nucleus in influenza virus-infected cells. A549 (**A**) or 293T (**B**) cells were infected at a m.o.i. of 10 pfu/cell with the WSN-PB2-HA virus (upper panels) or mock-infected (lower panels). At 8 hpi (**A**) or 6 hpi (**B**), cells were fixed, permeabilized, and stained with antibodies specific for the HA tag (PB2), and for the p23 and the Hsp90 proteins. Samples were analyzed under a fluorescence microscope (Zeiss Axioplan 2 Imaging - Zeiss ApoTome). A merge of the signals corresponding to DAPI (blue), HA (green) and p23 (red) is shown. Data are representative of three independent experiments.

Hsp90 proteins. The anti-HA antibody did not recognize the WSN hemagglutinin, as expected from the fact that the YPYDVPDY sequence of the HA tag is not present in this hemagglutinin, and as demonstrated by the background levels of fluorescence measured on control cells infected with the wild-type WSN virus (Figure S2). In uninfected A549 and 293T cells, p23 and Hsp90 were predominantly detected in the cytoplasm (Figure 4A and 4B, respectively, lower panels). In infected cells, relocalisation of p23 to the nucleus became detectable at 4 hpi (data not shown) and was very obvious at 6–8 hpi (Figure 4A and 4B, upper panels). Relocalisation of Hsp90 was also observed, in agreement with previously published data [5], but was less pronounced as compared to p23 relocalisation (Figure 4A and 4B, upper panels).

The subcellular localization of p23 was then examined in transfected cells transiently expressing the viral polymerase subunits. Relocalisation of p23 to the nucleus was clearly observed in A549 or 293T cells transiently expressing the PB2 subunit, either alone or in combination with the PB1 and PA subunits (Figure 5A and 5B, respectively). Nuclear relocalisation of p23 was

also observed in 293T cells expressing the PA subunit alone but not in cells expressing the PB1 subunit alone (data not shown), which was consistent with the fact that unlike PA, PB1 is not efficiently imported in the nucleus when expressed on its own [26]. Nuclear relocalisation of p23 was not observed in cells expressing the viral nucleoprotein, although the nucleoprotein was detected in the nucleus as well as in the cytoplasm of transfected cells (Figure S3). Overall, these observations supported the hypothesis that the specific association of p23 with the viral polymerase subunits is driving p23 relocalisation to the nucleus in infected cells.

Glucocorticoid-receptor mediated signalling is impaired in influenza virus infected cells

As a component of the Hsp90 chaperone complex, p23 plays a complex role in the maturation and function of the glucocorticoid receptor (GR) (reviewed in [16]). In p23-deficient cells, the GR-mediated gene transactivation is impaired, which coincides with a delayed nuclear translocation of the GR in response to dexamethasone [21]. We hypothetized that the strong relocalisa-

A

B

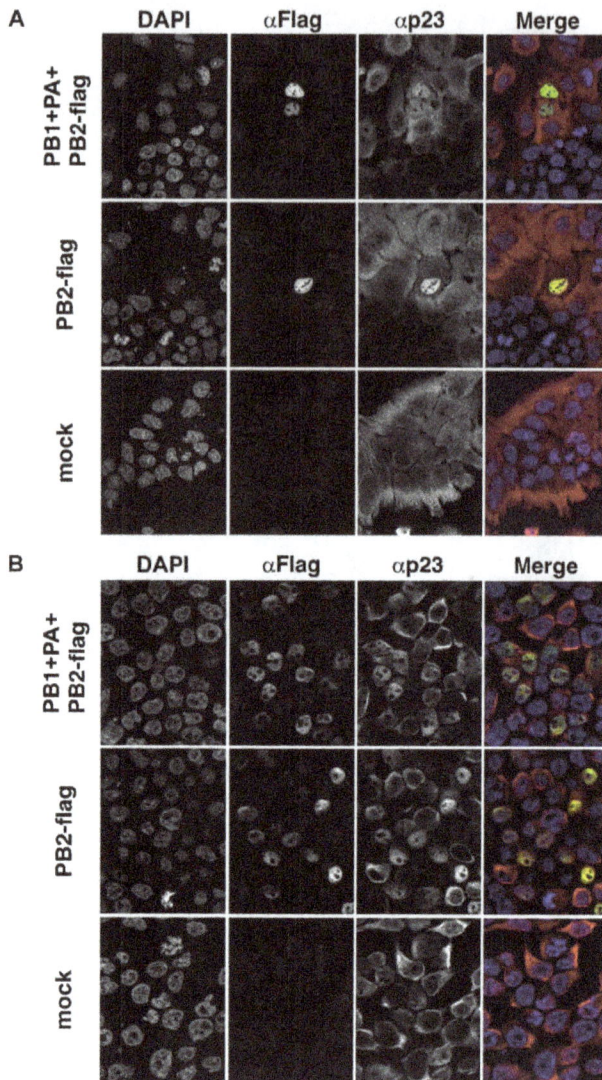

Figure 5. Relocalization of p23 to the nucleus of cells transiently expressing influenza virus polymerase subunits. A549 (**A**) or 293T (**B**) cells were transfected with a WSN-PB2-Flag expression plasmid alone or in combination with PB1 and PA expression plasmids, or mock-transfected. At 24 hours post-transfection, cells were fixed, permeabilized, and stained with antibodies specific for the Flag tag (PB2) and for the p23 protein. Samples were analyzed under a fluorescence microscope (Zeiss Axioplan 2 Imaging - Zeiss ApoTome). A merge of the signals corresponding to DAPI (blue), Flag (green) and p23 (red) is shown. Data are representative of two independent experiments.

tion of p23 observed in influenza-virus infected cells might have an impact on GR signalling. To evaluate GR-mediated gene transactivation in influenza-infected *vs* mock-infected cells, 293T cells were cotransfected with a GR expressing plasmid, a reporter plasmid containing the *Firefly*-luciferase gene under the control of a minimal TK promoter and GR-responsive elements, and a *Renilla*-luciferase expressing construct. At 48 hours post-transfection, they were infected with WSN at a m.o.i. of 5 pfu/ml, or mock-infected. After one hour of adsorption, the viral inoculum was removed, and replaced with fresh medium either supplemented with dexamethasone or not. After 10 hours of stimulation, cell lysates were prepared and *Firefly*-luciferase activities were determined and

normalized with respect to *Renilla*-luciferase activities. As shown in Figure 6A, the dexamethasone-induced transactivation of the *Firefly*-luciferase gene in infected cells (12- and 19-fold at 1 nM and 10 nM dexamethasone, respectively) was reduced as compared to in mock-infected cells (28- and 25-fold at 1 nM and 10 nM dexamethasone, $p < 0.02$ and $p < 0.05$, respectively). The subcellular localisation of the GR was examined in WSN-PB2-HA- and in mock-infected 293T cells, upon incubation in the absence or in the presence of 10 nM dexamethasone. An indirect immunoassay was performed at 5 hpi, using a mixture of an anti-HA and an anti-GR antibody. Uninfected cells generally showed cytoplasmic or cytoplasmic and nuclear GR staining in the absence of dexamethasone (Figure 6B, panel a), and predominantly nuclear GR upon stimulation with dexamethasone (Figure 6B, panel c). Strikingly, infected cells showed nuclear relocalisation of the GR in the absence as well as in the presence of dexamethasone (Figure 6B, panels b and d, respectively). Sequestration of the GR in the nucleus in its hormone-free conformation could contribute to the impairment of GR-mediated signalling by reducing the pool of cytoplasmic GR available for hormone recognition.

We finally asked whether the observed reduction of GR-mediated gene transactivation in influenza-infected *vs* mock-infected cells was mediated by p23. To this end, the luciferase reporter assay described above was repeated using $p23^{-/-}$ MEFs, either transfected with a p23 expression plasmid or mock-transfected. Upon infection, cells were incubated in the presence of 10 to 100 nM dexamethasone. In mock-infected cells, transactivation of the *Firefly*-luciferase gene increased with the dose of dexamethasone and was stronger in the presence of the p23 expression plasmid (Figure 7, white bars), which was in agreement with the known functions of p23 in GR-mediated signalling [21,27,28,29]. A negative effect of viral infection on transactivation of the *Firefly*-luciferase gene in response to dexamethasone was clearly observed, in the presence as well as in the absence of the p23 expression plasmid (Figure 7, grey bars). These data indicated that the observed viral effect could occur through a p23-independent pathway.

Discussion

We used a recombinant influenza virus expressing a PB2 protein fused to a Strep-tag for the co-purification and identification of interacting host factors during the course of viral infection. The Strep-tag has been described as an appropriate tag to purify protein complexes from crude extracts under mild elution conditions and with good yields [23]. Indeed, PB2-Strep viruses allowed co-purification of PB2 and PB2-associated viral proteins such as PB1, PA and NP (this study, and [24]), as well as a number of cellular proteins that have already been identified as cellular interactors of the viral polymerase or nucleoprotein, such as the RNA polymerase II large subunit [10,24], Hsp90 (this study), Hsp70, and actin (data not shown). The PB2-Strep virus is potentially a useful tool to explore the spatial and temporal dynamics of these protein interactions.

We found that the p23 cochaperone of Hsp90 was associated with PB2 in cytoplasmic extracts from 293T cells infected with the WSN-PB2-Strep virus. A transient co-expression/purification assay confirmed that a GST-p23 fusion protein, but not a control GST-EF1α fusion protein, bound to each of the PB1, PB2 and PA polymerase subunits. In both experimental systems, the elution samples containing the p23 and polymerase subunit(s) also contained the Hsp90 chaperone, in agreement with existing data showing PB2-Hsp90 and p23-Hsp90 interactions [5,16]. Whether

A

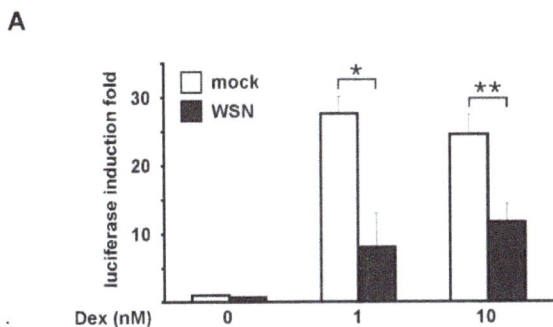

B

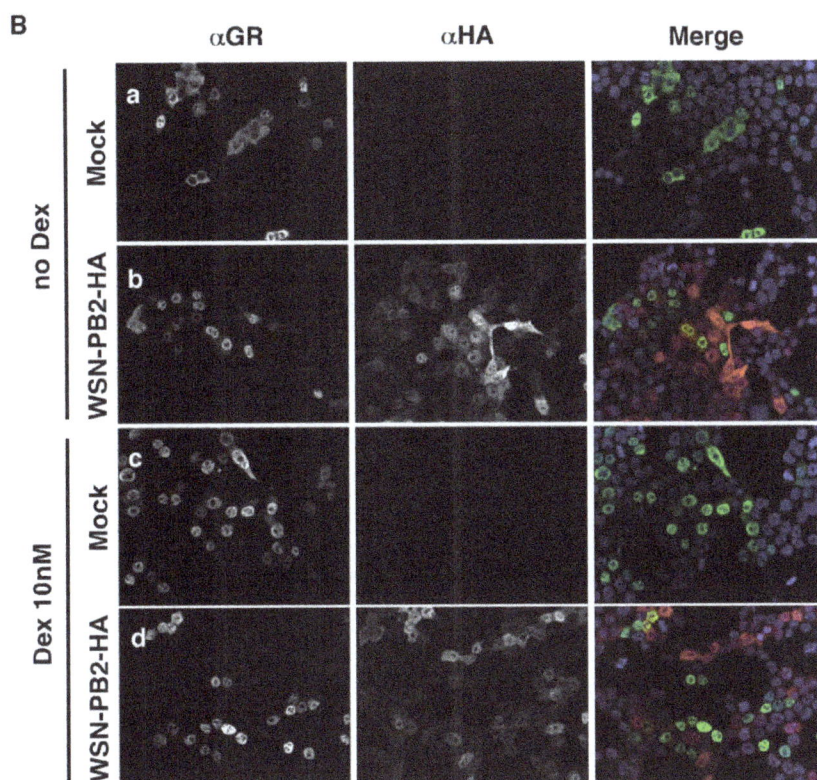

Figure 6. Altered glucocorticoid receptor-mediated transcriptional response and glucocorticoid receptor localization in influenza virus-infected cells. A. 293T cells were co-transfected with a GR expressing plasmid, a reporter plasmid containing the *Firefly*-luciferase gene under the control of GR-responsive elements, and a *Renilla*-luciferase expressing plasmid. At 48 hours post-transfection, cells were infected with the WSN virus at a m.o.i. of 5 pfu/ml (grey bars) or mock-infected (white bars), and incubated for 10 hours in the presence of dexamethasone at the indicated concentrations. *Firefly*-luciferase activities were measured in cell lysates and normalized with respect to *Renilla*-luciferase activities. The results are expressed as the mean ± SD of four independent experiments performed in duplicate, and as fold induction of *Firefly*-luciferase activity relative to the untreated uninfected control. * $p < 0.05$; ** : $p < 0.02$ (Student's *t* test). **B.** 293T cells were transfected with a GR expressing plasmid or mock-transfected. At 24 hours post-transfection, cells were infected with the WSN-PB2-HA virus at a m.o.i. of 5 pfu/ml (panels b and d) or mock-infected (panels a and c). At 5 hpi, they were incubated for one hour in the absence (panels a and b) or in the presence of 10 nM dexamethasone (panels c and d). The cells were then fixed, permeabilized, and stained with antibodies specific for the HA tag (PB2) and for the GR. Samples were analyzed under a fluorescence microscope (Zeiss Axioplan 2 Imaging - Zeiss ApoTome). A merge of the signals corresponding to DAPI (blue), HA (red) and GR (green) is shown. Data are representative of two independent experiments.

p23 is directly or indirectly binding to influenza polymerase subunits thus remains unclear. p23 was found in complexes with Hsp90 and a variety of client proteins, including hepatitis B virus polymerase [30], but whether p23 is able to interact directly with these proteins has not been established. Since Hsp90 does not bind efficiently to PA [5, Chase and Schwemmle, unpublished observations], the p23-PA association suggests that p23 can associate with the influenza polymerase, at least partially,

independently of Hsp90. We observed relocalization of p23 in the nucleus of infected cells, which is consistent with the biochemical interaction data as the viral polymerase accumulates in the nuclear compartment. Nuclear retention was more pronounced for p23 than for Hsp90, which might be indicative of some Hsp90-independent interaction between p23 and influenza polymerase occuring in the nucleus. Relocalization of p23 in the nucleus was also observed in cells that transiently co-

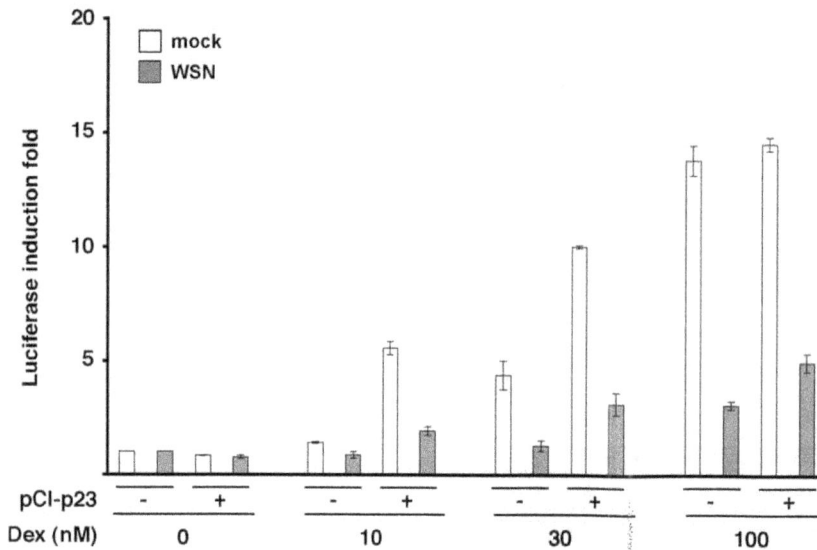

Figure 7. Altered glucocorticoid receptor-mediated transcriptional response in influenza virus-infected p23$^{-/-}$ mouse embryonic fibroblasts. p23$^{-/-}$ MEFs were co-transfected with a GR expressing plasmid, a reporter plasmid containing the *Firefly*-luciferase gene under the control of GR-responsive elements, and a *Renilla*-luciferase expressing plasmid, together with the pCI-p23 plasmid (+) or the control pCI plasmid (−). At 24 hours post-transfection, cells were infected with the WSN virus at a m.o.i. of 5 pfu/ml (grey bars) or mock-infected (white bars), and incubated for 10 hours in the presence of dexamethasone at the indicated concentrations. *Firefly*-luciferase activities were measured in cell lysates and normalized with respect to *Renilla*-luciferase activities. The results are expressed as the mean ± SD of duplicate assays, and are representative of 2 independent experiments performed in duplicates.

expressed the three viral polymerase subunits as well as in cells that expressed the PB2 or PA subunit alone, but not in cells that expressed the viral NP. These observations further demonstrated that the interaction between p23 and influenza virus polymerase was specific and did not require the presence of other viral proteins. Nuclear sequestration of p23 may alter some of p23 and Hsp90 functions in influenza virus-infected cells.

Whereas Hsp90 is thought to play a role in the import and assembly of newly synthetized influenza polymerase subunits [5,31], we show here that p23 depletion has no impact on viral multiplication efficiency in cultured murine embryonic fibroblasts or 293T cells. The chaperoning activity of Hsp90 is regulated by ATP and by a large variety of cofactors, which control Hsp90's shuttling between open and closed conformations [32]. p23 is considered a general cochaperone of Hsp90 client proteins which acts by stabilizing the ATP-bound closed conformation of Hsp90 [33,34]. However, p23 was found to be an enhancing but not an essential factor for several Hsp90 client proteins, and might be dispensable for some of them [16]. Functional redundancy beween p23 and other cochaperone(s) of Hsp90 cannot be excluded [35], and could also account for our observations.

The usually observed nucleo-cytoplasmic shuttling of p23 is related to its complex role in glucocorticoid signalling. In the absence of hormone, glucocorticoid receptors (GRs) are mainly located in the cytoplasm, and p23 promotes their folding into a hormone-binding conformation by stabilizing GR-Hsp90-p60-Hsp70 complexes [27]. Upon hormone binding, GRs rapidly accumulate in the nucleus and upregulates the transcription of a large array of genes, such as IκBα or GC-induced leucine zipper, which are thought to be involved in the GC-mediated anti-inflammatory effects [36]. Nuclear translocation of the GR in response to hormonal stimulation is delayed in p23-deficient cells [21], and recent data suggest that the p23 and p60 co-chaperones play a role in the nuclear import of GRs [28]. Furthermore, p23 acts independently of Hsp90 in the nucleus by mediating the

disassembly of transcriptional regulatory complexes formed by intra-nuclear hormone-bound GRs [37].

This complex regulatory function of p23 at various steps of the GR signalling pathway is likely to be disrupted by the strong relocalisation of p23 in the nucleus of influenza-virus infected cells. Indeed, we found that the GR sub-cellular localisation is altered and the GR-mediated gene transactivation is impaired in influenza virus-infected cells. Viral infection still shows a negative effect on GR-mediated gene transactivation in cells that are defective for p23. This observation, although it does not rule out a contribution of p23, indicates that viral-induced inhibition of GR-mediated signalling can occur through a p23-independent and redundant pathway. A possible approach to unravel the contribution of p23 would be to identify influenza variants defective for p23 binding and to compare their impact on GR signalling.

Our observation of an impaired response to glucocorticoids in influenza infected cells adds to few previously published data showing alterations of the GR activity upon viral infections (reviewed in [38]). A recent study reports repression of GR-mediated gene transactivation upon infection with the Respiratory Syncitial Virus [39]. Very little is known about the interaction of influenza virus and the GR signalling pathway. In vitro, influenza viruses are usually grown in the absence of serum and thus in the absence of glucocorticoids. Any potential downstream effects of an altered GR activity upon influenza infection have therefore most likely been overlooked. Influenza virus infection in mice was shown to result in a sustained increase in serum glucocorticoid levels [40] and a transcriptional induction of two GR-regulated genes, metallothionein I (MT-I) and II (Mt-II) [41]. Our data suggest that, besides the systemic activation of the hypothalamic-pituitary-adrenal axis with resulting release of glucocorticoids, the intensity of the glucocorticoid response to influenza infection could be limited by intracellular viral-induced mechanisms. A better understanding of these mechanisms may have implications for the therapeutic treatment of severe cases of influenza in which the balance between pro-inflammatory and anti-inflammatory cytokines is a major physiopathological parameter [42].

Supporting Information

Figure S1   Subcellular localisation of the PB2 protein upon influenza virus infection of p23$^{-/-}$ and wild-type mouse embyonic fibroblasts. p23$^{-/-}$ and wild-type p23$^{+/+}$ mouse embryonic fibroblasts (MEFs) were infected at a m.o.i. of 10 pfu/cell with the WSN-PB2-HA virus. At 5 hpi, cells were fixed, permeabilized and stained with antibodies specific for the HA tag (PB2) and for the Hsp90 protein. Samples were analyzed under a fluorescence microscope (Zeiss Axioplan 2 Imaging - Zeiss ApoTome). A merge of the signals corresponding to DAPI (blue), HA (red) and Hsp90 (green) is shown.

Figure S2   Specific recognition of the HA-tag and not the WSN virus hemagglutinin by the anti-HA antibody. A549 (**A**) or 293T (**B**) cells were infected at a m.o.i. of 10 pfu/cell with the WSN-PB2-HA virus (upper panels) or the WSN wild-type virus (lower panels). At 8 hpi (**A**) or 6 hpi (**B**), cells were fixed, permeabilized, and stained with antibodies specific for the HA tag (PB2) and for the p23 protein. Samples were analyzed under a fluorescence microscope (Zeiss Axioplan 2 Imaging - Zeiss ApoTome). A merge of the signals corresponding to DAPI (blue), HA (green) and p23 (red) is shown.

Figure S3   Subcellular localisation of p23 in 293T cells transiently expressing the viral PB2 or NP protein. 293T cells were transfected with a plasmid encoding NP (middle pannel), PB2-Flag (lower panel) or mock-transfected (upper panel). At 24 hpi cells were fixed, permeabilized, and stained with antibodies specific for the Flag tag (PB2) or the NP protein, together with an anti-p23 antibody. Samples were analyzed under a fluorescence microscope (Zeiss Axioplan 2 Imaging - Zeiss ApoTome). A merge of the signals corresponding to DAPI (blue), Flag or NP (green) and p23 (red) is shown.

Acknowledgments

We are grateful to G. Brownlee (Oxford University, UK), J. Ortin (Centro Nacional de Biotecnologia, Madrid, Spain), Y. Jacob (Institut Pasteur, Paris, France) and D. Toft (Mayo Clinic, Rochester, USA) for providing plasmids and reagents. We thank P. Lenormand at the Plateforme de Protéomique of Institut Pasteur for mass spectrometry analysis, the Plateforme de séquençage and Plateforme d'Imagerie Dynamique at Institut Pasteur for their expertise, and S. van der Werf for her support.

Author Contributions

Conceived and designed the experiments: M-AR-W EG GC ESA NN. Performed the experiments: XG M-AR-W EG GC ESA NN. Analyzed the data: XG M-AR-W EG GC EdSA DP MS NN. Contributed reagents/materials/analysis tools: DP MS NN. Wrote the paper: NN M-AR-W.

References

1. Engelhardt OG, Fodor E (2006) Functional association between viral and cellular transcription during influenza virus infection. Rev Med Virol 16: 329–345.
2. Deng T, Engelhardt OG, Thomas B, Akoulitchev AV, Brownlee GG, et al. (2006) Role of ran binding protein 5 in nuclear import and assembly of the influenza virus RNA polymerase complex. J Virol 80: 11911–11919.
3. Tarendeau F, Boudet J, Guilligay D, Mas PJ, Bougault CM, et al. (2007) Structure and nuclear import function of the C-terminal domain of influenza virus polymerase PB2 subunit. Nat Struct Mol Biol 14: 229–233.
4. Gabriel G, Herwig A, Klenk HD (2008) Interaction of polymerase subunit PB2 and NP with importin alpha1 is a determinant of host range of influenza A virus. PLoS Pathog 4: e11.
5. Naito T, Momose F, Kawaguchi A, Nagata K (2007) Involvement of Hsp90 in assembly and nuclear import of influenza virus RNA polymerase subunits. J Virol 81: 1339–1349.
6. Plotch SJ, Bouloy M, Ulmanen I, Krug RM (1981) A unique cap(m7GpppXm)-dependent influenza virion endonuclease cleaves capped RNAs to generate the primers that initiate viral RNA transcription. Cell 23: 847–858.
7. Dias A, Bouvier D, Crepin T, McCarthy AA, Hart DJ, et al. (2009) The cap-snatching endonuclease of influenza virus polymerase resides in the PA subunit. Nature 458: 914–918.
8. Guilligay D, Tarendeau F, Resa-Infante P, Coloma R, Crepin T, et al. (2008) The structural basis for cap binding by influenza virus polymerase subunit PB2. Nat Struct Mol Biol 15: 500–506.
9. Yuan P, Bartlam M, Lou Z, Chen S, Zhou J, et al. (2009) Crystal structure of an avian influenza polymerase PA(N) reveals an endonuclease active site. Nature 458: 909–913.
10. Engelhardt OG, Smith M, Fodor E (2005) Association of the influenza A virus RNA-dependent RNA polymerase with cellular RNA polymerase II. J Virol 79: 5812–5818.
11. Shih SR, Krug RM (1996) Novel exploitation of a nuclear function by influenza virus: the cellular SF2/ASF splicing factor controls the amount of the essential viral M2 ion channel protein in infected cells. Embo J 15: 5415–5427.
12. Read EK, Digard P (2010) Individual influenza A virus mRNAs show differential dependence on cellular NXF1/TAP for their nuclear export. J Gen Virol 91: 1290–1301.
13. Schneider J, Wolff T (2009) Nuclear functions of the influenza A and B viruses NS1 proteins: do they play a role in viral mRNA export? Vaccine 27: 6312–6316.
14. Elton D, Simpson-Holley M, Archer K, Medcalf L, Hallam R, et al. (2001) Interaction of the influenza virus nucleoprotein with the cellular CRM1-mediated nuclear export pathway. J Virol 75: 408–419.
15. Neumann G, Hughes MT, Kawaoka Y (2000) Influenza A virus NS2 protein mediates vRNP nuclear export through NES-independent interaction with hCRM1. Embo J 19: 6751–6758.
16. Felts SJ, Toft DO (2003) p23, a simple protein with complex activities. Cell Stress Chaperones 8: 108–113.
17. Fodor E, Devenish L, Engelhardt OG, Palese P, Brownlee GG, et al. (1999) Rescue of influenza A virus from recombinant DNA. J Virol 73: 9679–9682.
18. Dos Santos Afonso E, Escriou N, Leclercq I, van der Werf S, Naffakh N (2005) The generation of recombinant influenza A viruses expressing a PB2 fusion protein requires the conservation of a packaging signal overlapping the coding and noncoding regions at the 5′ end of the PB2 segment. Virology 341: 34–46.
19. Crescenzo-Chaigne B, Naffakh N, van der Werf S (1999) Comparative analysis of the ability of the polymerase complexes of influenza viruses type A, B and C to assemble into functional RNPs that allow expression and replication of heterotypic model RNA templates in vivo. Virology 265: 342–353.
20. Bunone G, Briand PA, Miksicek RJ, Picard D (1996) Activation of the unliganded estrogen receptor by EGF involves the MAP kinase pathway and direct phosphorylation. Embo J 15: 2174–2183.
21. Grad I, McKee TA, Ludwig SM, Hoyle GW, Ruiz P, et al. (2006) The Hsp90 cochaperone p23 is essential for perinatal survival. Mol Cell Biol 26: 8976–8983.
22. Vignuzzi M, Gerbaud S, van der Werf S, Escriou N (2001) Naked RNA immunization with replicons derived from poliovirus and Semliki Forest virus genomes for the generation of a cytotoxic T cell response against the influenza A virus nucleoprotein. J Gen Virol 82: 1737–1747.
23. Schmidt GM, Skerra A (2007) The Strep-tag system for one-step purification and high-affinity detection or capturing of proteins. Nature Protocols 2: 1528–1535.
24. Rameix-Welti MA, Tomoiu A, Dos Santos Afonso E, van der Werf S, Naffakh N (2009) Avian Influenza A virus polymerase association with nucleoprotein, but not polymerase assembly, is impaired in human cells during the course of infection. J Virol 83: 1320–1331.
25. Robb NC, Chase G, Bier K, Vreede FT, Shaw PC, et al. (2011) The influenza A virus NS1 protein interacts with the nucleoprotein of viral ribonucleoprotein complexes. J Virol 85: 5228–5231.
26. Fodor E, Smith M (2004) The PA subunit is required for efficient nuclear accumulation of the PB1 subunit of the influenza A virus RNA polymerase complex. J Virol 78: 9144–9153.
27. Dittmar KD, Demady DR, Stancato LF, Krishna P, Pratt WB (1997) Folding of the glucocorticoid receptor by the heat shock protein (hsp) 90-based chaperone machinery. The role of p23 is to stabilize receptor.hsp90 heterocomplexes formed by hsp90.p60.hsp70. J Biol Chem 272: 21213–21220.
28. Echeverria PC, Mazaira G, Erlejman A, Gomez-Sanchez C, Piwien Pilipuk G, et al. (2009) Nuclear import of the glucocorticoid receptor-hsp90 complex through the nuclear pore complex is mediated by its interaction with Nup62 and importin beta. Mol Cell Biol 29: 4788–4797.
29. Lovgren AK, Kovarova M, Koller BH (2007) cPGES/p23 is required for glucocorticoid receptor function and embryonic growth but not prostaglandin E2 synthesis. Mol Cell Biol 27: 4416–4430.

30. Hu J, Toft D, Anselmo D, Wang X (2002) In vitro reconstitution of functional hepadnavirus reverse transcriptase with cellular chaperone proteins. J Virol 76: 269–279.
31. Chase G, Deng T, Fodor E, Leung BW, Mayer D, et al. (2008) Hsp90 inhibitors reduce influenza virus replication in cell culture. Virology 377: 431–439.
32. Pearl LH, Prodromou C (2006) Structure and mechanism of the Hsp90 molecular chaperone machinery. Annu Rev Biochem 75: 271–294.
33. Ali MM, Roe SM, Vaughan CK, Meyer P, Panaretou B, et al. (2006) Crystal structure of an Hsp90-nucleotide-p23/Sba1 closed chaperone complex. Nature 440: 1013–1017.
34. Karagoz GE, Duarte AM, Ippel H, Uetrecht C, Sinnige T, et al. (2011) N-terminal domain of human Hsp90 triggers binding to the cochaperone p23. Proc Natl Acad Sci U S A 108: 580–585.
35. Caplan AJ (2003) What is a co-chaperone? Cell Stress Chaperones 8: 105–107.
36. Clark AR (2007) Anti-inflammatory functions of glucocorticoid-induced genes. Mol Cell Endocrinol 275: 79–97.
37. Freeman BC, Yamamoto KR (2002) Disassembly of transcriptional regulatory complexes by molecular chaperones. Science 296: 2232–2235.
38. Webster JI, Sternberg EM (2004) Role of the hypothalamic-pituitary-adrenal axis, glucocorticoids and glucocorticoid receptors in toxic sequelae of exposure to bacterial and viral products. J Endocrinol 181: 207–221.
39. Hinzey A, Alexander J, Corry J, Adams KM, Claggett AM, et al. (2010) Respiratory Syncytial Virus Represses Glucocorticoid Receptor-Mediated Gene Activation. Endocrinology.
40. Jamieson AM, Yu S, Annicelli CH, Medzhitov R (2010) Influenza virus-induced glucocorticoids compromise innate host defense against a secondary bacterial infection. Cell Host Microbe 7: 103–114.
41. Ghoshal K, Majumder S, Zhu Q, Hunzeker J, Datta J, et al. (2001) Influenza virus infection induces metallothionein gene expression in the mouse liver and lung by overlapping but distinct molecular mechanisms. Mol Cell Biol 21: 8301–8317.
42. Peiris JS, Hui KP, Yen HL (2010) Host response to influenza virus: protection versus immunopathology. Curr Opin Immunol 22: 475–481.

14

Posterior Cingulate Cortex-Related Co-Activation Patterns: A Resting State fMRI Study in Propofol-Induced Loss of Consciousness

Enrico Amico[1,2]*, **Francisco Gomez[1]**, **Carol Di Perri[7]**, **Audrey Vanhaudenhuyse[1,6]**, **Damien Lesenfants[1]**, **Pierre Boveroux[1,4]**, **Vincent Bonhomme[1,4,5]**, **Jean-François Brichant[4]**, **Daniele Marinazzo[2]**, **Steven Laureys[1,3]**

1 Coma Science Group, Cyclotron Research Centre, University of Liège, Liège, Belgium, 2 Faculty of Psychology and Educational Sciences, Department of Data Analysis, Ghent University, Ghent, Belgium, 3 Department of Neurology, University of Liège, Liège, Belgium, 4 Department of Anesthesia and Intensive Care Medicine, CHU Sart Tilman Hospital, University of Liège, Liège, Belgium, 5 Department of Anesthesia and Intensive Care Medicine, CHR Citadelle, University of Liège, Liège, Belgium, 6 Department of Algology and Palliative Care, CHU Sart Tilman Hospital, University of Liège, Liège, Belgium, 7 Department of Neuroradiology, National Neurological Institute C. Mondino, Pavia, Italy

Abstract

Background: Recent studies have been shown that functional connectivity of cerebral areas is not a static phenomenon, but exhibits spontaneous fluctuations over time. There is evidence that fluctuating connectivity is an intrinsic phenomenon of brain dynamics that persists during anesthesia. Lately, point process analysis applied on functional data has revealed that much of the information regarding brain connectivity is contained in a fraction of critical time points of a resting state dataset. In the present study we want to extend this methodology for the investigation of resting state fMRI spatial pattern changes during propofol-induced modulation of consciousness, with the aim of extracting new insights on brain networks consciousness-dependent fluctuations.

Methods: Resting-state fMRI volumes on 18 healthy subjects were acquired in four clinical states during propofol injection: wakefulness, sedation, unconsciousness, and recovery. The dataset was reduced to a spatio-temporal point process by selecting time points in the Posterior Cingulate Cortex (PCC) at which the signal is higher than a given threshold (i.e., BOLD intensity above 1 standard deviation). Spatial clustering on the PCC time frames extracted was then performed (number of clusters = 8), to obtain 8 different PCC co-activation patterns (CAPs) for each level of consciousness.

Results: The current analysis shows that the core of the PCC-CAPs throughout consciousness modulation seems to be preserved. Nonetheless, this methodology enables to differentiate region-specific propofol-induced reductions in PCC-CAPs, some of them already present in the functional connectivity literature (e.g., disconnections of the prefrontal cortex, thalamus, auditory cortex), some others new (e.g., reduced co-activation in motor cortex and visual area).

Conclusion: In conclusion, our results indicate that the employed methodology can help in improving and refining the characterization of local functional changes in the brain associated to propofol-induced modulation of consciousness.

Editor: Yong He, Beijing Normal University, Beijing, China

Funding: This research was supported by the Belgian Funds for Scientific Research (FRS), European Commission (DECODER), Belgian Science Policy (CEREBNET), McDonnell Foundation, European Space Agency, Wallonia-Brussels Federation Concerted Research Action Mind Science Foundation, University of Liège. The funders had no role in study design, data collection and analysis, decision to publish, or preparation of the manuscript.

* Email: eamico@ulg.ac.be

Introduction

Functional magnetic resonance imaging (fMRI) technique has been widely used in the investigation of brain connectivity patterns at rest [1,2]. Blood-oxygen-level dependent (BOLD) signal activity at rest is organized in correlated spatial patterns, which are called "resting state networks" (i.e. RSNs). These networks have been increasingly investigated and their modulation or disruption has been associated to several pathophysiological conditions [3,4], together with the importance of these RSNs to provide informa-

tion about brain dynamic organization, as a complement to structural information.

In particular, in altered states of consciousness it's important to see which functional connections remain unaltered and which ones are modified or disrupted [5,6]. In this regards, functional connectivity studies of RSNs in induced sedation through anesthesia, have shown widespread changes in fronto-parietal networks, compared with the relative preservation of sensory networks, suggesting a major role of higher-order frontoparietal associative network activity in the loss of consciousness phenom-

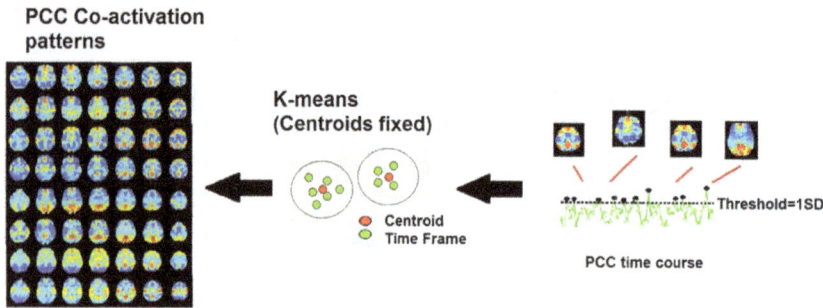

Figure 1. Co-activation patterns (CAPs). The approach is similar to the ones proposed in [16] and [15]. After the extraction of a seed region, in this case Posterior Cingulate Cortex (PCC), a threshold equal to 1 standard deviation(SD) was applied, as to consider only the time points corresponding to peaks in the BOLD signal; next, the spatial maps (namely, time frames), associated with these time points are collected and clusterized using k-means, with a number of clusters fixed to 8. The centroids were kept fixed as well, to allow cluster comparison between the different clinical conditions. The within-cluster time frames were then averaged to obtain 8 spatial PCC-related co-activation patterns. Finally, the computation was iterated over the 4 different states of consciousness (wakefulness, sedation, unconsciousness, recovery), obtaining 8 PCC-related co-activation patterns for each state.

ena [7,8]. Moreover, functional impairment of highly connected frontoparietal areas seems to have greater repercussions on global brain function than on less centrally connected sensorimotor areas [9,10].

Additionally, recent studies have been shown that functional connectivity of cerebral areas is not a static phenomenon, but exhibits spontaneous fluctuations over time [11–13]. Previously, fluctuations of functional connectivity have been thought to reflect changing levels of vigilance, task switching or conscious processing. There is evidence that fluctuating connectivity is an intrinsic phenomenon of brain dynamics that persists even during anesthesia [11]. Fluctuations of functional connectivity within an attention network in macaques have been demonstrated and interpreted as mechanistically important network information [14]. Still, the relationship between changes of consciousness and network dynamics is not understood yet.

Lately, a new approach in exploring functional brain connectivity, using point process analysis, has been proposed by Tagliazucchi et al. [15]. The main idea in this work is that important features of brain functional connectivity at rest can be obtained from BOLD fluctuations, isolating the periods in which the signal crosses some amplitude threshold. In this way the study of the dynamics of a continuous BOLD time series is reduced to the exploration of a discretized one (a point process), defined by time and location of BOLD signal threshold crossings. Through point process analysis, Tagliazucchi and colleagues showed that much of the information regarding a specific RSN is actually contained in a fraction of critical time points (i.e. BOLD signal peaks) of a resting state dataset. This idea has next been adopted by Liu et al. [16], in a study showing that seed-based RSNs extracted from fMRI BOLD signal are averages of multiple distinct spatial co-activations patterns (CAPs) at different time points, and that the analysis of these patterns might provide more fine-grained information on brain functional network organization.

In the present study we want to extend and apply this methodology for the investigation of fMRI resting state spatial pattern changes during propofol-induced modulation of consciousness, with the central aim of extracting new information regarding brain networks consciousness-dependent fluctuations.

Materials and Methods

Ethics Statement

The study was approved by the Ethics Committee of the Medical School of the University of Liège (University Hospital, Liège, Belgium). The subjects provided written informed consent to participate in the study.

Clinical Protocol

The present work is a reanalysis of previous published data [7,8]. Eighteen healthy right-handed volunteers participated in the study. Subjects fasted for at least 6 h from solids and 2 h from liquids before sedation. During the study and the recovery period, electrocardiogram, blood pressure, pulse oxymetry (SpO2), and breathing frequency were continuously monitored (Magnitude 3150M; Invivo Research, Inc., Orlando,FL). Propofol was infused through an intravenous catheter placed into a vein of the right hand or forearm. An arterial catheter was placed into the left radial artery. Throughout the study, the subjects breathed spontaneously, and additional oxygen (5 l/min) was given through a loosely fitting plastic facemask. The level of consciousness was evaluated clinically throughout the study with the scale used by Ramsay et al. [17].

The subject was asked to strongly squeeze the hand of the investigator. She/he was considered fully awake or to have recovered consciousness if the response to verbal command (squeeze my hand) was clear and strong (Ramsay 2), in sedation if the response to verbal command was clear but slow (Ramsay 3), and in unconsciousness if there was no response to verbal command (Ramsay 5–6). For each consciousness level assessment, Ramsay scale verbal commands were repeated twice. Functional MRI acquisitions consisted of resting-state functional MRI volumes repeated in four clinical states: normal wakefulness (Ramsay 2), sedation (Ramsay 3), unconsciousness (Ramsay 5), and recovery of consciousness (Ramsay 2). The typical scan duration was half an hour in each condition. The number of scans per session (197 functional volumes) was matched in each subject to obtain a similar number of scans in all four clinical states. Functional images were acquired on a 3 Tesla Siemens Allegra scanner (Siemens AG, Munich, Germany; Echo Planar Imaging sequence using 32 slices; repetition time = 2460 ms, echo time = 40 ms, field of view = 220 mm, voxel size = $3.45 \times 3.45 \times 3$ mm^3, and matrix size = $64 \times 64 \times 32$).

Table 1. Stereotactic coordinates of peak voxels in clusters of PCC-CAPs showing a linear correlation with propofol-induced changes in consciousness.

CAP 1	x	y	z	Z-value	FDR-p
Right Superior Frontal Gyrus	18	42	48	5.41	0.002
Left Superior Medial Frontal Gyrus	−9	60	30	5.12	0.002
Left Mid Orbital Gyrus	0	57	−9	4.65	0.004
Right Superior Medial Frontal Gyrus	9	57	36	4.06	0.016
CAP 2	**x**	**y**	**z**	**Z-value**	**FDR-p**
Left Superior Medial Frontal Gyrus	−3	60	9	6.55	<0.001
Left Superior Frontal Gyrus	−15	60	24	6.55	<0.001
Right Precuneus	3	−54	36	5.54	<0.001
Left Middle Cingulate Cortex	0	−36	39	3.09	0.011
Right ParaHippocampal Gyrus	24	−21	−18	4.47	<0.001
Right Angular Gyrus	60	−63	33	3.97	<0.001
Left Middle Temporal Gyrus	−63	−15	−24	3.38	0.005
CAP 3	**x**	**y**	**z**	**Z-value**	**FDR-p**
Left Anterior Cingulate Cortex	0	39	15	5.23	0.003
Thalamus	0	−12	0	4.48	0.012
CAP 5	**x**	**y**	**z**	**Z-value**	**FDR-p**
Right Superior Medial Frontal Gyrus	3	57	12	6.55	<0.001
Left Superior Medial Frontal Gyrus	0	57	3	6.55	<0.001
Left Precentral Gyrus	−39	−18	60	5.47	<0.001
Right Cerebellum	27	−33	−33	5.053	<0.001
Hippocampus	15	−33	−9	3.47	0.011
Right Precuneus	3	−57	21	4.83	<0.001
Left Middle Temporal Gyrus	−66	−15	−21	4.75	<0.001
Right Inferior Occipital Gyrus	48	−81	−6	4.03	0.002
Left Superior Frontal Gyrus	−21	30	48	4.51	<0.001
Right Postcentral Gyrus	57	−15	48	4.28	<0.001
Right Precentral Gyrus	48	−15	60	3.64	0.006
Left Precuneus	−9	−45	39	3.61	0.007
CAP 6	**x**	**y**	**z**	**Z-value**	**FDR-p**
Left Middle Frontal Gyrus	−24	30	54	7.52	<0.001
Right Superior Frontal Gyrus	27	27	54	7.11	<0.001
Right Middle Frontal Gyrus	45	18	48	5.68	<0.001
Right Precuneus	9	−54	15	6.12	<0.001
Left Hippocampus	−15	−33	−6	5.09	<0.001
Left Middle Temporal Gyrus	−57	−18	−24	5.55	<0.001
Right Fusiform Gyrus	30	−27	−21	4.71	<0.001
Right ParaHippocampal Gyrus	30	−36	−9	3.69	0.005
CAP 7	**x**	**y**	**z**	**Z-value**	**FDR-p**
Left Thalamus	6	−12	9	5,48	<0.001
Right Thalamus	6	−12	0	5,48	<0.001
Left Anterior Cingulate Cortex	0	48	9	5,25	<0.001
Left Precuneus	−15	−60	21	4,67	0,001
Right Precuneus	12	−51	15	4,43	0,002
Right Calcarine Gyrus	12	−60	15	4,37	0,002
Right Middle Frontal Gyrus	33	30	45	4,19	0,003
Right Superior Frontal Gyrus	24	33	54	3,61	0,012
Right Inferior Temporal Gyrus	54	3	−39	3,93	0,006

Table 1. Cont.

CAP 7	x	y	z	Z-value	FDR-p
Left Middle Cingulate Cortex	0	−33	48	3,86	0,007
Hippocampus	−24	−9	−21	3,84	0,007
Right Inferior Frontal Gyrus	48	39	15	3,74	0,009
Right Inferior Parietal Lobule	51	−51	57	3,47	0,016

CAP 8	x	y	z	Z-value	FDR-p
Left Postcentral Gyrus	−54	−18	54	6,58	<0.001
Right Postcentral Gyrus	63	−12	42	4,86	0,001
Right Precentral Gyrus	48	−6	60	3,91	0,011
Right Middle Temporal Gyrus	60	−12	−24	4,76	0,002
Left Superior Medial Frontal Gyrus	0	57	6	3,82	0,013
Left Anterior Cingulate Cortex	−12	45	0	3,65	0,018
Left Middle Temporal Gyrus	−57	−6	−18	4,43	0,005
Left Rolandic Operculum	−39	0	15	4,32	0,005
Left Insula Lobe	−42	−9	3	3,84	0,012
Right Rolandic Operculum	48	−12	21	4,15	0,007
Left Amygdala	−27	−3	−24	3,95	0,011
Right Hippocampus	30	−3	−24	3,95	0,011

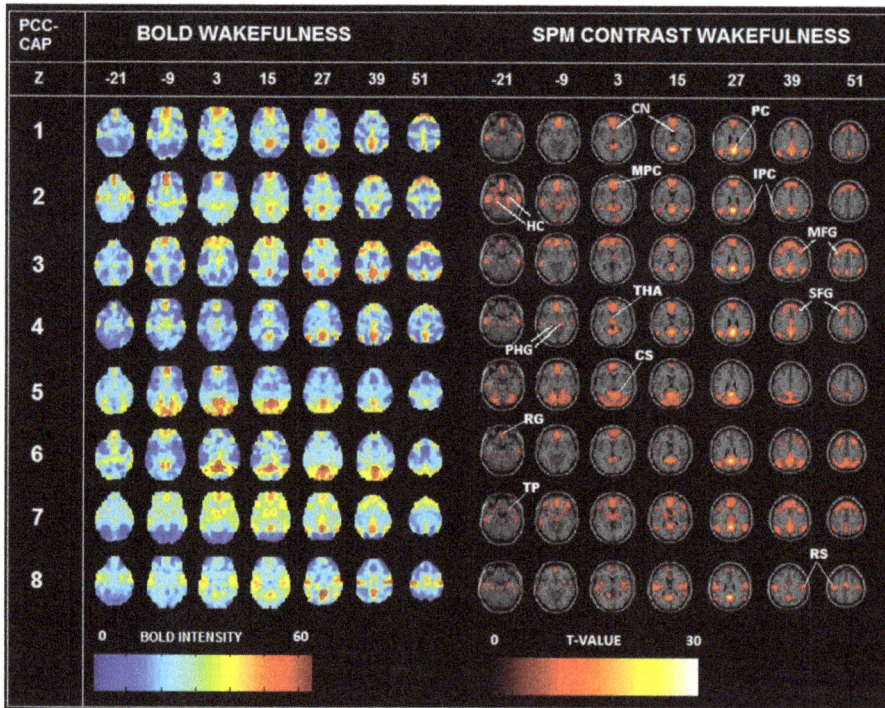

Figure 2. PCC-CAPs in wakefulness. Left: PCC co-activation patterns in wakefulness (colormap normalized by BOLD intensity), current dataset (18 subjects). Note the similarity of these patterns with the ones showed in Fig. 2 of [16]. Right: t-test on the same CAPs in the awake state showing statistically significant PCC co-activations. The seven slices shown in the maps are at Z = −21, −9, 3, 15, 27, 39, 51, respectively. The activation of precuneus (PC) appears in all 8 CAPs (see Z = 27); superior frontal gyrus (SFG) is co-activated in CAPs 1, 2, 3, 4, 6, 7 (Z = 39 and 51); the mesial prefrontal cortex (MPC) in CAPs 1, 2, 3, 4, 5, 6, 7 (Z = 3); rectus gyrus (RG) in CAPs 1, 2, 3,4, 5, 6, 7 (Z = −21); thalamus(THA) in CAPs 4 and 7 (Z = 3); caudate nucleus (CN) in CAPs 1, 3, 7 (Z = 15); temporal pole (TP) in all CAPs (slice Z = −21); hippocampus(HC) in CAPs 2, 4, 6, 8 (Z = −21); parahippocampus gyrus(PHG) in CAPs 2 and 4 (Z = −9); intraparietal cortex(IPC) all CAPs (Z = 27); medial frontal gyrus(MFG) in CAPs 3, 6, 7 (Z = 39); cuneus(CS) in CAPs 4 and 5 (Z = 3); rolandic stripe(RS) in CAPs 5 and 8 (Z = 51). Note how all these region-specific PCC co-activations survive to the t-test (e.g. HC for CAPs 2, 4, 6, 8; MFG for CAPs 3, 6, 7; PHG for CAPs 2, 4 etc.)

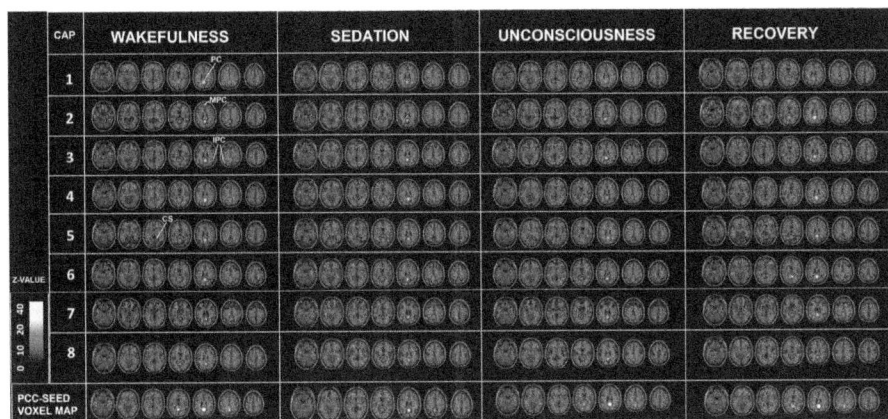

Figure 3. CAPs at different levels of consciousness. Co-activation patterns (t-contrast) in wakefulness (left), sedation (middle-left), unconsciousness (middle-right), recovery (right), corrected at FDR p<0.05. Lower panel shows PCC seed-voxel correlation maps for each state. The seven slices shown in the maps are at Z = −21, −9, 3, 15, 27, 39, 51, respectively. Spatial patterns in wakefulness and recovery do not significantly differ from each other. Precuneal (PC) activations are preserved in all CAPs in all conditions (Z = 27 and Z = 39); mesial prefrontal (MPC) cortical activity is preserved in CAPs 1, 2, 3, 4 and 7 during wakefulness, sedation and recovery (Z = 27); intraparietal cortex (IPC) activation is preserved in CAPs 1, 2, 3, 4, 6 and 7 in all conditions (Z = 39); cuneus(CS) in CAPs 4 and 5 in all conditions (Z = 3). Note that PCC-CAPs add spatial region-specific information to the network characterization across the different stages of consciousness, when compared to the equivalent PCC seed-based contrast (last row), which exhibit a prominent drop of frontal activation during sedation and unconsciousness.

fMRI preprocessing

The fMRI data were preprocessed using Statistical Parametric Software (SPM8), performing the typical preprocessing steps of functional connectivity analysis. These steps included motion correction, spatial smoothing (FWHM = 8 mm), temporal filtering with a bandpass filter (0.005 to 0.1 Hz), and the removal of linear and quadratic temporal trends. In addition, the brain-averaged signal, the time series of regions of interest in the white matter and cerebrospinal fluid, and six affine motion parameters were regressed out from the dataset. The fMRI data of each subject was first spatially coregistered to high-resolution anatomical images and then to the 152-brain Montreal Neurological Institute (MNI) space. It has recently been shown that even after standard motion correction, residual head movements can still inflate connectivity measures [18]. In order to evaluate the extent of these residual motion artifact in CAPs, for each subject and for each state of consciousness, we computed the two indices proposed by [18], i.e. Framewise Displacement (FD) and DVARS: D referring to temporal derivative of timecourses, VARS referring to root mean square (RMS) variance over voxels. FD is a scalar quantity that expresses instantaneous head motion, while DVARS is a measure of how much the intensity of a brain image changes in comparison to the previous timepoint [18]. Secondly, we defined as motion corrupted the frames in which FD and DVARS values were both above 0.5 mm for FD and 0.5% Bold for DVARS, as suggested in the same paper. Next, for each state of consciousness, we checked if there were corrupted time frames in our PCC-CAPs, and the percentage of these frames over the whole sample (see also Figure S4). We noticed that the percentage of corrupted time frames in wakefulness was 5% of the total number of frames collected; in sedation 3%; in unconsciousness 8%; in recovery 1%. However, there was no significant difference between CAPs calculated with or without artifact removal. Additionally, the preprocessed fMRI data were resampled to $3 \times 3 \times 3$ mm^3 in the MNI space, and the signal of each voxel was demeaned and normalized by its temporal standard deviation (SD).

Co-activation patterns construction

After preprocessing, the dataset was reduced to a spatio-temporal point process [15] by selecting time points in the seed region at which the signal is higher than a given threshold. In this work we used a $6 \times 6 \times 6$ mm^3 cube centered at the posterior cingulate cortex (i.e. PCC, [0, 53, 26] in MNI coordinates, identical to Liu et al. [16]). We chose PCC as seed to study default mode network (DMN) variability during consciousness modulation, since PCC is widely known as a central node in the DMN [19,20]. CAPs construction can then be summarized in three steps (Fig. 1):

1. First, we collected all the points in the normalized PCC time course where the BOLD signal was above threshold. In our study we fixed the threshold at 1 SD, roughly the 15% of the whole dataset. This percentage did not significantly vary across the four levels of consciousness. For each of these points in the PCC, and for each of the 4 levels of consciousness, we collected the relative spatial maps (Fig. 1). These spatial maps, or time frames [16], represent whole-brain patterns of functional activations correlated to PCC BOLD peaks, previously extracted using this thresholding approach.

2. In order to achieve a spatio-temporal mapping of correlated activity we clustered all the time frames which were significantly co-activated with PCC, in the same way as described in [16]. The sorting of the time frames was performed by K-means clustering, a machine learning classification method able to group unlabeled data into clusters. Once that the desired number of clusters has been fixed, K-means iteratively optimizes the position of the centers in order to minimize the total variance within each cluster [21]. We performed K-means (number of clusters fixed at 8) over all the spatial maps collected to classify the time frames based on their spatial similarity, and then averaging them within-cluster to extract 8 different spatial PCC-related co-activation patterns (i.e. CAPs [16]). Here, since we also aimed to compare different PCC-CAPs between different conditions (i.e. 4 different levels of consciousness), we added an extra step. With the purpose of

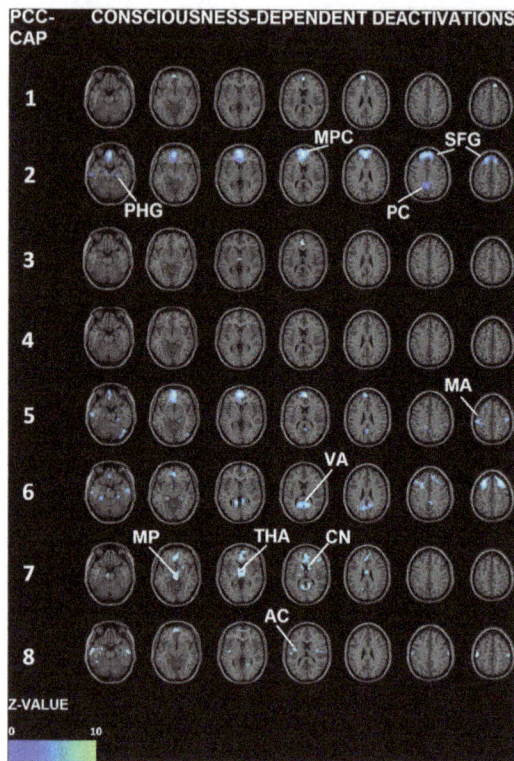

Figure 4. Decreases in CAPs. This figure shows the local decreases in co-activation from wakefulness to unconsciousness, using the same t-contrast as in [7]. All the images report contrast which are significant at p<0.05, FDR corrected. The seven slices shown in the maps are at Z = −21, −9, 3, 15, 27, 39, 51, respectively. CAPs consciousness-dependent deactivations appear in mesial prefrontal cortex (MPC), CAPs 1, 2, 5 (see Z=15); superior fontal gyrus (SFG) in CAP 2 (Z=39 and 51); thalamus (THA) in CAPs 3 and 7 (Z=3); mesencephalon (MP) in CAP 7 (Z=−9); motor area (MA) in CAP 5 and CAP 8 (Z=51); parahippocampal gyrus (PHG) in CAPs 2, 5, 6 (Z=−21); caudate nucleus (CN) in CAP 7 (Z=15); visual area (VA) in CAP 6 (Z=15); auditory cortex (AC) in CAP 8 (Z=15) and precuneus (PC) in CAP 2 (Z=39). For details see also Fig. 5 and Table 1.

obtaining a robust benchmark baseline against which to track modifications related to level of consciousness, we first ran k-means clustering over the PCC time frames collected on an independent dataset from the 1000 Functional Connectome Project (FCP, www.nitrc.org/projects/fcon_1000/), which includes wakefulness resting-state functional magnetic resonance imaging (fMRI) collected at multiple sites (247 subjects), as used by Liu and colleagues [16].

3. The eight PCC-CAPs centroids obtained from the clustering of the 1000 Functional Connectome Project dataset (FCP, www.nitrc.org/projects/fcon_1000/) were then kept fixed, and spatial clustering on the PCC time frames extracted from our propofol dataset, for each condition (i.e. wakefulness, sedation, unconsciousness, recovery), was then performed around these centroids, averaging the within-cluster spatial maps to obtain 8 different PCC-CAPs for each level of consciousness. The clustering with centroid fixed allowed us to compare PCC-CAPs between states (i.e. CAP1 in wakefulness with CAP1 in sedation, etc.), and to follow thus the fluctuation of each PCC-CAP over the course of consciousness modulation.

Statistical analysis

All statistical analyses were carried out using SPM8. For each CAP, individual time frames were entered in a second-level analysis, corresponding to a random effects model in which subjects are considered random variables. These second-level analyses consisted of analyses of variance (repeated measures analysis of variance) with the four clinical conditions as factors: normal wakefulness, sedation, unconsciousness, and recovery of consciousness. The error covariance was not assumed to be independent between regressors, and a correction for non-sphericity was applied. We used one-sided T contrasts, as implemented in Statistical Parametric Mapping software, to test for significant effects in all our analyses. After model estimation, a first T contrast searched for areas co-activated with the PCC during normal wakefulness, sedation, unconsciousness and recovery. Afterwards, in a second analysis a linear one-tailed T contrast was computed for each CAP, searching for a linear relationship between PCC co-activation patterns and the level of consciousness of the subjects across the four conditions (i.e., normal wakefulness, sedation, unconsciousness, and recovery of consciousness, SPM contrast [1.5 −0.5 −1.5 0.5], as previously described in [7]).

It should here be noted that during the recovery of consciousness subjects showed residual plasma propofol levels and lower reaction times scores (table 1 in [7]). Therefore we fixed different SPM contrast values for wakefulness (1.5) and recovery (0.5).

Results were considered significant at p<0.05, corrected for multiple comparisons with False Discovery Rate (FDR [22]), as in [7].

Results

We studied PCC-CAPs in our 18 subjects fMRI resting state dataset, for all the 4 different states of consciousness acquired, i.e. normal wakefulness, sedation, unconsciousness, recovery (see **Material and Methods** section for details). Fig. 2 shows the CAPs obtained in our study, before and after t-contrast on the significant co-activations. These spatial patterns are well reproduced in our smaller cohort (compared to the one obtained from the 1000 Functional Connectome Project dataset, depicted in Fig. 2 of [16]), and they also appear to be statistically significant(see Legend Fig. 2 for details).

Fig. 3 illustrates significant PCC co-activations in wakefulness, sedation, unconsciousness and recovery. The coarse core of the patterns throughout the consciousness modulation seem to be preserved (see Legend Fig. 3 for details). The comparison with the common seed-voxel analysis (bottom) helps to understand the advantage of this methodology, that is the ability to differentiate spatially the activation, adding fine grained information [16].

Preserved CAPs aside, some regions are no longer co-activated with the PCC in states of propofol-reduced consciousness. As to better quantify this phenomenon we decided to use a contrast that correlates with levels of consciousness. Fig. 4 illustrates the regions in each PCC-CAP where activity follows consciousness modulation. Interestingly, results show several region specific drops in CAPs activation that we are able to differentiate thanks to the employed methodology, some of them already shown in literature, some others not. In Fig. 4, CAP 1, 2 5 and 7 show drop in the prefrontal cortex, CAP 3 and 7 isolates the thalamic drop, the auditory and motor cortex decreases come up in CAP 8 and 5, drop of the visual area in CAP 6 (see also Fig. 5 and Table 1 for details).

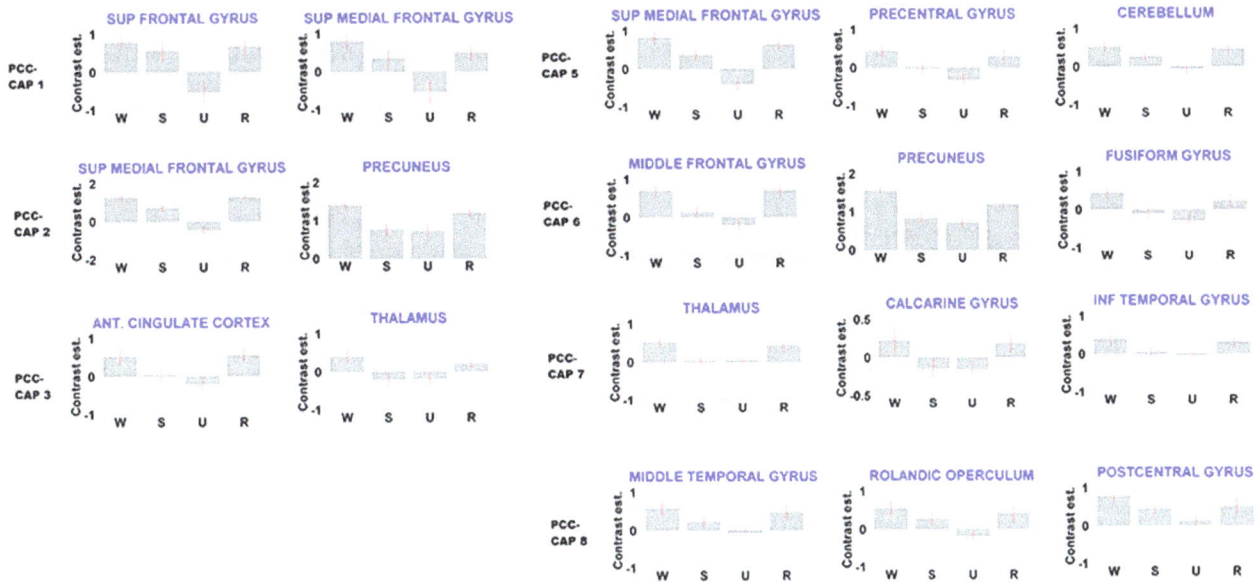

Figure 5. Region specific consciousness modulation in CAPs. Parameters estimates for the t-contrast employed, identical as in [7], for some indicative regions where PCC-related activation correlates with propofol-induced changes in consciousness. (mean ± SE; x axis labels: W = wakefulness; S = sedation; U = unconsciousness; R = recovery). Note how PCC co-activation in these regions significantly follows consciousness modulation (see also Table 1).

Discussion

With the aim to investigate changes in global and local brain activity, in this study we assessed propofol-induced changes in PCC co-activation functional patterns, during wakefulness, sedation, unconsciousness, and wakefulness recovery. Our results contribute to a growing literature addressing the changes in functional connectivity accompanying the loss of consciousness [23–26]. The approach proposed, based on the clustering of instantaneous PCC-related spatial maps, helps in the refinement and the differentiation in the spatial modulation of the default mode network when switching from wakefulness to unconsciousness.

Two key aspects of the methodology proposed in [16], and extended here, are worth discussing. One is the choice of the threshold, that is a crucial step for the construction of a spatio-temporal point process from BOLD time series. We decided to fix our threshold at 1 SD, as in [15], rather than address the threshold in terms of time frame similarity with the seed-based correlation map (see Fig. 1B in [16]). The hypothesis behind this choice is that BOLD signal point processing can help in the spatial characterization of functional connectivity patterns, better than standard correlation analysis (see also Figure S2 and S3). This data-driven evidence is independent of the assumption that BOLD signal peaks may or may not reflect cortical activations [15,27]. In this study we simply focused on spatial clustering of point processed BOLD time series, which allowed us to better characterize functional spatial interaction with the PCC during modulation of consciousness. On the other hand, the employed point process methodology is not purely dominated by hemodynamics. Indeed, co-activations patterns obtained after deconvolving the hemodynamic response function (HRF) at rest as in [27], are not qualitatively different from the ones presented in Fig. 2 (see also Figure S1).

Furthermore, the results from our PCC coactivation patterns seem in line with the ones obtained by Liu [16], in a different cohort and with a different choice of the threshold. This comes out on the side of point process methodology and of the importance of these BOLD signal peaks in spatial differentiation of network co-activations. Also, the use of clustering with centroid fixed, that is new with respect to the approach proposed in [16], can be an useful benchmark for statistical comparison of functional changing patterns between conditions (conscious states in this case, but it could also be used in pathological conditions, etc.).

A primary result is that the core of PCC-CAPs is preserved in anesthesia (Fig. 3). This is in line with other studies [7,14], where, using standard seed-based functional connectivity, the preservation of a core network of correlated regions independent on the level of consciousness was confirmed. The origin of these functional networks could be related to the fixed structural connection present in the awake brain, albeit anesthetized. This partial preservation of functional connectivity in the absence of consciousness has been suggested to possibly reflect preserved anatomical connections dissociated from higher cognitive functions [28].

Also, this approach adds new information on region specific drops in connectivity between the seeds in the DMN area and whole brain connectivity, correlating with levels of consciousness (Fig. 4 and Fig. 5): prefrontal drops (CAP 1, 2, 5, 7) are in line with previous findings in the field, showing widespread changes in prefrontal connectivity [7,9,10]: at the cortical level, hypnotic anesthetic agents have traditionally been considered to decrease activity in a widespread bilateral frontoparietal network. The primary action of hypnotic anesthetic agents would be to functionally disconnect different parts of the cortex, which would probably impair the ability to integrate information [8,23,29]. A recent electroencephalography study similarly suggests the presence of some anterior-posterior functional uncoupling in the brain, during anesthesia-induced loss of consciousness [30].

The disconnection of the thalamic area, already noted in [31,32], is highlighted in CAP 3 and 7. Using positron emission tomography, thalamic metabolism has been shown to decrease significantly during anesthesia-induced unconsciousness [24]. Furthermore, a model has been suggested in which the thalamus orchestrates the commonly observed increased and coherent alpha frequency activity in the frontal cortex during propofol-induced unconsciousness. This steady thalamic alpha rhythm could impede conduction and thus responsiveness to external stimuli [33].

Decrease of activation in the visual area (CAP 6) during anesthesia has previously been studied in monkeys [34,35], where it has been shown how local and global processing in the visual area might depend gradually on the depth of anesthesia. It may also critically depend on information integration mechanisms that function properly only in the awake and perceiving animal [34]. Here, this disconnection is shown in fMRI resting state on humans: thus, this approach seem to enlighten instantaneous spatial connectivity changes between DMN and other external areas, unlikely to be seen with other commonly used correlation analysis (e.g. seed-based functional connectivity).

Similarly, the PCC-related primary motor disconnection is pointed out here (CAP 5 and 8) on fMRI resting state data. These results are in line with previous transcranial magnetic stimulation (TMS) and electroencephalographic (EEG) studies, that indicate intracortical inhibition of central motor circuitry during incremental suppression by a potentiator of GABA agonist (propofol) in a dose-dependent manner [36,37]. The decrease in auditory cortex PCC-coactivation (CAP8) is in agreement with previous findings, in animals [38] and humans [39]. Our finding of decreased auditory cortex co-activation could be related to the hypothesis that propofol bilaterally attenuates the auditory-induced BOLD signal activation of the auditory cortex in a dose-dependent manner [40]. However, it should be noted that activation studies and resting state acquisitions offer different assessments of the underlying neurophysiological activity, in response to external stimulation or during resting conditions, respectively.

A limitation to this approach is the choice of the seed, that needs to be based on a strong priori hypothesis: whole brain connectivity analysis can improve research in this direction. Finally, since it has recently been shown that EEG directional connectivity shows characteristic changes during propofol-induced unconsciousness [41], the nature of BOLD peaks and their correlation with cortical activity needs to be explored using combined fMRI-EEG recordings.

In conclusion, our result show that functional changes in the brain associated to propofol-induced modulation of consciousness can be efficiently revealed by tracking the patterns of co-activation in the Posterior Cingulate Cortex, an area with a central role in the dynamical connectivity at rest. This methodology, based on point process analysis, can help in refining the characterization of local functional disconnections following the partial or total loss of consciousness.

Supporting Information

Figure S1 CAPs from BOLD and deconvolved BOLD signal. To avoid the possibility that the PCC-coactivation patterns were only due to different hemodynamic response functions in the different areas of the brain, we applied the approach proposed in Wu et al. [27], where point process is used to deconvolve the HRF at rest from the BOLD signal. As shown above, the CAPs obtained from the BOLD signal reported in the manuscript are confirmed when obtained from the deconvolved BOLD, suggesting a connection between spatial functional co-activations and neuronal brain response.

Figure S2 CAPs from negative BOLD peaks. CAPs obtained using positive threshold crossing (left) and negative threshold crossing (right), during wake resting state (CAPs colormap in absolute Z-value, to make patterns comparable). After the clustering, the specificity of the spatial patterns obtained using positive peaks in BOLD is not reproducible using negative peaks; positive BOLD peaks allow to reconstruct a richer variety of patterns.

Figure S3 Sliding window correlation vs CAPs. PCC co-activation patterns in wakefulness (left) compared to the 8 patterns obtained after spatial clustering of the N PCC-correlation maps computed using sliding window correlation, with window size varying from 5 time points (i.e. 12 s window, TR = 2.46 s) to 20 time points (i.e. 50 s window). Note that the region-specific patterns obtained with point process on the BOLD peaks are not recovered by using sliding window correlation. This approach seems to add more refined information in the spatial differentiation of functional networks.

Figure S4 Motion correction in CAPs. Example of the procedure discussed in **Materials and Methods**, for one subject, for each level of consciousness (i.e. wakefulness, sedation, unconsciousness, recovery). In order to evaluate the extent of these residual motion artifact in CAPs, for each subject and for each state of consciousness, we computed the two indices proposed by [18], i.e. Framewise Displacement (FD) and DVARS. FD is a scalar quantity that expresses instantaneous head motion, while DVARS is a measure of how much the intensity of a brain image changes in comparison to the previous time point [18]. Secondly, we defined as motion corrupted the frames (ArtFrames in the figure) in which FD and DVARS values were both above 0.5 mm for FD and 0.5.

Author Contributions

Conceived and designed the experiments: DM SL EA. Performed the experiments: AV DL PB JB VB CD. Analyzed the data: EA FG. Wrote the paper: EA DM SL.

References

1. Greicius MD, Krasnow B, Reiss AL, Menon V (2003) Functional connectivity in the resting brain: a network analysis of the default mode hypothesis. Proceedings of the National Academy of Sciences 100: 253–258.
2. Fox MD, Snyder AZ, Vincent JL, Corbetta M, Van Essen DC, et al. (2005) The human brain is intrinsically organized into dynamic, anticorrelated functional networks. Proceedings of the National Academy of Sciences of the United States of America 102: 9673–9678.
3. Fox MD, Raichle ME (2007) Spontaneous uctuations in brain activity observed with functional magnetic resonance imaging. Nature Reviews Neuroscience 8: 700–711.

4. Fox MD, Greicius M (2010) Clinical applications of resting state functional connectivity. Frontiers in systems neuroscience 4: 19–24.
5. Boly M, Tshibanda L, Vanhaudenhuyse A, Noirhomme Q, Schnakers C, et al. (2009) Functional connectivity in the default network during resting state is preserved in a vegetative but not in a brain dead patient. Human brain mapping 30: 2393–2400.
6. Vanhaudenhuyse A, Noirhomme Q, Tshibanda LJF, Bruno MA, Boveroux P, et al. (2010) Default network connectivity reects the level of consciousness in non-communicative brain-damaged patients. Brain 133: 161–171.
7. Boveroux P, Vanhaudenhuyse A, Bruno MA, Noirhomme Q, Lauwick S, et al. (2010) Breakdown of within-and between-network resting state functional

magnetic resonance imaging connectivity during propofol-induced loss of consciousness. Anesthesiology 113: 1038–1053.

8. Schrouff J, Perlbarg V, Boly M, Marrelec G, Boveroux P, et al. (2011) Brain functional integration decreases during propofol-induced loss of consciousness. Neuroimage 57: 198–205.

9. Martuzzi R, Ramani R, Qiu M, Rajeevan N, Constable RT (2010) Functional connectivity and alterations in baseline brain state in humans. NeuroImage 49: 823–834.

10. Deshpande G, Kerssens C, Sebel PS, Hu X (2010) Altered local coherence in the default mode network due to sevoflurane anesthesia. Brain research 1318: 110–121.

11. Hutchison RM, Womelsdorf T, Allen EA, Bandettini PA, Calhoun VD, et al. (2013) Dynamic functional connectivity: Promises, issues, and interpretations. NeuroImage 80: 360–368.

12. Allen EA, Damaraju E, Plis SM, Erhardt EB, Eichele T, et al. (2012) Tracking whole-brain connectivity dynamics in the resting state. Cerebral Cortex : bhs352.

13. Chang C, Glover GH (2010) Time–frequency dynamics of resting-state brain connectivity measured with fmri. Neuroimage 50: 81–98.

14. Hutchison RM, Womelsdorf T, Gati JS, Everling S, Menon RS (2012) Resting-state networks show dynamic functional connectivity in awake humans and anesthetized macaques. Human brain mapping 34: 2154–2177.

15. Tagliazucchi E, Balenzuela P, Fraiman D, Chialvo DR (2012) Criticality in large-scale brain fmridynamics unveiled by a novel point process analysis. Frontiers in Physiology 3: 15–25.

16. Liu X, Duyn JH (2013) Time-varying functional network information extracted from brief instances of spontaneous brain activity. Proceedings of the National Academy of Sciences 110: 4392–4397.

17. MacLaren R, Plamondon JM, Ramsay KB, Rocker GM, Patrick WD, et al. (2000) A prospective evaluation of empiric versus protocol-based sedation and analgesia. Pharmacotherapy: The Journal of Human Pharmacology and Drug Therapy 20: 662–672.

18. Power JD, Barnes KA, Snyder AZ, Schlaggar BL, Petersen SE (2012) Spurious but systematic correlations in functional connectivity mri networks arise from subject motion. Neuroimage 59: 2142–2154.

19. Fransson P, Marrelec G (2008) The precuneus/posterior cingulate cortex plays a pivotal role in the default mode network: Evidence from a partial correlation network analysis. Neuroimage 42: 1178–1184.

20. Leech R, Kamourieh S, Beckmann CF, Sharp DJ (2011) Fractionating the default mode network: distinct contributions of the ventral and dorsal posterior cingulate cortex to cognitive control. The Journal of Neuroscience 31: 3217–3224.

21. Hastie T, Tibshirani R, Friedman J, Hastie T, Friedman J, et al. (2009) The elements of statistical learning, volume 2. Springer.

22. Genovese CR, Lazar NA, Nichols T (2002) Thresholding of statistical maps in functional neuroimaging using the false discovery rate. Neuroimage 15: 870–878.

23. Alkire MT, Hudetz AG, Tononi G (2008) Consciousness and anesthesia. Science 322: 876–880.

24. Fiset P, Paus T, Daloze T, Plourde G, Meuret P, et al. (1999) Brain mechanisms of propofolinduced loss of consciousness in humans: a positron emission tomographic study. The Journal of neuroscience 19: 5506–5513.

25. Boveroux P, Bonhomme V, Boly M, Vanhaudenhuyse A, Maquet P, et al. (2008) Brain function in physiologically, pharmacologically, and pathologically altered states of consciousness. International anesthesiology clinics 46: 131–146.

26. Sanders RD, Tononi G, Laureys S, Sleigh J (2012) Unresponsiveness≠unconsciousness. Anesthesiology 116: 946.

27. Wu GR, Liao W, Stramaglia S, Ding JR, Chen H, et al. (2013) A blind deconvolution approach to recover effective connectivity brain networks from resting state fmri data. Medical image analysis 17: 365–374.

28. Peigneux P, Orban P, Balteau E, Degueldre C, Luxen A, et al. (2006) Offline persistence of memoryrelated cerebral activity during active wakefulness. PLoS biology 4: e100.

29. Lee U, Mashour GA, Kim S, Noh GJ, Choi BM (2009) Propofol induction reduces the capacity for neural information integration: implications for the mechanism of consciousness and general anesthesia. Consciousness and cognition 18: 56–64.

30. John ER, Prichep LS (2005) The anesthetic cascade: a theory of how anesthesia suppresses consciousness. Anesthesiology 102: 447–471.

31. Ying SW, Goldstein PA (2005) Propofol-block of sk channels in reticular thalamic neurons enhances gabaergic inhibition in relay neurons. Journal of neurophysiology 93: 1935–1948.

32. Guldenmund P, Demertzi A, Boveroux P, Boly M, Vanhaudenhuyse A, et al. (2013) Thalamus, brainstem and salience network connectivity changes during propofol-induced sedation and unconsciousness. Brain connectivity 3: 273–285.

33. Vijayan S, Ching S, Purdon PL, Brown EN, Kopell NJ (2013) Thalamocortical mechanisms for the anteriorization of alpha rhythms during propofol-induced unconsciousness. The Journal of Neuroscience 33: 11070–11075.

34. Lamme VA, Zipser K, Spekreijse H (1998) Figure-ground activity in primary visual cortex is suppressed by anesthesia. Proceedings of the National Academy of Sciences 95: 3263–3268.

35. Tenenbein PK, Lam AM, Klein M, Lee L (2006) Effects of sevoflurane and propofol on ash visual evoked potentials. Journal of Neurosurgical Anesthesiology 18: 310.

36. Ziemann U, Lönnecker S, Steinhoff B, Paulus W (1996) Effects of antiepileptic drugs on motor cortex excitability in humans: a transcranial magnetic stimulation study. Annals of neurology 40: 367–378.

37. Kalkman CJ, Drummond JC, Ribberink AA, Patel PM, Sano T, et al. (1992) Effects of propofol, etomidate, midazolam, and fentanyl on transcranial electrical or magnetic motor evoked responses in humans. Anesthesiology 76: 502–509.

38. Gaese BH, Ostwald J (2001) Anesthesia changes frequency tuning of neurons in the rat primary auditory cortex. Journal of neurophysiology 86: 1062–1066.

39. Plourde G, Belin P, Chartrand D, Fiset P, Backman SB, et al. (2006) Cortical processing of complex auditory stimuli during alterations of consciousness with the general anesthetic propofol. Anesthesiology 104: 448–457.

40. Dueck M, Petzke F, Gerbershagen H, Paul M, Hesselmann V, et al. (2005) Propofol attenuates responses of the auditory cortex to acoustic stimulation in a dose-dependent manner: A fmri study. Acta anaesthesiologica scandinavica 49: 784–791.

41. Untergehrer G, Jordan D, Kochs EF, Ilg R, Schneider G (2014) Fronto-parietal connectivity is a non-static phenomenon with characteristic changes during unconsciousness. PloS one 9: e87498.

15

Neuromodulatory Control of a Goal-Directed Decision

Keiko Hirayama[2¤a], **Leonid L. Moroz**[1¤b], **Nathan G. Hatcher**[1¤c], **Rhanor Gillette**[1,2*]

1 Department of Molecular & Integrative Physiology, University of Illinois, Urbana, Illinois, United States of America, 2 The Neuroscience Program, University of Illinois, Urbana, Illinois, United States of America

Abstract

Many cost-benefit decisions reduce to simple choices between approach or avoidance (or active disregard) to salient stimuli. Physiologically, critical factors in such decisions are modulators of the homeostatic neural networks that bias decision processes from moment to moment. For the predatory sea-slug *Pleurobranchaea*, serotonin (5-HT) is an intrinsic modulatory promoter of general arousal and feeding. We correlated 5-HT actions on appetitive state with its effects on the approach-avoidance decision in *Pleurobranchaea*. 5-HT and its precursor 5-hydroxytryptophan (5-HTP) augmented general arousal state and reduced feeding thresholds in intact animals. Moreover, 5-HT switched the turn response to chemosensory stimulation from avoidance to orienting in many animals. In isolated CNSs, bath application of 5-HT both stimulated activity in the feeding motor network and switched the fictive turn response to unilateral sensory nerve stimulation from avoidance to orienting. Previously, it was shown that increasing excitation state of the feeding network reversibly switched the turn motor network response from avoidance to orienting, and that 5-HT levels vary inversely with nutritional state. A simple model posits a critical role for 5-HT in control of the turn network response by corollary output of the feeding network. In it, 5-HT acts as an intrinsic neuromodulatory factor coupled to nutritional status and regulates approach-avoidance via the excitation state of the feeding network. Thus, the neuromodulator is a key organizing element in behavioral choice of approach or avoidance through its actions in promoting appetitive state, in large part via the homeostatic feeding network.

Editor: Vladimir Brezina, Mount Sinai School of Medicine, United States of America

Funding: This work was supported by NSF IOB 04-47358 and NIH R21 DA023445. The funders had no role in study design, data collection and analysis, decision to publish, or preparation of the manuscript.

Competing Interests: The authors have declared that no competing interests exist.

* Email: rhanor@illinois.edu

¤a Current address: Wolfram Inc., Champaign, Illinois, United States of America
¤b Current address: The Whitney Laboratory for Marine Bioscience, University of Florida, St. Augustine, Florida, United States of America
¤c Current address: Merck & Co., Inc., West Point, Pennsylvania, United States of America

Introduction

Major decisions in foraging behavior concern the approach or avoidance of salient stimuli in the environment. Such decisions are generally made on a cost-benefit basis where decision is informed by the moment-to-moment integration of sensation, internal state and memory. Foraging behavior is regulated by animal arousal state and appetite, themselves organized by neuromodulatory systems that regulate homeostatic neuronal networks and the sensory and motor ensembles that serve them. Documenting and testing the roles of neuromodulation in decision are significant to understanding and modeling the neural and behavioral economics of foraging.

The opisthobranch and pulmonate gastropod molluscs offer model organisms in which the neuromodulatory players in arousal and appetitive state can be addressed directly. For these molluscs serotonin (5-HT) is the most prominent neuromodulator yet found to affect arousal and appetitive state through its stimulatory effects on behavior and neural activity when applied to intact animals or to the isolated CNS [1–4]. In particular, Palovcik et al. [5] showed that injected 5-HT promoted arousal and appetitive state in terms of general activity and reduced sensory thresholds and latencies for eliciting feeding behaviors in the predatory sea-slug *Pleurobranchaea*. 5-HT is a central, and possibly the main, neuromodulatory factor regulating arousal and appetitive state through its likely roles in mediating circadian activity rhythms [6,7] and satiation [8].

Appetitive state, the readiness for expressing appetitive behavior, represents the integration of sensation, internal state, and memory. Hirayama and Gillette [9] found that appetitive state in *Pleurobranchaea* is expressed directly in the excitatory state of the feeding motor network, which sums effects of sensation, satiety and learning into the intensity and configuration of neuronal activity. It was of particular interest to find that the excitatory state of the feeding network controlled the switch between approach and avoidance behavior, converting avoidance turn responses to orienting with increasing excitation. A potential significant role for 5-HT in the decision process was suggested by its actions as an intrinsic modulator of the feeding CPG network and diverse other neuronal circuits [10,11].

We addressed how 5-HT might influence the choice of approach-avoidance in behavioral choice of intact animals and in the fictive turn responses of their isolated CNSs. The results are consistent with the role of 5-HT as a potent neuromodulator that promotes the excitation of the feeding motor network. The enhanced excitatory state biased the switching of the motor output of the turn network from avoidance to orienting responses to sensory stimuli. These results add to the known role of 5-HT as a central organizing factor in gastropod behavior and provide a novel example of the neuromodulatory regulation of a homeostatic decision.

Materials and Methods

Specimens of *Pleurobranchaea californica*, 80–1000 ml volume, were obtained by trawl or trapping through Sea Life Supply, Sand City, CA and Monterey Abalone, Inc., Monterey, CA. and maintained in artificial seawater at 12–13°C until use.

Appetitive state, measured as behavioral readiness-to-feed, in *Pleurobranchaea* is controlled by sensation, nutritional state, learning, reproductive condition and health. Readiness-to-feed here is quantified in terms of feeding thresholds measured as the minimal concentrations of appetitive stimuli to elicit proboscis extension and active biting. Feeding thresholds were measured as previously described [12,13] in response to squid homogenate or betaine (trimethylglycine; Sigma-Aldrich) solutions in seawater with 10 mM MOPS buffer (3-(N-morpholino)propanesulfonic acid) at pH 8.0, applied in 1.5 ml volumes to the oral veil with a hand-held Pasteur pipette over 10 seconds in a series of ascending concentrations in ten-fold steps. Squid homogenate was prepared as a fresh 1:1 squid-seawater cheesecloth filtrate, assigned a value of 10^0, and ten-fold dilutions were prepared down to 10^{-6}. Betaine was freshly prepared as 10^{-1} M in seawater and dilutions were prepared down to 10^{-6} M. Parameters recorded were those concentrations at which animals showed proboscis extension and biting. When specimens failed to respond to the highest concentration (10^0 squid homogenate or 10^{-1} M betaine) the next highest values, 10^1 or 10^0 for squid and betaine, respectively, were assigned. Tests began with a control sea-water application assigned a value of 10^{-7}. These conventions assign conservative finite values to essentially infinitely high or low thresholds. Threshold data were analyzed and presented as the logarithms of the dilutions; thus, 10^{-1} is -1.0 and so on.

Results were analyzed using non-parametric methods for the non-Gaussian distribution of the data. Friedman's non-parametric repeated measures ANOVA was used to detect differences in treatments across multiple tests. Wilcoxon matched-pairs signed-ranks tests were used to compare repeated measurements to assess whether control or experimental population mean ranks differed with time. Kruskal–Wallis ANOVA was used to compare groups of unequal size. The Mann-Whitney test was used to test for significant differences in control vs. experimental thresholds. Population thresholds are presented as medians, and errors are presented as interquartile range (+/− IQR). Data are presented in box and whisker charts where the ends of the whisker are set at 1.5*IQR above the third quartile (Q3) and 1.5*IQR below the first quartile (Q1). When Minimum or Maximum values are outside this range, they are shown as outliers.

Taurine for behavioral testing was made as a 10^{-2} M solution in artificial sea-water (pH 8.0). 5-hydroxytryptamine creatine sulfate (5-HT; Sigma-Aldrich) solutions were prepared for hemocoele injection as 1 mM in artificial saline (below) and as 2.5, 5 and 50 μM solutions for bath application to isolated CNSs. The 5-HT precursor 5-hydroxytryptophan (5-HTP; Sigma-Aldrich) was prepared for hemocoele injections as a 1 mM solution in artificial saline. For estimation of final dilutions after injections, animal volumes were measured prior to injections and hemolymph volumes were estimated at 65% of total volume. Animals were satiated in some experiments by feeding strips of squid flesh until they stopped eating, having consumed quantities of 10–35% body weight.

For electrophysiological recordings animals were anesthetized by cooling to 4°C. CNSs, consisting of interconnected cerebro-pleural, pedal, visceral and buccal ganglia, were dissected out and pinned in a Sylgard dish under artificial saline (in mM) 460 NaCl, 10 KCl, 25 MgCl$_2$, 25 MgSO$_4$, 10 CaCl$_2$, and 10 MOPS buffer at pH 7.5 and 12–13°C. Suction electrodes recorded activity in buccal ganglion motor nerve root 3 (R3), which displays both rhythmic and non-rhythmic output of the feeding central motor pattern generator, and from the bilateral lateral body wall nerves (LBWNs) which are motor outputs for the turn network.

Fictive turns were induced by brief stimulation of one of the bilateral pair of large oral veil nerves (LOVNs; 15 Hz, 2 msec pulse duration; [14]). Data were captured and analyzed with Chart 5 Pro (AD Instruments). Spikes were counted at threshold levels above spontaneous noise and spike frequencies were normalized to counts for 20 seconds prior to the stimulus event and plotted in 2–3 second bins. Fictive turn events were assessed by comparing mean spike frequencies in LBWNs [9,14] and by comparing the ratios of relative spike frequencies across bins in the ipsilateral vs. contralateral turn nerves. Kruskal–Wallis ANOVA was used to assess variations across ratio medians, and the two-tailed Dunn's Multiple Comparisons Test was used to compare ratio differences between control and experimental (5-HT) conditions. P values were calculated by comparing the spike counts in ipsilateral and contralateral LBWNs for 30 seconds from the first steep inflection following the initial peak. The initial peak corresponds to a fictive withdrawal preceding the turn, as in intact animals [14]. Criteria for assigning "fictive avoidance" vs. "fictive orienting" to LBWNs' activities were significant differences of at least $p<0.05$ for bilateral spike counts [9], and values for ratios of ipsilateral/contralateral nerves spike frequencies of less than or greater than 1.0, respectively. To assess effects of 5-HT on turn direction, measured volumes of 1 mM 5-HT in saline were added to the recording chamber by pipette and gently mixed to final concentrations of 5–50 μM.

Results

Orienting and avoidance turns have been well described in intact animals [14,15]. Strong avoidance turn responses to transient noxious stimuli are relatively stereotypic, mediated by contraction of longitudinal body wall muscles and body flexion away from the stimulus to 45–250°, accompanied by suppression of locomotion and feeding, and are generally complete in 30–40 seconds. Orienting turns tend to be of smaller angles, slower, and do not always interrupt locomotion. Turn stimuli induce a transient withdrawal (around 10 seconds) preceding avoidance turns and sometimes orienting turns as well. These characters are reflected in the fictive behavior of the isolated CNS.

5-HT Reduces Feeding Thresholds and Biases Turn Choice to Orienting in Intact Animals

Injecting animals with the 5-HT precursor 5-HTP (50 μM estimated internal dilution) significantly reduced feeding thresholds for proboscis extension and biting at 7 hours post-injection; measured effects peaked at 10 hours post-injection (Fig. 1). The appearance of spontaneous locomotor activity, spontaneous local mantle contractures, handling-induced biting and escape swimming were consistent with a state of general arousal. Our field observations suggest that these features are also characteristic of naturally very hungry animals freshly captured in trawls. In contrast, saline-injected control animals showed slightly elevated feeding thresholds, which are characteristic of handling effects [16].

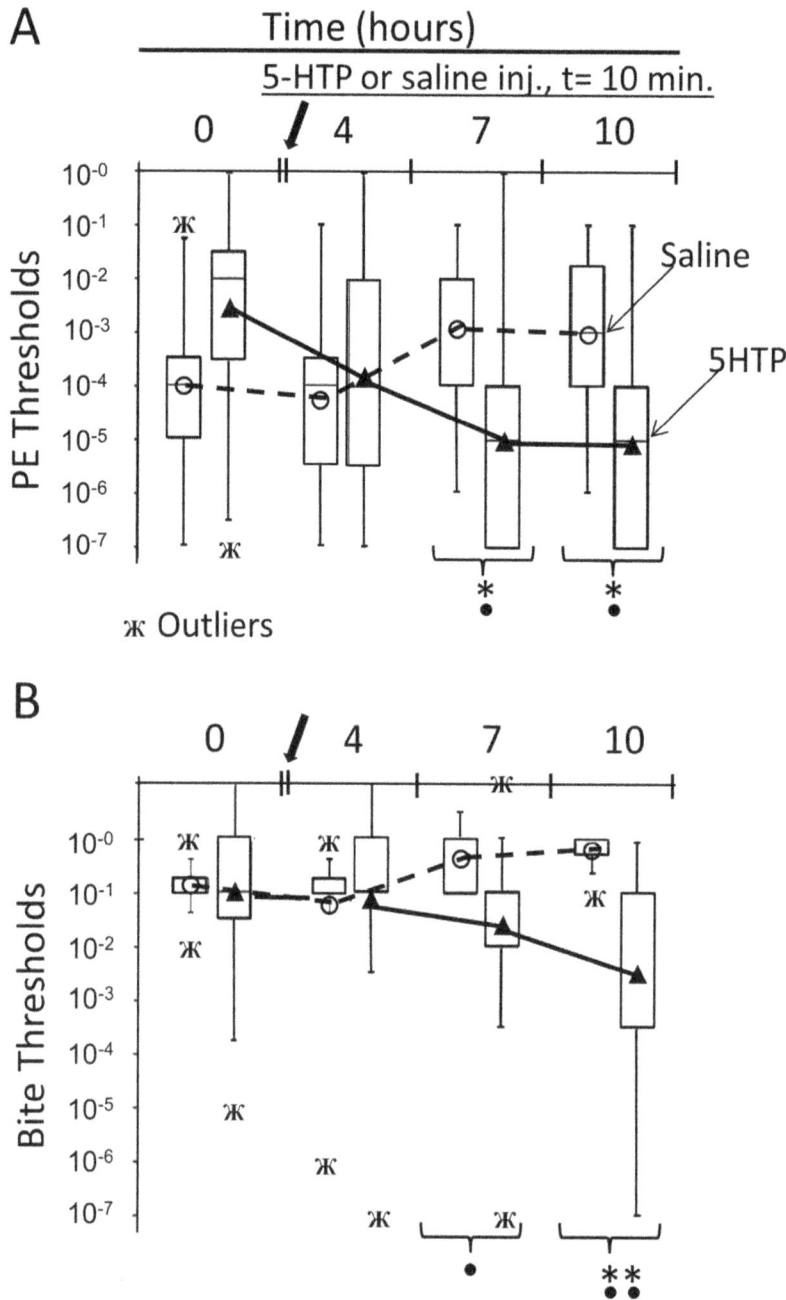

Figure 1. 5-HTP injection reduced thresholds for both proboscis extension (A) and biting (B). Following initial threshold measures at t = 0 with squid homogenate dilutions, animals were injected with 5-HTP (50 μM estimated internal dilution) at t = 10 min. (○, group mean experimentals; N = 15) or isotonic saline (▲, group mean controls; N = 8) and measured at intervals over 10 hours. Proboscis extension (PE) and bite thresholds differed significantly over trials in the 5-HTP injected groups (Friedman's non-parametric repeated measures ANOVA, $\chi^2 = 21.744$ (PE), $\chi^2 = 12.830$ (Bite), $p < 0.0001$ and $p < 0.005$, respectively). Experimentals' PE thresholds were significantly reduced starting at 7 and 10 hours (Wilcoxon matched-pairs signed-ranks tests: $W = -101$, *$p < 0.0005$). Bite thresholds were significantly reduced at 10 hours (**$p < 0.0001$). 5-HTP injected experimentals differed over time from saline injected controls (Kruskal-Wallis Non-parametric ANOVA, $H = 19.315$ (PE), $H = 14.838$ (Bite), $p < 0.01$ and $p < 0.04$ for PE and Bite thresholds, respectively). Threshold differences between experimentals and controls were significant at 7 and 10 hours (Mann-Whitney tests, •$p < 0.02$). Bite threshold increased over the experiment in saline injected controls (Friedman's non-parametric repeated measures ANOVA, $\chi^2 = 8.882$, $p < 0.02$), suggesting handling effects [16], but the individual increases were non-significant.

Subsequently, we tested effects of 5-HTP on satiation. Eight animals were fed to satiation, raising averaged biting threshold 100-fold. Injecting 4 animals with 5-HTP lowered thresholds to pre-satiation values ($p < 0.03$; Fishers Exact test) and increased general arousal state as above, although crops and stomachs remained visibly full of squid, as seen through the translucent mantle. Saline-injected controls retained high thresholds.

Injections of 5-HT caused behavioral effects similar to the 5-HTP precursor, but with much shorter latency. Twenty-three animals were injected with sufficient 1 mM 5-HT for an estimated hemolymph dilution of 2.5 μM. This treatment lowered the averaged thresholds for inducing proboscis extension and biting with betaine by 27- and 15-fold, respectively, and significantly reduced median biting thresholds when animals were tested at 12 minutes post-injection (Fig. 2A). General behavioral arousal, as seen with 5-HTP, also appeared quickly and effects lasted over 40 minutes. Control injections of saline alone given to the animals on the days previous and following 5-HT injection caused no significant changes. Injections of a much larger amount of 5-HT (50 μM final dilution) into 15 different animals over-dosed them into 40–60 minutes of seeming locomotor paralysis accompanied by spasmodic waves of local mantle contracture, transient (5–10 minutes) penis eversion and non-responsiveness to mechanical and appetent chemical sensory inputs. Such effects recall the inverted U-shaped function typical of the relation for performance and arousal [17], where performance is diminished at higher arousal states. On eventual recovery of sensory responsiveness and locomotor ability, animals entered a state of general activity as above for an hour or more. Thus 5-HT stimulated arousal state in general, and readiness to feed in particular.

5-HT reduces avoidance and promotes appetitive behavior to a mildly noxious stimulus like that observed in untreated animals with high readiness to feed.Turning responses to taurine were also altered at 12 min. after 5-HT injection (2.5 μM final hemolymph concentration). Taurine is a deterrent stimulus that induces skin acid secretion, which itself is aversive to the animal [15]. Unilateral application of 10^{-2} M taurine to the oral veil normally induces avoidance responses in animals with mid- to high-level feeding thresholds. However, in animals with lower feeding thresholds, taurine, acidified sea-water and moderate mechanical stimuli induce feeding attack [12]. We tested 20 animals with higher feeding thresholds (biting at or above 10^{-1} M betaine) and found that 18 animals avoided the taurine stimulus and 2 animals showed orienting responses. 12 minutes after the 5-HT injection, turn responses ceased in 11 subjects, orienting turns were elicited

in 6, and only 3 animals continued to show avoidance turns (Fig. 2B).

5-HT Promotes Fictive Orienting Turn Choice and Excitation in the Feeding Network of Isolated CNSs

Choice of fictive turn response, avoidance or orienting, in isolated CNSs responding to unilateral sensory nerve stimuli was previously found to correlate with donor animals' feeding thresholds, and to be regulated by the excitation state of the feeding network [9]. Thus, we assayed effects of 5-HT on fictive turn choice in CNSs from four donor animals with high feeding thresholds (betaine thresholds 10^{-1} M and above) that responded initially with fictive avoidance to unilateral stimulation of the sensory LOVN. Tested within 5 minutes after bath application of 5 μM 5-HT, all four CNSs showed fictive orienting to the LOVN stimulation (Fig. 3, Table 1), significant at $p < 0.03$ (two-sided Fisher's Exact Test). Increased overall spiking activities were observed in both turn and feeding motor nerves soon after 5-HT application and gradually declined over 10–20 minutes.

It was shown that artificially increasing the excitatory state of the feeding network can cause the switch from fictive avoidance to orienting turns [9]. Thus, we tested effects of 5-HT on the feeding network. No robust differences were observed in the sensitivity to 5 μM 5-HT in CNSs from 5 high- and 5 low-threshold animals (not shown). However, 5-HT had dose-dependent excitatory effects on the feeding network at concentrations of 5–50 μM, with lesser and more variable effects at the lower concentrations (Fig. 4).

Discussion

These observations directly demonstrate regulation of a homeostatic (feeding) network by an intrinsic neuromodulatory factor, thereby directing goal-seeking behavior. The results support a central role for 5-HT in regulating appetitive state in the molluscan CNS, and they extend the neuromodulator's known

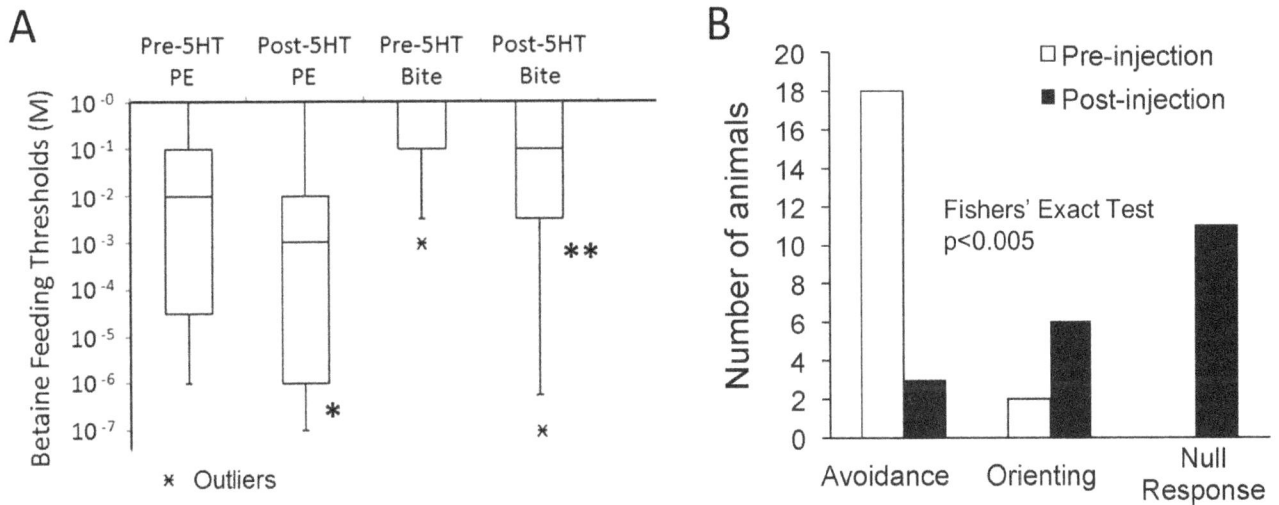

Figure 2. 5-HT injections reduced feeding thresholds, suppressed avoidance, and promoted orienting turn responses to a noxious stimulus in intact animals. A. Injection of 23 animals with 5-HT (1–2.5 μM final hemolymph dilution) significantly reduced median feeding thresholds to betaine measured 12 minutes later (Wilcoxon matched-pairs signed-ranks tests, PE: W = −28, *p<0.02; Bite: W = −36, **p<0.01). Control saline injections were ineffective. B. Responses to noxious unilateral taurine application (10^{-2} M) to the tentacle/oral veil were compared before and after 5-HT injection to an estimated final hemolymph concentration of 2.5 μM. Among 20 animals tested, 18 initially showed avoidance and 2 animals showed orienting responses to taurine application. 12 minutes after 5-HT injection, avoidance was replaced by null responses in 11 animals and orienting turns were observed in 6 (p<0.005, Fishers' Exact Test); only 3 animals continued to show avoidance.

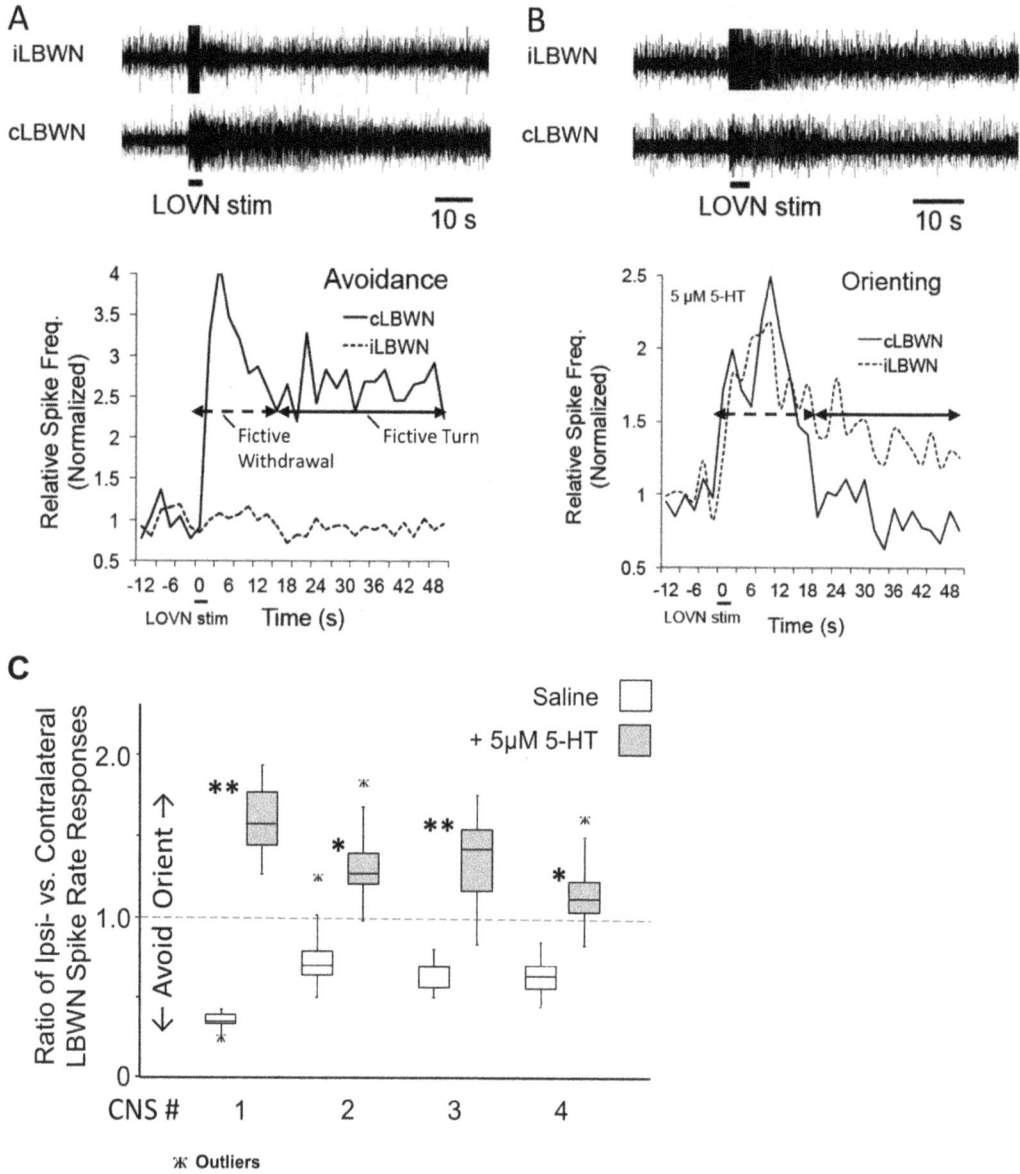

Figure 3. 5-HT altered fictive turn preference from avoidance to orienting. Application of 5 μM 5-HT to isolated CNS from each of 4 donors changed fictive turn preference from avoidance to orienting. The figure shows a fictive avoidance turn (A) changed to fictive orienting (B) within 5 minutes following 5-HT addition. Fictive turn direction is shown in differing relative spike rates of the LBWNs following stimulation of the ipsilateral LOVN (short horizontal bar at bottom) [9]. Fictive turns (solid double arrows) are measured following transient fictive withdrawal responses (dashed double arrows). C. Box and whiskers plot of ratios of spike frequencies for the LBWNs calculated across bins to assess orienting vs. avoidance turns in control vs. 5-HT conditions. Variations across ratio medians were significant (Kruskal–Wallis ANOVA; $p < 0.0001$). Ratios of spike frequencies in 5-HT were significantly different from controls (two-tailed Dunn's Multiple Comparisons Test; *$p < 0.01$; **$p < 0.001$; Table 1).

Table 1. Ratios of relative spike rate responses of contralateral vs. ipsilateral turn nerves to unilateral LOVN stimulation.

Experiment	Initial Avoidance Response: ipsilateral/ contralateral LBWN spike frequencies	5-HT Induced Orienting Response: ipsilateral/ contralateral LBWN spike frequencies	Two-Sided Fisher's Exact Test: Significance of the 5-HT Effect
1	0.349	1.592**	P = 0.0286
2	0.739	1.328*	
3	0.616	1.350**	
4	0.628	1.140*	

Dunn's Multiple Comparison Test; *$p < 0.01$, **$p < 0.001$. Avoidance turns are characterized by ratios < 1.0, and orienting turns by ratios > 1.0. Fisher's Exact Test supports a significant effect of 5-HT in changing avoidance responses to orienting in the four experiments of Figure 3.

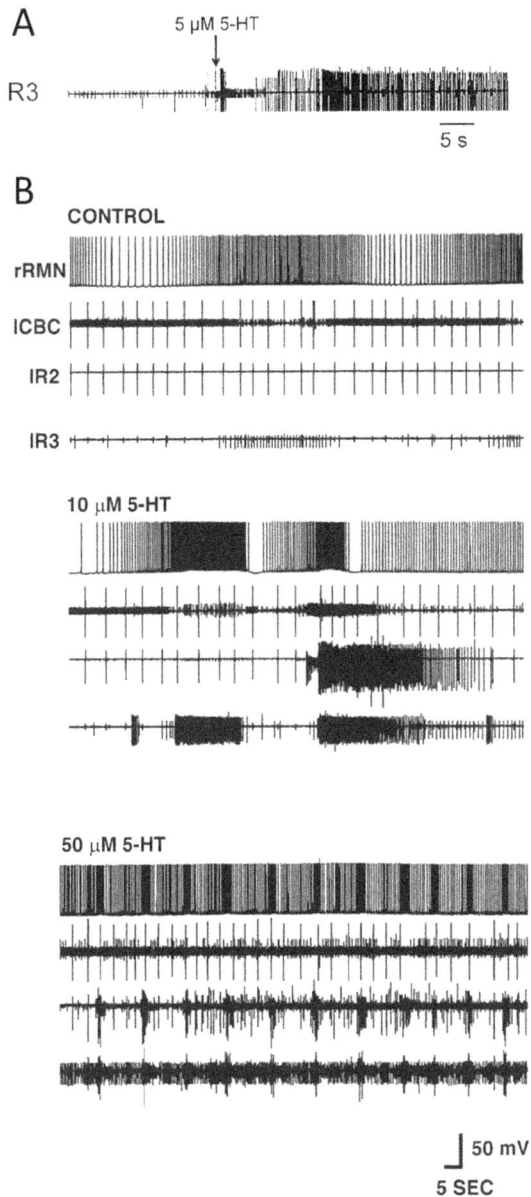

Figure 4. 5-HT stimulates general excitation state of the feeding motor network in isolated CNSs. Similar stimulation of the feeding network by driving command neurons or gastroesophageal stimulation converts fictive avoidance turn responses to orienting [9]. A. 5 μM 5-HT induces spike activity in nerve root 3 (R3) of the buccal ganglion. B. A separate experiment in which sequential applications of 10 and 50 μM 5-HT show dose-dependence of induced spiking activity recorded intracellularly in a right retraction phase buccal motorneuron (rRMN) and extracellularly in a left cerebrobuccal connective (lCBC), and left nerve roots 2 and 3 (lR2, lR3).

functions beyond general arousal mechanisms and plasticity to an elemental, value-based decision: the goal-directed turn.

5-HT is a well-recognized regulator of appetitive state and arousal in lophotrochozoan (mollusc and leech) model systems. This is well documented across molluscan species: for the sea-butterfly *Clione limacina* [18], the pond snails *Helisoma trivolvis* [19], *Lymnaea stagnalis* [20], and *Planorbis corneus* [21], the sea-hare *Aplysia californica* [22], and the side-gilled sea-slug *Pleurobranchaea californica* [5,8]. In particular, the work of C.

M. Lent and collaborators [23,24] indicated that satiation-related changes in levels of 5-HT might modulate homeostatic decision in the leech, where increasing CNS levels would promote prey search, attack and feeding, while decreasing 5-HT levels accompanied quiescence and crypsis. Similar observations in *Pleurobranchaea* [8] suggested a role for 5-HT in mediating cost-benefit decisions for approach and avoidance, and spurred our investigations.

The main findings of this study were three: 1) Exogenous 5-HT and its 5-HTP precursor enhanced expressions of appetitive state in both the intact animal and the isolated CNS; 2) 5-HT increased overall excitation state in the feeding motor network; and 3) Avoidance turns expressed in intact animals and fictively in isolated CNS could be converted to orienting by exogenous 5-HT, paralleling expression of appetitive state in feeding thresholds of intact animals and spontaneous activity in the feeding motor network.

The effects of 5-HT as a global modulator of behavioral state were confirmed and were extended to show that 5-HTP, the precursor of 5-HT, had stimulatory effects in the intact animal similar to native 5-HT. The action of 5-HTP in enhanced stimulation of molluscan neuronal circuitry has been related to increased presynaptic 5-HT content and release [25–27].

Behavioral effects of 5-HT were further extended to approach-avoidance responses to a noxious stimulus, taurine. Taurine at concentrations of 10^{-5} to 10^{-2} M induces acid secretion in the skin of *Pleurobranchaea*, which is normally a defensive chemical response that also acts as an auto-irritant to potentiate aversive behavior [15]. However, animals with lower feeding thresholds can respond to noxious stimuli like taurine and acidified sea-water with appetitive behavior [12]. This may be an adaptive behavioral response, where mildly painful stimuli reinforce attack behavior in the hungry predators to deal with struggling prey [12]. 5-HT injections changed taurine-avoidance responses to either orienting or null responses in a significant number of subjects tested, showing a stimulating action of 5-HT on appetitive state.

5-HT stimulates the excitation state of sensory pathways and multiple motor networks in the molluscan nervous system, among them the feeding motor network. In particular, the excitation state of the feeding motor network directs the approach-avoidance decision of the goal-directed turn [9], and these results connect the actions of 5-HT in the feeding motor network to regulation of the turn motor network in behavioral choice. The conversion of fictive turn decision from avoidance to orienting by 5-HT is consistent with the neuromodulator's action in promoting feeding network excitation, and resembles the effects of direct stimulation of the feeding CPG by driving feeding command neurons or feeding nerves [9].

A model for the role of 5-HT in approach-avoidance choice is based on regulation of basal excitation state in the feeding motor network (Fig. 5A). The model combines the present results with previous findings that resting excitation state in the feeding network of the isolated CNS is proportionate to donors' feeding thresholds, where excitation state is significantly higher in animals with lower thresholds [9]. The turn network responds by default to unilateral, somatotopically mapped sensory input from the oral veil [28] with avoidance turns, and increasing feeding network activity switches turn responses to orienting [9]. The model posits that variations in endogenous 5-HT in the feeding network regulate excitability, based on findings that 5-HT content in serotonergic neurons of the feeding motor network varies inversely with satiation state [8]. Thus, higher levels of endogenous 5-HT in the feeding networks of more ready-to-feed animals may underlie

A

B

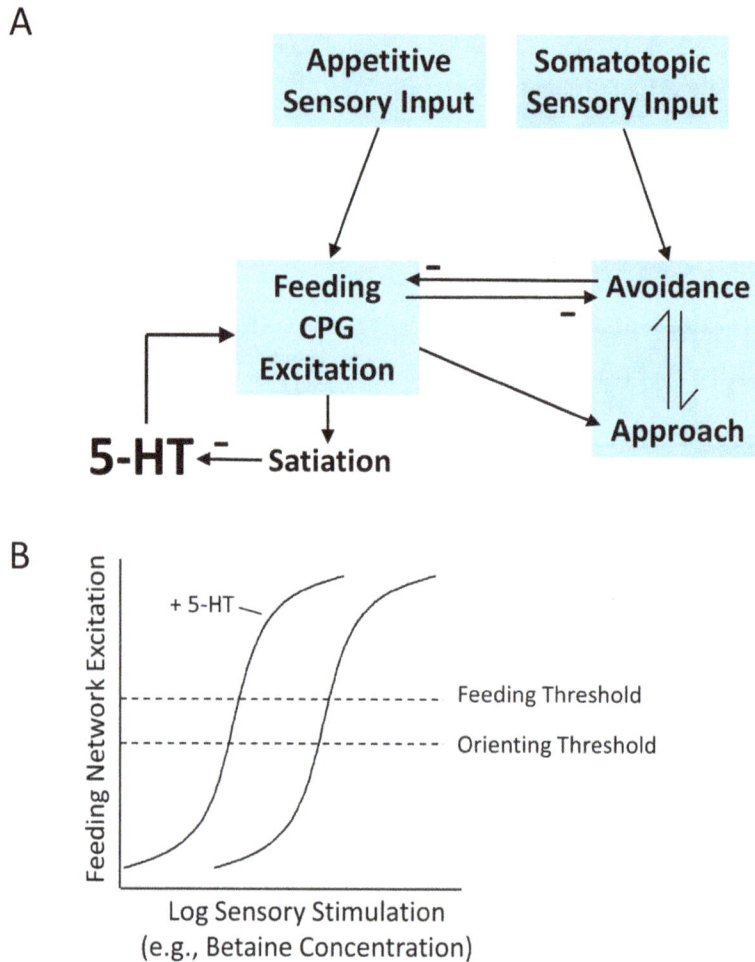

Figure 5. A model for regulation of appetitive state and behavioral choice by satiation via serotonin. A. The model builds on the relation that the default turn response to somatotopically mapped stimuli from the oral veil is avoidance, and that corollary outputs of the feeding network can change this response to orienting. The resting excitation state of the feeding motor network is set by endogenous 5-HT level, which is an inverse function of satiation state. Thus, network excitation state sums effects of satiation and appetitive sensory inputs (including effects of learned values of different prey odors). At increasing levels of feeding network excitation the turn response is switched from avoidance to approach. B. Increasing levels of 5-HT, through decline of satiation or by exogenous addition, increase feeding CPG excitation and thereby reduce the sensory thresholds for orienting and active feeding.

their enhanced appetitive states, lower feeding thresholds, and their consequent biases toward orienting turns (Fig. 5B).

We speculate that endogenous 5-HT acts in the feeding network within a neuromodulatory positive feedback loop, where temporal decline in primary satiation factors (e.g., gut stretch) would result in a sharpened appetite due to the excitatory action of recovering 5-HT activity. Thus, in modulating gastropod appetitive state, 5-HT may act much as the hypothalamic orexin/hypocretin peptides do in mammals [29], and is similarly regulated by more primary satiation factors. In gastropods, gut stretch is the primary satiation factor, and acts in *Pleurobranchaea* to bias the rhythmic radular protraction/retraction cycle of the feeding motor CPG towards the retraction phase, thereby suppressing feeding (reviewed in ref. 11). Possibly, satiation-induced decrease in 5-HT levels in modulatory feeding neurons might be caused by use-dependent effects of decreased activity in the feeding network. This suggestion is supported by an early observation of an increase with depolarization of a 5-HT-like intracellular voltammetry signal in a homologous neuron of the gastropod *Aplysia* [30]. Otherwise, an effect of some other, as yet unidentified, satiation factor could mediate effects on 5-HT levels.

Serotonergic neurons in the gastropod nervous system are embedded in motor networks as intrinsic neuromodulatory elements and they are loosely coupled across the CNS to form a distributed serotonergic network important in behavioral arousal, sensitization, and learning [11,27,31,32]. In the vertebrates, 5-HT has similar neuromodulatory roles in excitatory arousal of sensory and motor circuits, consistent with evolutionary conservation of function. However, its vertebrate arousal functions are secondary and subservient to the hypothalamic neuropeptide orexin/hypocretin and a neuromodulatory network of other peptides in regulating arousal and appetitive state. This relationship has been related to a relative lack of communication between the CNS and nutritional stores in those lophotrochozoans that have been studied [11], unlike the complex regulation of appetite in vertebrates by hormonal communication with CNS from nutritional stores (fat, glucose and glycogen) and the gut via the hypothalamic peptidergic network [33]. Thus, animals like *Pleurobranchaea* with simpler behavioral economies use minimal systems of neuromodulatory controls of appetitive state and cost-benefit approach/avoidance decisions that may well resemble those built upon in vertebrate evolution.

Pleurobranchaea readily learns the values of environmental stimuli by experience [16], and the effects of learning are integrated into appetitive state along with sensation and satiation in the feeding network [9,34,35]. Thus, approach/avoidance decision in the directed turn is an elemental, goal-directed cognitive choice that embodies expected utility and risk. The neuromodulatory role of 5-HT as a central regulator of homeostatic decision offers an example for homeostatic regulation of goal-directed decision that can be readily pursued in this and similar systems.

References

1. Kupfermann I, Cohan JL, Mandelbaum DE, Schonberg M, Susswein AJ, et al. (1979) Functional role of serotonergic neuromodulation in *Aplysia*. Fed Proc 38: 2095–2102.
2. Satterlie RA, Norekian TP (1996) Modulation of swimming speed in the pteropod mollusc, *Clione limacina*: role of a compartmental serotonergic system. Invert Neurosci. 2: 157–165.
3. Marinesco S, Wickremasinghe N, Kolkman KE, Carew TJ (2004) Serotonergic modulation in *Aplysia*. II. Cellular and behavioral consequences of increased serotonergic tone. J Neurophysiol 92: 2487–2496.
4. Katz PS, Frost WN (1995) Intrinsic neuromodulation in the *Tritonia* swim CPG: serotonin mediates both neuromodulation and neurotransmission by the dorsal swim interneurons. J Neurophysiol 74: 2281–2294.
5. Palovcik RA, Basberg BA, Ram JL (1982) Behavioral state changes induced in *Pleurobranchaea* and *Aplysia* by serotonin. Behav Neural Biol 35: 383–394.
6. Corrent G, McAdoo DJ, Eskin A (1978) Serotonin shifts the phase of the circadian rhythm from the *Aplysia* eye. Science 202: 977–979.
7. Stuart JN, Ebaugh JD, Copes AL, Hatcher NG, Gillette R, et al. (2004) Systemic serotonin sulfate in opisthobranch mollusks. J Neurochem 90, 734–742.
8. Hatcher NG, Zhang X, Stuart JN, Moroz LL, Sweedler JV, et al. (2007) 5-HT and 5-HT-SO$_4$, but not tryptophan or 5-HIAA levels in single feeding neurons track animal hunger state. J Neurochem 104: 1358–1363.
9. Hirayama K, Gillette R (2012) A neuronal network switch for approach/avoidance toggled by appetitive state. Current Biol 22: 118–123.
10. Gillette R, Davis WJ (1977) The role of the metacerebral giant neuron in the feeding behavior of *Pleurobranchaea*. J Comp Physiol 116: 129–159.
11. Gillette R (2006) Evolution and function in serotonergic systems. Integ Comp Biol 46: 838–846.
12. Gillette R, Huang RC, Hatcher N, Moroz LL (2000) Cost-benefit analysis potential in feeding behavior of a predatory snail by integration of hunger, taste, and pain. Proc Natl Acad Sci USA 97: 3585–3590.
13. Davis WJ, Mpitsos GJ (1971) Behavioral choice and habituation in the marine mollusk *Pleurobranchaea californica* MacFarland (Gastropoda, Opisthobranchia). Z vergl Physiol 75: 207–232.
14. Jing J, Gillette R (2003) Directional avoidance turns encoded by single interneurons and sustained by multifunctional serotonergic cells. J Neurosci 23: 3039–3051.
15. Gillette R, Saeki M and Huang R-C (1991) Defense mechanisms in notaspidean snails: Acid humor and evasiveness. J Exp Biol 156, 335–347.
16. Noboa V, Gillette R (2013) Selective prey avoidance learning in the predatory sea-slug *Pleurobranchaea californica*. J Exp Biol 216: 3231–3236.
17. Yerkes RM, Dodson JD (1908) The relation of strength of stimulus to rapidity of habit-formation. J Comp Neurol Psychol 18: 459–482.
18. Kabotyanski EA, Sakharov DA (1991) Neuronal correlates of the serotonin-dependent behavior of the pteropod mollusc *Clione limacina*. Neurosci Behav Physiol 21: 422–435.
19. Murphy AD (2001) The neuronal basis of feeding in the snail, *Helisoma*, with comparisons to selected gastropods. Prog Neurobiol 63: 383–408.
20. Straub VA, Benjamin PR (2001) Extrinsic modulation and motor pattern generation in a feeding network: a cellular study. J Neurosci 21: 1767–1778.
21. Berry MS, Pentreath VW (1976) Properties of a symmetric pair of serotonin-containing neurones in the cerebral ganglia of *Planorbis*. J Exp Biol 65: 361–380.
22. Kupfermann I, Cohen JL, Mandelbaum DE, Schonberg M, Susswein AJ, et al. (1979) Functional role of serotonergic neuromodulation in *Aplysia*. Fed Proc 38: 2095–2102.
23. Lent CM, Dickinson MH, Marshall CG (1989) Serotonin and leech feeding behavior: obligatory neuromodulation. Am Zool 29: 1241–1254.
24. Lent CM, Zundel D, Freedman E, Groome JR (1991) Serotonin in the leech central nervous system: anatomical correlates and behavioral effects. J Comp Physiol A 168: 191–200.
25. Fickbohm DJ, Katz PS (2000) Paradoxical actions of the serotonin precursor 5-hydroxytryptophan on the activity of identified serotonergic neurons in a simple motor circuit. J Neurosci 20: 1622–1634.
26. Marinesco S, Carew TJ (2002) Serotonin release evoked by tail nerve stimulation in the CNS of *Aplysia*: Characterization and relationship to heterosynaptic plasticity. J Neurosci 22: 2299–2312.
27. Marinesco S, Kolkman KE, Carew TJ (2004) Serotonergic modulation in Aplysia. I. Distributed serotonergic network persistently activated by sensitizing stimuli. J Neurophysiol 92: 2468–2486.
28. Yafremava LS, Gillette R (2011) Putative lateral inhibition in sensory processing for directional turns. J Neurophysiol 105: 2885–2890.
29. Willie JT, Chemelli RM, Sinton CM, Yanagisawa M (2001) To eat or to sleep? Orexin in the regulation of feeding and wakefulness. Annu Rev Neurosci 24: 429–458.
30. Meulemans A, Poulain B, Baux G, Tauc L (1987) Changes in serotonin concentration in a living neurone: a study by on-line intracellular voltammetry. Brain Res 414: 158–162.
31. Norekian TP, Satterlie RA (1996) Cerebral serotonergic neurons reciprocally modulate swim and withdrawal neural networks in the mollusk *Clione limacina*. J Neurophysiol 75: 538–546.
32. Jing J, Gillette R (2000) Escape swim network interneurons have diverse roles in behavioral switching and putative arousal in *Pleurobranchaea*. J Neurophysiol 83: 1346–1355.
33. Wynne K, Stanley S, McGowan B, Bloom S (2005) Appetite Control. J Endocrinol 184: 291–318.
34. Davis WJ, Gillette R (1978) Neural correlates of behavioral plasticity in command neurons in *Pleurobranchaea*. Science 199: 801–804.
35. Davis WJ, Gillette R, Kovac MP, Croll RP, Matera EM (1983) Organization of synaptic inputs to paracerebral feeding command interneurons of *Pleurobranchaea californica* III. Modifications induced by experience. J Neurophysiol 49: 1557–1572.

Acknowledgments

Part of this work was conducted with the hospitality of Friday Harbor Laboratories, University of Washington, and its then director, A.O.D. Willows.

Author Contributions

Conceived and designed the experiments: RG LLM KH NGH. Performed the experiments: RG LLM KH NGH. Analyzed the data: RG LLM KH NGH. Contributed reagents/materials/analysis tools: RG. Wrote the paper: RG KH.

16

VPA Alleviates Neurological Deficits and Restores Gene Expression in a Mouse Model of Rett Syndrome

Weixiang Guo[1]❾¤, Keita Tsujimura[2]❾, Maky Otsuka I.[3], Koichiro Irie[2], Katsuhide Igarashi[3]*, Kinichi Nakashima[2]*, Xinyu Zhao[1]*

1 Department of Neuroscience and Waisman Center, School of Medicine and Public Health, University of Wisconsin, Madison, Wisconsin, United States of America, **2** Department of Stem Cell Biology and Medicine, Graduate School of Medical Sciences, Kyushu University, Fukuoka, Japan, **3** Life Science Tokyo Advanced Research center (L-StaR), Hoshi University School of Pharmacy and Pharmaceutical Science, Tokyo, Japan

Abstract

Rett syndrome (RTT) is a devastating neurodevelopmental disorder that occurs once in every 10,000–15,000 live female births. Despite intensive research, no effective cure is yet available. Valproic acid (VPA) has been used widely to treat mood disorder, epilepsy, and a growing number of other disorders. In limited clinical studies, VPA has also been used to control seizure in RTT patients with promising albeit somewhat unclear efficacy. In this study we tested the effect of VPA on the neurological symptoms of RTT and discovered that short-term VPA treatment during the symptomatic period could reduce neurological symptoms in RTT mice. We found that VPA restores the expression of a subset of genes in RTT mouse brains, and these genes clustered in neurological disease and developmental disorder networks. Our data suggest that VPA could be used as a drug to alleviate RTT symptoms.

Editor: Nicoletta Landsberger, University of Insubria, Italy

Funding: This work was supported by grants from the National Institutes of Health (NIH) (R01MH080434 and R01MH078972 to X. Zhao), the International Rett Syndrome Foundation (IRSF, 2755 to X. Zhao), and a Center grant from the NIH to the Waisman Center (P30HD03352 to X. Zhao). W. Guo was funded by a postdoctoral fellowship from University of Wisconsin Center for Stem Cells and Regenerative Medicine. This work was also supported in part by a Grant-in-Aid for Scientific Research (A) (to K. Nakashima), a Grant-in-Aid for Scientific Research on Innovative Areas: Foundation of Synapse and Neurocircuit Pathology (to K. Nakashima), all from the Ministry of Education, Culture, Sports, Science and Technology of Japan, and by an Intramural Research Grant (24-12) for Neurological and Psychiatric Disorders of NCNP (to K. Nakashima). This work was also supported in part by a Grant-in-Aid for Challenging Exploratory Research and a Grant-in-Aid for Scientific Research (B) (to K. Igarashi). The funders had no role in study design, data collection and analysis, decision to publish, or preparation of the manuscript.

Competing Interests: The authors have declared that no competing interests exist.

* Email: xzhao69@wisc.edu (XZ); kin1@scb.med.kyushu-u.ac.jp (KN); k-igarashi@hoshi.ac.jp (KI)

❾ These authors contributed equally to this work.

¤ Current address: State Key Laboratory of Molecular Developmental Biology, Institute of Genetics and Developmental Biology, Chinese Academy of Sciences, Beijing, China

Introduction

Rett syndrome (RTT) is a devastating neurodevelopmental disorder that occurs once in every 10,000–15,000 live female births. RTT patients develop normally until 6 to 18 months of age, but then regress rapidly, experiencing a wide range of neurological symptoms, including seizures, ataxia, and stereotypical hand movements with impairment of communication and cognition [1]. Seizure activity is common and reportedly occurs in up to 80% of patients.

RTT results largely from functional mutations in the X-linked *MECP2* gene [2], which encodes a methylated CpG-binding protein that regulates transcription via epigenetic mechanisms [3]. Mutations and duplications of MeCP2 are also found in several other developmental disorders, including autism, demonstrating the functional importance of MeCP2 [4,5]. *Mecp2* null mutant (KO) mice develop similar symptoms as those seen in RTT patients; these mice have been used widely to study the etiology of human RTT [6,7,8]. Using RTT mice, we and others have shown that MeCP2 deficiency leads to altered expression of downstream effectors, resulting in impaired neuronal differentiation and maturation [9,10,11]. During the past decade, there have been extensive efforts devoted to understanding and treating RTT. However, for the most part we still lack effective and safe treatments.

Valproic acid (VPA) has been used clinically for decades as a treatment for mood disorders and seizures [12,13,14]. It was later also found to be an inhibitor for histone deacetylases, which are known to repress the expression of many genes [15,16]. Therefore, VPA could potentially affect a large number of genes, although its impact might be specific to different cell types. Despite the fact that its mechanism of action is not fully clear, VPA has been used or considered as a drug for a number of neurological diseases, including spinal muscular atrophy (SMA), Parkinson's disease, Huntington's disease, migraine, and dementia, as well as other diseases such as cancer and HIV infection. Since VPA exhibits broad efficacy but only mild and transient side effects, to date it has been used in more than 200 clinical trials for various diseases [12].

VPA has also been used to treat RTT patients, but mostly for seizure control [17]. Although one study found no beneficial effects [18], another study demonstrated a significant reduction in seizures in RTT patients by VPA [19]. Some limited data have also revealed that VPA can improve behavioral deficits other than seizure in RTT, including verbal fluency [20] and decreased risk of fracture [21]. However, whether VPA can improve neurological symptoms has not been systematically assessed. VPA is known to restore MeCP2 deficiency-induced protein changes in a cultured cell system [22], yet whether VPA treatment can restore gene expression in MeCP2-deficient brains has not been tested.

In this study, we aimed to evaluate the therapeutic effect of VPA on symptomatic RTT mice. We treated Mecp2 KO mice with VPA at a peak of neurological symptoms and found that VPA could alleviate RTT-associated neurological symptoms. In addition, VPA partially restores global gene expression changes in MeCP2 KO mice. Interestingly, VPA specifically affects genes in the pathway related to neurological diseases. Thus our data support a potential therapeutic role for VPA in the treatment of RTT.

Materials and Methods

Ethics Statement

All animal procedures were performed according to protocols approved by the University of New Mexico and University of Wisconsin Animal Care and Use Committee. The *Mecp2* KO mice (*Mecp2$^{tm1.1Jae}$*) used in this study were created by deleting exon 3 containing the MBD domain of Mecp2 [23]. These mice have been bred over 40 generations on the ICR background. They start to show neurological symptoms between 5 and 7 weeks of age, and many die before 10 weeks of age, although some live as long as 17 weeks of age.

VPA Treatment

When mice reached 6 weeks old, they received daily injections of VPA (300 mg/kg; make 50 mg/ml VPA in saline) for 2 weeks (Fig 1). Three batches of mice were used. The first batch of mice included 3 groups of mice: WT control (n = 3), KO treated with VPA (KO+VPA, n = 5), and KO treated with saline (KO+saline, n = 4). We first did behavioral assessments during the VPA injection period. Immediately after the last injection, we dissected the brains from 3 mice per group and froze them in liquid N_2 for RNA isolation. The rest of the mice were used for survival analysis. The second and third batches of mice included KO+VPA (n = 4) and KO+saline (n = 5); we did behavioral assessments during the injection period, and then we recorded the survival of mice. Therefore, total 9 KO+VPA and 9 KO+saline mice were assessed for behavioral symptom (Figure 1B) and 6 KO+VPA and 6 KO+saline mice were assessed for survival (Figure 1C).

Neurological Symptom Assessment

This assessment was carried out based on a published method [24]. We evaluated 6 core symptoms of RTT and scored the severity of symptoms: Score 0 indicated an absence of symptoms (wild-type all had 0); Score 1 indicated the presence of symptoms; Score 2 designated severe symptoms. Mice were also weighed at each scoring session. The sum of scores in all categories was used to represent the severity of symptoms. The symptoms we assessed and scoring criteria are as follow:

Mobility: The mouse is observed when placed on a bench, then when handled gently. Score 0 = same as wild-type. Score 1 = reduced movement when compared to wild-type: extended freezing period when first placed on bench and longer periods spent immobile. Score 2 = no spontaneous movement when placed on the bench; mouse can move in response to a gentle prod or a

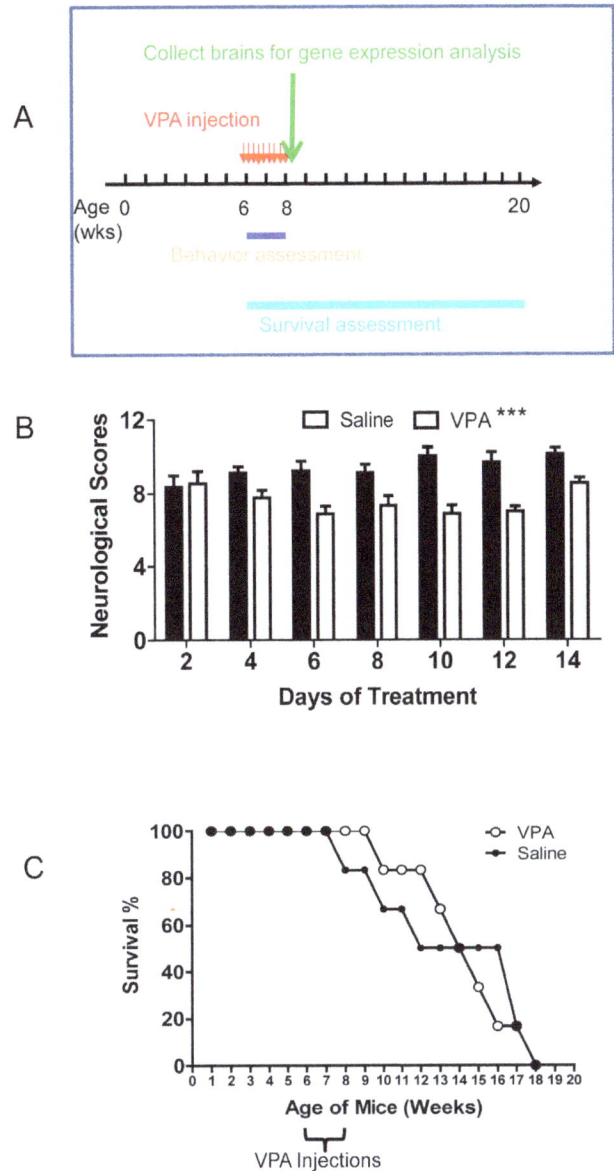

Figure 1. VPA treatment rescues certain neurological symptoms in MeCP2 KO mice. (A) Schematic drawing shows the timeline of experiments. (B) Neurological symptom scores of saline (control) and VPA-treated MeCP2 KO mice (n = 9 per group, two-way ANOVA with repeated measure, time and treatment interaction: $F_{6,96} = 3.079$, p = 0.0084; VPA treatment: $F_{1,96} = 28.22$, p < 0.0001). (C) VPA treatment has small but noticeable effects on the lifespan of MeCP2 KO mice. ***, p < 0.001

food pellet placed nearby. (Note: mice may become more active when in their own cage environment.)

Gait: Score 0 = same as wild-type. Score 1 = hind legs are spread wider than wild-type when walking or running with reduced pelvic elevation, resulting in a "waddling" gait. Score 2 = more severe abnormalities: tremor when feet are lifted, walks backwards or "bunny hops" by lifting both rear feet at once.

Hind limb clasping: Mouse observed when suspended by holding base of the tail. Score 0 = legs splayed outwards. Score 1 = hind limbs are drawn towards each other (without touching) or one leg is drawn in to the body. Score 2 = both legs are pulled in tightly, either touching each other or touching the body.

Tremor: Mouse observed while standing on the flat palm of the hand. Score 0 = no tremor. Score 1 = intermittent mild tremor. Score 2 = continuous tremor or intermittent violent tremor.

Breathing: Movement of flanks observed while animal is standing still. Score 0 = normal breathing. Score 1 = periods of regular breathing interspersed with short periods of more rapid breathing or with pauses in breathing. Score 2* = very irregular breathing: gasping or panting.

General condition: Mouse observed for indicators of general wellbeing, such as coat condition, eyes, body stance. Score 0 = clean shiny coat, clear eyes, normal stance. Score 1 = eyes dull, coat dull/un-groomed, somewhat hunched stance. Score 2* = eyes crusted or narrowed, piloerection, hunched posture.

Gene Expression Microarray Analysis

Half of the brain tissues from the first batch of mice (n = 3 mice/condition) were used for microarray analysis. Microarray analysis was performed following the manufacturer's instructions. First, total RNAs were purified using an RNeasy Mini kit (Qiagen) from half brains. First strand cDNAs were synthesized by incubating 5 µg of total RNA with SuperScript II reverse transcriptase (Invitrogen). After second-strand synthesis, the double-stranded cDNAs were purified using a MinElute Reaction Cleanup Kit (Qiagen) and labeled by in vitro transcription using a BioArray High Yield RNA transcript labeling kit (Enzo Life Sciences, Farmingdale, NY, USA). The labeled cRNA was then purified using an RNeasy Mini kit (Qiagen) and treated with fragmentation buffer at 94°C for 35 min. For hybridization to a GeneChip Mouse Genome 430 2.0 Array (Affymetrix), 7.5 µg of fragmented cRNA probe was incubated with 50 pM control oligonucleotide B2, 1x eukaryotic hybridization control (1.5 pM BioB, five pM BioC, 25 pM BioD and 100 pM Cre), 0.1 mg/mL herring sperm DNA, 0.5 mg/mL acetylated BSA, and 1X manufacturer-recommended hybridization buffer in a 45°C rotator for 16 h. Washing and staining were performed in a GeneChip Fluidics Station (Affymetrix). The phycoerythrin-stained arrays were scanned as digital image files that were then analyzed with GeneChip Operating Software (Affymetrix). We selected the probe sets with the fold change of MeCP2KO-saline to wild-type more than 1.2 and a p-value under 0.05. Pathway analysis was performed using the Ingenuity Pathways Analysis software (Ingenuity Systems). Gene Ontology (GO) analyses were performed using Genespring software (Agilent Technologies)

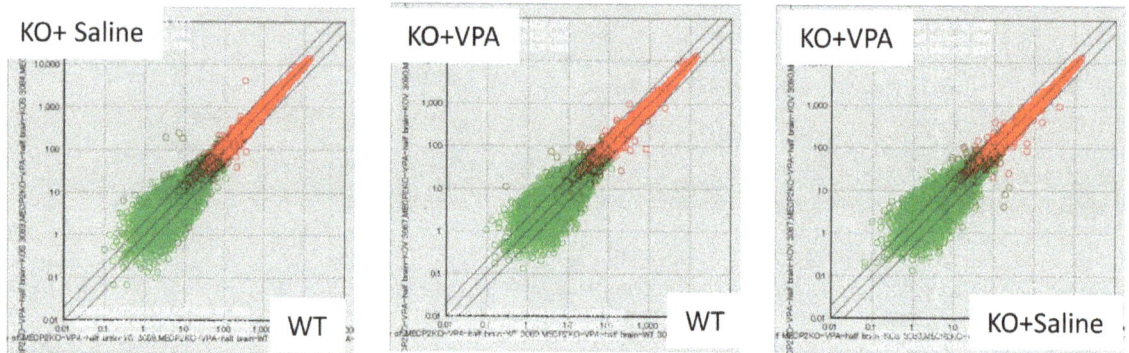

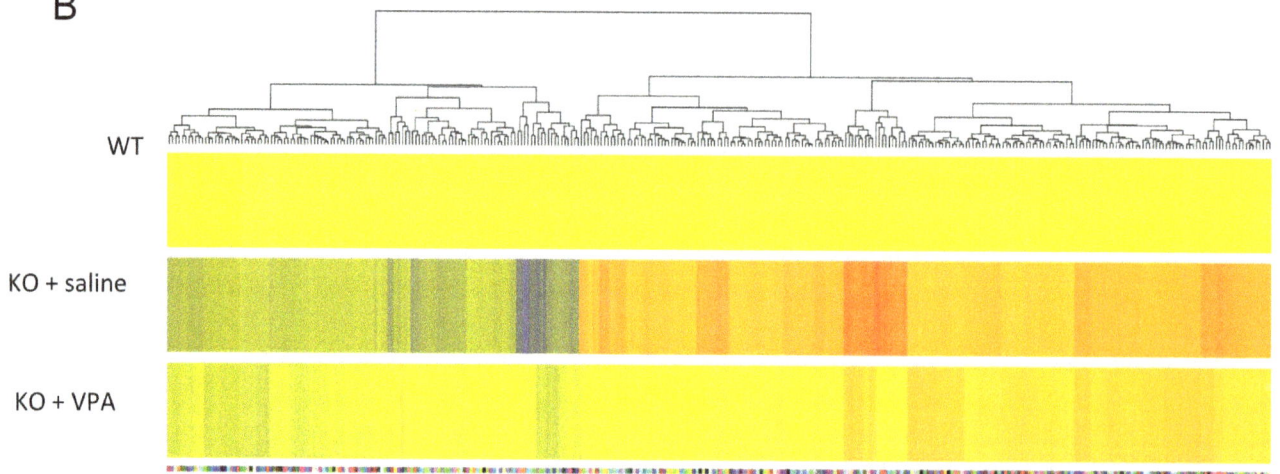

Figure 2. VPA treatment restores the expression of a subset of genes in MeCP2 KO brains. (A) Scatter plots showing differential gene expression profiles among experimental conditions. (B) Heatmap showing 33 genes with >1.2-fold changes in the MeCP2 KO compared to WT brains and that were restored to <1.2-fold changes upon VPA treatment.

A Neurological Diseases

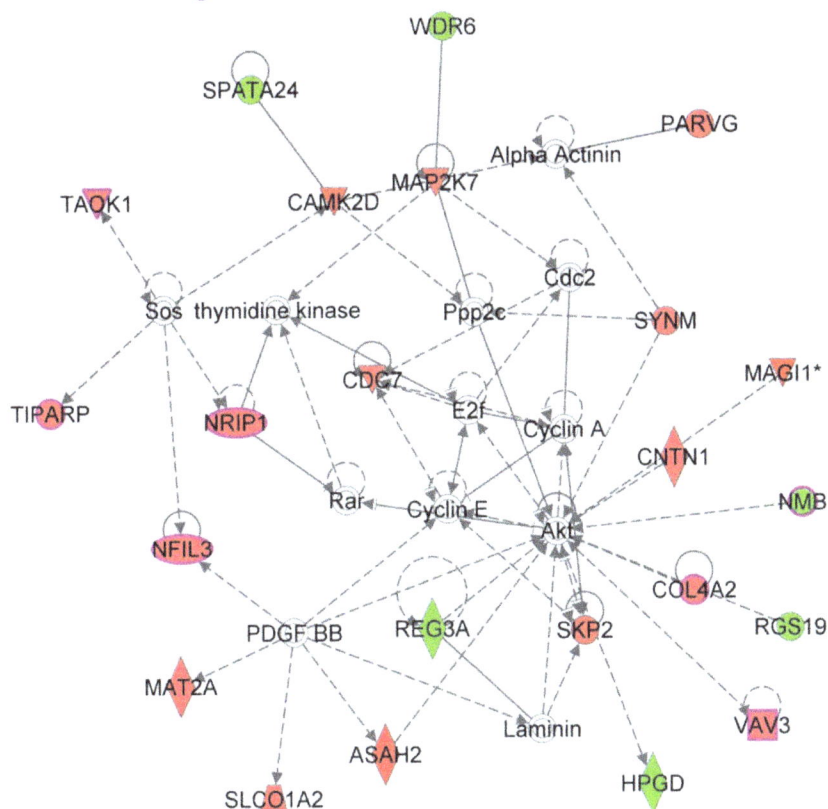

B Nervous System Development and Function

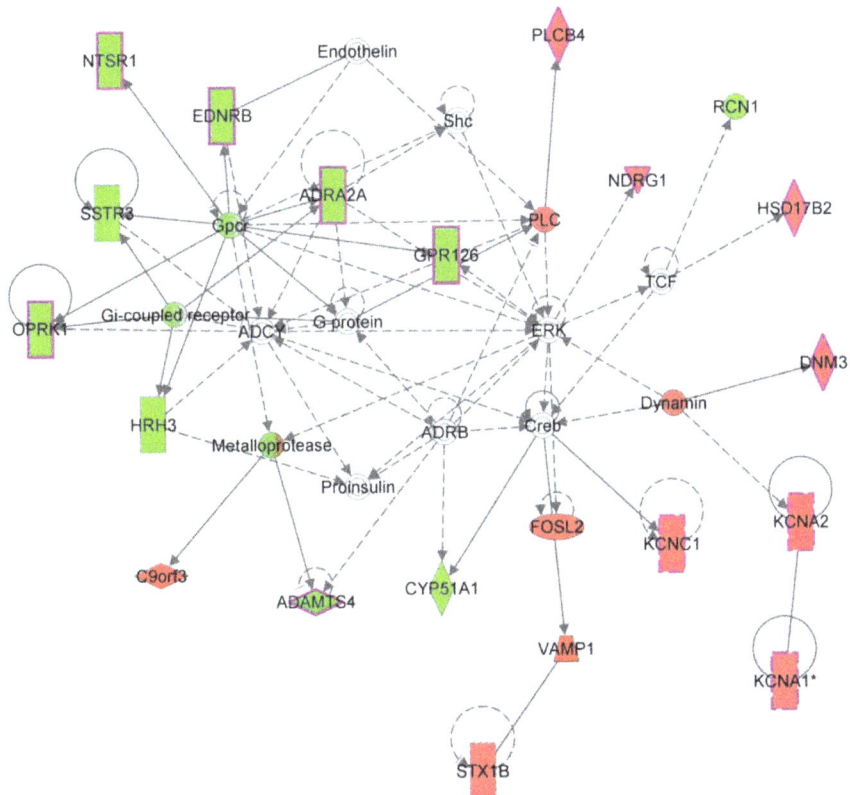

Figure 3. Ingenuity Pathway Analysis showing the two top networks restored by VPA in MeCP2 KO brains. The 310 gene restored by VPA in MeCP2 KO brains are mostly categorized into two networks: Neurological Disease network (A) and Nervous System Development and Function network (B). The colors indicate the direction of gene changes. Red, KO is higher than WT. Green, KO is lower than WT. The shapes of the boxes represent the functional categories of the genes. Inverted triangle: Kinase; Horizontally oval: Transcription Regulator, Vertical diamond: Enzyme, Square: Cytokine; Circle: Other; Bordered circle: Complex/Group, Vertically rectangle: G-protein Coupled Receptor; Horizontally diamond: Peptidase, Triangle: Phospatase.

Real-time PCR

Total RNAs from half brains (n = 3/condition) were prepared by using RNA purification kits (Qiagen). Real-time RT-PCR TaqMan probes and reaction reagents were purchased from Applied Biosystems. Reactions were performed according to manuals from the manufacturer by using StepOnePlus Real-time PCR system (Applied Biosystems). All results were normalized to levels of the GAPDH gene. Catalog numbers for the probes are: GAPDH (Mm03302249_g1), zinc finger with KRAB and SCAN domains 1 (Zkscan1) (Mm00551752_m1), AE binding protein 2 (Aebp2) (Mm01267857_m1), contactin 1 (Cntn1) (Mm00514374_m1), and potassium inwardly-rectifying channel, subfamily J, member 16 (Kcnj16) (Mm04208325_m1).

Data deposition

The datasets that were generated and reported in this paper have been deposited into the National Center for Biotechnology Information GEO database through accession number GSE56780.

Results

VPA treatment can alleviate neurological symptoms in MeCP2-deficient mice

Since Mecp2 mutant mice on C57B/L6 background are difficult to breed, we bred the Mecp2 mutant (Jaenisch/MIT) line [23] onto ICR background for over 40 generations. The Mecp2 heterozygote ICR female mice gave birth to significantly more surviving pups compared to their C57B/L6 counterparts therefore we used ICR mice for this study. Mecp2 KO male mice on the ICR genetic background started showing symptoms at about 5 weeks of age, and many of them died between 8 and 10 weeks of age, which is similar to Mecp2 KO mice on C57B/L6 background. However, some of the Mecp2 KO ICR males lived up to 17 weeks, which is significantly longer than their C57B/6 counterparts. To determine whether VPA treatment might have a therapeutic effect on symptomatic KO mice, we decided to treat mice between 6 to 8 weeks of age, when all of them were showing clear RTT symptom, but before they were too sick to receive Intraperitoneal (i.p.) injections (Fig. 1A). Before daily injection of VPA, we first assessed the severity of neurological symptoms that are characteristics of RTT, including mobility, gait, hind limb clasping, tremor, breathing, and their general condition. We applied a published scoring system by setting the severity scale from 0 to 2: 0 is absent, 1 is present, and 2 is severe for each symptom [24]. Based on these criteria, all wild-type (WT) mice showed no symptoms, and therefore scored as 0. We found that the severity of neurological symptoms in saline-injected KO mice did not change significantly during the 2-week assessment and injection period (Figure 1B, black bar, one-way ANOVA with repeated measure, $F_{6,48} = 2.085$, p = 0.0724). On the other hand, the neurological scores of VPA-treated KO mice exhibited significant changes during the 2-week period (Figure 1B, white bar, one-way ANOVA with repeated measure, $F_{6,48} = 2.685$, p = 0.025), suggesting effects from VPA treatment on symptom development. More importantly, VPA treatment led to a

significant reduction in the neurological severity scores compared to saline-treated KO mice (Fig. 1B, two-way ANOVA with repeated measure, time and treatment interaction: $F_{6,96} = 3.079$, p = 0.0084; VPA treatment: $F_{1,96} = 28.22$, p<0.0001). Among all six symptoms analyzed, gait ($F_{1,96} = 8.544$, p = 0.01), tremor ($F_{1,96} = 16.42$, p = 0.0009), breathing ($F_{1,96} = 14.22$, p = 0.0017), and general health condition ($F_{1,96} = 5.511$, p = 0.0321) showed significant improvement in VPA treated KO mice (Figure S1 in File S1). Mobility showed strong time and treatment interaction ($F_{6,96} = 5.657$, p<0.0001) without significant effect by treatment alone. There was no significant difference in body weight between the treatment groups. We also assessed the survival of these mice both during and after the 2-week VPA treatment period. We found that although VPA treatment delayed the death of some of these KO mice, it had no significant effect on the overall lifespan of KO mice (Fig. 1C). Therefore, a short 2-week VPA treatment during the peak symptomatic period can reduce several key RTT neurological symptoms in a RTT mouse model.

VPA can rescue gene expression changes

To determine the molecular basis of symptom improvement, we collected brains from Mecp2 KO mice treated with VPA (KO+VPA) or saline (KO+Saline) and WT mice at one day after the last VPA injection. We isolated RNA from these brains and subjected them to microarray analysis. The biological triplicates within the same experimental groups showed excellent reproducibility (Figure S2 in File S1).

Comparison among different experimental groups revealed significant expression changes in subsets of genes resulting from MeCP2 deficiency (KO+saline vs. WT), as well as restoration by VPA (KO+VPA vs. WT) (Table S1). To evaluate whether VPA could restore gene expression caused by MeCP2 deficiency, we selected genes that are significantly altered in MeCP2 KO mice (KO+saline vs WT:>1.2-fold, p<0.05), but are restored by VPA treatment (KO+VPA vs. WT:<1.2-fold). The heat map demonstrates that 310 genes presented by 333 probe sets met these criteria (Fig 2B). Expression of some of these genes, such as *Zkscan1*, was reduced to near WT levels by VPA. Therefore, VPA can normalize the expression of a subset of genes to nearly WT levels in MeCP2-deficient brains.

Table 1. Top Networks Restored by VPA Treatment.

ID	Top Diseases and Functions	Score
1	Cancer, Neurological Disease, Connective Tissue Disorders	40
2	Organismal Injury and Abnormalities, Cellular Growth and Proliferation, Cellular Movement	35
3	Nervous System Development and Function, Molecular Transport, Behavior	35
4	Cellular Function and Maintenance, Hematological System Development and Function, Inflammatory Response	32
5	Cellular Assembly and Organization, Cellular Function and Maintenance, Cell Morphology	30

Table 2. Top Disease and Bio Function Groups Restored by VPA.

Diseases and Disorders

Name	p-value #	Molecules
Neurological Disease	3.34E-08-1.74E-02	83
Cancer	5.18E-07-1.71E-02	150
Cardiovascular Disease	2.98E-06-1.71E-02	44
Organismal Injury and Abnormalities	2.69E-05-1.71E-02	42
Psychological Disorders	3.12E-05-1.33E-02	43

Molecular and Cellular Functions

Name	p-value #	Molecules
Cell Morphology	9.35E-06-1.82E-02	69
Molecular Transport	1.05E-04-1.59E-02	60
Lipid Metabolism	1.45E-04-1.57E-02	29
Small Molecule Biochemistry	1.45E-04-1.57E-02	45
Cellular Assembly and Organization	1.79E-04-1.61E-02	58

Physiological System Development and Function

Name	p-value #	Molecules
Behavior	1.43E-07-1.34E-02	45
Cardiovascular System Development and Function	2.33E-04-1.81E-02	43
Organismal Survival	2.34E-04-5.76E-03	65
Organismal Development	3.66E-04-1.82E-02	60
Nervous System Development and Function	4.78E-04-1.82E-02	62

VPA treatment restores expression of a subset of genes involved in neurological disorders

To determine the types of genes whose expression was restored by VPA in the context of MeCP2 deficiency, we subjected these 310 genes to Ingenuity Pathway Analysis and found that the top networks affected by VPA (Table 1 and Table S2) include Neurological Diseases (Fig 3A) and Nervous System Development and Function (Fig 3B). When we analyzed the biological functions of these 310 genes, they were categorized into three main biological function groups: "Diseases and Disorders," "Molecular and Cellular Functions," and "Physiological System Development and Function" (Table 2). Interestingly, the "Diseases and Disorders" group contains the largest number of genes, with 83 genes in the category of "Neurological Disease" (Table 3). A Gene Ontology (GO) analysis also showed many of these genes are involved in important cellular functions (Table S3). Thus VPA restored genes in MeCP2-deficient brains mainly in the category of neurological disease and brain development.

We next used quantitative PCR to assess the expression levels of some of these VPA-restored genes (Figure 2B and Table S1). We confirmed that VPA treatment indeed restored the expression levels of Zkscan1, a transcription factor important for cell differentiation, and Cntn1, a cell adhesion protein with a central role in neuronal growth cones and axon guidance (Fig 4). We then selected a few interesting genes that also showed VPA restoration, but were just below the cut-off of our stringent data analysis criteria. Among these candidates that also showed restoration by VPA were Aebp2, a DNA-binding epigenetic regulator, and

Kcnj16, a potassium channel (Figure S3 in File S1). Therefore, in MeCP2-defiicent brains, VPA could restore the expression of a subset of genes involved in neurological disease and brain development.

Discussion

In this study we explored whether VPA treatment could alleviate neurological symptoms of RTT. We discovered that VPA treatment during the symptomatic stage of disease significantly reduced neurological deficits in RTT mice. We also showed that VPA can restore the expression of a subset of neurological disease-related genes resulting from MeCP2 deficiency.

Although VPA has been used to treat seizures in a small number of RTT patients, its effect on neurological symptoms has not been well documented. The fact that treatment with VPA during the peak symptomatic stage of the disease could significantly improve neurological symptoms in MeCP2 KO mice is exciting. Our data suggest VPA may be a promising drug for the treatment of RTT. One remaining question is whether VPA treatment either before or during the early onset of symptoms may lead to additional improvements. Moreover, we only treated mice for two weeks. It is possible that longer treatment might bring more relief of symptoms and a longer lifespan. However, i.p. injection at the symptomatic stage may cause more stress to the animals, so the VPA injection route will have to be optimized (e.g. oral administration).

Since VPA inhibits HDACs, which are known to be involved in the suppression of many genes, we expected to detect a great many genes whose expression level is altered by VPA in the brain; however, we could only find 310 genes with a significant restoration of their expression levels in response to the VPA treatment. This could be due in part to the fact that we used brain tissues containing different cell types, which may respond to VPA differently. It is also likely that the brain's compensatory changes may mask the effect of VPA. Nevertheless, it is worth noting that the 310 genes restored by VPA are clustered in the network of Neurological Disease and Nervous System Development (Figure 3, Table 1, Table S2), and 83 of these genes are in the Disease and Disorder functional group (Table 2). Many of these genes have been linked to human diseases. For example, a mutation in CNTN1, a neural adhesion protein, leads to a familial form of lethal congenital myopathy [25]. Transcription factor FOXP1 deletion and overexpression are both linked to autism [26,27], and transcription factor ZKSCAN1 is associated with Wolf-Hirschhorn syndrome with intellectual disability (www.genecards.org). The molecular and cellular biological function group restored by VPA included molecular transport, lipid metabolism, small molecule biochemistry, and cell morphology. The restoration of cell morphology may be an important application for rescuing the impaired dendritic development in MeCP2-deficient brains that we and others have observed [9]. The potential action of VPA in molecular transport, metabolism, and biochemistry is also very interesting because MeCP2 was recently found to play a role in RNA splicing [28,29] and nuclear size determination [30]. In addition, as a next step, it would be interesting to explore the cell type-specific changes of some of the candidate genes we have discovered. We also believe we may have missed some other genes restored by VPA due to the stringency of our data analysis. For example, Aebp2, an epigenetic DNA-binding protein involved in Hirschsprung's disease and Waardenburg syndrome [31], and Kcnj16, a potassium channel involved in respiratory response to hypoxia during breathing [32], showed VPA-restored expression changes, but the p value was greater than 0.05. It is likely that

Table 3. Neurological Disease Genes Restored by VPA.

Gene Symbol	Gene Title
2010111I01Rik	RIKEN cDNA 2010111I01 gene
Adamts4	a disintegrin-like and metallopeptidase (reprolysin type) with thrombospondin type 1 motif, 4
Adamtsl1	ADAMTS-like 1
Adra2a	adrenergic receptor, alpha 2a
Bcl11a	B cell CLL/lymphoma 11A (zinc finger protein)
Bub3	budding uninhibited by benzimidazoles 3 homolog (S. cerevisiae)
Cdc14b	CDC14 cell division cycle 14B
Cds1	CDP-diacylglycerol synthase 1
Chrna6	cholinergic receptor, nicotinic, alpha polypeptide 6
Cntn1	contactin 1
Col3a1	collagen, type III, alpha 1
Col4a2	collagen, type IV, alpha 2
Col5a2	collagen, type V, alpha 2
Crym	crystallin, mu
Cyp51	cytochrome P450, family 51
Dab1	disabled 1
Dnajc1	DnaJ (Hsp40) homolog, subfamily C, member 1
Dusp5	dual specificity phosphatase 5
Ednrb	endothelin receptor type B
Efna5	ephrin A5
Fat4	FAT tumor suppressor homolog 4 (Drosophila)
Fbln1	fibulin 1
Fhdc1	FH2 domain containing 1
Fos	FBJ osteosarcoma oncogene
Foxp1	forkhead box P1
Gabra3	gamma-aminobutyric acid (GABA) A receptor, subunit alpha 3
Galnt7	UDP-N-acetyl-alpha-D-galactosamine: polypeptide N-acetylgalactosaminyltransferase 7
Glra1	glycine receptor, alpha 1 subunit
Gpr126	G protein-coupled receptor 126
Hcn1	hyperpolarization-activated, cyclic nucleotide-gated K+1
Hrh3	histamine receptor H3
Ier5	immediate early response 5
Kazn	kazrin, periplakin interacting protein
Kcna1	potassium voltage-gated channel, shaker-related subfamily, member 1
Kcna2	potassium voltage-gated channel, shaker-related subfamily, member 2
Kcnc1	potassium voltage gated channel, Shaw-related subfamily, member 1
Krit1	KRIT1, ankyrin repeat containing
Ldlr	low density lipoprotein receptor
Lgals1	lectin, galactose binding, soluble 1

Gene Symbol	Gene Title
Malat1	metastasis associated lung adenocarcinoma transcript 1 (non-coding RNA)
Marcksl1	MARCKS-like 1
Met	met proto-oncogene
Mtmr9	myotubularin related protein 9

Table 3. Cont.

Gene Symbol	Gene Title
Ndrg1	N-myc downstream regulated gene 1
Nfatc2	nuclear factor of activated T cells, cytoplasmic, calcineurin dependent 2
Nfil3	nuclear factor, interleukin 3, regulated
Nmb	neuromedin B
Nppa	natriuretic peptide type A
Nrip1	nuclear receptor interacting protein 1
Ntrk3	neurotrophic tyrosine kinase, receptor, type 3
Oprk1	opioid receptor, kappa 1
Paqr6	progestin and adipoQ receptor family member VI
Pclo	piccolo (presynaptic cytomatrix protein)
Pcsk1	proprotein convertase subtilisin/kexin type 1
Pim3	proviral integration site 3
Plcb4	phospholipase C, beta 4
Pnkd	paroxysmal nonkinesiogenic dyskinesia
Ppargc1a	peroxisome proliferative activated receptor, gamma, coactivator 1 alpha
Ppp1r1a	protein phosphatase 1, regulatory (inhibitor) subunit 1A
Prdm2	PR domain containing 2, with ZNF domain
Prkcg	protein kinase C, gamma
Rims3	regulating synaptic membrane exocytosis 3
Scn1a	sodium channel, voltage-gated, type I, alpha
Sema3f	sema domain, immunoglobulin domain (Ig), short basic domain, secreted, (semaphorin) 3F
Skp2	S-phase kinase-associated protein 2 (p45)
Slc16a2	solute carrier family 16 (monocarboxylic acid transporters), member 2
Slco3a1	solute carrier organic anion transporter family, member 3a1
Smpx	small muscle protein, X-linked
Sst	somatostatin
Sstr3	somatostatin receptor 3
Sv2c	synaptic vesicle glycoprotein 2c
Taok1	TAO kinase 1
Thbs3	thrombospondin 3
Tiparp	TCDD-inducible poly(ADP-ribose) polymerase
Tnc	tenascin C
Tnnt1	troponin T1, skeletal, slow
Trps1	trichorhinophalangeal syndrome I (human)
Tubb2b	tubulin, beta 2B class IIB
Vamp1	vesicle-associated membrane protein 1
Vav3	vav 3 oncogene
Vcam1	vascular cell adhesion molecule 1

changes in other genes were masked by the complexity of brain tissues we used. Previous studies have found hundreds of genes are changed in the hypothalamus or cerebellum of MeCP2 KO mice [33,34]. A recent study has identified 127 genes were altered in the striatum of MeCP2 KO mice [35]. A comparison of our data and these data showed a small percentage of the genes are shared. For example, among 383 genes altered in the hypothalamus of Mecp KO mice[34], 8 of them are in the 621 genes we found altered in

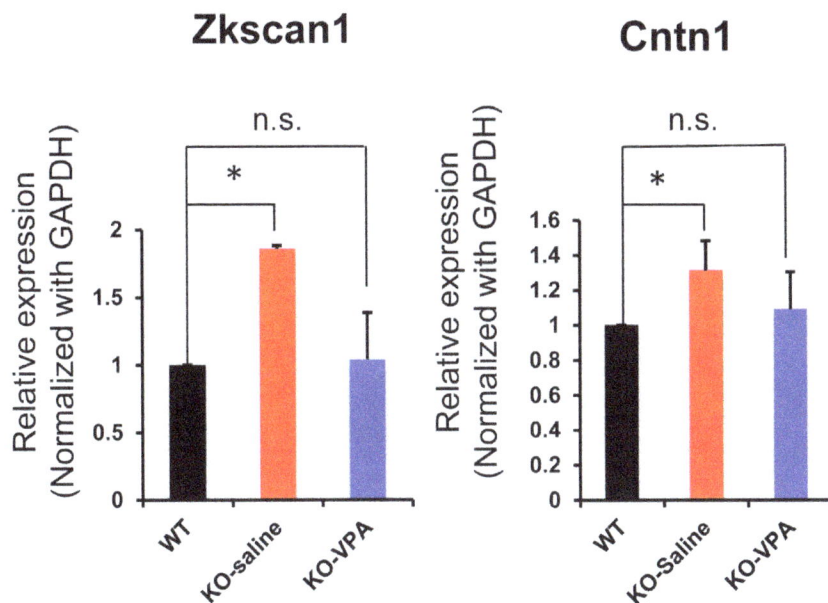

Figure 4. Quantitative PCR data showing restoration to WT levels of Zkscan1 and Cntn1 in MeCP2 KO brains by VPA treatment. The levels of Zkscan1 and Cntn1 mRNA were reduced to the WT levels by VPA treatment. *, $p < 0.05$ (n = 3).

the whole brain of Mecp2 KO mice and 5 of them are found in the 310 genes restored by VPA. It is not surprising that only small percentage of genes overlap among these data sets given the different original of the tissues and mixed composition of cells in these brain regions. Future studies using pure populations of cells will likely reduce false negatives and uncover more VPA-restored genes in specific brain cell types. VPA may affect different sets of genes in specific cell types, which will be a valuable avenue of study to pursue in the future.

Supporting Information

Table S1   VPA restored Genes in MeCP2 KO Brains.

Table S2   Top Networks and Genes Restored by VPA Treatment.

Table S3   Gene Ontology Analysis of VPA-Restored Genes in MeCP2 KO Brains.

File S1   This file contains 3 supplemental figures (Figure S1, Figure S2, and Figure S3). Figure S1. VPA treatment rescues certain pathological symptoms in MeCP2 KO mice. **Figure S2**. Scatter plots showing reproducibility in gene expression profiles among biological triplicates within each experimental condition. **Figure S3**. Quantitative PCR data showing restoration of Aebp2 and Kcnj16 genes in MeCP2 KO brains by VPA treatment.

Author Contributions

Conceived and designed the experiments: XZ KN. Performed the experiments: WG KT K. Irie. Analyzed the data: WG KT MOI K. Igarashi KN XZ. Wrote the paper: KN XZ K. Igarashi. Final approval of the version to be published: KN XZ K. Igarashi.

References

1. Kriaucionis S, Bird A (2003) DNA methylation and Rett syndrome. Hum Mol Genet 12 Suppl 2: R221–R227.
2. Amir RE, Van den Veyver IB, Wan M, Tran CQ, Francke U, et al. (1999) Rett syndrome is caused by mutations in X-linked MECP2, encoding methyl- CpG-binding protein 2. Nat Genet 23: 185–188.
3. Bird A (2002) DNA methylation patterns and epigenetic memory. Genes Dev 16: 6–21.
4. Amir RE, Van den Veyver IB, Wan M, Tran CQ, Francke U, et al. (1999) Rett syndrome is caused by mutations in X-linked MECP2, encoding methyl-CpG-binding protein 2. Nat Genet 23: 185–188.
5. Neul JL (2012) The relationship of Rett syndrome and MECP2 disorders to autism. Dialogues in clinical neuroscience 14: 253–262.
6. Guy J, Hendrich B, Holmes M, Martin JE, Bird A (2001) A mouse Mecp2-null mutation causes neurological symptoms that mimic Rett syndrome. Nat Genet 27: 322–326.
7. Chen RZ, Akbarian S, Tudor M, Jaenisch R (2001) Deficiency of methyl-CpG binding protein-2 in CNS neurons results in a Rett-like phenotype in mice. Nat Genet 27: 327–331.
8. Shahbazian M, Young J, Yuva-Paylor L, Spencer C, Antalffy B, et al. (2002) Mice with truncated MeCP2 recapitulate many Rett syndrome features and display hyperacetylation of histone H3. Neuron 35: 243–254.
9. Smrt RD, Eaves-Egenes J, Barkho BZ, Santistevan NJ, Zhao C, et al. (2007) Mecp2 deficiency leads to delayed maturation and altered gene expression in hippocampal neurons. Neurobiol Dis 27: 77–89.
10. Smrt RD, Pfeiffer RL, Zhao X (2011) Age-dependent expression of MeCP2 in a heterozygous mosaic mouse model. Human molecular genetics 20: 1834–1843.
11. Szulwach KE, Li X, Smrt RD, Li Y, Luo Y, et al. (2010) Cross talk between microRNA and epigenetic regulation in adult neurogenesis. J Cell Biol 189: 127–141.
12. Chiu CT, Wang Z, Hunsberger JG, Chuang DM (2013) Therapeutic potential of mood stabilizers lithium and valproic acid: beyond bipolar disorder. Pharmacological reviews 65: 105–142.
13. Chateauvieux S, Morceau F, Dicato M, Diederich M (2010) Molecular and therapeutic potential and toxicity of valproic acid. Journal of biomedicine & biotechnology 2010.
14. Koch-Weser J, Browne TR (1980) Drug therapy: Valproic acid. The New England journal of medicine 302: 661–666.
15. Gottlicher M (2004) Valproic acid: an old drug newly discovered as inhibitor of histone deacetylases. Annals of hematology 83 Suppl 1: S91–92.
16. Grozinger CM, Schreiber SL (2002) Deacetylase enzymes: biological functions and the use of small-molecule inhibitors. Chem Biol 9: 3–16.

17. Faulkner MA, Singh SP (2013) Neurogenetic disorders and treatment of associated seizures. Pharmacotherapy 33: 330–343.
18. Huppke P, Kohler K, Brockmann K, Stettner GM, Gartner J (2007) Treatment of epilepsy in Rett syndrome. European journal of paediatric neurology: EJPN: official journal of the European Paediatric Neurology Society 11: 10–16.
19. Krajnc N, Zupancic N, Orazem J (2011) Epilepsy treatment in Rett syndrome. Journal of child neurology 26: 1429–1433.
20. Al Keilani MA, Carlier S, Groswasser J, Dan B, Deconinck N (2011) Rett syndrome associated with continuous spikes and waves during sleep. Acta neurologica Belgica 111: 328–332.
21. Leonard H, Downs J, Jian L, Bebbington A, Jacoby P, et al. (2010) Valproate and risk of fracture in Rett syndrome. Archives of disease in childhood 95: 444–448.
22. Vecsler M, Simon AJ, Amariglio N, Rechavi G, Gak E (2010) MeCP2 deficiency downregulates specific nuclear proteins that could be partially recovered by valproic acid in vitro. Epigenetics: official journal of the DNA Methylation Society 5: 61–67.
23. Chen RZ, Akbarian S, Tudor M, Jaenisch R (2001) Deficiency of methyl-CpG binding protein-2 in CNS neurons results in a Rett-like phenotype in mice. Nature genetics 27: 327–331.
24. Guy J, Gan J, Selfridge J, Cobb S, Bird A (2007) Reversal of neurological defects in a mouse model of Rett syndrome. Science 315: 1143–1147.
25. Compton AG, Albrecht DE, Seto JT, Cooper ST, Ilkovski B, et al. (2008) Mutations in contactin-1, a neural adhesion and neuromuscular junction protein, cause a familial form of lethal congenital myopathy. American journal of human genetics 83: 714–724.
26. Palumbo O, D'Agruma L, Minenna AF, Palumbo P, Stallone R, et al. (2013) 3p14.1 de novo microdeletion involving the FOXP1 gene in an adult patient with autism, severe speech delay and deficit of motor coordination. Gene 516: 107–113.
27. Chien WH, Gau SS, Chen CH, Tsai WC, Wu YY, et al. (2013) Increased gene expression of FOXP1 in patients with autism spectrum disorders. Molecular autism 4: 23.
28. Young JI, Hong EP, Castle JC, Crespo-Barreto J, Bowman AB, et al. (2005) Regulation of RNA splicing by the methylation-dependent transcriptional repressor methyl-CpG binding protein 2. Proceedings of the National Academy of Sciences of the United States of America 102: 17551–17558.
29. Maunakea AK, Chepelev I, Cui K, Zhao K (2013) Intragenic DNA methylation modulates alternative splicing by recruiting MeCP2 to promote exon recognition. Cell research.
30. Yazdani M, Deogracias R, Guy J, Poot RA, Bird A, et al. (2012) Disease modeling using embryonic stem cells: MeCP2 regulates nuclear size and RNA synthesis in neurons. Stem Cells 30: 2128–2139.
31. Kim H, Kang K, Ekram MB, Roh TY, Kim J (2011) Aebp2 as an epigenetic regulator for neural crest cells. PLoS One 6: e25174.
32. Trapp S, Tucker SJ, Gourine AV (2011) Respiratory responses to hypercapnia and hypoxia in mice with genetic ablation of Kir5.1 (Kcnj16). Experimental physiology 96: 451–459.
33. Ben-Shachar S, Chahrour M, Thaller C, Shaw CA, Zoghbi HY (2009) Mouse models of MeCP2 disorders share gene expression changes in the cerebellum and hypothalamus. Human molecular genetics 18: 2431–2442.
34. Chahrour M, Jung SY, Shaw C, Zhou X, Wong ST, et al. (2008) MeCP2, a key contributor to neurological disease, activates and represses transcription. Science 320: 1224–1229.
35. Zhao YT, Goffin D, Johnson BS, Zhou Z (2013) Loss of MeCP2 function is associated with distinct gene expression changes in the striatum. Neurobiology of disease 59: 257–266.

17

Neural Correlates of Advantageous and Disadvantageous Inequity in Sharing Decisions

Berna Güroğlu[1,2]*[9], **Geert-Jan Will**[1,2]9, **Eveline A. Crone**[1,2]

1 Institute of Psychology, Leiden University, Leiden, the Netherlands, **2** Leiden Institute for Brain and Cognition (LIBC), Leiden University, Leiden, the Netherlands

Abstract

Humans have a strong preference for fair distributions of resources. Neuroimaging studies have shown that being treated unfairly coincides with activation in brain regions involved in signaling conflict and negative affect. Less is known about neural responses involved in violating a fairness norm ourselves. Here, we investigated the neural patterns associated with inequity, where participants were asked to choose between an equal split of money and an unequal split that could either maximize their own (advantageous inequity) or another person's (disadvantageous inequity) earnings. Choosing to divide money unequally, irrespective who benefited from the unequal distribution, was associated with activity in the dorsal anterior cingulate cortex, anterior insula and the dorsolateral prefrontal cortex. Inequity choices that maximized another person's profits were further associated with activity in the ventral striatum and ventromedial prefrontal cortex. Taken together, our findings show evidence of a common neural pattern associated with both advantageous and disadvantageous inequity in sharing decisions and additional recruitment of neural circuitry previously linked to the computation of subjective value and reward when violating a fairness norm at the benefit of someone else.

Editor: Hengyi Rao, University of Pennsylvania, United States of America

Funding: This research was supported by the Netherlands Organization for Scientific Research (NWO; VENI grant number 451-10-021 to BG and FES grant number 056-34-010 to EC). The funders had no role in study design, data collection and analysis, decision to publish, or preparation of the manuscript.

Competing Interests: The authors have declared that no competing interests exist.

* Email: bguroglu@fsw.leidenuniv.nl

9 These authors contributed equally to this work.

Introduction

Although economic models assume that the maximization of personal gains is the main motivation when distributing resources, investigations of actual decision-making have shown that fairness concerns play an important role in social interactions [1–6]. Indeed, the evidence is overwhelming: people have a preference for fair outcomes and, all else being equal, acting fairly is generally the expected social norm [1–8] and equality is often used as a cognitive heuristic in decision-making [9]. In search of proximate mechanisms it has been shown that equal distributions are perceived as rewarding, both indicated by self-reported ratings of fair divisions of resources as well as reward-related neural activation patterns associated with these choices [7,8,10,11]. Further, being treated unfairly leads to anger [10–14] and has been associated with activation of neural networks involved in conflict and negative affect [12–16]. Finally, when confronted with unfair treatment and given the power to retaliate, people generally reject inequitable distributions of resources, even when this is costly for them [2,15,16].

Despite this strong preference for equity and the aversion towards inequity, people often make inequity choices, such as when inequity is more advantageous for the self. For example, people aim to increase relative advantage over others [2,17,18] and when a high social position is experimentally induced they become more selfish and display higher levels of immoral

behavior, such as cheating and lying [19–22]. It is thus crucial to gain a better understanding of the neural mechanisms underlying inequity decisions in order to better understand when and why we decide to divide resources in an unequal fashion. The current study aimed to investigate the neural responses associated with inequity in sharing decisions when maximization of outcomes for the self or another person is in conflict with the equity norm.

Using allocation tasks such as the "Dictator Game" where participants divide a certain amount of rewards (i.e., the stake) between themselves and another player without sanctions or reputation-related consequences, many studies have shown that people often give away a nontrivial amount of the stake to anonymous others, with an equitable 50–50 split being the most frequent allocation [17,18,21,23,24]. Nonetheless, such a preference for fairness is highly sensitive to different aspects of the (social) context in which they occur [19,21,22,25,26]. For example, a preference for equity decreases when the costs of establishing equal outcomes increase, supporting the crucial role of self-outcome maximization in fairness considerations. Furthermore, people seem to be less tolerant to receiving less than other people (i.e., disadvantageous inequity) compared to receiving more than others (i.e., advantageous inequity) [7,12–14,21,23,24,27]. In other words, fairness considerations are not solely shaped by other-regarding preferences and prosocial intentions, but also by self-outcome maximization and aversion to disadvantageous inequity [12,25,26].

Studies investigating the neural mechanisms associated with inequity have predominantly focused on the *perception and receipt* of unfair treatment [7,12–14,27,28]. These studies have consistently shown involvement of the dorsal anterior cingulate cortex (dACC) and the anterior insula in perceiving unfairness. Interestingly, studies have shown heightened anterior insula activity when people themselves are the target of unfair treatment [12] and when they see someone else receiving an unfair offer [28]. Based on anterior insula's domain general role in providing anticipatory emotional signals in decision-making [29–31] and the ACC and insula's involvement in neural representations of bodily arousal states [29,32–34], it has been argued that the ACC and anterior insula play an important role in guiding our social behavior to follow social norms [35]. Behaviors in response to unfairness have been consistently associated with activation in the dorsolateral prefrontal cortex (dlPFC), which has been suggested to reflect increased regulation of a default prepotent reaction to unfair offers [13,27,36–40]. Although these findings overall support the idea that equity is perceived as a social norm, fewer studies have investigated how neural responses to unfairness might be different when *making* inequity decisions. Two studies investigating allocation of resources to others who had previously excluded the participants from a social interaction have shown the involvement of the ACC – insula network when sharing unequally with those excluders [41,42]. In the current study, we aimed to investigate whether inequity choices are processed differently than equity choices and how this depends on the benefit for the self and the other. For this purpose, we investigated inequity choices in different experimental conditions that aimed to disentangle inequity that is advantageous for the self from inequity that is advantageous for another person (while leaving the decision-maker's own outcome unaffected).

First, based on previous findings, we expected higher insula and dACC activity when making inequity choices in general [29,33]. A central question was whether the insula and dACC response subserves a general role through acting as a "social alarm system" that is activated in response to both advantageous and disadvantageous inequity, i.e. regardless of whether the participants themselves or another person benefits from the inequity. If equity were perceived as the social norm, we would expect higher levels of insula and dACC activity in making inequity choices across different conditions that differ in relative outcomes for self and other. However, if other-regarding (prosocial) outcomes were perceived as the social norm, we would expect increased levels of activation in this network when making choices that ensure equity, but also lead to less optimal outcomes for others.

Second, we tested the hypothesis that inequity choices that lead to benefit of others is associated with activation in neural circuitry previously linked to reward-processing. This hypothesis is based on prior studies wherein participants were the allocators of resources and that showed that neural regions implicated in the computation of subjective value and reward play an important role in resource distribution [29,33]. Although the paradigms used in these studies differed considerably, these prior studies showed that reward-related brains regions [e.g. the striatum and ventromedial PFC (vmPFC)] were associated with choosing outcomes that maximized the amount of joint resources. However, paradigms in these studies did not investigate two core processes of fairness considerations, namely, choices that incur costs to the self [29] and a fair alternative to making inequity choices [33]. In the current study, we included similar experimental conditions that involved a fair alternative to inequity and that also differed in respective possible

costs and benefits for the self and the other. We expected that choices indicating other-regarding preferences through a maximization of the other's outcomes would result in increased activation in reward-related brain regions, such as the striatum and the vmPFC.

Methods

Participants and procedure

Twenty-eight young adults ($M = 20.7$ years, $SD = 1.91$; 11 male) were recruited through local advertisements. All participants were right-handed and did not report any contraindications for fMRI. Before scanning participants were familiarized with the scanner environment using a mock scanner. After scanning, they filled out a battery of questionnaires, and received €25 for their participation and an additional amount of money, which was told to be determined by their decisions in the allocation games. In reality everyone received an additional €2. The current study was conducted in accordance with the ethical standards of the American Psychological Association as expressed in the Declaration of Helsinki. All participants provided written informed consent for the study. The study was approved by the Leiden University Medical Center (LUMC) ethics committee. A radiologist reviewed all anatomical scans; no anomalies were reported.

fMRI task description

Participants played the role of the allocator in a set of three modified dictator games [21]. In each game the participants were asked to distribute coins between themselves and an anonymous other player based on preset dichotomous choices. One of the two options was always a fair (equal) distribution of coins, i.e. one coin for the self and one coin for the other (1/1). The alternative distribution in the three games were as follows: i) one coin for the self and zero coins for the other (i.e., 1/0) in the *Advantageous Competitive Inequity* game, where the inequity choice maximized the difference between self and other without gains relative to the equity choice, ii) two coins for the self and zero coins for the other (i.e., 2/0) in the *Advantageous Self-maximizing Inequity* game, where the inequity choice maximized outcomes for the self, and iii) one coin for the self and two coins for the other (i.e., 1/2) in the *Disadvantageous Prosocial Inequity* game, where the inequity choice signified other-regarding (i.e., prosocial) concerns.

Each trial started with a jittered fixation cross (mean = 1540 ms, min = 550 ms, max = 4950 ms; optimized with Opt-Seq2, surfer.nmr.mgh.harvard.edu/optseq/; [43]). On the left hand side of this screen, participants were also presented with the name of the other player (see Fig. 1A). This was followed by the decision screen where participants were presented with two distributions (i.e., two buckets with coins in them) they could choose between. In each distribution coins for the self were indicated in red and coins for the other were indicated in blue. Participants had 4000 ms to make a choice. Upon making a choice, the bucket of their choice was encircled in red and this was displayed until the end of 5000 ms in total. In case of no response within the 4000 ms period, participants were presented a screen with 'Too late!' for the duration of 1000 ms. Trials without a response consisted of less than 1% of all trials and were excluded from further analyses. Prior to scanning participants were provided with instructions (see Text S1) and practiced the game (6 trials) on a computer. During the scanning session participants played a total of 60 trials, with 20 trials of each game, in randomized order. The location of the equal distribution was counterbalanced across trials. All trials were presented in one block lasting about 8 minutes.

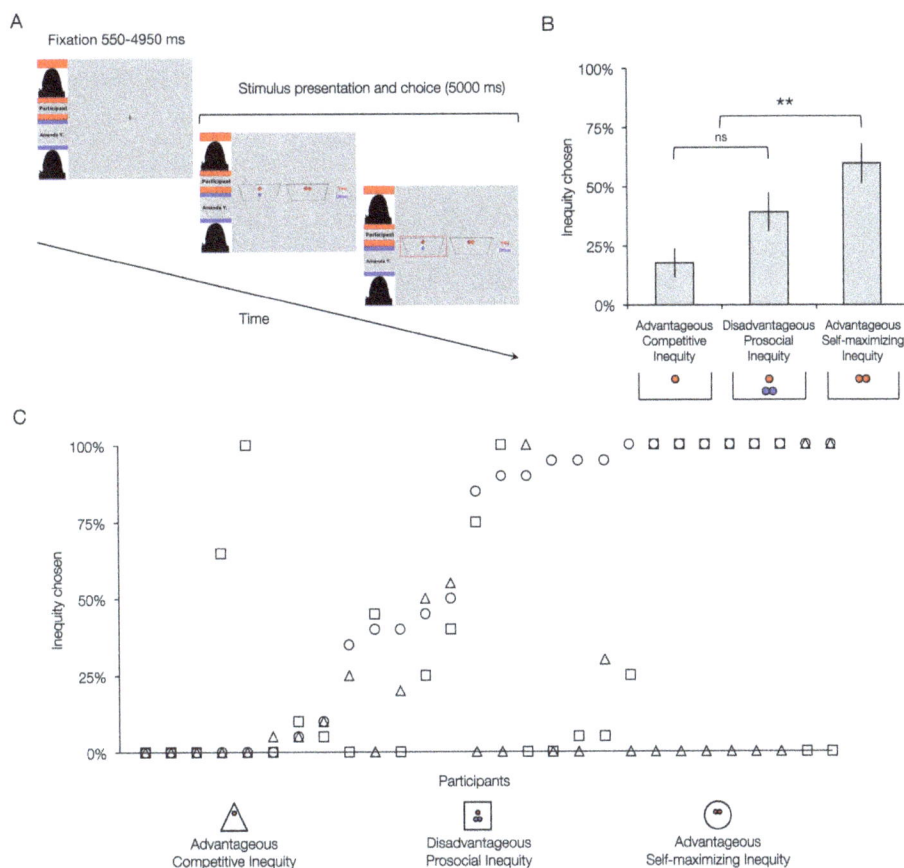

Figure 1. Visual display of the fMRI task and frequency of inequity choices. (A) Visual display of events presented in the one trial of the fMRI task. Each trial started with a jittered fixation cross lasting 550–4950 ms. The following screen displayed the name of the participant in red (here 'Participant') and the name of the recipient (here 'Amanda Y.'). This screen also presented the available choice options for distributing the coins (here Advantageous Self-Maximizing Inequity game; 1/1 vs 2/0) with red and blue coins indicating the share for the participant and the recipient, respectively. The participant had a maximum response time of 4000 ms to make a choice. Upon response, the chosen distribution was encircled in red (here 1/1) until the end of the 5000 ms. (B) Percentage of inequity choices made in each of the three games. **$p<.001$, *$p<.05$. (C) Percentage of inequity choices made by each participant in each of the three games.

On each trial, the first name and the first letter of the surname of both the participant and the recipient were displayed on screen to ensure anonymity, but also to emphasize the notion that participants would play each trial with a new player (see Figure 1A). Participants were told that random trials would be selected and their choices on these trials would determine their final earnings in the task. Prior to the experiment, participants were explained that the recipients were participants in the study and it was also emphasized that their decisions would have consequences for the other players' earnings. None of the participants reported disbelief in the cover story that their offers influenced other players' outcomes.

fMRI data acquisition

Scanning was carried out at the University Medical Centre using a 3.0 T Philips Achieva. The scanning procedure included: i) a localizer scan, ii) T2*-weighted whole-brain echo planar images (EPI) measuring the bold-oxygen-level-dependent (BOLD) signal (TR = 2.2 s, TE = 30 ms, slice matrix = 80×80, slice thickness = 2.75 ms, slice gap = 0.28 mm, field of view (FOV) = 220 mm), iii) high-resolution T1- and T2- weighted matched bandwidth anatomical images with the same slice prescriptions as the EPIs. Functional data were acquired in a

single functional run of 210 volumes; the first two volumes were discarded to allow for equilibration of T1 saturation effects. The task was programmed in E-prime and was projected onto a screen that was viewed through a mirror fastened upon the head coil assembly. Head movement was restricted by the use of foam inserts around the head.

MRI data analysis

Image pre-processing and analysis was conducted using SPM8 software (www.fil.ion.ucl.ac.uk/spm). Pre-processing included slice-time correction, realignment, spatial normalization to EPI templates, and smoothing with a Gaussian filter of 8 mm full-width at half maximum. Movement parameters in all directions were below 1.08 mm for all participants and all scans. The fMRI time series were modeled by a series of events convolved with a canonical hemodynamic response function (HRF). The data were modeled at stimulus onset of the decision screen with zero duration and based on the game (3 levels: Advantageous Competitive Inequity, Advantageous Self-maximizing Inequity and Disadvantageous Prosocial Inequity) and participant's choice (2 levels: equity or inequity), resulting in a 3×2 full factorial model that included six regressors. The participant-specific contrast images were obtained at the subject level and were then submitted to group level analyses at the second level, where participants served as a random effect in a repeated measures ANOVA. The full factorial ANOVA had an unbalanced design with varying number of participants in each cell of the model due to the fact that not all participants chose all options. The number of participants included in each cell of the design is as follows: Advantageous Competitive Inequity Game Equity choice (n = 25), Advantageous Competitive Inequity Game Inequity choice (n = 11), Advantageous Self-maximizing Inequity Game Equity choice (n = 19), Advantageous Self-maximizing Inequity Game Inequity choice (n = 22), Disadvantageous Prosocial Inequity Game Equity choice (n = 20), and Disadvantageous Prosocial Inequity Game Inequity choice (n = 18). We also conducted follow-up analyses examining the t-contrasts of Inequity > Equity for each game separately. Mean percentage of inequity offers in each game was used in regression analyses to test for brain-behavior relations in a GLM model based on the game (collapsed across choices; 3 levels: Advantageous Competitive Inequity, Advantageous Self-maximizing Inequity and Disadvantageous Prosocial Inequity). The fMRI analyses were conducted at the threshold of $p<.001$ uncorrected with a voxel threshold of 10 functional voxels to balance between Type 1 and Type 2 errors [44]. Regions of interest (ROI) analyses were further conducted on the regions obtained from the whole-brain analyses using the MARSBAR tool in SPM8 [45]. All results are reported in the MNI305 (Montreal Neurological Institute) stereotactic space.

Results

Behavioral results

An examination of response patterns of the participants showed that they had strong preferences for equity or inequity choices, which depended on the costs for self and other (see Table 1). A detailed overview of these choices per participant can be seen in Figure 1C. Percentage of inequity choices across the three conditions was compared using a repeated measure ANOVA, which yielded a significant main effect of Game ($F(2,54) = 8.4$, $p = .001$, $\eta_p^2 = .24$; Fig. 1B). Participants chose the inequity distribution more often in the Advantageous Self-maximizing Inequity condition ($M = .60$, $SD = .43$) than in the Disadvantageous Prosocial Inequity condition ($M = .39$, $SD = .44$; F (1, 27) = 4.90, $p<.05$, $\eta_p^2 = .15$) and in the Advantageous Competitive Inequity condition ($M = .18$, $SD = .33$; F (1, 27) = 21.98, $p< .001$, $\eta_p^2 = .45$). Inequity choices in the latter two conditions did not differ significantly from each other ($p = .09$, $\eta_p^2 = .10$). There was also a significant correlation between inequity choices in the Disadvantageous Prosocial Inequity and the Advantageous Competitive Inequity conditions (r (28) = −.41, $p<.05$).

Neuroimaging results

In order to examine the neural correlates of equity and inequity choices, we conducted the Inequity > Equity and reverse contrasts

within the 3 (Game) ×2 (Choice) ANOVA. The Inequity > Equity t-contrast revealed a network of regions comprising bilateral insula (x/y/z coordinates: −30, 21, −12; 19 voxels and 27, 24, −9; 95 voxels), right IFG (54, 21, 18; 12 voxels), dorsal ACC (6, 39, 21; 46 voxels and 0, 24, 36; 61 voxels), and dorsolateral (27, 45, 36; 22 voxels) and ventrolateral PFC (30, 54, −3; 49 voxels) ($t(109) = 3.17$; Figure 2; activation levels obtained from ROI analyses in right insula is plotted for demonstration purposes in a bar graph of activation per game and offer). The reverse contrast (Equity>Inequity) did not yield any clusters of activation and the game by choice interaction also did not result in significant activation. Thus, insula, ACC and dlPFC were activated in response to choosing an unequal distribution of resources, regardless of the consequences of this distribution for self or other in terms of maximizing outcomes or costs.

Next, in order to examine inequity related neural responses in more depth, we focused on the Inequity > Equity and reverse contrasts in the context of each of the three games separately using t-tests. The Equity > Inequity contrast did not yield activation in any of the three games. We also did not detect any regions for the Inequity > Equity contrasts in the Advantageous Competitive (n = 8) and the Advantageous Self-maximizing (n = 13) games at the chosen threshold, but note that the effects reported above are partially replicated at a more lenient threshold (see Table S1).

The Inequity > Equity contrast in the Disadvantageous Prosocial Inequity condition (n = 10) yielded increased activation in the vmPFC (6, 48, 0; 62 voxels), ventral striatum (12, 21, 0; 11 voxels), and right anterior insula (45, 15, −6; 53 voxels) during inequity choices than equity choices (Figure 3; activation levels obtained from ROI analyses in ventral striatum and vmPFC are plotted for demonstration purposes in a bar graph of activation per game and offer). Importantly, here the inequity choices were not only disadvantageous for the self relative to the other player, but also beneficial for the other player. Post-hoc ROI analyses showed that higher activation in these regions during inequity than equity was specific for the Disadvantageous Prosocial Inequity game; inequity and equity related activity in the Advantageous Competitive and Advantageous Self-maximizing Inequity games did not differ significantly in any of the regions (all $p>.25$).

Finally, we examined brain-behavior relations by conducting whole-brain regressions where inequity choice frequency was included as a regressor in activations involved in the Disadvantageous Prosocial Inequity Game (collapsed across choices) – null contrast (n = 28). This approach enabled us to examine the relation between frequency of inequity choices and brain activation across the complete sample of 28 participants, whereas the previously reported inequity vs. equity and reverse contrasts could be examined only among the 10 participants who had made both equity and inequity choices in the Disadvantageous Prosocial Inequity condition. This analysis resulted in a set of regions in which activation correlated positively with inequity choices, including the precuneus (−9, −57, −48; 25 voxels), ventromedial

Table 1. Frequency (and percentage) of participants making 100% equity, 100% inequity or both choices across the trials per game.

Game	100% Equity	100% Inequity	Both
Disadvantageous Prosocial Inequity (1/2)	10 (37.5%)	8 (28.6%)	10 (37.5%)
Advantageous Competitive Inequity (1/0)	17 (60.7%)	3 (10.7%)	8 (28.6%)
Advantageous Self-maximizing Inequity (2/0)	6 (21.4%)	9 (32.1%)	13 (46.4%)

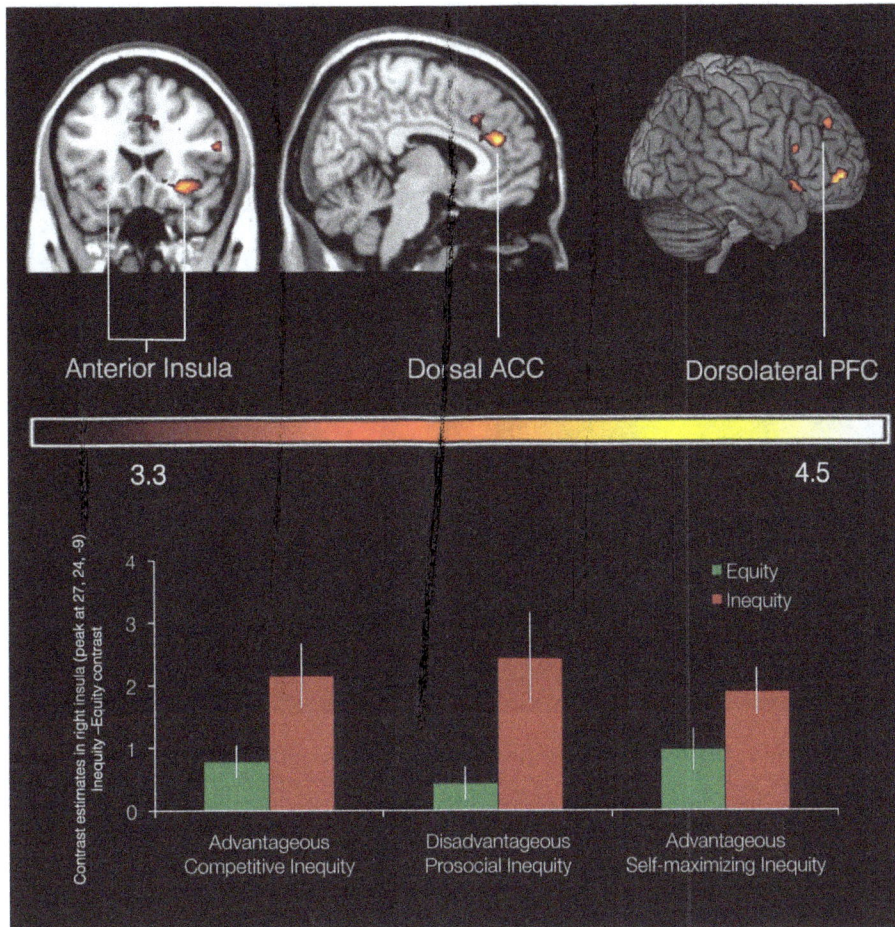

Figure 2. Neural network associated with inequity. Network of brain regions from the Inequity > Equity contrast in the 3 (Game) ×2 (Choice) full factorial ANOVA; $p < .001$, 10 voxel threshold. Bar graph displays contrast estimates obtained from ROI analysis in right anterior insula (MNI 27, 24, −9) for inequity and equity choices in the three conditions. Error bars indicate SEM.

PFC (15, 45, 0; 23 voxels), and dlPFC (MNI 24, 39, 42; 33 voxels) (Figure 4; the relation between DLPFC activation and frequency of inequity offers is demonstrated in a scatterplot). There was no activation in brain regions of interest in the brain-behavior correlations for the other two games (see Table S2).

Discussion

The current study set out to investigate the common and distinct neural responses associated with inequity decisions involved in maximizing outcomes for the self or another person. Our behavioral results demonstrate that participants more often chose unequal distributions in situations where their own profits could be maximized relative to alternatives where they could maximize the other person's profits. The neuroimaging findings showed that choosing inequity regardless of whether it entails benefits for the other is associated with increased activation in the anterior insula, dACC and dlPFC. In addition, decisions to distribute resources unequally, but in a way that benefits another person's profits additionally coincided with increased activation in ventral striatum, vmPFC, precuneus and dlPFC. Taken together, our findings show that there is a common neural response to making advantageous and disadvantageous inequity choices, which resembles the pattern of neural activity previously associated with being treated unfairly [12–14,28]. Furthermore,

we show a distinct neural response associated with prosocial inequity, which suggests that violating a fairness norm in order to increase another person's outcomes is processed differently on a neural level compared to selfish violations of a fairness norm.

Our behavioral findings show that participants adjusted their behavior depending on the available alternatives to an equal split. In doing so, it seems that different principles interact to guide decision-making when distributing resources: a social norm of equity, (possible) costs for the self, and a concern for outcomes of others *relative* to the self. Whereas an equal distribution was the most preferred option when it did not involve possible costs to the allocator (i.e., the participant), equal distributions became less preferred when it was costly to establish them. This finding is in line with previous studies on fairness preferences, which show that, although an equal split is used as a cognitive heuristic, contextual factors related to the relevance of self-interest systematically shifts preferences away from an equal split [9]. Preference for an equal distribution was not only influenced by *absolute* costs, as in the Advantageous Self-maximizing Inequity condition, but also in terms of *relative* costs compared to the other player, as in the Disadvantageous Prosocial Inequity condition. This latter finding demonstrates that a preference for equal outcomes does not necessarily have to be grounded in a prosocial motivation, but might also result from the desire to avoid receiving lower payoffs than another person [2,28,46,47].

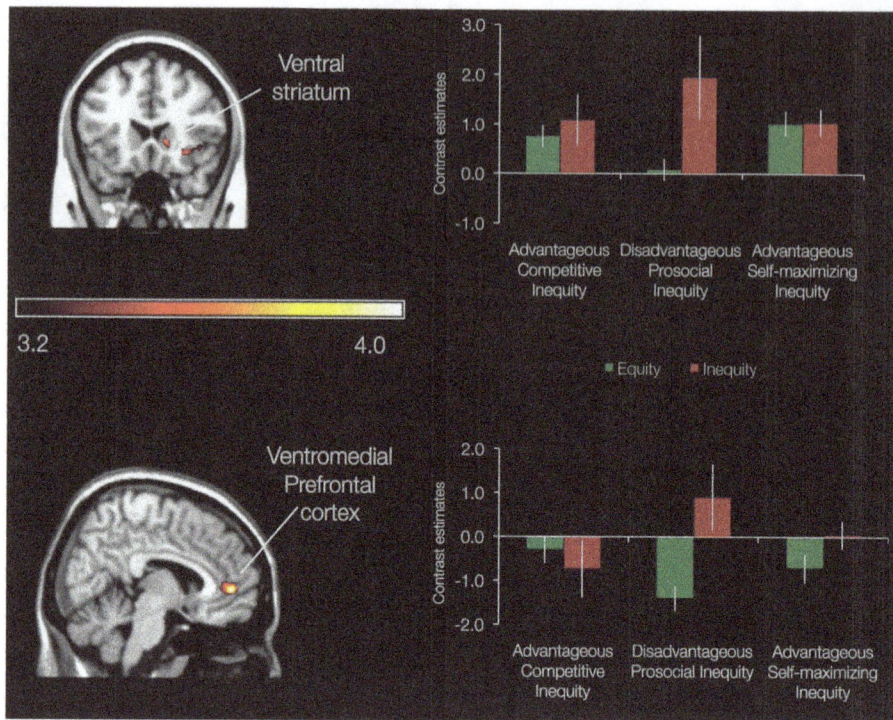

Figure 3. Neural network involved in Disadvantageous Prosocial Inequity. Ventral striatum (MNI 12, 21, 0) and ventromedial PFC (MNI 6, 48, 0) from the Inequity > Equity contrast in the Disadvantageous Prosocial Inequity condition; $p<.001$, 10 voxel threshold. Bar graphs display contrast estimates obtained from ROI analyses for inequity and equity choices in the three conditions. Error bars indicate SEM.

Neuroimaging results further show that there is a common neural response in dACC, bilateral anterior insula and dlPFC to both advantageous and disadvantageous inequity. This suggests that a general neural mechanism is implicated in signaling deviations from a fairness norm in sharing decisions, regardless of who benefits from the unequal distribution of goods. Our findings corroborate previous findings showing that both advantageous and disadvantageous inequity were associated with anterior insula activity [48] and a heightened medial frontal negativity [49], which has been interpreted as suggesting the involvement of the insula-ACC network in norm and associated expectancy violations. The dACC and the anterior insula are part of a "salience network" that serves an important domain general role in integrating cognitive and emotional signals when processing motivationally salient information [47,50]. Activation in this network has been associated with error processing [51], uncertainty [52], conflict [53] and violations of a social norms [28,46,47,54,55]. We extend previous research by showing that the insula and dACC are also activated when creating inequity in choices that involve possible costs to the self and a fair alternative to inequity, both of which are core components of fairness considerations previously not investigated using fMRI.

Increased dlPFC activity during both advantageous and disadvantageous inquity choices relative to equity choices fits with findings from a recent study showing dlPFC involvement in both advantageous and disadvantageous inequity in a game in which participants received less or more money than another person after performing a perceptual task [56]. Based on its role in cognitive control and goal-directed behavior it has been argued that dlPFC activity in social decision-making tasks reflects increased control over prepotent responses that are aimed to maximize self-gain [27,36,39,57,58]. Our results suggest that dlPFC activity might

reflect higher levels of executive control required to violate a salient social norm regardless of whether this maximizes gains for the self or someone else. The notion that this is not restricted to maximizing outcomes for the self was supported by our individual differences analyses that showed that participants who more often chose outcomes that maximize the profits of the other over an equal distribution recruit the dlPFC to a greater extent when doing so.

In addition to a common neural pattern associated with inequity, we also found that violations of a fairness norm in the Disadvantageous Prosocial Inequity condition were associated with activation in the striatum and the vmPFC. Activation in these regions associated with such prosocial behavior that leads to better outcomes for another person is in line with prior findings showing that the striatum not only responds to primary rewards, but also to social rewards such as charitable donations [59,60], maximizing another person's outcomes [33,61,62], and mutual cooperation in a prisoner's dilemma paradigm [21,26,61,63]. Moreover, individual differences analyses showed that the more frequent people showed this other-outcome maximizing behavior, the more they activated the vmPFC and the precuneus. The vmPFC is not only important for the encoding the subjective value of rewards [64,65], but is also part of a network, including the precuneus, dorsomedial prefrontal cortex and the temporo-parietal junction [66,67] important for mental state-reasoning [14,41,68,69] and perspective-taking [60]. Moreover activation in the mPFC has been shown to be associated with processing one's own and other people's actions and intentions in economic games [61,62]. Acting in a way that does not necessarily benefit outcomes for the self, but is beneficial to another person's gains might thus possibly require increased levels of perspective-taking. It would be recommended for future studies to assess self-reported subjective value associated

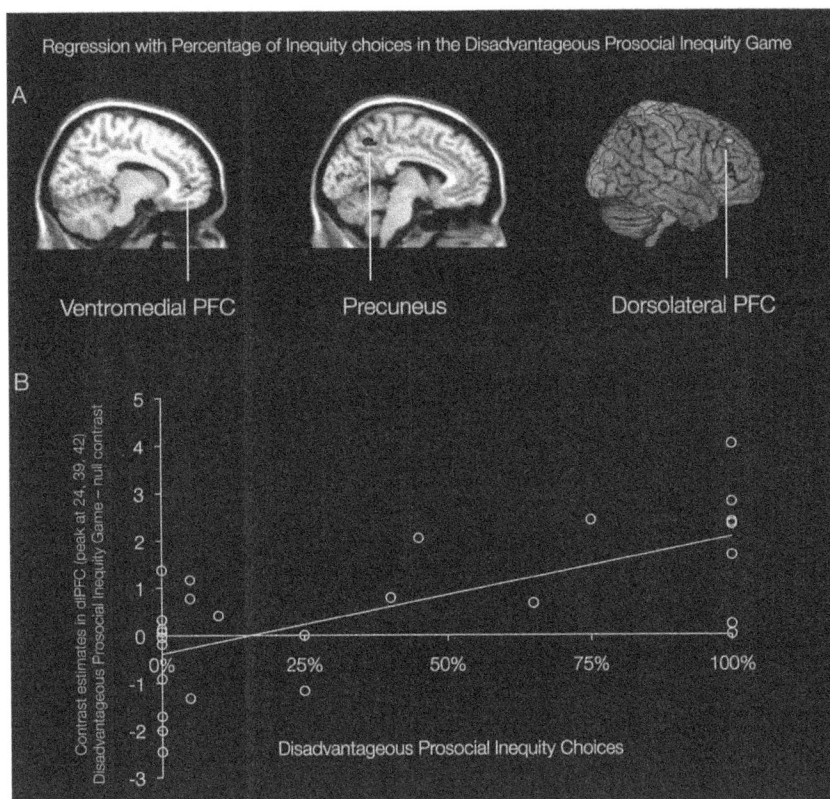

Figure 4. Neural network related to frequency of inequity choices. Brain regions from the regression of neural activity during the Disadvantageous Prosocial Inequity game with frequency of inequity choices. (A) Activation in the ventromedial PFC (MNI 15, 45, 0), precuneus (MNI -9, -57, -48), and dorsolateral prefrontal cortex (dlPFC; MNI 24, 39, 42) correlates positively with the frequency of inequity choices in the Disadvantageous Prosocial Inequity condition; $p<.001$, 10 voxel threshold. (B) Scatter plot displays contrast estimates for the Disadvantageous Prosocial Inequity condition on the y-axis and behavior (% inequity) on the x-axis (N = 28).

with individuals' choices of advantageous and disadvantageous inequity in order to be able to examine how experience of reward is related to the neural signal associated with these choices.

Several limitations of the current study should be noted. One of the main challenges of the current research design is related to individual differences in observed behavior. As indicated by the behavioral patterns (see Figure 1C), the majority of participants were consistent in their choices within a certain condition, which might be considered desired given that this consistency reflects stable individual preferences and implies that participants did not choose randomly. However, this resulted in relatively small numbers of observations in several neuroimaging analyses where choice-related neural activation was examined based on contrasts of inequity versus equity choices per condition. For example, although there was a main effect of the Inequity > Equity contrast across conditions, these effects could not be observed when this contrast was examined per condition separately at the chosen threshold, but was only evident at more lenient threshold levels. In addition, the results may represent the neural activity of individuals who are ambiguous about equity choices, and in future research it should be examined whether these also represent choices of individuals with strict equity norms. Previous behavioral studies using the three allocation games have also examined profiles of individual behavior patterns [21,26]. In the current study, our sample size did not allow us to examine the neural correlates of individual behavioral profiles. Future studies employing larger sample sizes should aim to examine individual differences in neural activation related to profiles of behavior.

The individual differences in behavior also resulted in an unbalanced design in our fMRI analysis. In other words, due to the fact that not all participants made all choices in each game, it was not possible to conduct a balanced full-factorial analysis with the same number of observations in each cell of the design. Future studies can aim to manipulate the study design in order to obtain a more balanced response pattern or, as indicated above, aim for larger sample sizes that will enable to examine individual differences based on choice profiles.

Furthermore, the current study did not employ self-report explicit measures about cognitive and affective processes related to making (inequity) choices. Future research should include measures about beliefs on fairness norms, affect related to inequity choices or autonomic measurements, such as heart rate, which can provide the researchers with additional measures in interpreting behavioral and neural findings.

The current results offer a number of avenues for future research. For example, our current design did not allow for a dissociation between joint-outcome maximization and maximization of another person's outcomes in the disadvantageous inequity (1/2) choices. Future studies could include a condition where the 1/1 option is pitted against a 2/1 distribution, in which the latter choice would both be self- and joint outcome maximization [70]. A contrast between the 2/1 and 1/2 choices could disentangle joint outcome maximization from person-specific (self vs. other) outcome maximization. Furthermore, using the same set of three allocation tasks [21,26] and other paradigms [71,72] it has been shown that across development children and adolescents increasingly start enforcing equality between the ages of 3 and 13. Recent developmental work has shown that developmental changes in late maturing brain regions such as regions of the mentalizing network and the lateral PFC are associated with developmental increases in intentionality understanding and strategic considerations in fairness decisions [14,37]. It would be of great interest to relate behavioral changes in both advantageous and disadvantageous inequity choices to brain development, because taking a developmental perspective has the potential to enhance not only our understanding of social development, but could also provide insights into adult social decision-making and its underlying mechanisms.

Taken together, the current results further inform our understanding of an important aspect of human social behavior, that is, when and why we decide to divide resources unequally. We show that violations of an equity norm, both with selfish (i.e., advantageous) and prosocial (i.e., disadvantageous) outcomes, are associated with a common neural response in the "salience network". Furthermore, prosocial violations of a simple fairness norm were associated with activation in brain regions that code for primary and more complex social rewards [29,33] and switching attention to another person's perspective [60–62]. These findings show that neural networks implicated in social cognition, domain general cognitive functions and emotional processes are important for both following social norms and for violating such norms when these violations serve a more prosocial purpose than the norm itself.

References

1. Kahneman D, Knetsch JL, Thaler RH (1986) Fairness and the Assumptions of Economics. The Journal of Business 59: S285–S300.
2. Fehr E, Schmidt K (1999) A theory of fairness, competition, and cooperation*. Quarterly journal of Economics 114: 817–868.
3. Turillo CJ, Folger R, Lavelle JJ, Umphress EE, Gee JO (2002) Is virtue its own reward? Self-sacrificial decisions for the sake of fairness. Organizational Behavior and Human Decision Processes 89: 839–865.
4. Fehr E, Fischbacher U (2004) Social norms and human cooperation. Trends Cogn Sci (Regul Ed) 8: 185–190. doi:10.1016/j.tics.2004.02.007.
5. Henrich J, Boyd R, Bowles S, Camerer C, Fehr E, et al. (2005) "Economic man" in cross-cultural perspective: Behavioral experiments in 15 small-scale societies. Behav Brain Sci 28: 795–814.
6. Tabibnia G, Lieberman MD (2007) Fairness and Cooperation Are Rewarding: Evidence from Social Cognitive Neuroscience. Annals of the New York Academy of Sciences 1118: 90–101. doi:10.1196/annals.1412.001.
7. Tabibnia G, Satpute AB, Lieberman MD (2008) The sunny side of fairness preference for fairness activates reward circuitry (and disregarding unfairness activates self-control circuitry). Psychological science: a journal of the American Psychological Society/APS 19: 339–347.
8. Tricomi E, Rangel A, Camerer CF, O'doherty JP (2010) Neural evidence for inequality-averse social preferences. Nature 463: 1089–1091. doi:10.1038/nature08785.
9. Civai C, Rumiati RI, Rustichini A (2013) More equal than others: Equity norms as an integration of cognitive heuristics and contextual cues in bargaining games. Acta Psychol (Amst) 144: 12–18. doi:10.1016/j.actpsy.2013.05.002.
10. Pillutla MM, Murnighan JK (1996) Unfairness, anger, and spite: Emotional rejections of ultimatum offers. Organizational Behavior and Human Decision Processes 68: 208–224.
11. Srivastava J, Espinoza F, Fedorikhin A (2009) Coupling and decoupling of unfairness and anger in ultimatum bargaining. Journal of Behavioral Decision Making 22: 475–489. doi:10.1002/bdm.631.
12. Sanfey AG, Rilling JK, Aronson JA, Nystrom LE, Cohen JD (2003) The neural basis of economic decision-making in the ultimatum game. Science 300: 1755–1758. doi:10.1126/science.1082976.
13. Güroğlu B, Van Den Bos W, Rombouts SA, Crone EA (2010) Unfair? It depends: neural correlates of fairness in social context. Social Cognitive and Affective Neuroscience 5: 414–423. doi:10.1093/scan/nsq013.
14. Güroğlu B, Van Den Bos W, van Dijk E, Rombouts SARB, Crone EA (2011) Dissociable brain networks involved in development of fairness considerations: understanding intentionality behind unfairness. NeuroImage 57: 634–641. doi:10.1016/j.neuroimage.2011.04.032.
15. Guth W, Schmittberger R, Schwarze B (1982) An experimental analysis of ultimatum bargaining. Journal of Economic Behavior and Organization 3: 367–388.
16. Straub PG, Murnighan JK (1995) An experimental investigation of ultimatum games: Information, fairness, expectations, and lowest acceptable offers. Journal of Economic Behavior and Organization 27: 345–364.
17. Forsythe R, Horowitz J, Savin N, Martin S (1994) Fairness in Simple Bargaining Experiments. Games and Economic Behavior 6: 347–369.
18. Camerer C, Thaler RH (1995) Anomalies: Ultimatums, dictators and manners. The Journal of Economic Perspectives 9: 209–219.
19. Bardsley N (2008) Dictator game giving: altruism or artefact? Exp Econ 11: 122–133. doi:10.1007/s10683-007-9172-2.
20. Piff PK, Stancato DM, Côté S, Mendoza-Denton R, Keltner D (2012) Higher social class predicts increased unethical behavior. Proceedings of the National Academy of Sciences 109: 4086–4091. doi:10.1073/pnas.1118373109/-/DCSupplemental.
21. Fehr E, Bernhard H, Rockenbach B (2008) Egalitarianism in young children. Nature 454: 1079–1083. doi:10.1038/nature07155.
22. Koch AK, Normann H-T (2008) Giving in dictator games: Regard for others or regard by others? Southern Economic Journal: 223–231.
23. Fehr E, Gächter S (2002) Altruistic punishment in humans. Nature 415: 137–140.
24. Raihani NJ, McAuliffe K (2012) Does inequity aversion motivate punishment? Cleaner fish as a model system. Social Justice Research 25: 213–231. doi:10.1007/s11211-012-0157-8.
25. Güroğlu B, Van Den Bos W, Crone EA (2009) Fairness considerations: Increasing understanding of intentionality during adolescence. Journal of Experimental Child Psychology 104: 398–409. doi:10.1016/j.jecp.2009.07.002.
26. Steinbeis N, Singer T (2013) The effects of social comparison on social emotions and behavior during childhood: the ontogeny of envy and Schadenfreude predicts developmental changes in equity-related decisions. Journal of Experimental Child Psychology 115: 198–209. doi:10.1016/j.jecp.2012.11.009.
27. Wright ND, Symmonds M, Fleming SM, Dolan RJ (2011) Neural segregation of objective and contextual aspects of fairness. Journal of Neuroscience 31: 5244–5252. doi:10.1523/JNEUROSCI.3138-10.2011.
28. Corradi-Dell'Acqua C, Civai C, Rumiati RI, Fink GR (2013) Disentangling self- and fairness-related neural mechanisms involved in the ultimatum game: an fMRI study. Social Cognitive and Affective Neuroscience 8: 424–431. doi:10.1093/scan/nss014.
29. Hsu M, Anen C, Quartz SR (2008) The Right and the Good: Distributive Justice and Neural Encoding of Equity and Efficiency. Science 320: 1092–1095. doi:10.1126/science.1153651.
30. Kuhnen CM, Knutson B (2005) The neural basis of financial risk taking. Neuron 47: 763–770. doi:10.1016/j.neuron.2005.08.008.
31. Dosenbach NUF, Visscher KM, Palmer ED, Miezin FM, Wenger KK, et al. (2006) A core system for the implementation of task sets. Neuron 50: 799–812. doi:10.1016/j.neuron.2006.04.031.

Supporting Information

Table S1 Regions of neural activation from the Inequity > Equity contrast per allocation game.

Table S2 Regions of neural activation from whole-brain regression analyses with frequency of inequity choices per game as a regressor.

Text S1 Task instructions for the allocation game.

Acknowledgments

The authors would like to thank the Cédric Koolschijn, Anneke de Gier, Eduard Klapwijk, Marthe de Jong and Sandy Overgaauw for their support during the data collection.

Author Contributions

Conceived and designed the experiments: BG EC. Performed the experiments: BG GJW. Analyzed the data: BG GJW. Contributed reagents/materials/analysis tools: BG GJW EC. Contributed to the writing of the manuscript: BG GJW EC.

32. Craig AD (2003) Interoception: the sense of the physiological condition of the body. Curr Opin Neurobiol 13: 500–505. doi:10.1016/S0959-4388(03)00090-4.

33. Zaki J, Mitchell JP (2011) Equitable decision making is associated with neural markers of intrinsic value. Proceedings of the National Academy of Sciences 108: 19761–19766. doi:10.1073/pnas.1112324108/-/DCSupplemental.

34. Critchley HD (2005) Neural mechanisms of autonomic, affective, and cognitive integration. J Comp Neurol 493: 154–166. doi:10.1002/cne.20749.

35. Rilling JK, Sanfey AG (2011) The neuroscience of social decision-making. Annu Rev Psychol 62: 23–48. doi:10.1146/annurev.psych.121208.131647.

36. van t Wout M, Kahn RS, Sanfey AG, Aleman A (2005) Repetitive transcranial magnetic stimulation over the right dorsolateral prefrontal cortex affects strategic decision-making. NeuroReport 16: 1849–1852.

37. Knoch D, Pascual-Leone A, Meyer K, Treyer V, Fehr E (2006) Diminishing reciprocal fairness by disrupting the right prefrontal cortex. Science 314: 829–832. doi:10.1126/science.1129156.

38. Knoch D, Nitsche MA, Fischbacher U, Eisenegger C, Pascual-Leone A, et al. (2008) Studying the neurobiology of social interaction with transcranial direct current stimulation–the example of punishing unfairness. Cereb Cortex 18: 1987–1990. doi:10.1093/cercor/bhm237.

39. Spitzer M, Fischbacher U, Herrnberger B, Groen G, Fehr E (2007) The neural signature of social norm compliance. Neuron 56: 185–196. doi:10.1016/j.neuron.2007.09.011.

40. Knoch D, Gianotti LR, Baumgartner T, Fehr E (2010) A neural marker of costly punishment behavior. Psychological science: a journal of the American Psychological Society/APS 21: 337–342. doi:10.1177/0956797609360750.

41. Gunther Moor B, Güroğlu B, Op de Macks Z, Rombouts S, Van der Molen M, et al. (2012) Social exclusion and punishment of excluders: Neural correlates and developmental trajectories. NeuroImage 59: 708–717.

42. Will GJW, Crone EA, Güroğlu B (in press) Acting on social exclusion: Neural correlates of punishment and forgiveness of excluders. Social Cognitive and Affective Neuroscience.

43. Dale AM (1999) Optimal experimental design for event-related fMRI. Hum Brain Mapp 8: 109–114.

44. Lieberman MD, Cunningham WA (2009) Type I and Type II error concerns in fMRI research: Re-balancing the scale. Social Cognitive and Affective Neuroscience 4: 423–428. doi:10.1093/scan/nsp052.

45. Brett M, Anton JL, Valabregue R, Poline JB (2002) Abstract presented at the 8th International Conference on Functional Mapping of the Human Brain, June 2, Sendai, Japan.

46. Klucharev V, HytOnen K, Rijpkema M, Smidts A, Fernández G (2009) Reinforcement learning signal predicts social conformity. Neuron 61: 140–151. doi:10.1016/j.neuron.2008.11.027.

47. Montague P, Lohrenz T (2007) To Detect and Correct: Norm Violations and Their Enforcement. Neuron 56: 14–18. doi:10.1016/j.neuron.2007.09.020.

48. Yu R, Calder AJ, Mobbs D (2013) Overlapping and distinct representations of advantageous and disadvantageous inequality. Hum Brain Mapp 35: 3290–3301. doi:10.1002/hbm.22402.

49. Wu Y, Hu J, van Dijk E, Leliveld MC, Zhou X (2012) Brain activity in fairness consideration during asset distribution: Does the initial ownership play a role? PLoS One 7(6): e39627. doi:10.1371/journal.pone.0039627.

50. Botvinick M, Cohen J, Carter C (2004) Conflict monitoring and anterior cingulate cortex: an update. Trends Cogn Sci (Regul Ed) 8: 539–546. doi:10.1016/j.tics.2004.10.003.

51. de Bruijn ERA, de Lange FP, von Cramon DY, Ullsperger M (2009) When errors are rewarding. J Neurosci 29: 12183–12186. doi:10.1523/JNEUROSCI.1751-09.2009.

52. Singer T, Critchley HD, Preuschoff K (2009) A common role of insula in feelings, empathy and uncertainty. Trend Cogn Sci 13: 334–340. doi:10.1016/j.tics.2009.05.001.

53. Shenhav A, Botvinick MM, Cohen JD (2013) The expected value of control: An integrative theory of anterior cingulate cortex function. Neuron 79: 217–240. doi:10.1016/j.neuron.2013.07.007.

54. Chang LJ, Yarkoni T, Khaw MW, Sanfey AG (2013) Decoding the role of the insula in human cognition: functional parcellation and large-scale reverse inference. Cerebral Cortex 23: 739–749. doi:10.1093/cercor/bhs065.

55. Civai C, Crescentini C, Rustichini A, Rumiati RI (2012) Equality versus self-interest in the brain: Differential roles of anterior insula and medial prefrontal cortex. NeuroImage 62: 102–112. doi:10.1016/j.neuroimage.2012.04.037.

56. Fliessbach K, Philipps CB, Trautner P, Schnabel M, Elger CE, et al. (2012) Neural responses to advantageous and disadvantageous inequity. Front Hum Neurosci 6: 1–9. doi:10.3389/fnhum.2012.00165.

57. Steinbeis N, Bernhardt BC, Singer T (2012) Impulse Control and Underlying Functions of the Left DLPFC Mediate Age-Related and Age-Independent Individual Differences in Strategic Social Behavior. Neuron 73: 1040–1051. doi:10.1016/j.neuron.2011.12.027.

58. Grecucci A, Giorgetta C, Van't Wout M, Bonini N, Sanfey AG (2013) Reappraising the ultimatum: an fMRI study of emotion regulation and decision making. Cerebral Cortex 23: 399–410. doi:10.1093/cercor/bhs028.

59. Harbaugh WT, Mayr U, Burghart DR (2007) Neural responses to taxation and voluntary giving reveal motives for charitable donations. Science 316: 1622–1625. doi:10.1126/science.1140738.

60. Lamm C, Batson CD, Decety J (2007) The neural substrate of human empathy: effects of perspective-taking and cognitive appraisal. J Cogn Neurosci 19: 42–58. doi:10.1162/jocn.2007.19.1.42.

61. Rilling J (2004) The neural correlates of theory of mind within interpersonal interactions. NeuroImage 22: 1694–1703. doi:10.1016/j.neuroimage.2004.04.015.

62. Halko M-L, Hlushchuk Y, Hari R, Schürmann M (2009) Competing with peers: Mentalizing-related brain activity reflects what is at stake. NeuroImage 46: 542–548. doi:10.1016/j.neuroimage.2009.01.063.

63. Rilling J, Gutman D, Zeh T, Pagnoni G, Berns G, et al. (2002) A neural basis for social cooperation. Neuron 35: 395–405.

64. Rangel A, Hare T (2010) Neural computations associated with goal-directed choice. Curr Opin Neurobiol 20: 262–270. doi:10.1016/j.conb.2010.03.001.

65. Levy DJ, Glimcher PW (2012) The root of all value: a neural common currency for choice. Curr Opin Neurobiol 22: 1027–1038. doi:10.1016/j.conb.2012.06.001.

66. Saxe R, Carey S, Kanwisher N (2004) Understanding Other Minds: Linking Developmental Psychology and Functional Neuroimaging. Annu Rev Psychol 55: 87–124. doi:10.1146/annurev.psych.55.090902.142044.

67. Saxe RR, Whitfield-Gabrieli S, Scholz J, Pelphrey KA (2009) Brain Regions for Perceiving and Reasoning About Other People in School Aged Children. Child Development 80: 1197–1209.

68. Blakemore S-J, Ouden Den H, Choudhury S, Frith C (2007) Adolescent development of the neural circuitry for thinking about intentions. Social Cognitive and Affective Neuroscience 2: 130–139. doi:10.1093/scan/nsm009.

69. Moriguchi Y, Ohnishi T, Mori T, Matsuda H, Komaki G (2007) Changes of brain activity in the neural substrates for theory of mind during childhood and adolescence. Psychiatry Clin Neurosci 61: 355–363. doi:10.1111/j.1440-1819.2007.01687.x.

70. Meuwese R, Crone EA, de Rooij M, Güroğlu B (in press) Development of equity preferences in boys and girls across adolescence. Child Dev.

71. Blake PR, McAuliffe K (2011) "I had so much it didn't seem fair": Eight-year-olds reject two forms of inequity. Cognition 120: 215–224. doi:10.1016/j.cognition.2011.04.006.

72. Shaw A, Olson KR (2012) Children discard a resource to avoid inequity. Journal of Experimental Psychology: General 141: 382–395. doi:10.1037/a0025907.

18

Neural Network Cascade Optimizes MicroRNA Biomarker Selection for Nasopharyngeal Cancer Prognosis

Wenliang Zhu[1]*, Xuan Kan[2]

1 Institute of Clinical Pharmacology, the Second Affiliated Hospital of Harbin Medical University, Harbin, China, **2** Department of Otolaryngology, the Second Affiliated Hospital of Harbin Medical University, Harbin, China

Abstract

MicroRNAs (miRNAs) have been shown to be promising biomarkers in predicting cancer prognosis. However, inappropriate or poorly optimized processing and modeling of miRNA expression data can negatively affect prediction performance. Here, we propose a holistic solution for miRNA biomarker selection and prediction model building. This work introduces the use of a neural network cascade, a cascaded constitution of small artificial neural network units, for evaluating miRNA expression and patient outcome. A miRNA microarray dataset of nasopharyngeal carcinoma was retrieved from Gene Expression Omnibus to illustrate the methodology. Results indicated a nonlinear relationship between miRNA expression and patient death risk, implying that direct comparison of expression values is inappropriate. However, this method performs transformation of miRNA expression values into a miRNA score, which linearly measures death risk. Spearman correlation was calculated between miRNA scores and survival status for each miRNA. Finally, a nine-miRNA signature was optimized to predict death risk after nasopharyngeal carcinoma by establishing a neural network cascade consisting of 13 artificial neural network units. Area under the ROC was 0.951 for the internal validation set and had a prediction accuracy of 83% for the external validation set. In particular, the established neural network cascade was found to have strong immunity against noise interference that disturbs miRNA expression values. This study provides an efficient and easy-to-use method that aims to maximize clinical application of miRNAs in prognostic risk assessment of patients with cancer.

Editor: Raffaele A. Calogero, University of Torino, Italy

Funding: This work was supported by National Natural Science Foundation of China (No. 31301136). The funder had no role in study design, data collection and analysis, decision to publish, or preparation of the manuscript.

Competing Interests: The authors have declared that no competing interests exist.

* Email: wenzwl@yeah.net

Introduction

MicroRNAs (miRNAs) belong to a class of small ($\sim$22 nt) endogenous non-coding RNA molecules. MiRNAs play vital roles in regulating mRNA expression and fine-tuning protein levels posttranscriptionally [1,2]. Substantial evidence has shown that miRNAs may serve as promising therapeutic targets for clinical cancer treatment in the near future [3–5]. Meanwhile, the potential clinical applications of diagnostic and prognostic biomarkers are also widely studied and strongly suggest the utility of measuring circulating and biopsy tissue miRNAs [6–8]. Due to continual technological innovations in the past years, high-throughput methods such as miRNA microarray have been successful in the identification of potential biomarkers from thousands of mature miRNAs in humans [9,10]. As a result, such efforts have led to an increasing accumulation of miRNA expression data in the public Gene Expression Omnibus (GEO) database [11].

Simultaneous detection of many miRNAs generates a huge dataset of biological data that requires significant computational analysis. Although the current miRNA detection technologies are already very well established, there is still no widely recognized method for analyzing the massive amount of data obtained by high-throughput methods [12]. The vast majority of previous studies assumed a linear relationship between miRNA expression and disease phenotype [13–15]. This led to wide application of straightforward statistical methods such as Student's t-test or the analysis of variance test for between-group comparison of miRNA expression values. However, this assumption has not been specifically tested, or shown to be valid. Alternatively, rather than a linear relationship, we speculated that a nonlinear association may be possible between miRNA expression and disease phenotype. This assumption is primarily based on the knowledge that miRNAs play multi-faceted and complex roles in many biological processes [16]. If the nonlinear relationship is valid, it may imply that traditional miRNA expression data processing, analyzing, and modeling with linear methods are insufficient.

The improper selection of statistical or modeling methods may harm the potential performance of miRNAs as biomarkers and result in poor discrimination of patients [17,18]. We propose one feasible way to address this issue through transforming miRNA expression values into a linear variable before establishing a diagnostic or prognostic model. Using this proposed method, the present study aims to provide a holistic and generic solution for miRNA biomarker selection and prediction model construction. In recent years, artificial neural network (ANN) modeling has been successfully applied in cancer diagnosis and management [19–21]. Herein, a novel artificial neural network (ANN) modeling method was established for this purpose: the neural network cascade (NNC), an extensible and pyramid-like cascade of small ANN units. Each small ANN unit has simple network architecture and is limited to dealing with only one task, such as data transformation, data integration, or prediction output. In theory, an NNC model can simultaneously accommodate and process large amounts of information in parallel. Even if a single input has poor predictive performance, as long as sufficient input information is given, an accurate final prediction is guaranteed. The number of input parameters included in the model depends on the accuracy requirements placed on the final prediction.

To better illustrate our method, we developed an NNC prognostic model for death risk assessment in patients with nasopharyngeal carcinoma (NPC) using a miRNA expression dataset retrieved from GEO (dataset ID: GSE32960). Our results suggest a nonlinear association between miRNA expression and the death risk of patients diagnosed with NPC. The established NNC model showed good prediction performance by accurately identifying high-risk patients, even in the case where miRNA expression levels were artificially disturbed. In summary, such an effort aims to analytically enhance the utility of miRNAs as clinical biomarkers for achieving accurate diagnosis and individualized cancer treatment. Our successful case study analysis of NPC prognosis using the novel NNC model suggests that this model will also be applicable to diagnosis and prognosis of other human diseases.

Materials and Methods

miRNA expression data: acquisition and pre-processing

The miRNA expression dataset for patients with NPC (GSE32960) was retrieved from GEO. Only the 312 NPC samples were included in our study. We downloaded the preprocessed microarray expression values for 873 miRNAs for each sample and recorded the survival status (alive: 0 or dead: 1) of the corresponding patient. The original microarray expression values of each miRNA were then normalized as numbers between 0 and 1 as calculated below:

$$\text{Normalized value} = \frac{(Value - MIN\_Value)}{(Max\_Value - MIN\_Value)}$$

Max_Value and Min_Value are the maximum and minimum original miRNA expression values in the whole collection of samples, respectively. After that, the samples were randomly divided into two sets: a model training set (n = 208) and an external validation set (n = 104). For samples in the training set, the ANN software STATISTICA Neural Networks (SNN, Release 4.0E) was used to build ANN units, which transform miRNA expression values into miRNA scores for each of the 873 miRNAs. The ANN units have three layers: the input variable, output variable, and a function to connect the two. We used the imported normalized miRNA expression values as the input variable and survival status as the output variable. For the middle layer, the advanced version of Intelligent Problem Solver (IPS) tool was applied to build a radial basis function (RBF)-ANN with 11 hidden units. Network output values were referred to as miRNA scores, which were thought to be linearly associated with the death risk of patients. The nonparametric Spearman correlation coefficient (Spearman R) was calculated to assess the linear relationship between the normalized miRNA score and survival status for each patient.

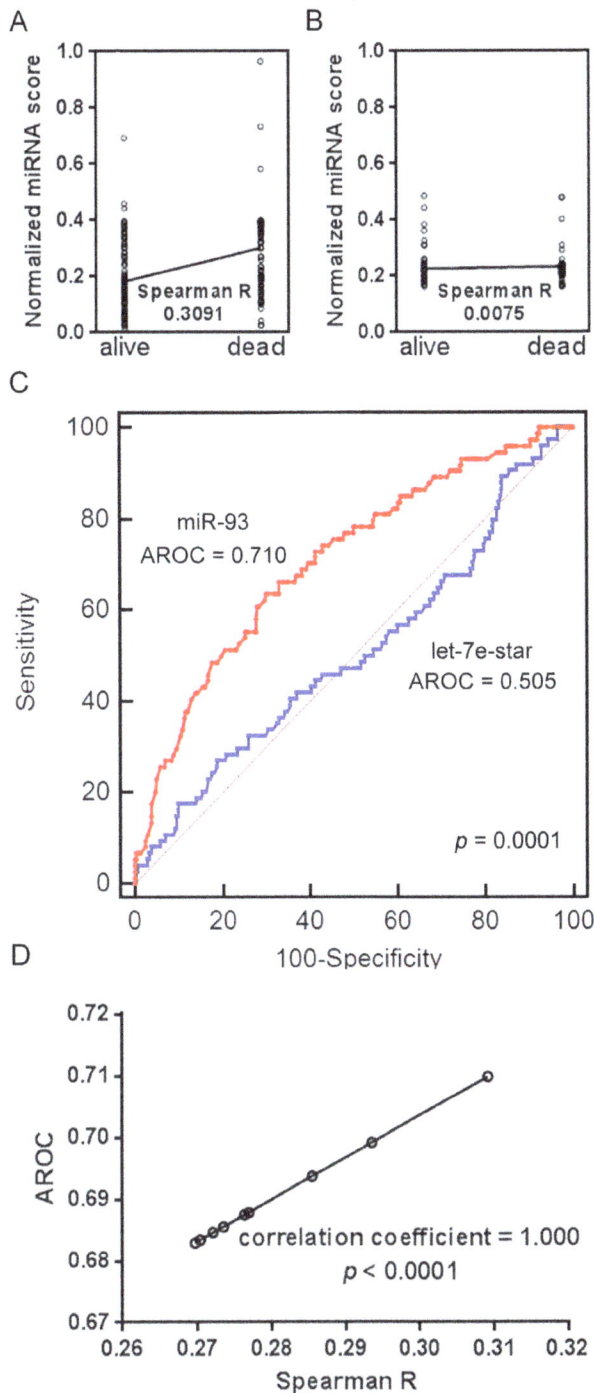

Figure 1. miRNA biomarker selection results. A) A significant linear relationship exists between the normalized miR-93 scores and patient survival status. Spearman R = 0.3091; $p<0.0001$. **B)** No significant linear relationship was found between normalized let-7e-star scores and patient survival status. Spearman R = 0.0075; $p<0.895$. **C)** AUROC comparison between the death risk prediction models using miR-93 and let-7e-star scores. A significant difference was observed ($p = 0.0001$). **D)** A perfect linear correlation relationship was found between Spearman R values and AUROCs (n = 9). $p<0.0001$.

miRNA biomarker selection and ANN model building

Putative miRNAs biomarkers were ranked and selected on the basis of Spearman R values. In this study, we chose to retain only

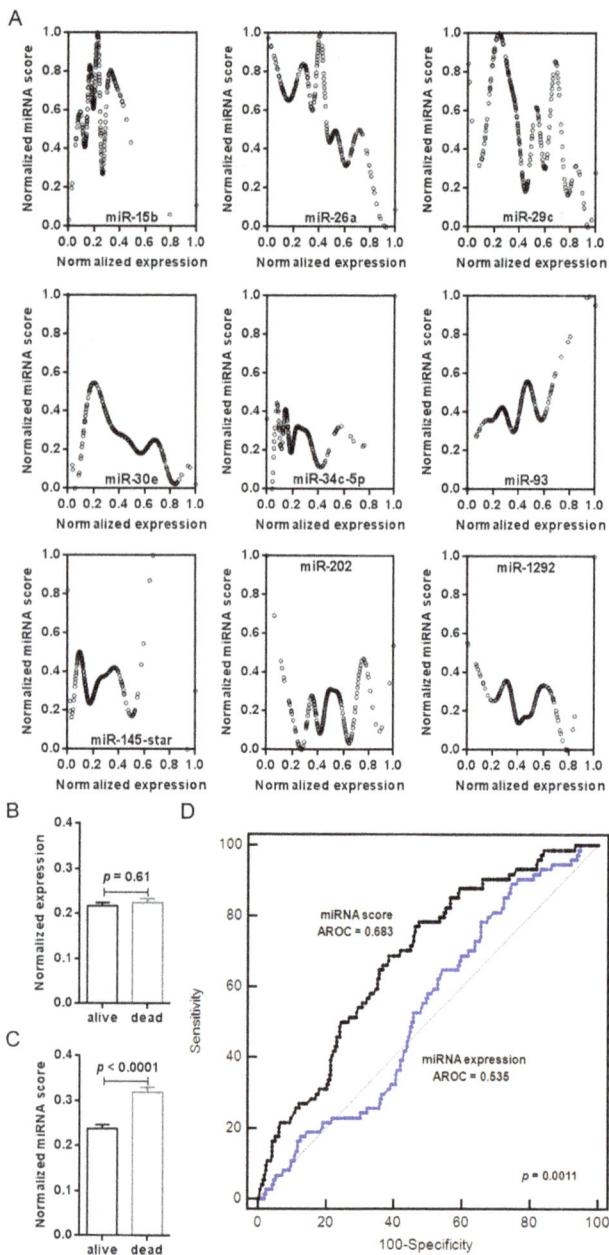

Figure 2. miRNA expression is non-linearly related with NPC patient death risk. A) Illustration of the relationship between normalized miRNA expression and normalized miRNA scores of the selected nine miRNA biomarkers. **B)** No significant difference was observed in normalized miR-15b expression between patients with survival statuses of 'alive' and 'dead'. Mean ± SEM; $p = 0.61$. **C)** The miRNA scores of miR-15b were significantly different when patients with survival statuses of 'alive' and 'dead' were compared. Mean ± SEM; $p < 0.0001$. **D)** AUROC comparison between the death risk prediction models using miRNA expression and miRNA scores of miR-15b, respectively. A significant difference was found ($p = 0.0011$).

the nine miRNAs with the highest R values and discard the others. The normalized miRNA expression values and normalized miRNA scores of three miRNAs with the best Spearman R values (miR-29c, miR-34c-5p, and miR-93) were used to build the untransformed neural network models (UNN) and transformed neural network (TNN), respectively. Both models had the same

network architecture (3-11-1). All of the miRNA scores of the nine miRNAs were then used for building the novel ANN model, which we named the neural network cascade (NNC). An NNC is composed of many ANN units. Each ANN unit is an independent ANN model. In an NNC model, the primary nine ANN units were used for the selected nine miRNAs to transform them from miRNA expression levels into miRNA scores. Each unit had a 1-11-1 network architecture. After that, a secondary ANN unit with a 3-11-1 framework was then built to integrate the outputs of the three data transformation units. A total of three such secondary units were needed for the nine miRNAs. Finally, a tertiary ANN unit was built to combine the outputs of the above three secondary ANN units. The ultimate output is a numerical prediction of the death risk of patients with NPC based on their miRNA gene expression signatures. Notably, we named all model outputs as miRNA scores, regardless of their origin from the ANN units or the composite models. Additionally, a detailed description of NNC model building was provided in Text S1.

Internal and external validation

The holdout cross-validation method was used to conduct internal validation for each ANN unit by using the default settings of the IPS tool. The 208 training model samples were randomly divided into three sets, including training set, verification set, and testing set in a ratio of 2:1:1. Linear regression was used to assess the consistency of the training and testing set outputs. Similar correlation coefficients for the training and testing sets implies the given ANN unit has good generalization ability and *vice versa*. Furthermore, an independent set that consisted of 104 samples was used to perform external validation of the prediction accuracies of the NNC model. In addition to linear regression, a receiver operating characteristic (ROC) curve analysis was also performed to assess the prediction effects of the UNN, TNN, and NNC models by using the software MedCalc (version 13.0). The positive predictive value (PV) at each miRNA score criterion was calculated and used to estimate the probability of poor prognosis for the 104 patients in the external validation set.

Statistical analysis

Student's *t*-test was used for comparisons between two survival status groups of patients with NPC from various aspects, including miRNA expression, miRNA score, and probability of poor prognosis. Analysis of the area under the ROC curve (AUROC) was used to compared each risk prediction performance by miRNA scores of different miRNAs, miRNA expression, and scores of the same miRNA, or final outputs of different ANN models [22]. Differences were considered as statistically significant when $p < 0.05$ for all the statistical methods used in this study.

Results

Nine miRNAs were selected as NPC prognostic biomarkers from the 873 measured miRNAs

First, we normalized and processed the original miRNA expression values that were downloaded from the GEO dataset of gene expression in patients with NPC (GSE32960). Next, the 312 patient samples were randomly divided into a model training set and an external validation set at a ratio of 2:1. In the model training set, small ANN models with network architecture of 1-11-1 was applied to convert miRNA expression values into miRNA scores for each miRNA analyzed. The software GraphPad Prism 6.0 was then used to calculate the Spearman R between miRNA scores and patient survival status for each of the 873 miRNAs. Finally, among the 873 miRNAs, nine miRNAs with the highest

A

B

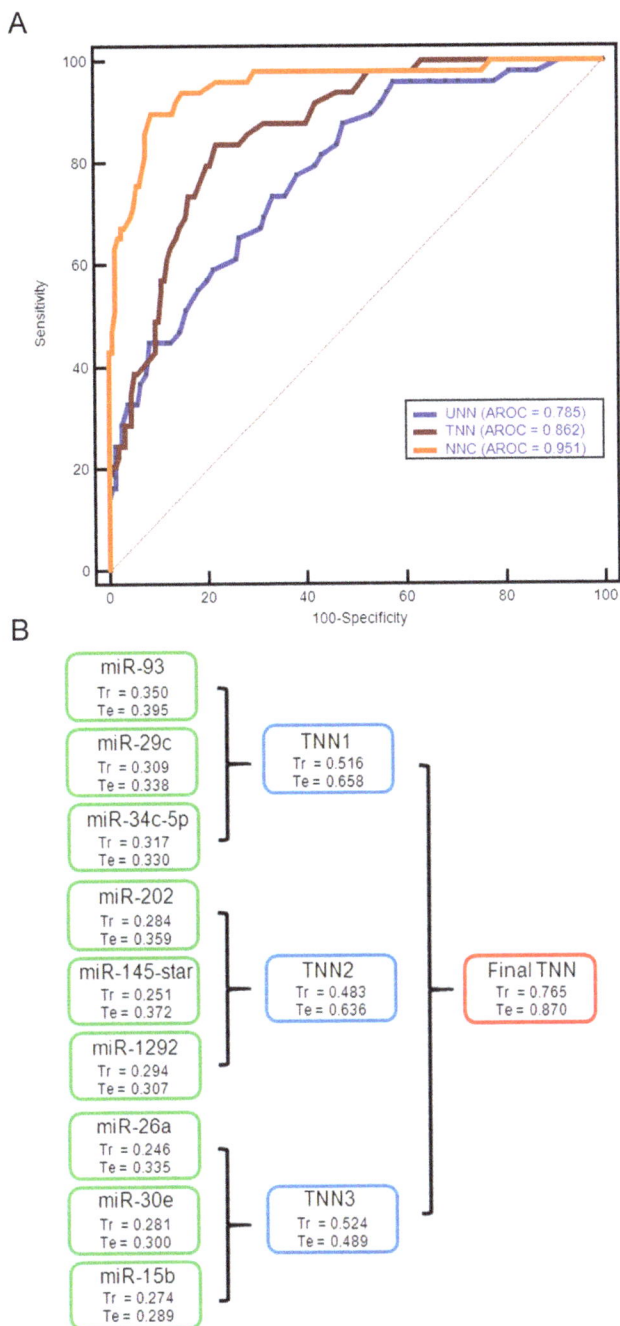

Figure 3. AUROC comparison of three ANN models (A) and results of internal validation of the NNC prediction model (B). UNN: untransformed neural network; TNN: transformed neural network; NNC: neural network cascade. Tr and Te represent correlation coefficients between the output variable and miRNA score of training set and testing set in each ANN unit, respectively.

Spearman R values were highlighted: miR-93, miR-29c, miR-34c-5p, miR-202, miR-145-star, miR-1292, miR-26a, miR-30e, and miR-15b (in descending order of Spearman R value). The miR-93 miRNA score showed the best linear correlation with survival status (Figure 1A, Spearman R = 0.3091). Comparably, the let-7-star miRNA score was found to be unrelated with NPC patient survival (Figure 1B, Spearman R = 0.0075). This result was further confirmed by our ROC analysis (Figure 1C). The AUROC of the

prediction model using the miR-93 miRNA score was significantly higher than that of the prediction model using the miRNA score of let-7e-star ($p = 0.0001$). Furthermore, we calculated AUROCs for the other eight miRNAs that were selected as potential biomarkers for NPC prognosis. A stringent correlation relationship was revealed between the values of Spearman R and those of AUROCs (Figure 1D). This result suggests calculating Spearman R or AUROC leads to similar effectiveness in the ability to detect preferred biomarkers from miRNA microarray experiments.

Expression of nine candidate miRNAs biomarkers was nonlinearly related with survival status

Scatter plots were drawn to illustrate the relationship between miRNA expression and miRNA scores (Figure 2A). As a result, no linear relationship was detected between miRNA expression and miRNA scores for the nine selected candidate miRNA biomarkers. As the miRNA score is a linear variable assessing the death risk of patients with NPC, such a result indicates a nonlinear relationship between miRNA expression and patient survival statuses. This finding also implies that direct between-patient comparison of miRNA expression may not be suitable for predicting prognosis. The miRNA miR-15b was used to further examine this point. According to the Spearman R value, miR-15b was selected as one of the nine preferred miRNA biomarkers indicating NPC prognosis. However, we did not find any difference in miR-15b expression between the two patient groups with different survival statuses by Student's t-test (Figure 2B). In contrast, our method of transforming miRNA gene expression values into the miRNA score enabled us to successfully distinguish between the two patient groups (Figure 2C). Compared with miRNA expression, the miRNA score gave a positive prediction, which was further verified by the ROC analysis (Figure 2D). Similar results were also observed in miR-34c-5p, miR-145-star, miR-202, and miR-1292 (Figure S1).

The NNC model showed the best prediction of patient death risk

In this study, we built three ANN models to further demonstrate the significance of linear transformation of miRNA expression values into a miRNA score. The UNN model was a traditional ANN model with a 3-11-1 network framework constructed using the normalized miRNA expression values of miR-29c, miR-34c-5p, andmiR-93 as input variables. With the same network framework, the TNN model used the normalized miRNA scores of these three miRNAs as input variables. ROC analysis reveals a better predictive performance of the TNN model than that of the UNN model (Figure 3A). The last ANN model we built was an NNC model, which had the most complex network framework, incorporating 13 ANN units as shown in Figure 3B. The NNC model has an AUROC of 0.951, which indicates this model has the best predictive ability to distinguish patients with different survival statuses (Figure 3A). Internal validation indicates that it has good generalization ability for prognosis prediction of patients beyond the modeling training set (Figure 3B).

The NNC model showed strong immunity against disturbed miRNA expression

Scatter plots more clearly display the discriminative effect of different ANN models (Figure 4A). Compared with UNN or TNN, it is easy to identify that NNC had the best performance, despite the fact that all three models could significantly distinguish patients with the survival status of "dead" from those with the "alive" status ($p < 0.0001$). The high predictive performance of

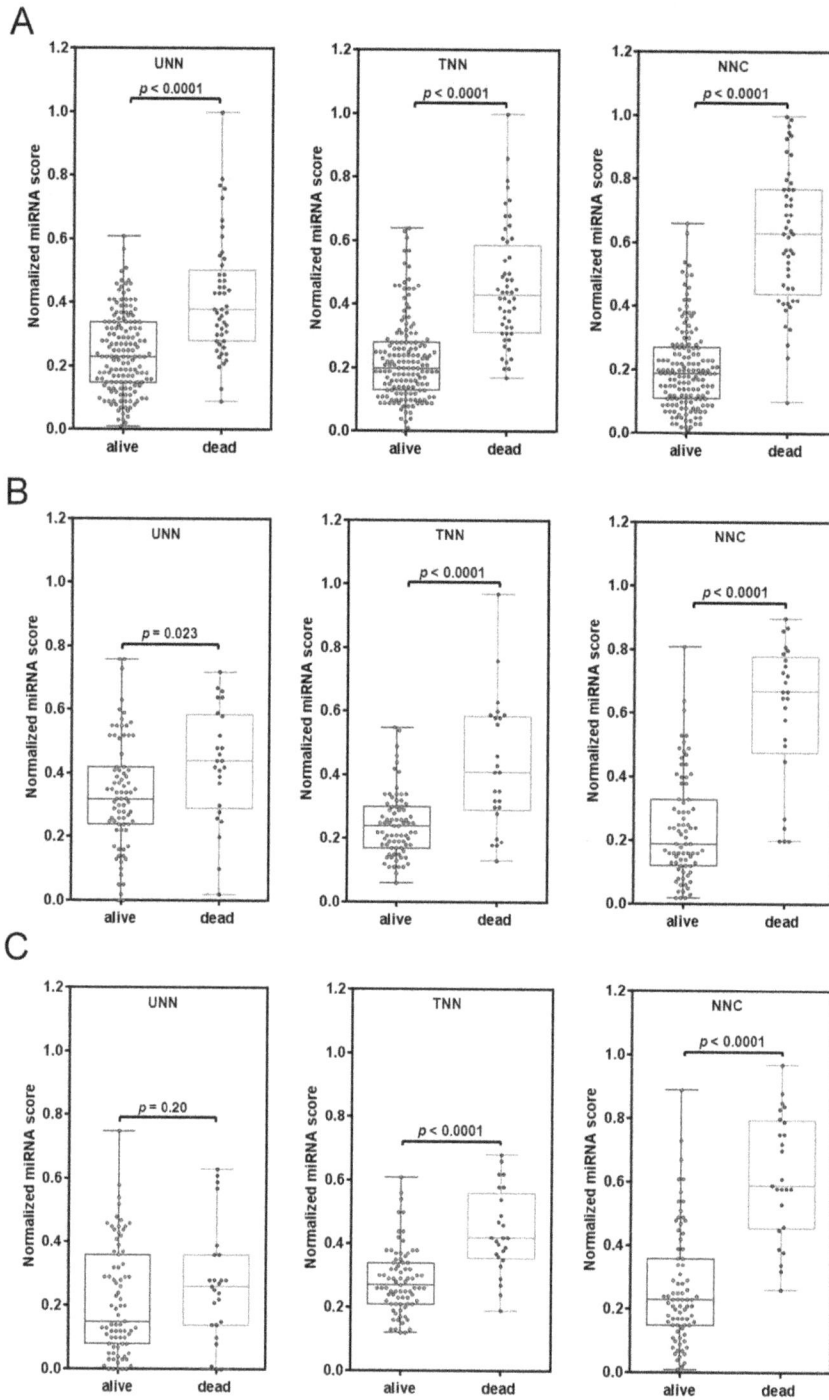

Figure 4. Scatter plots of miRNA scores exported from different ANN models (normalized). Comparisons of miRNA scores were performed between patients with different survival statuses in the model training set (**A**) and the external validation sets with normal miR-93 expression input (**B**) and with disturbed miR-93 expression input (**C**). UNN: untransformed neural network; TNN: transformed neural network; NNC: neural network cascade.

NNC was confirmed when tested on the 104 patients used for external validation (Figure 4B). Further ROC analysis showed that the prediction accuracy was 83% for identifying high-risk patients by using the NNC model established here. Considering the diversity of the actual patients in the clinic, we also investigated the anti-interference capability of different models by replacing the miR-93 miRNA expression values with those of let-7e-star. In this

study, the let-7e-star miRNA score had shown no relationship to the death risk of patients diagnosed NPC (Figure 1B and C). The result of this swap found that the UNN could not survive if the miR-93 expression values were seriously disturbed (Figure 4C). There is no significant difference in miRNA scores between two patient groups in this model ($p = 0.20$). Comparably, the other two

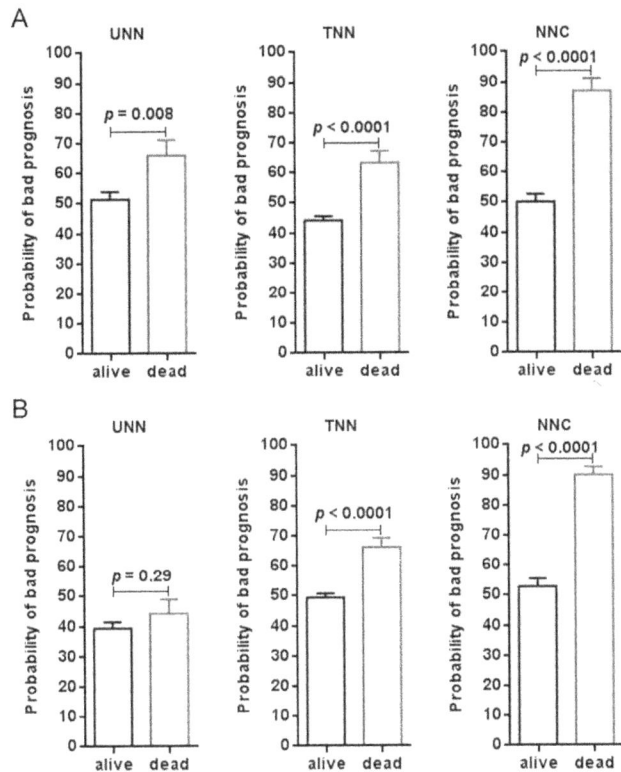

Figure 5. Comparison of bad prognosis likelihood between external validation patients with different survival statuses. A) Normal miR-93 expression input. **B)** Disturbed miR-93 expression input. UNN: untransformed neural network; TNN: transformed neural network; NNC: neural network cascade. All data are expressed as mean ± SEM.

models, especially the NNC model, still showed robust performance in distinguishing patients' status.

Additionally, we evaluated the probability of a bad prognosisfor each patient with NPC. The mean probability of the patients with the survival status of 'alive' was 0.50, indicating that the death risk still exists for this group of patients (Figure 5A). Compared with UNN or TNN, NNC most accurately estimated the death risk of patients with the survival status of 'dead', even in the situation where the expression of miR-93 was seriously disturbed (Figure 5B). This finding suggests that the NNC model may have strong immunity against noise interference caused by unknown factors.

Discussion

MiRNAs are widely thought to be the most promising class of endogenous substances for clinical diagnostic and prognostic biomarkers for cancer [23]. This conviction has prompted researchers worldwide to perform disease-specific miRNA expression profiling in an extensive field of cancer research [24,25]. In this study, we attempt for the first time to present a generic method for translating miRNA expression data into clinically relevant language, such as the possibility of having cancer or the risk of bad prognosis due to suffering from cancer. Briefly, a computational model was constructed by integrating many small single-function ANN units into a cascaded network system. We named it the neural network cascade. We demonstrated that the neural network cascade was efficient for identifying the death risk of patients diagnosed with NPC.

The theoretical cornerstone for the NNC model established here is the assumption that miRNA expression may not be linearly associated with clinical phenotype indicators. This hypothesis is reasonable and realistic given the complexity of miRNAs involvement in human biology [16,26,27]. Based on this assumption, miRNA expression should be transformed into a linear variable before using it to evaluate the possibility of clinical consequences, such as that whether a patient is at high risk of death due to cancer. Our results support the validity of the hypothesis. We found a nonlinear relationship between miRNA expression and the death risk of patients with NPC. This finding implies the importance of miRNA expression data preprocessing before any miRNA-based clinical decisions are made.

Distinct from traditional artificial neural networks previously used in cancer diagnosis and management [19–21], the NNC did not directly use miRNA expression. Rather, the NNC first transforms miRNA gene expression into an miRNA score, a linear variable for assessing clinical phenotype. As a result, the miRNA score instead of miRNA expression was used for the purpose of selecting potential miRNA biomarkers and final decision-making. In the NNC model, the transformation and integration of data and final prediction output was achieved stepwise. This ensures overall computational simplification of the model's operation. Another advantage of the NNC is that every miRNA is assigned an independent channel for information input. By such a design, if more miRNAs are needed for better prediction, one may expand the scale of the NNC model without increasing the network complexity of a single unit. This makes the NNC model freely expandable according to specific requirements. Expression data of different miRNAs can be considered as diverse information contributing to our existing knowledge of the death risk of patients. In our study, inclusion of more miRNAs was resulted in better predictions. The TNN contained three miRNAs and had an AUROC of 0.862. In contrast, the NNC model had an AUROC of 0.951, which contained 9 miRNAs. However, it is also possible that a larger NNC model for NPC prognosis could contain more than nine miRNAs. The nine miRNAs used in the NNC model here simply served as a methodology illustration.

Our external validation results of UNN and TNN indicate that linear transformation of miRNA expression notably improves the prediction effect of the model. Importantly, this procedure did not increase the number of miRNA biomarkers required, implying the advantage of using a cascaded structure of ANNs. Additionally, we found that the cascaded ANN constitution had a more robust performance than the traditional ANN model, where unexplained variability in miR-93 expression caused one ANN unit malfunction. Although unable to estimate the degree of such interference on disease prognosis in actual clinical settings, it remains possible that this variability will be an important factor that hinders miRNA-based prediction models in practice. Comparison of the TNN and NNC models suggests that inclusion of more miRNAs would increase robustness of the established ANN model against noise disturbance.

In conclusion, our study provided a rational and feasible method for miRNA biomarker selection and prediction model establishment. The advantage of a cascaded construction of small artificial neural network units is reflected from several aspects, including scalable capacity and flexible combination of miRNA expression inputs, better prediction with robust stability, and greater opportunities for meaningful modeling if the number of miRNA biomarkers is unrestricted. In the future, more attempts should be made to further validate the application of our approach by translating miRNA expression data into clinically relevant information for the diagnosis and prognosis of cancer.

Supporting Information

Figure S1 Comparison of miRNA expression and miRNA scores between the two patient groups with different survival statuses. A) miR-26a; **B)** miR-29b; **C)** miR-30e; **D)** miR-34c-5p; **E)** miR-93; **F)** miR-145-star; **G)** miR-202; **H)** miR-1292. All data are expressed as mean ± SEM.

Text S1 A step-to-step procedure for NNC model building.

Author Contributions

Conceived and designed the experiments: WZ. Performed the experiments: WZ. Analyzed the data: WZ. Contributed reagents/materials/analysis tools: WZ. Contributed to the writing of the manuscript: WZ XK.

References

1. Selbach M, Schwanhäusser B, Thierfelder N, Fang Z, Khanin R, et al. (2008) Widespread changes in protein synthesis induced by microRNAs. Nature. 455: 58–63.
2. Baek D, Villén J, Shin C, Camargo FD, Gygi SP, et al. (2008) The impact of microRNAs on protein output. Nature. 455: 64–71.
3. Trang P, Weidhaas J B, Slack F J. (2008) MicroRNAs as potential cancer therapeutics. Oncogene. 27: S52–S57.
4. Pereira DM, Rodrigues PM, Borralho PM, Rodrigues CM. (2013) Delivering the promise of miRNA cancer therapeutics. Drug Discov Today. 18: 282–289.
5. van Rooij E, Kauppinen S. (2014) Development of microRNA therapeutics is coming of age. EMBO Mol Med. 6: 851–864.
6. Mitchell PS, Parkin RK, Kroh EM, Fritz BR, Wyman SK, et al. (2008) Circulating microRNAs as stable blood-based markers for cancer detection. Proc Natl Acad Sci U S A. 105: 10513–10518.
7. Kosaka N, Iguchi H, Ochiya T. (2010) Circulating microRNA in body fluid: a new potential biomarker for cancer diagnosis and prognosis. Cancer Sci. 101: 2087–2092.
8. Shen J, Stass SA, Jiang F. (2013) MicroRNAs as potential biomarkers in human solid tumors. Cancer Lett. 329: 125–136.
9. de Planell-Saguer M, Rodicio MC. (2011) Analytical aspects of microRNA in diagnostics: a review. Anal Chim Acta. 699: 134–152.
10. Pritchard CC, Cheng HH, Tewari M. (2012) MicroRNA profiling: approaches and considerations. Nat Rev Genet. 13: 358–369.
11. Barrett T1, Wilhite SE, Ledoux P, Evangelista C, Kim IF, et al. (2013) NCBI GEO: archive for functional genomics data sets–update. Nucleic Acids Res. 41: D991–D995.
12. De Cecco L, Dugo M, Canevari S, Daidone MG, Callari M. (2013) Measuring microRNA expression levels in oncology: from samples to data analysis. Crit Rev Oncog. 18: 273–287.
13. Wang JL, Hu Y, Kong X, Wang ZH, Chen HY, et al. (2013) Candidate microRNA biomarkers in human gastric cancer: a systematic review and validation study. PLoS One. 8: e73683.
14. Okugawa Y, Toiyama Y, Goel A. (2014) An update on microRNAs as colorectal cancer biomarkers: where are we and what's next? Expert Rev Mol Diagn. 28: 1–23.
15. Zhou X, Wang X, Huang Z, Wang J, Zhu W, et al. (2014) Prognostic value of miR-21 in various cancers: an updating meta-analysis. PLoS One. 9: e102413.
16. Boettger T, Braun T. (2012) A new level of complexity: the role of microRNAs in cardiovascular development. Circ Res. 110: 1000–1013.
17. Liu N, Chen NY, Cui RX, Li WF, Li Y, et al. (2012) Prognostic value of a microRNA signature in nasopharyngeal carcinoma: a microRNA expression analysis. Lancet Oncol. 13: 633–641.
18. Luque A, Farwati A, Crovetto F, Crispi F, Figueras F, et al. (2014) Usefulness of circulating microRNAs for the prediction of early preeclampsia at first-trimester of pregnancy. Sci Rep. 4: 4882.
19. Lisboa PJ, Taktak AF. (2006) The use of artificial neural networks in decision support in cancer: a systematic review. Neural Netw. 19: 408–415.
20. Abbod MF, Catto JW, Linkens DA, Hamdy FC. (2007) Application of artificial intelligence to the management of urological cancer. J Urol. 178: 1150–1156.
21. Hu X, Cammann H, Meyer HA, Miller K, Jung K, Stephan C. (2013) Artificial neural networks and prostate cancer–tools for diagnosis and management. Nat Rev Urol. 10: 174–182.
22. Hastie T, Tibshirani R, Friedman J. (2009) Elements of statistical learning. Second ed. New York: Springer. 600 p.
23. Calin GA, Croce CM. (2006) MicroRNA signatures in human cancers. Nat Rev Cancer. 6: 857–866.
24. Cho WC. (2010) MicroRNAs: potential biomarkers for cancer diagnosis, prognosis and targets for therapy. Int J Biochem Cell Biol. 42: 1273–1281.
25. Iorio MV, Croce CM. (2012) MicroRNA dysregulation in cancer: diagnostics, monitoring and therapeutics. A comprehensive review. EMBO Mol Med. 4: 143–159.
26. Winter J, Jung S, Keller S, Gregory RI, Diederichs S. (2009) Many roads to maturity: microRNA biogenesis pathways and their regulation. Nat Cell Biol. 11: 228–234.
27. Filipowicz W, Bhattacharyya SN, Sonenberg N. (2008) Mechanisms of post-transcriptional regulation by microRNAs: are the answers in sight? Nat Rev Genet. 9: 102–114.

19

Arrays of MicroLEDs and Astrocytes: Biological Amplifiers to Optogenetically Modulate Neuronal Networks Reducing Light Requirement

Rolando Berlinguer-Palmini[1], Roberto Narducci[2], Kamyar Merhan[1], Arianna Dilaghi[2], Flavio Moroni[2], Alessio Masi[2], Tania Scartabelli[3], Elisa Landucci[3], Maria Sili[2], Antonio Schettini[3], Brian McGovern[4], Pleun Maskaant[5], Patrick Degenaar[1], Guido Mannaioni[2]*

1 School of Electric and Electronic Engineering – Institute of Neuroscience, Newcastle University, Newcastle, United Kingdom, 2 Department of Neuroscience, Psychology, Drug Research and Child Health Section of Pharmacology and Toxicology, University of Florence, Florence, Italy, 3 Department of Health Science, Section of Clinical Pharmacology and Oncology, University of Florence, Florence, Italy, 4 Institute of Biomedical Engineering, Imperial College, London, United Kingdom, 5 Tyndall National Institute of Technology, Cork, Ireland

Abstract

In the modern view of synaptic transmission, astrocytes are no longer confined to the role of merely supportive cells. Although they do not generate action potentials, they nonetheless exhibit electrical activity and can influence surrounding neurons through gliotransmitter release. In this work, we explored whether optogenetic activation of glial cells could act as an amplification mechanism to optical neural stimulation via gliotransmission to the neural network. We studied the modulation of gliotransmission by selective photo-activation of channelrhodopsin-2 (ChR2) and by means of a matrix of individually addressable super-bright microLEDs (μLEDs) with an excitation peak at 470 nm. We combined Ca^{2+} imaging techniques and concurrent patch-clamp electrophysiology to obtain subsequent glia/neural activity. First, we tested the μLEDs efficacy in stimulating ChR2-transfected astrocyte. ChR2-induced astrocytic current did not desensitize overtime, and was linearly increased and prolonged by increasing μLED irradiance in terms of intensity and surface illumination. Subsequently, ChR2 astrocytic stimulation by broad-field LED illumination with the same spectral profile, increased both glial cells and neuronal calcium transient frequency and sEPSCs suggesting that few ChR2-transfected astrocytes were able to excite surrounding not-ChR2-transfected astrocytes and neurons. Finally, by using the μLEDs array to selectively light stimulate ChR2 positive astrocytes we were able to increase the synaptic activity of single neurons surrounding it. In conclusion, ChR2-transfected astrocytes and μLEDs system were shown to be an amplifier of synaptic activity in mixed corticalneuronal and glial cells culture.

Editor: Shumin Duan, Zhejiang University School of Medicine, China

Funding: PD received funding from the European Commission (http://ec.europa.eu/) under project OptoNeuro, project number 249867 (www.optoneuro.eu). The funders had no role in study design, data collection and analysis, decision to publish, or preparation of the manuscript.

Competing Interests: The authors have declared that no competing interests exist.

* Email: guido.mannaioni@unifi.it

Introduction

The traditional view of astrocytes is that their primary purpose is to provide biochemical support of the nerve cells, including trophic support, metabolic regulation, and regulating neurotransmitter concentrations in the synaptic cleft [1]. However, astrocytes also actively participate in synaptic transmission through gliotransmitter release [2,3]. The understanding and the modulation of these processes could have particular translational impact to the pharmacology and neuroprosthesis communities as well as for neuro-computational studies. Fundamentally, indirect stimulation of astrocytes may lower operational power requirements of brain machine interfaces. Optogenetics is now a decade old genetic manipulation technique which can render nerve cells light sensitive [4]. The great advantages of the technique has been to provide genetically targeted excitatory [5] and inhibitory [6]

control of neural circuitry with millisecond precision. The key issue for the neuroprosthesis community has been an intense light requirement of typically 10^{15}–10^{19} photons/cm^2 at 480 nm (instantaneous pulsed irradiance) [7,8] which is close to the photochemical damage threshold of nerve cells [9], but also makes it challenging to create stimulation optoelectronics. High radiance optoelectronic arrays for specific use in retinal prosthesis have been previously developed [10]. However, in implantable systems, local thermal dissipation becomes an increasing issue [11]. Therefore, we aimed to study ChR2-transfected astrocytes as a potential amplifier of neuronal signalling by means of increasing gliotransmission. For this reason, we wanted to explore the potential for optogenetically transfected astrocytes to influence the excitatory state of nerve cells, and thus bring down the threshold requirements for optoelectronic stimuli.

Materials and Methods

Ethical Statement

All animal manipulations were carried out according to the European Community guidelines for animal care (DL 116/92, application of the European Communities Council Directive 86/609/EEC). Formal approval to conduct the experiments described has been obtained from Italian Ministry of Health, according to DL 116/92. All efforts were made to minimize animal sufferings and to use only the number of animals necessary to produce reliable scientific data. No alternatives to animal experimentation are available for this type of experiments.

μLED optoelectronic illuminator

Electronically driven μLEDs were fabricated as part of the OptoNeuro FP7 project (www.optoneuro.eu) and transferred to the researchers on this project. These are fundamentally a micro-LED chip bonded to a CMOS (Complementary Metal Oxide Semiconductor) control chip. The array comprises of a 16×16 array of 20 μm diameter micro-emitters with a centre-to-centre pitch of 150 μm. The LEDs chip was fabricated from Gallium Nitride and the CMOS was fabricated from a standard 0.35 μm foundry process [12]. Bonding was achieved via flip-chip process, and the resulting die was packaged in ceramic pin grid array which was then placed on a PCB board and controlled by a PC via a MBED microcontroller.

μLEDs controlling software

The CMOS driven optoelectronic array does not have a USB interface, so we have used a MBED microcontroller to act as an interface between a PC and the chip. This was programmed using the online software development kit from mbed.org. On the PC side, a software interface has been developed to provide intuitive functionality for the electrophysiology experiments. The software/hardware control can independently tune pulse widths of each of the micro-emitters down to 1 ms and is stable for many hours of recording. A hardware/software interface with standard patch-clamp electrophysiology software has also been developed via an in-house-designed trigger box for sending and receiving monitoring signals.

Optical characterization

The emission spectrum of the optoelectronic array was measured by placing a USB2000 spectrometer (Ocean Optics) directly above the emitters. In order to measure radiance and efficiency, we used a Newport UV-818 calibrated photodiode and a Keithley Source Measure Unit 2612 (Keithley Instruments Inc.), with the diode placed just above the LED array. Variability in the emission power was tested by driving the μLEDs both individually and as part of a group. The on-sample emission powers were measured by placing the calibrated photodiode on the sample plane.

Rat cortical cell cultures

Cultures of mixed cortical cells containing both neuronal and glial elements were prepared as previously described in detail [13] and used at 5–25 days in vitro (DIV). Pure neuronal cultures were prepared as previously described in detail [14] by seeding cortical cells (re-suspended in Neurobasal medium with B-27 supplement, GIBCO) onto poly-l-lysine-coated wells, used at 5–25 DIV. Either male and female animals were used.

Plasmid amplification and cell transfection

Plasmid DNA encoding adeno-associated viral vector with light sensitive channelrhodopsin-2 under GFAP promoter (pAAV-GFP- hChR2 (H134R)-EYFP) or CatCh plasmid (pcDNA3.1(-)-chop2(1-309)[L132C]-EYFP) were purified using Plasmid Midi Kit (Qiagen) in according to the manufacturer's instruction. After 48 hours in culture at 70% confluence, astrocytes were transfected with 1 μg vector using Lipofectamine 2000 (Invitrogen) according to the manufacturer's manual. CatCh or ChR-2 expression in cortical neurons was achieved by electroporation (Lonza Biosciences Nucleofactor) using 2 μg of the construct.

Electrophysiology

The recording chamber was mounted on an upright microscope (Nikon Eclipse E600FN) equipped with IR-DIC optics, 20× and 60× water-immersion objectives (NA = 1.00 and 0.8 respectively) and an IR-camera (Hamamatsu) for visually guided experiments. Flow rate was 1 ml/min and driven by gravity. Whole-cell recordings were performed at room temperature between 5 and 28 DIV. The intracellular solution contained (in mM) K^+-gluconate (120), KCl (15), HEPES (10), EGTA (5), $MgCl_2$, (2), Na_2PhosphoCreatine (5), Na_2GTP (0.3), MgATP (2), resulting in a resistance of 3–4 MΩ in the bath. The external medium contained NaCl (150), KCl (3), $CaCl_2$ (2), $MgCl_2$ (1), glucose (10) and HEPES (10); the pH was adjusted to 7.30. Clampfit v10.1 was used for offline analysis. No whole cell compensation was used. Signals were sampled at 10 kHz, low-pass filtered at 10 kHz, acquired with an Axon Multiclamp 700B and digitized with a Digidata 1440 A and Clampex 10 (Axon).

Imaging of Fluo-3/Fura-2 fluorescence

Cultured cells were incubated in a solution containing (in mM): (150) NaCl, (10) Hepes, (3) KCl, (2) $CaCl_2$, (1) $MgCl_2$, (10) glucose (pH adjusted to 7.3) at 37°C for 30 min with the acetoxymethyl (AM) ester of fluo-3 and or fura-2 AM (5 μM, Molecular Probes). To aid solubilisation of fluo-3/fura-2 in aqueous medium, we added pluronic F-127 (1 mM, Molecular Probes). The dye was allowed to de-esterify for 30 min at room temperature. Coverslips containing fluo-3/fura-2-loaded cells were subsequently transferred to a continuously perfused microscope stage for imaging. Images were visualized with a 20× or 60× Fluor objective and acquired every 2 seconds. Exposure time was set to 200 ms and excitation was provided by a PE-1system (CoolLED) fitted with a 380±20 nm LED and a 470±30 nm LED. Fura-2 and fluo-3 fluorescence was recorded through (respectively) along pass filter (420 nm cut on) and aband pass filter (535±25 nm) with a Photometrics Coolsnap HP Camera set at −20°C. Fluorescence intensity was measured in cell bodies using Imaging Workbench 6 software (IndecBioSystem) and expressed as the ratio of (F−F0)/F0, where F0 is the baseline fluorescence intensity in cell bodies before any treatment. All measurements were corrected for the background fluorescence. Increases in fluorescence ratio greater than 0.1 were considered to be significant changes; baseline fluorescence values possessed a peak (F−F0)/F0 ratio of 0.01±0.01 on average. Experiments were performed at room temperature.

Statistics

Pooled data throughout the paper are presented as mean ± standard error (SEM) of n independent experiments. Unless otherwise specified, statistical difference between means is assessed with a Student t-Test for paired samples (GraphPad Prism 5.0). When single recordings are shown they are intended to represent

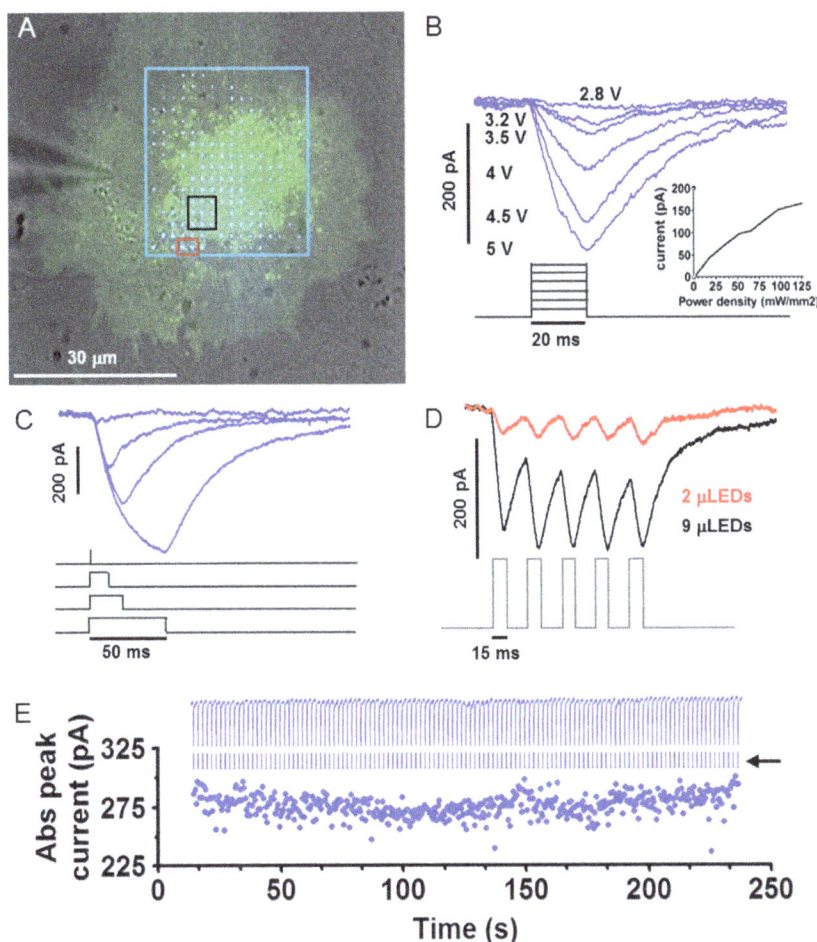

Figure 1. μLEDs finely modulate in time and space inward current in ChR2-transfected astrocytes. A,The ChR2+ astrocyte was stimulated with the whole matrix (blue box) or variable number of μLEDs (black and red boxes, 9 and 2 μLEDs, respectively) while recording the elicited inward currents in voltage clamp mode. Fine targeting and pulsing of the μLEDs on the cell was achieved overlaying in real time the fluorescent image to the μLEDs using a specific designed software. **B**, ChR-2 inward currents of different amplitude were recorded pulsing the whole matrix (blue box in **A**, pulse duration 20 ms) at different voltages (grey traces represent μLED stimulation pattern). Inset, mean inward current vs power density from different cells. **C**, μLEDs (blue box in **A**) can be finely modulated in time with submillisecond precision producing proportionally longer and larger ChR-2 currents (grey traces represent μLED stimulation pattern). **D**, Inward currents produced when 2 μLEDs (**A**, red box) or 9 μLEDs (**A**, black box) were pulsed 5 times at 33 Hz at different time on different locations (grey traces represent μLED stimulation pattern). **E**, The μLEDs irradiance is stable over time. When long term optogenetic light stimulation (central trace indicated by the black arrow, 200 ms pulse at 0.5 Hz, full led) is performed onChR-2 positive astrocyte the μLEDs produced stable current transients (Top trace) and peak inward currents (filled circles).

typical observations. Graphs, histograms and fittings were generated in GraphPad Prism 5.0. In Fig. S2 each response was normalised to a moving average of firing frequencies: average (all recordings) – average (preceding 4 readings and successive 4 readings).

Results

First, we tested the efficacy of the μLEDs array to elicit precise spatiotemporal current transients in ChR2-transfected glial cells. The μLEDs array was mounted on the microscope's camera port using a beam splitter allowing the μLEDs to be imagined onto the sample while observing it (Fig. 1A, S1). Whole cell patch clamp recordings were used to functionally verify the transfection and the capacity of μLEDs array to generate astrocytic ChR2-induced inward current. In each of the ChR2positive glial cells tested (n = 50), the μLEDs illumination produced inward currents using either the whole or partial array (Fig. 1A, whole array in white box

and different number of μLEDs tested in coloured boxes). We could finely modulate ChR2-induced astrocytic inward currents by either modulating μLEDs power density (Fig. 1B and inset), pulse width of the illumination (Fig. 1C) and the number of illuminating μLEDs (Fig. 1D and 1A). We were also able to produce inward currents using pulses as short as 1 ms (Fig. 1C, red trace; power density = 34.66 nW/μm^2@5V on cell, which equates to 34.66 pJ×pulse). In our previous paper we showed that the μLEDs irradiance is stable over time [15]. Here, we confirmed the array performance on a biological sample with long term light stimulation (200 ms pulse at 0.5 Hz, Fig. 1E, blue arrow) on ChR-2 positive astrocytes.The μLEDs produced stable current transients (Fig. 1E, black arrow) peaking at 275±20 pA (Fig. 1E bottom trace).

Then, we studied the optogenetic control of a glial network in culture via light stimulation of single ChR2 positive astrocytes in order to modulate surrounding ChR2 negative glial cells in pure astrocytic cultures by using calcium imaging as readout technique.

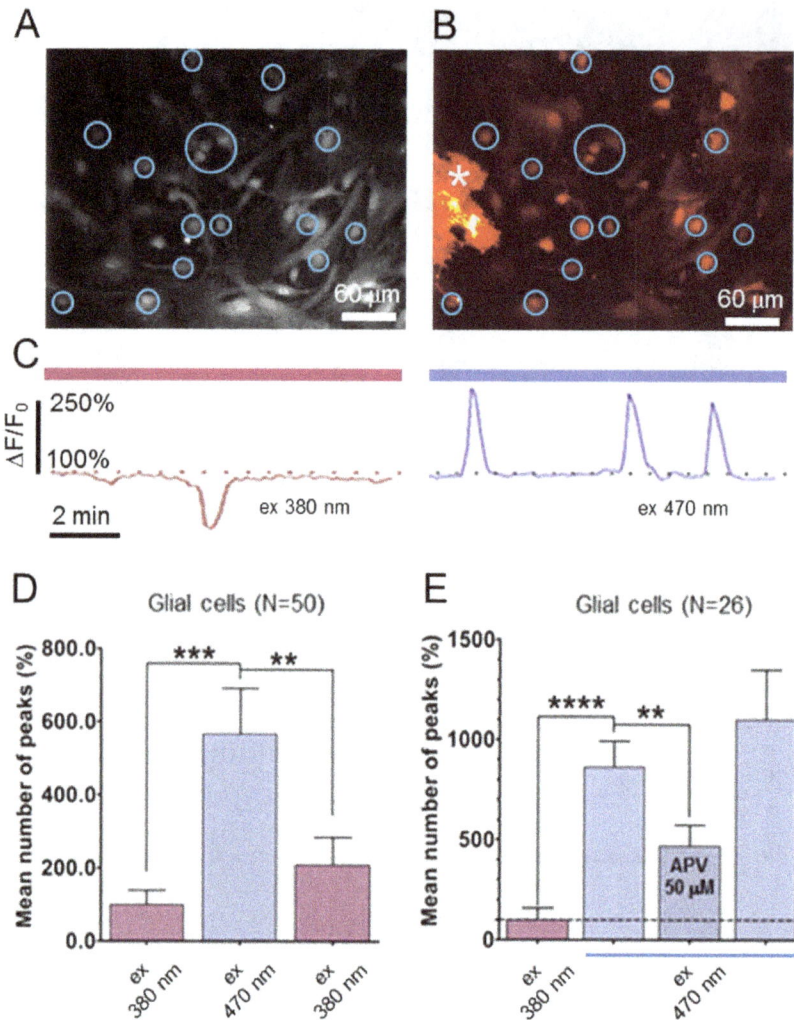

Figure 2. Stimulation ofChR2 positive astrocytesincreases glial cells calcium transients frequency. Cortical glial culture were co-incubated in fura-2-AM (**A**) and fluo-3-AM (**B**) and Ca^{2+} transients were monitored during UV [excitation (ex)380 ± 20 nm] and blue light [excitation (ex) 470 ± 20 nm] stimulation (200 ms light pulse @ 0.5 Hz; 10 min UV→10 min blue→10 min UV). The star (*) indicates the ChR-2 positive astrocyte. **C**, Time course of ChR-2 negative astrocyte during UV (left panel) and blue (right panel) illumination. Fura-2 downward peak indicates $[Ca^{2+}]_i$ increase, fluo-3 upward peak indicates $[Ca^{2+}]_i$ increase. **D**, Stimulation of the ChR-2 positive astrocyte with 470 nm light (blue column)increased calcium waves frequency to $566.7\%\pm124.2\%$ (UV vs Blue, paired t test p = 0.0002 – Blue vs UV, paired t test p = 0.0048). **E**,The increased Ca^{2+} waves frequency mediated by stimulation of ChR2 positive astrocyte was significantly reduced by APV 50 μM (UV vs Blue, paired t test p<0.0001 – Blue vs Blue+APV, paired t test p = 0.0019). Values are means ±SEM.

For this experiment, we used a CoolLED PE system (see methods) to stimulate all the transfected cells in the area imaged by the objective. Since ChR2 is only partially stimulated at 380 ± 20 nm (UV) [16], we used this wavelength as not-ratiometric Fura-2 exciting wavelength to assess the baseline activity of the culture (Fig. 2A and C, left panel).

We then compared this to the results obtained using Fluo-3/ ChR2 peak exciting wavelength (blue light) (470 ± 20 nm) to activate ChR2 positive astrocytes(Fig. 2B and C right panel) while recording the calcium activity of the surrounding ChR2-negative astrocytes (Fig. 2A and B, blue circles). Figure 2C shows a typical time course of a single ChR2 negative astrocyte excited at 380 and 470 nm, respectively. Stimulation at 470 nm increased calcium oscillation frequency in ChR2 negative astrocytes to $566.7\pm124.2\%$ (p = 0.0002) over baseline activity (Fig. 2C, D and E) and this effect was reverted by switching back to 380 nm light (Fig. 2D) ($208.1\%\pm75.5\%$ over the basal level; p = 0.0048).

In another set of cells we aimed to pharmacologically block the ChR2-induced calcium wave frequency increase. Addition of NMDA selective antagonist D-2-Amino-5-phosphonopentanoic acid (APV 50 μM) during 470 nm light stimulation (but after the calcium wave frequency increase was established reaching $862\pm128.6\%$ of the baseline level) reduced the induced increase to $469\%\pm23.2\%$(p = 0.0019) of the baseline level (Fig. 2E). This partial block was reversible and calcium wave frequency re-increased to the pre-drug treatment level following APV wash out (Fig. 2E).

After achieving optical modulation of glial cells network we then explored the interaction of optically modulated astrocytes and neurons. Initially, we stimulated ChR2 positive astrocytes by means of a CoolLED PE system while recording surrounding neuronal activity with calcium imaging technique (Fig. 3A). Figure 3B shows the time course of the mean calcium activity in 9 neurons during 380 and 470 nm stimulation (purple and blue),

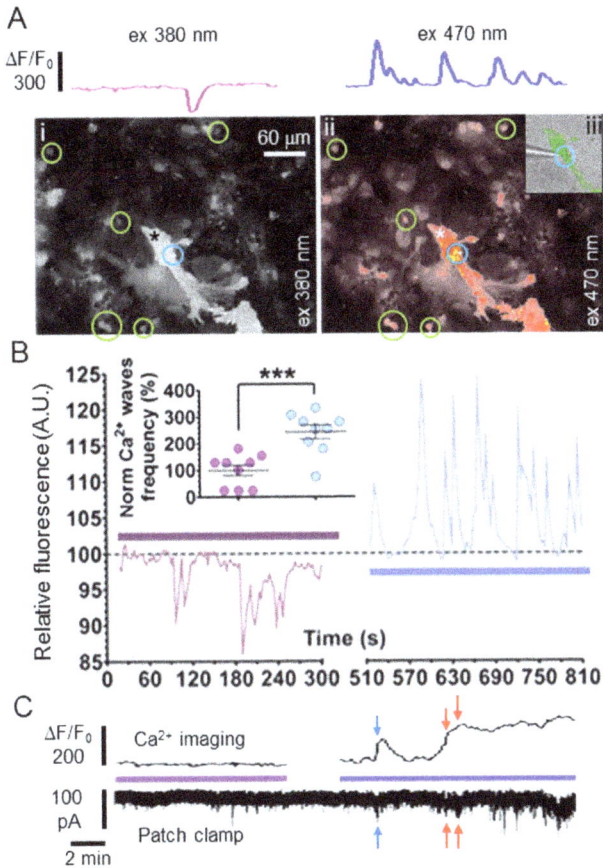

Figure 3. ChR2+ asctrocytic stimulation modulates neuronal calcium waves frequency. A, Bottom, snapshots from Ca^{2+} experiments during stimulation with 380 nm (**i**) and 470 nm (**ii**) light. Green circles indicate neurons, one of which (blue circle) was co-localized with the ChR-2 positive astrocyte (star). Top, time course of one of the not colocalized neurons (circled in green). **B**,Time course of all circled neurons mean relative fluorescence and (inset)single cell measurement of calcium wave frequency (paired t test p<0.0001). **C**, Concurrent patch clamp and Ca^{2+}imaging time course of the neuron circled in blue in **A(iii)**. The red arrow shows the first wave (top) syncronised with the first sEPSCs burst and the red arrows show following sEPSCs bursts concomitant to internal calcium concentration increase.

respectively.The modulatory effect on neuronal calcium wave frequency is shown in the inset and on a single cell in Fig. 3A (top).Moreover, in experiments where calcium imaging was coupled to concurrent patch clamp recordings (Fig. 3C), the increase in astrocytic intracellular Ca^{2+} concentration (blue and red arrows) was synchronized with spontaneous excitatory post synaptic currents (sEPSCs) burst of the colocalized neuron.

To further characterize the optical gliotransmission, we used the μLEDs array to selectively light stimulate ChR2 positive astrocytes while recordings synaptic activity of a single neuron surrounding it (Fig. 4A). μLEDs light stimulated ChR2 positive astrocyte for 5 min using 200 ms long light pulses at 0.5 Hz (Fig. 4B blue trace). Simultaneously, we recorded the neuronal activity before, during and after the μLEDs induced stimulus. Figure 4B upper panel shows a typical sEPSCs timecourse following μLEDs stimulation of ChR2 positive astrocyte.

The average sEPSCs frequency activity increased to 295.5±53.4% following μLEDs stimulus selectively directed on ChR2 positive astrocyte (Fig. 4C,D and S2). Interestingly, sEPSCs amplitude did not change significantly (103.3±4% versus 109.1±15.2%, in control and during μLEDs induced stimulation of ChR2 positive astrocyte, respectively; n = 13).

The addition of the glutamate (NMDA and AMPA) antagonists, APV (50 μM) and NBQX (20 μM)to the bath solution during light stimulation and after the excitation was successfully triggered, significantly reduced the increased sEPSCs frequency to 78.20±4.0% and 23.2%±5.5% of the pre-light stimulation level (100%), respectively. APV and NBQX co-application almost abolished μLEDs ChR2-induced increase ofsEPSCs frequency (3.8%±1.0% of the baseline level) (Fig. 4D).

Discussion

The data presented in this paper show that astrocytes can be finely tuned by ChR2 optogenetic stimulation and that the subsequent glutamate release rapidly affects the whole astrocytic network and the surrounding neurons. Perea and co-workers [17] have recently shown similar results in astrocytes of the primary visual cortex both for excitatory and inhibitory neurotransmission. The μLEDs system we previously tested in different cell lines [10,18] is able not only to finely modulate ChR2 current in a single astrocyte but also to increase neuronal sEPSCs frequency in mixed cortical astrocytic/neuronal primary cultures.Following neuronal activity, the activation of astrocytes is mediated by neurotransmitter released from synaptic terminals [19,20,21]. The subsequent release of gliotransmitters from astrocytes has been reported to depend upon Gq GPCR activation leading to astrocytic type-2 IP3 receptor (IP3R2) activation and Ca^{2+} release from the endoplasmic reticulum [reviewed in [22]]. While this pathway has been implicated in gliotransmitter release, the precise mechanisms of gliotransmission remains debated [21,23,24,2]. This is mainly due to our inability to selectively activate Ca^{2+} signals in astrocytes. Therefore, the exogenous generation of Ca^{2+} signals that mimic those evoked by neuronal stimuli should clarify the interactions between neurons and astrocytes and could finely modulate gliotransmission and the efficacy of neuroprosthetic devices.

For these reasons, we stimulated the astrocytes by means of ChR2-induced current showing that this direct astrocytic stimulation is cascaded onto the whole astrocytic network and increases neuronal spontaneous excitatory post synaptic current.

Interestingly, we also noticed that even if the currents elicited in Ca^{2+} translocating ChR2 (CatCh) positive astrocytes where on average 15 times larger than ChR2 (measured as area under the curve (AUC), Fig. S3) the neural network modulation was successfully achieved with ChR2, although previous reports suggest a better and stronger Ca^{2+} elevation by means of Ca^{2+}-permeable light-gated glutamate receptor (LiGluR) [25] and CatCh [25,26].

Recently, optogenetics elucidated the function of multiple neuronal circuits [27,4,28]. One of the most popular photo-switchable channel to activate neurons is the H314R channelrhodopsin 2 [ChR2(H134R)], a variant of the wild type ChR2 with reduced desensitization [29]. ChR2 is a cationic channel highly permeable to proton but weakly permeable to Ca^{2+} [30,31]. In neurons, its photoactivation triggers Ca^{2+}elevations which depend mainly on the secondary activation of voltage-gated Ca^{2+} channels (VGCC) [32,33].In astrocytes, the photoactivation of ChR2 can

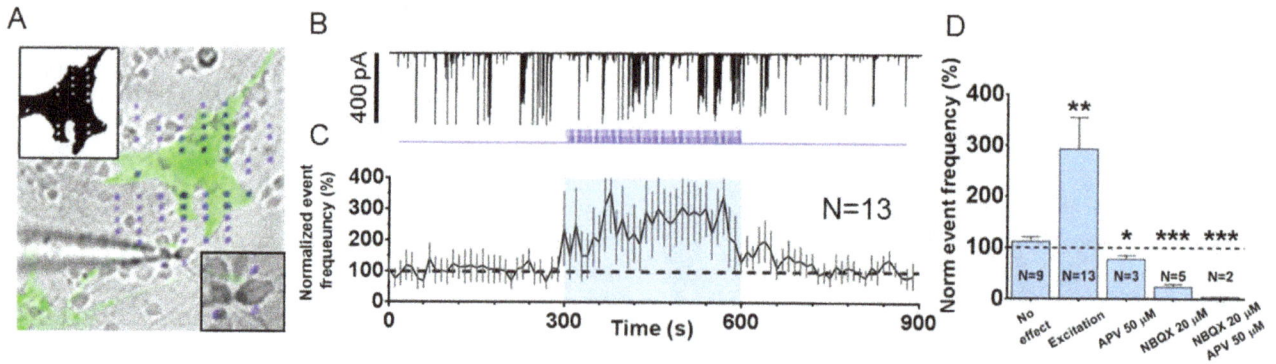

Figure 4. MicroLEDs-inducedChR2 positive astrocytes stimulation increases EPSCs frequency and is glutamate mediated. A, One of the ChR2 positive astrocyte in the field of view is light stimulated using 18 μLEDs (top left inset) while patch clamping from a nearby ChR2 negative neuron. Bottom right inset, a close-up of the ChR2-negative neuron showing that it is not illuminated by the μLEDs. **B**,Representative gap free patch clamp recording (black trace)performed on one of the 13 neurons that were modulated by the glial stimulationandstimulation pattern(blue trace)of the ChR2 positive astrocyte showing increase of synapticactivity following ChR2+ astrocytic light stimulation. **C**, Mean event frequency time course of the 13 neurons stimulated with the protocol as in **B** (blue trace) that showed a significant sEPSCs frequency increase over the baseline (black dashed line). **D**, The stimulation protocol was performed in 22 neurons, 13 of which showed a nearly 4-fold increase in the sEPSCs frequency. 9 out of the 22 neurons tested showed no significant sEPSCs frequency increase. Application of AMPA and NMDA receptor blockers after a significant increase of the sEPSCs frequency was established, reduced the latter to levels below the baseline level (all means paired t test vs control. No effect, p = 0.2635; Excitation, p = 0.0068; APV, p = 0.0371; NBQX, p = 0.0001; NBQX + APV, p = 0.0001.(Values are the means ± SEM).

trigger gliotransmitter release [34,35,36,37,17]. Indeed, in the rat brain stem retrotrapezoid nucleus, ChR2-expressing astrocytes reacted to long lasting (20–60 s) illumination by slow Ca^{2+} rises that lasted for minutes [35]. In the hippocampal CA1 region, blue light pulses induce rapid time-locked Ca^{2+} signals in astrocytes [37]. On the other end, mouse cortical astrocytes in culture showed a variable and weak Ca^{2+} elevations following ChR2 activation [25] while LiGluR and CatCh [7] evoked a reliable and robust Ca^{2+} signals in astrocytes [reviewed in [27] and [38]]. However, in our experimental conditions ChR2-transfected astrocytes showed a good efficacy in increasing $[Ca^{2+}]_i$ and in modulating glia to glia and glia to neurones transmission.

Unfortunately, due to the complexity of the astrocytic and neuronal network in cell cultures we could not discriminate the temporary resolution ofglial and neuronal cells stimulation. Pharmacological evidence showed that ChR2 non transfected astrocytes are partly stimulated through functional NMDA receptors activation which are present in cortical culture [39,40]. However, since the increased Ca2+ waves frequency mediated by stimulation of ChR2 positive astrocytes was significantly but not completely reduced by APV 50 μM (figure 2E), we could not rule out other gliotransmitter release such as ATP through connexin channels ("hemichannels") [41].

This study could have implications to the use of optogenetics for neuroprosthesis such as retinal prosthesis, visual brain prosthesis, brain and heart pacemakers. For practical application of optoelectronic prosthesis two platform technologies need to be optimized: 1) The biological expression – typically via viral vector of opsins with optimized biophysics. 2)The light generation and delivery mechanism to the optogenetically transfected cells [39].

In the case of the former, targeted delivery to specific cell types can allow for better communication and better sensitivity reducing the potential for long term photo-ionization damage [42]. In the case of the latter, a number of technologies are being developed including micro-light emitting diodes (μLEDs) [43] and optical delivery systems [44].

The μLEDs presented in this paper have delivered their light via microscope. If insulated, they could equally be placed against the

tissue for similar effect. However, as neural tissue scatters blue light strongly, the individual addressability gets lost after a few hundred microns. Thus, either some form of light delivery system such as an optrode [43] would need to be incorporated or the chip would need to be shaped into a penetrating structure [45] to get closer to the target cells. It is also possible to place such LEDs directly against the tissue. However light scattering effects would mean they lose spatial resolution.

In the case of light emissive optoelectronics, there is a direct inverse correlation between efficiency and intensity. As such, creating mechanisms which reduce the light requirement will improve the efficiency and thus battery performance. As batteries in current neural pacemakers are largely non-rechargeable and need to last at least 5 years, this is an important consideration. Furthermore, for implants in the brain, inefficiency leads to thermal emission, which could cause undesirable heating of the neural tissue.

Currently the literature indicates that implantable devices should dissipate no more than ~50 mW of thermal energy [11]. In this perspective, we demonstrated that ChR2transfection of astrocytes can be used to bring the requirement down in optogenetic systems, and this could have impact in future neuroprosthetic system design.

Supporting Information

Figure S1 System schematics.

Figure S2 A, Normalized moving average fit of the sEPSCs frequency time course. B, sEPSCs frequency during the relaxed and excited state and mean time (dA) to reach the excited state.

Figure S3 Example of current responses from a ChR2 positive astrocyte and a CatCh positive astrocyte elicited with a single 500 ms long pulse using the μLED array.

Acknowledgments

The authors thank Dr. Christian Bamann, Dr Andrea Lapucci and Prof. Ernst Bamberg.

References

1. Allen NJ, Barres BA (2009) NEUROSCIENCE Glia - more than just brain glue. Nature 457: 675–677.

2. Hamilton NB, Attwell D (2010) Do astrocytes really exocytose neurotransmitters? Nat Rev Neurosci 11: 227–238.

3. Berlinguer-Palmini R, Masi A, Narducci R, Cavone L, Maratea D, et al. (2013) GPR35 Activation Reduces Ca2+ Transients and Contributes to the Kynurenic Acid-Dependent Reduction of Synaptic Activity at CA3-CA1 Synapses. PloS one 8: e82180.

4. Fenno L, Yizhar O, Deisseroth K (2011) The development and application of optogenetics. Annu Rev Neurosci 34: 389–412.

5. Boyden ES, Zhang F, Bamberg E, Nagel G, Deisseroth K (2005) Millisecond-timescale, genetically targeted optical control of neural activity. Nat Neurosci 8: 1263–1268.

6. Li X, Gutierrez DV, Hanson MG, Han J, Mark MD, et al. (2005) Fast noninvasive activation and inhibition of neural and network activity by vertebrate rhodopsin and green algae channelrhodopsin. Proc Natl Acad Sci U S A 102: 17816–17821.

7. Kleinlogel S, Feldbauer K, Dempski RE, Fotis H, Wood PG, et al. (2011) Ultra light-sensitive and fast neuronal activation with the Ca2+-permeable channelrhodopsin CatCh. Nat Neurosci 14: 513–518.

8. Bi A, Cui J, Ma YP, Olshevskaya E, Pu M, et al. (2006) Ectopic expression of a microbial-type rhodopsin restores visual responses in mice with photoreceptor degeneration. Neuron 50: 23–33.

9. Degenaar P, Grossman N, Memon MA, Burrone J, Dawson M, et al. (2009) Optobionic vision-a new genetically enhanced light on retinal prosthesis. Journal of Neural Engineering 6.

10. Grossman N, Poher V, Grubb MS, Kennedy GT, Nikolic K, et al. (2010) Multisite optical excitation using ChR2 and micro-LED array. J Neural Eng 7: 16004.

11. Wolf PD (2008) Thermal Considerations for the Design of an Implanted Cortical Brain-Machine Interface (BMI). In: Reichert WM, editor. Indwelling Neural Implants: Strategies for Contending with the In Vivo Environment. Boca Raton (FL).

12. Chaudet L, Neil M, Degenaar P, Mehran K, Berlinguer-Palmini R, et al. (2013) Development of Optics with Micro-LED Arrays for Improved Opto-electronic Neural Stimulation. Optogenetics: Optical Methods for Cellular Control 8586.

13. Pellegrini-Giampietro DE, Cozzi A, Peruginelli F, Leonardi P, Meli E, et al. (1999) 1-Aminoindan-1,5-dicarboxylic acid and (S)-(+)-2-(3'-carboxybicyclo[1.1.1] pentyl)-glycine, two mGlu1 receptor-preferring antagonists, reduce neuronal death in vitro and in vivo models of cerebral ischaemia. Eur J Neurosci 11: 3637–3647.

14. Pellegrini-Giampietro DE, Peruginelli F, Meli E, Cozzi A, Albani-Torregrossa S, et al. (1999) Protection with metabotropic glutamate 1 receptor antagonists in models of ischemic neuronal death: time-course and mechanisms. Neuropharmacology 38: 1607–1619.

15. McGovern B, Palmini RB, Grossman N, Drakakis EM, Poher V, et al. (2010) A New Individually Addressable Micro-LED Array for Photogenetic Neural Stimulation. Ieee Transactions on Biomedical Circuits and Systems 4: 469–476.

16. Mattis J, Tye KM, Ferenczi EA, Ramakrishnan C, O'Shea DJ, et al. (2012) Principles for applying optogenetic tools derived from direct comparative analysis of microbial opsins. Nat Methods 9: 159–172.

17. Perea G, Yang A, Boyden ES, Sur M (2014) Optogenetic astrocyte activation modulates response selectivity of visual cortex neurons in vivo. Nat Commun 5: 3262.

18. Degenaar P, McGovern B, Berlinguer-Palmini R, Vysokov N, Grossman N, et al. Individually addressable optoelectronic arrays for optogenetic neural stimulation; 2010. IEEE. pp. 170–173.

19. Porter JT, McCarthy KD (1996) Hippocampal astrocytes in situ respond to glutamate released from synaptic terminals. J Neurosci 16: 5073–5081.

20. Wang X, Lou N, Xu Q, Tian GF, Peng WG, et al. (2006) Astrocytic Ca2+ signaling evoked by sensory stimulation in vivo. Nat Neurosci 9: 816–823.

21. Lee CJ, Mannaioni G, Yuan H, Woo DH, Gingrich MB, et al. (2007) Astrocytic control of synaptic NMDA receptors. J Physiol 581: 1057–1081.

22. Halassa MM, Fellin T, Haydon PG (2007) The tripartite synapse: roles for gliotransmission in health and disease. Trends Mol Med 13: 54–63.

23. Agulhon C, Petravicz J, McMullen AB, Sweger EJ, Minton SK, et al. (2008) What is the role of astrocyte calcium in neurophysiology? Neuron 59: 932–946.

24. Fiacco TA, Agulhon C, McCarthy KD (2009) Sorting out astrocyte physiology from pharmacology. Annu Rev Pharmacol Toxicol 49: 151–174.

25. Li D, Herault K, Isacoff EY, Oheim M, Ropert N (2012) Optogenetic activation of LiGluR-expressing astrocytes evokes anion channel-mediated glutamate release. J Physiol 590: 855–873.

26. Kleinlogel S, Feldbauer K, Dempski RE, Fotis H, Wood PG, et al. (2011) Ultra light-sensitive and fast neuronal activation with the Ca(2)+-permeable channelrhodopsin CatCh. Nat Neurosci 14: 513–518.

27. Szobota S, Isacoff EY (2010) Optical control of neuronal activity. Annu Rev Biophys 39: 329–348.

28. Miesenbock G (2011) Optogenetic control of cells and circuits. Annu Rev Cell Dev Biol 27: 731–758.

29. Nagel G, Brauner M, Liewald JF, Adeishvili N, Bamberg E, et al. (2005) Light activation of channelrhodopsin-2 in excitable cells of Caenorhabditis elegans triggers rapid Behavioral responses. Current Biology 15: 2279–2284.

30. Nagel G, Brauner M, Liewald JF, Adeishvili N, Bamberg E, et al. (2005) Light activation of channelrhodopsin-2 in excitable cells of Caenorhabditis elegans triggers rapid behavioral responses. Curr Biol 15: 2279–2284.

31. Lin JY, Lin MZ, Steinbach P, Tsien RY (2009) Characterization of engineered channelrhodopsin variants with improved properties and kinetics. Biophys J 96: 1803–1814.

32. Nagel G, Szellas T, Huhn W, Kateriya S, Adeishvili N, et al. (2003) Channelrhodopsin-2, a directly light-gated cation-selective membrane channel. Proc Natl Acad Sci U S A 100: 13940–13945.

33. Zhang YP, Oertner TG (2007) Optical induction of synaptic plasticity using a light-sensitive channel. Nat Methods 4: 139–141.

34. Gradinaru V, Mogri M, Thompson KR, Henderson JM, Deisseroth K (2009) Optical deconstruction of parkinsonian neural circuitry. Science 324: 354–359.

35. Gourine AV, Kasymov V, Marina N, Tang F, Figueiredo MF, et al. (2010) Astrocytes control breathing through pH-dependent release of ATP. Science (New York, N Y) 329: 571–575.

36. Sasaki T, Beppu K, Tanaka KF, Fukazawa Y, Shigemoto R, et al. (2012) Application of an optogenetic byway for perturbing neuronal activity via glial photostimulation. Proc Natl Acad Sci U S A 109: 20720–20725.

37. Chen J, Tan Z, Zeng L, Zhang X, He Y, et al. (2013) Heterosynaptic long-term depression mediated by ATP released from astrocytes. Glia 61: 178–191.

38. Li D, Agulhon C, Schmidt E, Oheim M, Ropert N (2013) New tools for investigating astrocyte-to-neuron communication. Front Cell Neurosci 7: 193.

39. Palygin O, Lalo U, Pankratov Y (2011) Distinct pharmacological and functional properties of NMDA receptors in mouse cortical astrocytes. British Journal of Pharmacology 163: 1755–1766.

40. Lalo U, Pankratov Y, Kirchhoff F, North RA, Verkhratsky A (2006) NMDA receptors mediate neuron-to-glia signaling in mouse cortical astrocytes. J Neurosci 26: 2673–2683.

41. Stout CE, Costantin JL, Naus CCG, Charles AC (2002) Intercellular calcium signaling in astrocytes via ATP release through connexin hemichannels. Journal of Biological Chemistry 277: 10482–10488.

42. Degenaar P, Grossman N, Memon MA, Burrone J, Dawson M, et al. (2009) Optobionic vision-a new genetically enhanced light on retinal prosthesis. J Neural Eng 6: 035007.

43. Nikolic K, Grossman N, Yan H, Drakakis E, Toumazou C, et al. (2007) A non-invasive retinal prosthesis - testing the concept. Conf Proc IEEE Eng Med Biol Soc 2007: 6365–6368.

44. Abaya TVF, Blair S, Tathireddy P, Rieth L, Solzbacher F (2012) A 3D glass optrode array for optical neural stimulation. Biomedical Optics Express 3.

45. McAlinden N, Massoubre D, Richardson E, Gu E, Sakata S, et al. (2013) Thermal and optical characterization of micro-LED probes for in vivo optogenetic neural stimulation. Optics Letters 38: 992–994.

Author Contributions

Conceived and designed the experiments: RB-P AM BM PM PD GM FM. Performed the experiments: RB-P RN KM AD AM TS EL MS. Analyzed the data: RB-P GM AS. Wrote the paper: RB-P PD GM.

20

Selective Vulnerability Related to Aging in Large-Scale Resting Brain Networks

Hong-Ying Zhang[1], Wen-Xin Chen[1], Yun Jiao[2], Yao Xu[3], Xiang-Rong Zhang[4], Jing-Tao Wu[1]*

1 Department of Radiology, Subei People's Hospital of Jiangsu Province, Yangzhou University, Yangzhou, China, 2 Jiangsu Key Laboratory of Molecular and Functional Imaging, Southeast University, Nanjing, China, 3 Department of Neurology, Subei People's Hospital of Jiangsu Province, Yangzhou University, Yangzhou, China, 4 Department of Psychiatry, Zhongda Hospital, Southeast University, Nanjing, China

Abstract

Normal aging is associated with cognitive decline. Evidence indicates that large-scale brain networks are affected by aging; however, it has not been established whether aging has equivalent effects on specific large-scale networks. In the present study, 40 healthy subjects including 22 older (aged 60–80 years) and 18 younger (aged 22–33 years) adults underwent resting-state functional MRI scanning. Four canonical resting-state networks, including the default mode network (DMN), executive control network (ECN), dorsal attention network (DAN) and salience network, were extracted, and the functional connectivities in these canonical networks were compared between the younger and older groups. We found distinct, disruptive alterations present in the large-scale aging-related resting brain networks: the ECN was affected the most, followed by the DAN. However, the DMN and salience networks showed limited functional connectivity disruption. The visual network served as a control and was similarly preserved in both groups. Our findings suggest that the aged brain is characterized by selective vulnerability in large-scale brain networks. These results could help improve our understanding of the mechanism of degeneration in the aging brain. Additional work is warranted to determine whether selective alterations in the intrinsic networks are related to impairments in behavioral performance.

Editor: Dante R. Chialvo, National Scientific and Technical Research Council (CONICET), Argentina

Funding: This work was supported in part by grant YZ2011087 from the Social Development and Scientific and Technology Project of Yangzhou; grants 81471642, 30870704, 81271739, and 91132727 from the National Natural Science Foundation of China; grants 2013CB733800, 2013CB733803, and 2010CB529602 from the National Program on Key Basic Research Project of China; and grant BK2012747 from Jiangsu Province Natural Science Foundation of China. The funders had no role in study design, data collection and analysis, decision to publish, or preparation of the manuscript.

Competing Interests: The authors have declared that no competing interests exist.

* Email: wujingtaodoctor@126.com

Introduction

The decline of functions such as memory, attention, problem-solving and sensorimotor ability is commonly experienced in old age. Such age-related cognitive decline may involve the selective deterioration of specific brain systems. Many hypotheses have been proposed to describe the aging process of the brain [1,2]. Studying the aged brain with respect to the networks that sustain brain functions may be helpful in understanding the complicated, age-related changes that occur in this organ.

Measuring synchronic low-frequency fluctuations (LFFs) among spatially distant brain regions using blood oxygen level-dependent (BOLD) functional magnetic resonance imaging (fMRI) signals is useful for mapping intrinsic neural networks in healthy and diseased subjects. Researchers have identified resting state neural network (RSN) architectures that are presumed to underlie the higher-order cognitive functions that are associated with memory, attention, execution and emotion processing [3–6] in addition to motor and sensory functions [7,8]. The corresponding higher-order networks include the following: 1) a default mode network (DMN), 2) a dorsal attention network (DAN), 3) an executive control network (ECN) and 4) a salience network (SN). The DMN is involved in internal and external environment alerts as well as memory- and self-related functions, and it presents temporospatial anti-correlations with other canonical networks during external-

ized cognitive tasks [5,9–11]. These canonical networks have been systemically measured in patients with neuropsychiatric disorders and have shown selective vulnerability in distinct neurodegenerative illnesses, such as Alzheimer's disease (AD) and frontotemporal dementia syndromes [12–15]. For instance, the DMN selectively disrupts the connectivity in patients with AD but enhances the connectivity in patients with behavioral variant frontotemporal dementia, whereas the SN shows enhanced activities in patients with AD and disrupted connectivity in patients with behavioral variant frontotemporal dementia [13]. These canonical networks are also differentially affected in schizophrenic patients compared to controls; schizophrenic patients demonstrate increased connectivity in the DMN, less connectivity in the ECN and DAN, and no difference in the salience network [16]. These findings indicate that the selective alterations in large-scale resting brain networks could represent a characteristic of neuropsychiatric disorders.

Aging, which could broadly affect multiple brain systems, is considered to be the primary risk factor for neurodegenerative disorders, such as sporadic AD. Numerous conventional task-based and resting-state fMRI investigations have been conducted to understand the effects of aging on brain function. In task-based studies, abnormally decreased or increased brain activation was found in normal elderly subjects during various cognitive processes, such as memory, attention and semantic judgments

[17–19]. The alterations in the balance between DMN and task-related activity could account for the increased vulnerability to distraction by irrelevant information among the elderly subjects [17]. Additional investigations revealed that aging is associated with changes in LFF correlations between different cortical regions during task performance and in the resting state [20–25]. Stronger resting-state network connectivity in older adults is associated with better performance in tests of executive function and processing speed, such as the Trail Making Test, the word frequency task and face-name associative memory task [20,24,25]. Accumulating evidence from neuroimaging studies has suggested that the decline in cognitive functions is accompanied by focal changes in activity in several brain regions, such as the prefrontal cortex [26–28], hippocampal formation [28–30], and parietal regions [19,27]. The evidence from graph theoretical analyses has indicated that older adults have decreased topological efficiency in small-world and modular organization of the entire brain [22,31,32]. In the present study, we investigated how the four canonical intrinsic networks underpinning cognitive functions change with aging.

Many studies have strongly indicated that resting-state functional connectivity provides relevant information regarding the effects of aging on brain functioning and cognition (for a review, see [33]). The most consistent age-related change is decreased resting-state connectivity in the DMN, which is crucial for memory [20–23,32,34]; another convergent finding is that the DAN is affected by the aging process [28,32,35]. Aging has a particular effect on the hub-related regions in the brain. The patterns of low-level anti-correlations between the DMN sub-networks and task-positive networks have also been demonstrated [23]. The findings noted from the topological analyses consistently suggest that the long-range connections mainly within the DMN and DAN regions are more vulnerable to aging effects compared with the short-range connections [31,32,36].

Age has a strong impact on the DMN throughout an individual's lifespan, and age-related changes in interregional functional connectivity exhibit spatially and temporally specific patterns [36,37]. In a broad spectrum of populations, resting-state fMRI studies have shown reliable and replicable results [38–40]. Particularly in healthy older adults, such reliability has been supported by a recent test-retest study that evaluated different methods for data processing, including seed-based, independent component analyses and graph theoretical approaches [41].

A majority of the studies have focused on the aging-related DMN and DAN, simultaneously ignoring several specified high-order networks. The ECN, which includes the anterior prefrontal cortex, insular and frontal opercular cortices, and the dorsal anterior cingulated cortex [11], is modulated by dopamine and is functionally involved in cognitive control, attention shift control and decision-making [11,42]. The behavioral theories of cognitive aging suggest that age-related decline in a range of cognitive tasks is mediated by selective impairment in executive processing functions [43–45]. Using neurobehavioral tests, such as an attention network test, previous studies have indicated that the executive effect is more significantly decreased with age than other functions, such as the alerting function and orienting attention function [46]. Although this observation indicates the existence of selective cognitive differences with advanced age, corresponding observations from neuroimaging are still required. Diffusion tensor MRI research provides a structural basis for the selective loss of executive functions by measuring the correlations between the changes in the frontal white matter integrity and the executive function performance assessed using the Trail Making Test [47]. A previous study demonstrated that moderate exercise attenuates the disruption of age-related resting brain connectivity between the

regions in the ECN and in the DMN [48]. Although there have been a few examinations of age-related disruption in intrinsic functional connectivity in the executive control and salience networks [47–49], much of the literature supports age-related decline in the performance of tasks implanted in the ECN (for reviews, see [33,45,50]).

Several studies have measured topological whole-brain connectivity by applying the graph theory, which demonstrated significant decreases in intermodular connections to the frontal modular regions in older groups and revealed that normal aging is associated with the functional segregation of large-scale brain systems [22,31,37]. One study indicated that aging impacts not only connectivity within networks but also connectivity between different functional networks [51]. Indeed, a specific brain network may have more relevance to a specific function than to other functions. However, whether aging has equivalent effects or selective effects on specific large-scale networks has not been established. Thus, the purpose of our study was to investigate the effects of aging on four canonical RSNs including the DMN, DAN, ECN and SN by comparing two groups consisting of younger and older adults. We hypothesize that the alterations in the canonical networks would vary across the networks; therefore, we are especially concerned with the degree to which the large-scale intrinsic networks are affected. Because previous studies have shown that reduced functional connectivity in the motor network is related to aging [52], we used the visual system network as a control.

Materials and Methods

Subjects and procedure

This study was approved by the Yangzhou University Research Ethics Committee. All the participants provided their written informed consent.

A total of 40 right-handed healthy subjects were recruited, including 18 younger subjects (age, 22–33 years; mean age, 23.9 ± 1.8 years; n = 9 males, 9 females) and 22 older adults (age, 60–80 years; mean age, 69.8 ± 5.8 years; n = 10 males, 12 females). Both groups were education- and gender-matched. None of the subjects had a history of head trauma, neuropsychiatric disorders, hypertensive disease or metabolic disorders. Additionally, none of the subjects showed abnormal findings in their structural brain MRIs. Each subject had a Mini-Mental State Examination (MMSE) score ranging between 28 and 30.

Imaging was performed using a 1.5T GE Signa Excite MR scanner (GE Healthcare Systems, Milwaukee, WI, USA) and a standard head coil. Before the fMRI scan, the subjects were instructed to lie quietly with their eyes closed and to avoid thinking of anything in particular. The functional images were obtained using a gradient echo-planar imaging (EPI) sequence (TR, 3000 ms; TE, 40 ms; flip angle, 90°; slice thickness, 6 mm; slice gap, 0 mm; FOV, 240 mm; and matrix, 64×64), and each frame included 18 contiguous slices that covered the entire cerebral volume. The slices were obtained parallel to the anterior/posterior commissures. The EPI scan lasted 6 min and 24 sec. Finally, a T1-weighted 3D fast spoiled gradient echo sequence was acquired (TR, 70 ms; TE, 4.2 ms; FOV, 240 mm; matrix, 256×256; slice thickness, 1 mm).

Data preprocessing and analysis

The fMRI data preprocessing was performed using DPARSF software V2.3 (http://www.restfmri.net), which is based on SPM8 (http://www.fil.ion.ucl.ac.uk/spm) and the Resting-State fMRI Data Analysis Toolkit (Beijing Normal University, Beijing, http://www.restfmri.net). The first four volumes were discarded. The images were corrected for slice timing and realigned for head movement correction. One young subject and two elderly subjects who failed to meet the study criterion were excluded because their head translation exceeded 1.5 mm or their head rotation exceeded 1.5°. There was no statistical significance between the groups for the movement parameters (two sample t test; the p values were 0.92, 0.93, and 0.55 for maximum, squared, and framewise displacement of the translation, respectively, and 0.60, 0.21, 0.12 for maximum, squared, and framewise displacement of the rotation, respectively). The functional images were normalized using DARTEL. The normalized volumes were re-sampled to a voxel size of 3 mm × 3 mm × 3 mm in MNI space, and the EPI images were spatially smoothed using an isotropic Gaussian filter (8 mm FWHM). The movement parameters (Friston 24-parameter model [53]) and signals of white matter, cerebrospinal fluid and global mean were regressed out. Linear detrending and temporal bandpass filtering (0.01–0.08 Hz) were applied.

The subsequent data processing and statistical analyses were performed using the Resting state fMRI data Analysis Toolkit (REST V1.8) (http://www.restfmri.net). For connectivity analysis, we created eight seed regions of interest (ROIs) with 6-mm radius spheres, which have been used in previous studies to identify the corresponding RSNs [11,16,54]. Each RSN and the seed ROI (in MNI coordinates) were as follows: DMN (PCC: −2, −54, 27; ventral medial prefrontal cortex: −2, 55, 6); ECN (left and right dorsolateral prefrontal cortex (dLPFC): −42, 34, 20/44, 36, 20); DAN (left and right superior parietal lobule (SPL): −25, −53, 52/ 25, −57, 52); and SN (left and right frontal-insular cortex (FI): −32, 26, −14/38, 22, −10). The positive Pearson correlation coefficients between the time series of each ROI and the time series in other voxels in the brain were calculated. A Fisher's z-transform was applied to improve the normality of these correlation coefficients. For the DMN, connectivity maps derived from the anterior and posterior seeds were averaged to create a single connectivity map; for the other canonical networks with bilateral ROI seeds, the connectivity maps derived from left and right ROI were averaged to create a single connectivity map, consistent with a prior study [16].

For the visual network, we selected two allelic seeds located approximately in the bilateral V2 primary cortex, which had been used in previous studies for mapping visual networks [35,55]. The two seeds are centered on MNI coordinates (19, −95, 2) and (−19, −95, 2) with a 6-mm radius. The mean time course was extracted and analyzed using correlation analysis.

One-sample t tests were performed on the individual z-maps to determine initial intra-group level network regions; the threshold was set at AlphaSim corrected $p < 0.01$, cluster size > 97. Considering the representation of other nodes within each RSN and the bias of the pre-defined seed approach, a dual regression process was performed (http://fsl.fmrib.ox.ac.uk/fsl/fslwiki/DualRegression). The dual regression process includes the following steps: 1) the initial group spatial maps are regressed into each subject's 4D dataset to give a set of time courses; 2) those time courses are regressed into the same 4D dataset to obtain a subject-specific set of spatial maps; 3) then, within-group and between-group analyses are performed based on the spatial maps acquired in the prior step. Dual regression has been applied in many brain network research studies [56–58]. Using dual regression, Wang et al. discovered that the network-wise temporal patterns for the majority of the RSNs (especially for the DMN) exhibited moderate-to-high test-retest reliability and reproducibility under different scan conditions [56]. For within-group statistics, a threshold adjustment method based on the Monte-Carlo

simulation correction was used with voxel wise $p < 0.8 \times 10^{-5}$, cluster size > 102 (2754 mm^3), and cluster connectivity criterion 4 rmm; this outcome yielded an AlphaSim correction threshold of $p < 0.005$. Before the group comparison of each map, the within-group threshold maps were combined across the young and elderly groups to create unified masks, which were then used to restrict the between-group analysis. The between-group two sample t test analysis was performed at an AlphaSim correction threshold of $p < 0.01$, cluster size > 97 (2619 mm^3), and cluster connectivity criterion 4 rmm based on Monte-Carlo simulation correction. The individual modulated gray matter volumes were entered as covariates to regress out the nuisance from the brain volume differences between groups.

Results

Within-group analyses of brain networks

As shown in Figure 1, the DMN consisted of the PCC, ventral medial prefrontal cortex (vmPFC), bilateral medial temporal cortex (MTC), hippocampus, pulvinars, precuneus and inferior parietal cortex. The regions of the bilateral insular cortex, dorsolateral prefrontal cortex (dlPFC), inferior parietal cortex and posterior middle temporal (area MT+) were involved in the ECN. The DAN consisted of the SPL/intraparietal sulcus (IPS), frontal eye fields (FEF), and extra-striate visual areas, and the SN included the orbital frontal-insular cortex, anterior cingulated cortex, superior temporal pole and subcortical paralimbic regions. The visual network spread across the bilateral primary and association visual cortex. A visual inspection of the RSNs indicated that the connectivity maps for both groups were similar and consistent with prior findings.

Between-group analyses of brain networks

Distinct alterations were noted in the four canonical networks between the younger and older groups when compared at the same statistical threshold level. In other words, the ECN was disrupted mainly in the older group, followed by the DAN; the DMN and SN showed limited functional connectivity disruption relative to the ECN and DAN.

For the ECN, 10 clusters (total of 2,668 voxels, 72,036 mm^3) presented significantly decreased connectivity in the older group, including regions of the bilateral dorsal frontal cortex, insular cortex, MT+ and right inferior parietal lobe, with a rightward hemisphere asymmetry. In the DAN, 6 clusters (total of 1,400 voxels, 37,800 mm^3) displayed reduced connectivity in the areas of the parietal postcentral gyrus, supplementary motor area and left mid-occipital gyrus, with a leftward asymmetry. For the DMN, 4 clusters (total of 612 voxels, 16,524 mm^3) involving the bilateral regions of vMPFC, PCC, pulvinars and bilateral dorsal MPFC presented significantly reduced connectivity. The SN showed the least connectivity reduction in the regions of the left frontal-insular cortex and right superior temporal cortex, with 3 clusters (310 voxels, 8,370 mm^3) (see Figure 2, details in Table 1). Significantly increased connectivity was not detected in any of the canonical networks in the older group.

In the control analysis, the visual networks did not demonstrate significant connectivity differences between the two experimental groups.

Considering that the canonical networks have different scales, the volume of connectivity decrease for each network was compared with the volume of each combined mask of the paired networks for the two groups (ratio of disruptive network volume) (Figure 3). For the ECN, DAN, DMN and SN, each disruptive network volume accounted for 25.7%, 12.7%, 5.7% and 4.9%,

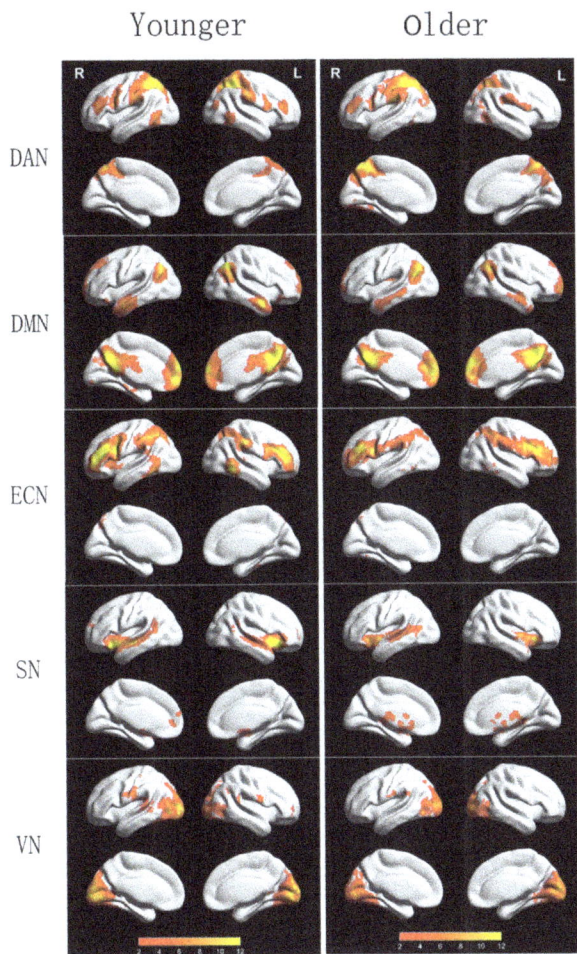

Figure 1. Intra-group maps of canonical networks in the resting brains of younger and older groups. DAN, dorsal attention network; DMN, default mode network; ECN, executive control network; SN: salience network; VN, visual network; R, right view; L, left view. The color bar denotes the T value. The statistical threshold was set at $p < 0.005$ and was corrected with AlphaSim.

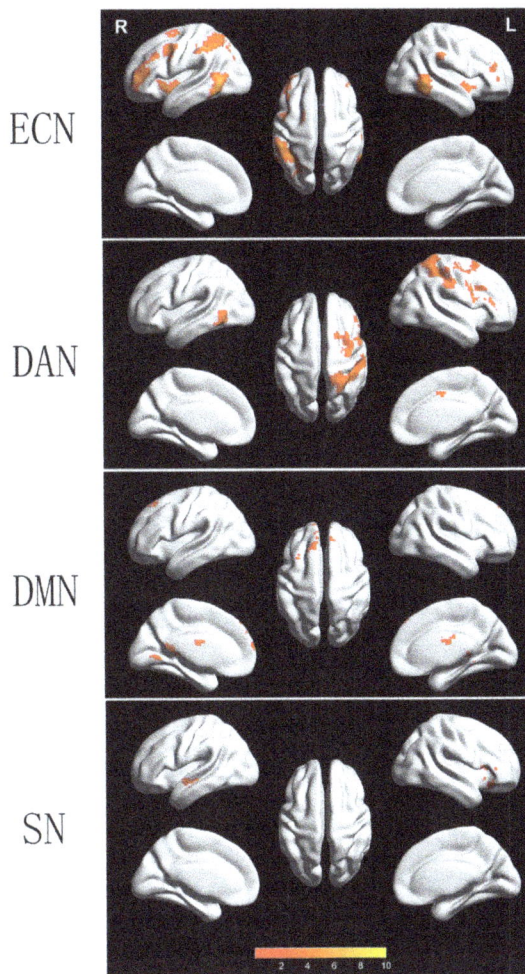

Figure 2. Comparisons of canonical networks between the younger and older groups. The visual network did not exhibit significant differences and is not shown on the map. The right and left lateralized disruptions are shown in the ECN and DAN, respectively. The threshold was set at $p < 0.01$ and was corrected with AlphaSim. ECN, executive control network; DAN, dorsal attention network; DMN, default mode network; SN, salience network; R, right view; L, left view. The color bar denotes the T value.

respectively, in each unified mask volume. Although the DAN had the largest volume, it was the second most impaired network in the older group. The map for the ratio of disruptive network volume can reflect the varying degree to which the canonical networks were affected.

Because there are debates concerning global signal regression, which could impact the resting-state fMRI inferences [59] and might reduce the effects of age-related differences on the connectivity in the blood flow, we estimated the results without global signal regression. We observed that the areas involved in each of the canonical networks exceeded the traditional network regions with positively biased correlations for the intra-group analyses, which is consistent with a recent study [60], and we found that the nuisance from the cerebrospinal fluid was incorporated into the maps for the inter-group analyses. DMN contrasting maps with and without global signal regression were used to illustrate the findings (Figure 4). The network maps without global signal regression for the intragroup and intergroup analyses are shown in Figure S1 and Figure S2. We believe that the global signal regression procedure might be appropriate in our study.

Discussion

Age-related functional brain changes have been extensively explored during tasks and during resting states; however, less is known regarding the effect of normal aging on large-scale brain networks. The present study analyzes the effects of aging on resting-state canonical networks. Our major finding is that selective vulnerability is present in large-scale resting brain networks in normal older adults. The functional connectivity in these canonical networks was selectively reduced as a function of age, even though these networks varied in size.

The most intensive connectivity disruption was demonstrated in the ECN, followed by the DAN and DMN. The salience network was minimally affected, and the visual network, which served as the control, was not significantly affected. These findings are similar to the common observation that age-related processes are characterized by the loss of neural specificity within distinct functional systems [61]. Reduced signal coordination within specific networks may imply less effective functional communication in that specific brain system.

Table 1. Primary clusters showing significant connectivity alterations in resting-state networks in younger and older groups.

Regions	Peak T	MNI Coordinates			Brodmann area
		x	y	z	
DMN					
bilateral MPFC	7.77	0	63	21	10,9,8
PCC	4.92	−3	−55	'9	30
left superior frontal gyrus	3.59	−27	21	54	6
right midfrontal gyrus	5.73	30	26	51	8
right superior frontal gyrus	3.97	11	43	51	9
DAN					
right midtemporal gyrus	4.78	54	−60	−9	37,19
left supramarginal gyrus	5.02	−60	−18	36	40
left postcentral gyrus	5.33	−34	−50	63	6,9
left inferior frontal gyrus	6.26	−59	14	26	46,9
left superior frontal gyrus	3.69	−23	12	63	8
supplementary motor area	4.39	9	3	45	24,6
ECN					
right MT+	4.68	63	−51	0	37,21
left MT+	4.99	−54	−57	3	37
right midfrontal gyrus	6.16	43	50	10	44,45,48
left midfrontal gyrus	4.34	−57	18	31	44
right inferior lobe	6.06	48	−49	53	40
left superior lobe	5.12	−45	44	59	40
right precentral gyrus	4.84	50	10	43	6,44
left supramarginal gyrus	3.93	−62	−26	35	2
Salience Network					
left frontal-insular gyrus	4.19	−33	24	−15	47
right superior temporal gyrus	3.41	56	−3	−8	22

Previous research has shown that clinical neurodegenerative syndromes involving AD, behavioral variant frontotemporal dementia, semantic dementia and progressive nonfluent aphasia each include distinct network vulnerability patterns. For example, the DMN is vulnerable in AD, and the behavioral variant frontotemporal dementia targets the SN [12–14]; schizophrenia-vulnerable networks include the ECN and DAN [16]. Our findings suggest that normal aging is also characterized by selective neuronal network vulnerability, with ECN as the first target.

Executive control function, which determines the manipulation and modulation of concrete information processing for many cognitive tasks, is thought to be a higher order cognitive activity that is critically dependent on the ECN. Cognitive tasks require segregated and integrated processing in these large-scale brain networks; for example, the ECN may flexibly couple with the DMN and DAN according to the task domain [5,10,62]. Connectivity disruption in the ECN implies that the communication signals between these higher order brain networks have been impaired. Neurobehavioral tests have suggested that normal aging is accompanied by a decline in a range of cognitive abilities that are thought to rely on executive functioning and that executive skills seem to be particularly vulnerable to the effects of aging [43–46,50]. By demonstrating that the ECN is impaired most severely among the canonical brain networks, our findings could provide support for the behavioral theories of cognitive aging.

Several studies have demonstrated the influence of aging on large-scale networks during various task states; for instance, during a semantic classification task, the DMN and DAN are markedly disrupted in advanced aging [35]. Grady et al. measured the connectivity within the DMN and task-positive networks during multiple cognitive tasks [63]. These authors noted that the functional connectivity in the DMN was reduced in older adults, whereas the pattern of task-positive network connectivity was equivalent in younger and older groups [63]. Task-directed age-comparative fMRI investigations showed that older adults have decreased and increased brain activation patterns and that these patterns can shift depending on the degree of the task demand [64–66]. Although the aging brain preserves the adaptive function for supporting explicit tasks, our findings indicated that the underlying brain networks were disrupted to varying degrees. Therefore, studying the aging brain using resting-state network connectivity measurements may be advantageous.

The DMN participates in episodic memory, presenting non-specific deactivation during externally directed tasks. The DMN is active when individuals are engaged in internally focused tasks, including retrieving autobiographical memory, envisioning the future, and conceiving the perspectives of others [3,9–11,67,68]. Disruption of the DMN implies impairment in these associated functions. Based on our findings, the DMN was mildly disrupted

Rate of disruptive networks volume

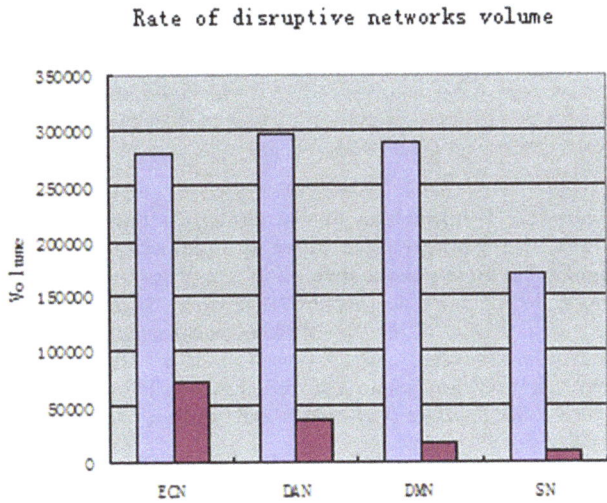

Figure 3. Histogram of the ratio of the disruptive network volume. The light blue bars represent each of the unified mask volumes in the canonical networks; the dark pink bars represent each of the disruptive network volumes in the canonical networks. In the older group, the network volumes were reduced by 25.7%, 12.7%, 5.7% and 4.9% compared with each unified mask for the DMN, DAN, ECN and SN, respectively. This histogram reflects the distinct influence of aging on the canonical networks.

distribution patterns of the ECN and DAN, the two models are not incompatible; e.g., the right lateralized disruption in the ECN may support the right hemi-aging model, and the left lateralized disruption in the DAN may support the HAROLD model. The aging brain models could depend on which network resource is more demanding.

The salience network was affected minimally in the older group, with decreased coordination between regions of the left FI and right superior temporal cortex. The salience network is involved in emotion processing, reward and interoceptive regulation [5,71,72]. Previous research has suggested that, on average, the emotional well-being of adults is stable and well maintained or even improved as they age, despite the fact that their physical health and cognitive abilities decline with age [73,74]. Our findings regarding SN changes in the elderly group could support this proposal.

The visual cortex, belonging to a low-order brain system, has broad fiber tracts connecting to the frontal and temporal lobes. Although the higher-order networks exhibit broadly reduced functional cooperation, our results showed that the visual network was spared during the aging process, which is consistent with previous findings [35]. According to supportive anatomical evidence, the occipital visual areas have the highest neuronal density and the most differential cytoarchitectonic structures in all cortices of the brain [75,76]. Although many studies indicated that the higher visual attentional function in older adults was impaired, our findings may only reflect the primary photic sense function in older adults.

Selective neuronal and molecular vulnerability could account for the selective network vulnerability in the aging brain. A pattern of selective loss of synapses and neurons in certain brain regions has been described during the aging process [77–79]. Genomic analyses have suggested that different molecular mechanisms exist in different neural subtypes that determine their survival or vulnerability to death, which is evidenced by several transgenic mouse model subsets [15].

According to our findings, the older group presented decreased resting functional connectivity within multiple networks rather than increased functional connectivity; therefore, we hypothesize that reduced brain functional cooperation could be a critical pattern as aging progresses.

relative to the ECN and DAN, even though the DMN was sensitive to aging, as previously documented.

Currently, there are two models of hemispheric asymmetry about aging brain: the right hemi-aging model and the hemispheric asymmetry reduction in older adults (HAROLD) model. The former model, which proposes that the right hemisphere shows greater age-related decline than the left hemisphere, is supported by behavioral studies in the domains of cognitive, affective, and sensorimotor processing; the latter model proposes that the prefrontal activity during cognitive performance, which tends to be less left-lateralized in older adults than in younger adults, is supported by evidence from task-directed fMRI [69,70]. In terms of our present observations on the asymmetric

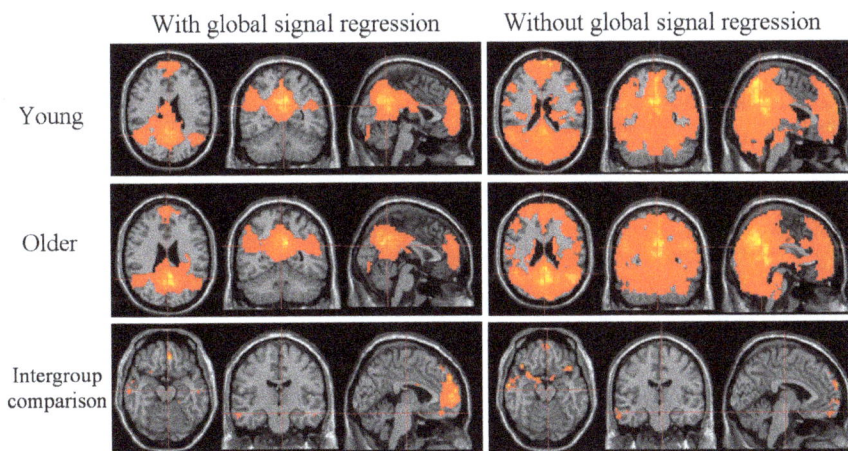

Figure 4. DMN contrasting maps with and without global signal regression for the two experimental groups. "Young" indicates the intra-group analyses with one t test for the younger adults. "Older" indicates the intra-group analyses with one *t* test for the older adults. The threshold for the intragroup and intergroup statistical analyses was set at $p<0.01$ and was corrected by AlphaSim. Note the positively biased correlations and the non-neural noise in the basilar cistern without global signal regression.

We acknowledge that the present study has several limitations. First, the relationship between the alteration of networks and behavioral performance requires additional investigation. Second, age-related preclinical atherosclerosis risks may have several effects on the brain's functional connectivity; for example, changes in interactions between the amygdala and rostral ACC have been implicated in an increased risk of atherosclerosis [80]. Thus, atherosclerosis co-variations should be quantified in the future. Additionally, the DMN is inhomogeneous and was decomposed into two or three sub-networks in previous studies [81,82]. The DMN was not further subdivided in our study.

In summary, our results suggest that the process of aging in the brain is characterized by selective vulnerability in large-scale brain systems. Specifically, the ECN, DAN and DMN are among the canonical networks that are sensitive to the effects of aging. Moreover, high-order brain networks are preferentially affected compared to low-order systems. These findings could provide insight to further our understanding of patterns in age-related decline in multiple cognitive functions.

Supporting Information

Figure S1 Intra-group maps of canonical networks without global signal regression in the resting brains of younger and older groups. DAN, dorsal attention network;

DMN, default mode network; ECN, executive control network; SN: salience network; VN, visual network; R, right view; L, left view. The color bar denotes the T value. The statistical threshold was set at $p<0.001$ and was corrected with AlphaSim. The map shows that the areas involved in each of the canonical networks exceed the traditional network regions.

Figure S2 Comparison of the canonical networks between the younger and older groups without global signal regression procedure. DAN, dorsal attention network; DMN, default mode network; ECN, executive control network; SN: salience network. Left is left. The color bar denotes the T value. The statistical threshold was set at $p<0.01$ and was corrected with AlphaSim. The prominent nuisance from the cerebrospinal fluid, arteries and veins can be noted, particularly on maps of the SN and DMN.

Author Contributions

Conceived and designed the experiments: HYZ JTW. Analyzed the data: HYZ YJ. Contributed reagents/materials/analysis tools: HYZ JTW. Wrote the paper: HYZ WXC YJ YX XRZ JTW. Contributed to data interpretation: HYZ WXC YJ YX XRZ JTW.

References

1. Hedden T, Gabrieli JD (2005) Healthy and pathological processes in adult development: new evidence from neuroimaging of the aging brain. Curr Opin Neurol 18: 740–747.
2. Silver H, Goodman C, Bilker W (2009) Age in high-functioning healthy men is associated with nonlinear decline in some 'executive' functions in late middle age. Dement Geriatr Cogn Disord 27: 292–300.
3. Greicius MD, Krasnow B, Reiss AL, Menon V (2003) Functional connectivity in the resting brain: a network analysis of the default mode hypothesis. Proc Natl Acad Sci U S A 100: 253–258.
4. Fox MD, Corbetta M, Snyder AZ, Vincent JL, Raichle ME (2006) Spontaneous neuronal activity distinguishes human dorsal and ventral attention systems. Proc Natl Acad Sci U S A 103: 10046–10051.
5. Seeley WW, Menon V, Schatzberg AF, Keller J, Glover GH, et al. (2007) Dissociable intrinsic connectivity networks for salience processing and executive control. J Neurosci 27: 2349–2356.
6. Hampson M, Driesen NR, Skudlarski P, Gore JC, Constable RT (2006) Brain connectivity related to working memory performance. J Neurosci 26: 13338–13343.
7. Biswal B, Yetkin FZ, Haughton VM, Hyde JS (1995) Functional connectivity in the motor cortex of resting human brain using echo-planar MRI. Magn Reson Med 34: 537–541.
8. Li SJ, Biswal B, Li Z, Risinger R, Rainey C, et al. (2000) Cocaine administration decreases functional connectivity in human primary visual and motor cortex as detected by functional MRI. Magn Reson Med 43: 45–51.
9. Fox MD, Snyder AZ, Vincent JL, Corbetta M, Van Essen DC, et al. (2005) The human brain is intrinsically organized into dynamic, anticorrelated functional networks. Proc Natl Acad Sci U S A 102: 9673–9678.
10. Spreng RN, Stevens WD, Chamberlain JP, Gilmore AW, Schacter DL (2010) Default network activity, coupled with the frontoparietal control network, supports goal-directed cognition. Neuroimage 53: 303–317.
11. Vincent JL, Kahn I, Snyder AZ, Raichle ME, Buckner RL (2008) Evidence for a frontoparietal control system revealed by intrinsic functional connectivity. J Neurophysiol 100: 3328–3342.
12. Seeley WW, Crawford RK, Zhou J, Miller BL, Greicius MD (2009) Neurodegenerative diseases target large-scale human brain networks. Neuron 62: 42–52.
13. Zhou J, Greicius MD, Gennatas ED, Growdon ME, Jang JY, et al. (2010) Divergent network connectivity changes in behavioural variant frontotemporal dementia and Alzheimer's disease. Brain 133: 1352–1367.
14. Seeley WW (2008) Selective functional, regional, and neuronal vulnerability in frontotemporal dementia. Curr Opin Neurol 21: 701–707.
15. Gotz J, Schonrock N, Vissel B, Ittner LM (2009) Alzheimer's disease selective vulnerability and modeling in transgenic mice. J Alzheimers Dis 18: 243–251.
16. Woodward ND, Rogers B, Heckers S (2011) Functional resting-state networks are differentially affected in schizophrenia. Schizophr Res 130: 86–93.
17. Grady CL, Springer MV, Hongwanishkul D, McIntosh AR, Winocur G (2006) Age-related changes in brain activity across the adult lifespan. J Cogn Neurosci 18: 227–241.
18. Ansado J, Monchi O, Ennabil N, Faure S, Joanette Y (2012) Load-dependent posterior-anterior shift in aging in complex visual selective attention situations. Brain Res.
19. Lustig C, Snyder AZ, Bhakta M, O'Brien KC, McAvoy M, et al. (2003) Functional deactivations: change with age and dementia of the Alzheimer type. Proc Natl Acad Sci U S A 100: 14504–14509.
20. Damoiseaux JS, Beckmann CF, Arigita EJ, Barkhof F, Scheltens P, et al. (2008) Reduced resting-state brain activity in the "default network" in normal aging. Cereb Cortex 18: 1856–1864.
21. Koch W, Teipel S, Mueller S, Buerger K, Bokde AL, et al. (2010) Effects of aging on default mode network activity in resting state fMRI: does the method of analysis matter? Neuroimage 51: 280–287.
22. Meunier D, Achard S, Morcom A, Bullmore E (2009) Age-related changes in modular organization of human brain functional networks. Neuroimage 44: 715–723.
23. Wu JT, Wu HZ, Yan CG, Chen WX, Zhang HY, et al. (2011) Aging-related changes in the default mode network and its anti-correlated networks: A resting-state fMRI study. Neurosci Lett 504: 62–67.
24. Goh JO (2011) Functional Dedifferentiation and Altered Connectivity in Older Adults: Neural Accounts of Cognitive Aging. Aging Dis 2: 30–48.
25. Wang L, Laviolette P, O'Keefe K, Putcha D, Bakkour A, et al. (2010) Intrinsic connectivity between the hippocampus and posteromedial cortex predicts memory performance in cognitively intact older individuals. Neuroimage 51: 910–917.
26. Logan JM, Sanders AL, Snyder AZ, Morris JC, Buckner RL (2002) Under-recruitment and nonselective recruitment: dissociable neural mechanisms associated with aging. Neuron 33: 827–840.
27. Madden DJ, Whiting WL, Provenzale JM, Huettel SA (2004) Age-related changes in neural activity during visual target detection measured by fMRI. Cereb Cortex 14: 143–155.
28. Cabeza R, Daselaar SM, Dolcos F, Prince SE, Budde M, et al. (2004) Task-independent and task-specific age effects on brain activity during working memory, visual attention and episodic retrieval. Cereb Cortex 14: 364–375.
29. Kukolja J, Thiel CM, Wilms M, Mirzazade S, Fink GR (2009) Ageing-related changes of neural activity associated with spatial contextual memory. Neurobiol Aging 30: 630–645.
30. Gutchess AH, Welsh RC, Hedden T, Bangert A, Minear M, et al. (2005) Aging and the neural correlates of successful picture encoding: frontal activations compensate for decreased medial-temporal activity. J Cogn Neurosci 17: 84–96.
31. Wang L, Li Y, Metzak P, He Y, Woodward TS (2010) Age-related changes in topological patterns of large-scale brain functional networks during memory encoding and recognition. Neuroimage 50: 862–872.
32. Tomasi D, Volkow ND (2012) Aging and functional brain networks. Mol Psychiatry 17: 471, 549–458.
33. Ferreira LK, Busatto GF (2013) Resting-state functional connectivity in normal brain aging. Neurosci Biobehav Rev 37: 384–400.

34. Sambataro F, Murty VP, Callicott JH, Tan HY, Das S, et al. (2010) Age-related alterations in default mode network: impact on working memory performance. Neurobiol Aging 31: 839–852.

35. Andrews-Hanna JR, Snyder AZ, Vincent JL, Lustig C, Head D, et al. (2007) Disruption of large-scale brain systems in advanced aging. Neuron 56: 924–935.

36. Cao M, Wang JH, Dai ZJ, Cao XY, Jiang LL, et al. (2014) Topological organization of the human brain functional connectome across the lifespan. Dev Cogn Neurosci 7: 76–93.

37. Wang L, Su L, Shen H, Hu D (2012) Decoding lifespan changes of the human brain using resting-state functional connectivity MRI. PLoS One 7: e44530.

38. Buckner RL, Sepulcre J, Talukdar T, Krienen FM, Liu H, et al. (2009) Cortical hubs revealed by intrinsic functional connectivity: mapping, assessment of stability, and relation to Alzheimer's disease. J Neurosci 29: 1860–1873.

39. Zuo XN, Di Martino A, Kelly C, Shehzad ZE, Gee DG, et al. (2010) The oscillating brain: complex and reliable. Neuroimage 49: 1432–1445.

40. Meindl T, Teipel S, Elmouden R, Mueller S, Koch W, et al. (2010) Test-retest reproducibility of the default-mode network in healthy individuals. Hum Brain Mapp 31: 237–246.

41. Guo CC, Kurth F, Zhou J, Mayer EA, Eickhoff SB, et al. (2012) One-year test-retest reliability of intrinsic connectivity network fMRI in older adults. Neuroimage 61: 1471–1483.

42. Diamond A, Briand L, Fossella J, Gehlbach L (2004) Genetic and neurochemical modulation of prefrontal cognitive functions in children. Am J Psychiatry 161: 125–132.

43. Braver TS, Barch DM (2002) A theory of cognitive control, aging cognition, and neuromodulation. Neurosci Biobehav Rev 26: 809–817.

44. Goh JO, Park DC (2009) Neuroplasticity and cognitive aging: the scaffolding theory of aging and cognition. Restor Neurol Neurosci 27: 391–403.

45. Bryan J, Luszcz MA (2000) Measurement of executive function: considerations for detecting adult age differences. J Clin Exp Neuropsychol 22: 40–55.

46. Zhou SS, Fan J, Lee TM, Wang CQ, Wang K (2011) Age-related differences in attentional networks of alerting and executive control in young, middle-aged, and older Chinese adults. Brain Cogn 75: 205–210.

47. O'Sullivan M, Jones DK, Summers PE, Morris RG, Williams SC, et al. (2001) Evidence for cortical "disconnection" as a mechanism of age-related cognitive decline. Neurology 57: 632–638.

48. Voss MW, Prakash RS, Erickson KI, Basak C, Chaddock L, et al. (2010) Plasticity of brain networks in a randomized intervention trial of exercise training in older adults. Front Aging Neurosci 2.

49. Onoda K, Ishihara M, Yamaguchi S (2012) Decreased functional connectivity by aging is associated with cognitive decline. J Cogn Neurosci 24: 2186–2198.

50. Park DC, Reuter-Lorenz P (2009) The adaptive brain: aging and neurocognitive scaffolding. Annu Rev Psychol 60: 173–196.

51. Geerligs L, Renken RJ, Saliasi E, Maurits NM, Lorist MM (2014) A Brain-Wide Study of Age-Related Changes in Functional Connectivity. Cereb Cortex.

52. Wu T, Zang Y, Wang L, Long X, Hallett M, et al. (2007) Aging influence on functional connectivity of the motor network in the resting state. Neurosci Lett 422: 164–168.

53. Friston KJ, Williams S, Howard R, Frackowiak RS, Turner R (1996) Movement-related effects in fMRI time-series. Magn Reson Med 35: 346–355.

54. Uddin LQ, Kelly AM, Biswal BB, Xavier Castellanos F, Milham MP (2009) Functional connectivity of default mode network components: correlation, anticorrelation, and causality. Hum Brain Mapp 30: 625–637.

55. Konishi S, Wheeler ME, Donaldson DI, Buckner RL (2000) Neural correlates of episodic retrieval success. Neuroimage 12: 276–286.

56. Wang X, Jiao Y, Tang T, Wang H, Lu Z (2013) Investigating univariate temporal patterns for intrinsic connectivity networks based on complexity and low-frequency oscillation: a test-retest reliability study. Neuroscience 254: 404–426.

57. Filippini N, MacIntosh BJ, Hough MG, Goodwin GM, Frisoni GB, et al. (2009) Distinct patterns of brain activity in young carriers of the APOE-epsilon4 allele. Proc Natl Acad Sci U S A 106: 7209–7214.

58. Washington SD, Gordon EM, Brar J, Warburton S, Sawyer AT, et al. (2014) Dysmaturation of the default mode network in autism. Hum Brain Mapp 35: 1284–1296.

59. Saad ZS, Gotts SJ, Murphy K, Chen G, Jo HJ, et al. (2012) Trouble at rest: how correlation patterns and group differences become distorted after global signal regression. Brain Connect 2: 25–32.

60. Hayasaka S (2013) Functional connectivity networks with and without global signal correction. Front Hum Neurosci 7: 880.

61. Reuter-Lorenz PA, Park DC (2010) Human neuroscience and the aging mind: a new look at old problems. J Gerontol B Psychol Sci Soc Sci 65: 405–415.

62. Bressler SL, Kelso JA (2001) Cortical coordination dynamics and cognition. Trends Cogn Sci 5: 26–36.

63. Grady CL, Protzner AB, Kovacevic N, Strother SC, Afshin-Pour B, et al. (2010) A multivariate analysis of age-related differences in default mode and task-positive networks across multiple cognitive domains. Cereb Cortex 20: 1432–1447.

64. Persson J, Nyberg L (2006) Altered brain activity in healthy seniors: what does it mean? Prog Brain Res 157: 45–56.

65. Smith EE, Geva A, Jonides J, Miller A, Reuter-Lorenz P, et al. (2001) The neural basis of task-switching in working memory: effects of performance and aging. Proc Natl Acad Sci U S A 98: 2095–2100.

66. Clapp WC, Rubens MT, Sabharwal J, Gazzaley A (2011) Deficit in switching between functional brain networks underlies the impact of multitasking on working memory in older adults. Proc Natl Acad Sci U S A 108: 7212–7217.

67. Buckner RL, Andrews-Hanna JR, Schacter DL (2008) The brain's default network: anatomy, function, and relevance to disease. Ann N Y Acad Sci 1124: 1–38.

68. Fransson P (2005) Spontaneous low-frequency BOLD signal fluctuations: an fMRI investigation of the resting-state default mode of brain function hypothesis. Hum Brain Mapp 26: 15–29.

69. Dolcos F, Rice HJ, Cabeza R (2002) Hemispheric asymmetry and aging: right hemisphere decline or asymmetry reduction. Neurosci Biobehav Rev 26: 819–825.

70. Cabeza R (2002) Hemispheric asymmetry reduction in older adults: the HAROLD model. Psychol Aging 17: 85–100.

71. Ongur D, Price JL (2000) The organization of networks within the orbital and medial prefrontal cortex of rats, monkeys and humans. Cereb Cortex 10: 206–219.

72. Menon V, Levitin DJ (2005) The rewards of music listening: response and physiological connectivity of the mesolimbic system. Neuroimage 28: 175–184.

73. Mather M (2012) The emotion paradox in the aging brain. Ann N Y Acad Sci 1251: 33–49.

74. Nashiro K, Sakaki M, Mather M (2012) Age differences in brain activity during emotion processing: reflections of age-related decline or increased emotion regulation? Gerontology 58: 156–163.

75. Zezula J, Cortes R, Probst A, Palacios JM (1988) Benzodiazepine receptor sites in the human brain: autoradiographic mapping. Neuroscience 25: 771–795.

76. la Fougere C, Grant S, Kostikov A, Schirrmacher R, Gravel P, et al. (2011) Where in-vivo imaging meets cytoarchitectonics: the relationship between cortical thickness and neuronal density measured with high-resolution [18F]flumazenil-PET. Neuroimage 56: 951–960.

77. Morrison JH, Hof PR (2007) Life and death of neurons in the aging cerebral cortex. Int Rev Neurobiol 81: 41–57.

78. Morrison JH, Hof PR (2002) Selective vulnerability of corticocortical and hippocampal circuits in aging and Alzheimer's disease. Prog Brain Res 136: 467–486.

79. Wang X, Michaelis ML, Michaelis EK (2010) Functional genomics of brain aging and Alzheimer's disease: focus on selective neuronal vulnerability. Curr Genomics 11: 618–633.

80. Gianaros PJ, Hariri AR, Sheu LK, Muldoon MF, Sutton-Tyrrell K, et al. (2009) Preclinical atherosclerosis covaries with individual differences in reactivity and functional connectivity of the amygdala. Biol Psychiatry 65: 943–950.

81. Uddin LQ, Kelly AM, Biswal BB, Castellanos FX, Milham MP (2009) Functional connectivity of default mode network components: correlation, anticorrelation, and causality. Hum Brain Mapp 30: 625–637.

82. Andrews-Hanna JR, Reidler JS, Sepulcre J, Poulin R, Buckner RL (2010) Functional-anatomic fractionation of the brain's default network. Neuron 65: 550–562.

21

Revealing a Brain Network Endophenotype in Families with Idiopathic Generalised Epilepsy

Fahmida A. Chowdhury[1,2☯¶], **Wessel Woldman**[3☯¶], **Thomas H. B. FitzGerald**[1,4], **Robert D. C. Elwes**[2], **Lina Nashef**[2], **John R. Terry**[3‡], **Mark P. Richardson**[1,2*‡]

1 Institute of Psychiatry, Psychology and Neuroscience, King's College London, London, United Kingdom, **2** Centre for Epilepsy, King's College Hospital, London, United Kingdom, **3** College of Engineering, Mathematics and Physical Sciences, University of Exeter, Exeter, United Kingdom, **4** Wellcome Trust Centre for Neuroimaging, UCL, London, United Kingdom

Abstract

Idiopathic generalised epilepsy (IGE) has a genetic basis. The mechanism of seizure expression is not fully known, but is assumed to involve large-scale brain networks. We hypothesised that abnormal brain network properties would be detected using EEG in patients with IGE, and would be manifest as a familial endophenotype in their unaffected first-degree relatives. We studied 117 participants: 35 patients with IGE, 42 unaffected first-degree relatives, and 40 normal controls, using scalp EEG. Graph theory was used to describe brain network topology in five frequency bands for each subject. Frequency bands were chosen based on a published Spectral Factor Analysis study which demonstrated these bands to be optimally robust and independent. Groups were compared, using Bonferroni correction to account for nonindependent measures and multiple groups. Degree distribution variance was greater in patients and relatives than controls in the 6–9 Hz band ($p = 0.0005$, $p = 0.0009$ respectively). Mean degree was greater in patients than healthy controls in the 6–9 Hz band ($p = 0.0064$). Clustering coefficient was higher in patients and relatives than controls in the 6–9 Hz band ($p = 0.0025$, $p = 0.0013$). Characteristic path length did not differ between groups. No differences were found between patients and unaffected relatives. These findings suggest brain network topology differs between patients with IGE and normal controls, and that some of these network measures show similar deviations in patients and in unaffected relatives who do not have epilepsy. This suggests brain network topology may be an inherited endophenotype of IGE, present in unaffected relatives who do not have epilepsy, as well as in affected patients. We propose that abnormal brain network topology may be an endophenotype of IGE, though not in itself sufficient to cause epilepsy.

Editor: Satoru Hayasaka, Wake Forest School of Medicine, United States of America

Funding: FAC was funded by a Clinical Research Training Fellowship from the Medical Research Council UK (G0701310, www.mrc.ac.uk). MPR was supported in part by the National Institute for Health Research Biomedical Research Centre at the South London and Maudsley NHS Foundation Trust (http://www.nihr.ac.uk/infrastructure/Pages/infrastructure_biomedical_research_centres.aspx). MPR and JRT are supported by a Medical Research Council UK Programme Grant (MR/K013998/1, www.mrc.ac.uk). The funders had no role in study design, data collection and analysis, decision to publish, or preparation of the manuscript.

Competing Interests: The authors have declared that no competing interests exist.

* Email: mark.richardson@kcl.ac.uk

☯ These authors contributed equally to this work.

¶ FAC and WW are first authors on this work.

‡ JRT and MPR also contributed equally to this work and are last authors on this work.

Introduction

Idiopathic generalised epilepsy (IGE) comprises a group of clinical syndromes which account for 15–20% of all epilepsies [1]. Although the classification scheme for the epilepsies is evolving, the concept of IGE remains robust, consisting of a set of epilepsy disorders characterised by specific well-recognised generalised seizure types. Although IGE may very rarely be a monogenic disorder in a few families [2], typically it has a complex inheritance suggesting susceptibility is associated with multiple genes [3].

Generalised spike-wave (GSW) seen in EEG is a hallmark of IGE, and reflects abnormal hypersynchronous electrical activity within brain networks. There is at present much interest concerning the structural and functional nature of brain networks

in which seizures arise [4] and how these factors give rise to specific seizure types or epilepsy syndromes. The complexity of the brain makes it challenging to study, but a well-developed approach to characterising complex networks, graph theory, has recently had a substantial impact on the investigation of data relating to brain networks [5]. Graph theory enables local and global characteristics of network connectivity to be computed and compared between subjects. Brain networks can be inferred from EEG by examining the patterns of association between EEG signals (correlation, synchronisation etc), based on the ability of EEG to capture information about multiple brain sources of activity. It is assumed that neuronal activity in distributed brain networks is reflected in multiple sources of independent activity detectable in scalp EEG, and that examining interactions between the signals obtained by different EEG electrodes is a reasonable proxy for examining interactions between the underlying sources which constitute the brain network. Graph theory can be used to summarize structural topological features of brain networks; these structural properties may have a key influence on the dynamics which the network can generate [4]. Abnormality of brain dynamics is evident in epilepsy as the paroxysmal occurrence of seizures, therefore it is logical to propose that these abnormal dynamics may be dependent on abnormal network topology. The aim of this study is to use graph theory applied to EEG to explore the hypothesis that abnormal properties of brain networks are a component of the inherited phenotype in IGE.

Investigations of the complex genetics of brain disorder have in some instances made important progress through investigating endophenotypes, heritable traits with a simpler genetic basis than the full disorder, which may be present in family members who do not have the disease [6]. Measures of network topology have been suggested as potential endophenotypes [5]. It is noteworthy that some basic EEG-derived network metrics obtained using graph theory, particularly clustering coefficient and average path length, show high heritability in healthy subjects, especially in the alpha frequency band [7,8]. Studies of the maturation of brain networks in children [9] suggest that normal development is characterised by a gradual alteration of the balance between the strength of local connectivity, presumably reflecting cortical localisation of function, and the strength of long-range connections which presumably reflects the functional integration between localised regions required for normal brain function. From a graph theoretic perspective, this balance is reflected in the small-world index. Given that IGE may often have onset in childhood and remit with maturation, we specifically hypothesise that brain networks in people with IGE and their relatives will show altered network properties compared to healthy controls, and that this may have a basis in aberrant development.

Interpretation of EEG in a clinical setting typically uses five broad frequency bands defined according to prominent features visible to an expert observer. A recent literature has sought to establish the frequency bands in which EEG oscillatory activity is maximally independent, hypothesising that such maximally-independent bands may represent different neurobiological generators, and may be optimally sensitive to differences between subjects or experimental manipulations. Although the conventional clinical EEG frequency bands relate to qualitative features seen in the EEG, it is not necessarily the case that these conventional bands optimally reflect the underlying generators. Furthermore, given that brain network features in the alpha band may show evidence of heritability [7,8], and that antiepileptic drug treatment my alter peak alpha frequency [10], we particularly focus on the alpha range through dividing into sub-bands. Here, we adopt the frequency bands defined by Spectral Factor Analysis (SFA) in two independent datasets of resting EEG activity [11], in which these bands were shown to be extremely robust to a range of methods used to determine the bands, artefact rejection schemes and scalp electrode positions.

Materials and Methods

Recruitment and selection of participants

Subjects with IGE were identified from five hospitals in London and outlying regions, and were a consecutive series that met the inclusion and exclusion criteria and were able to participate. Inclusion criteria for patients were age>18 years old, a diagnosis of IGE, and ≥ 2 family members with epilepsy according to self-

report. Twenty-eight families were recruited; in 16 families the reported presence of epilepsy in more than one family member was confirmed by us from history and investigation; in the other 12 families, the reportedly affected family members were not available for assessment. In addition to the affected probands, clinically unaffected first degree relatives were recruited from the 28 families. These unaffected relatives were interviewed in detail by a neurologist (FAC) and had no evidence of symptomatic seizures from detailed history. Furthermore, in addition to the EEG study carried out as part of this investigation, all unaffected relatives underwent diagnostic MRI which was in all cases normal. Healthy participants with no personal or family history of neurological or psychiatric diseases were recruited via a local research participant database. Participants were excluded if they had any other neuropsychiatric condition or a full scale IQ (FSIQ) <70. Ethical approval was obtained from King's College Hospital Research Ethics Committee (08/H0808/157). Written informed consent was obtained from all participants. We recently reported the neuropsychometric findings in this cohort of patients, relatives and controls [12].

EEG acquisition

Conventional 10–20 scalp EEG was collected using a NicoletOne system (Viasys Healthcare, San Diego, California, USA), 19 channels, sampling rate 256 Hz, bandpass filtered 0.3–70 Hz. EEG was carried out using the same system in the same recording room, undertaken by the same EEG technologist using conventional measurement techniques to determine electrode positions. Collection of subjects from the different groups was interleaved over the duration of the study. Ten minutes of awake EEG in all participants and 40 minutes of sleep was obtained where possible. Where specific consent was obtained, hyperventilation and photic stimulation were carried out. Here we examined only the awake EEG.

Conventional expert EEG analysis

The EEGs were reviewed independently by two reviewers (FC and RE). The following features were noted: presence of GSW; focal abnormalities including spikes, sharp waves and slow waves; response to photic stimulation; and normal variants.

Quantitative EEG analysis

EEG data was referenced to the channel average. A single 20 s epoch was selected which included continuous dominant background rhythm with eyes closed, without any artefacts, epileptiform abnormalities or patterns indicating drowsiness or arousal. Epoch selection for analysis was carried out by one investigator (TF) who was blinded to subject group. These EEG epochs were used for all the subsequent analysis methods described below. Our analyses used 5 frequency bands defined from previous literature applying SFA to resting EEG: 1–5 Hz, 6–9 Hz, 10–11 Hz, 12–19 Hz and 21–70 Hz. Although different from the conventional clinical EEG frequency bands, the bands we used here were shown to be extremely robust to a range of methods used to identify the maximally independent bands, artefact rejection schemes and scalp electrode positions [11].

Analyses were performed using a combination of EEGlab toolbox [13], the Brain Connectivity Toolbox [14], in addition to our own custom Matlab (Mathworks, Natick, Massachusetts, USA) scripts for band-pass filtering the EEG data to optimise the rectangular drop-off at the boundary between frequency bands.

Construction of weighted undirected graphs

The Hilbert transform was applied to the band-pass filtered EEG to generate instantaneous phase and amplitude estimates. For each electrode pair and each frequency band, we calculated the phase-locking factor (PLF) [15], a value between 0 and 1 reflecting the strength of synchronous activity between each pair. We assumed that each electrode is represented by a vertex in a graph with edge strength between vertices determined by the relevant PLF. All PLF analyses were carried out using custom scripts implemented in Matlab (available from authors on request). Note that we therefore construct weighted graphs, with each edge taking the value of the corresponding PLF.

Degree distribution, clustering coefficient, characteristic path length

For each individual, we characterise the degree distribution by establishing the strength of each vertex through summing the PLF values associated with the edges connected to that vertex and then using the mean and variance of these vertex strengths, denoted by K and D respectively. The clustering coefficient C indexes the tendency of a network to form local clusters; the path length L is a measure of how well the nodes of the network are interconnected [16]. C and L are sensitive to changes in network degree distribution [16,17]. To control for this, we calculated normalised metrics $\hat{C} = \frac{C}{C^{surr}}$ and $\hat{L} = \frac{L}{L^{surr}}$ where C^{surr} and L^{surr} are the mean clustering coefficient and characteristic path length of a distribution of 500 surrogate random networks [16,17]. We calculated $\hat{C}$ and $\hat{L}$ for each subject for each frequency band network. All network topology analyses were carried out using the Brain Connectivity Toolbox [14].

Statistical testing

To explore differences in the proportions of each group showing qualitative EEG abnormalities we used a Chi-squared test with significance threshold of $p = 0.05$ two-tailed, Bonferroni-corrected for three between-group comparisons.

Prior to testing, all quantitative measures were tested for normality and a non-normal distribution was observed. Thus a non-parametric Kruskal-Wallis test was used to examine for effects in each measure across the three groups and five frequency bands; results were declared significant at $p<0.05$ two-tailed, Bonferroni corrected for five frequency bands. Where the Kruskall-Wallis test was significant, we investigated further using Mann-Whitney tests to compare between pairs of groups for each frequency band. Results were declared significant when $p<0.05$ after Bonferroni correction for three between-group comparisons.

Results

We studied 117 participants: 40 normal controls (20 female, mean age 30.7 yrs), 35 patients with IGE (21 female, mean age 34.4 yrs), and 42 unaffected first-degree relatives of patients with IGE (19 female, mean age 36.0 yrs). The age and gender distributions of the groups were not significantly different (all $p>0.05$ uncorrected). Clinical details of the patients who participated in the study are presented in Table 1. Thirteen patients and 8 relatives refused photic stimulation because of the risk of provoking a seizure.

Qualitative Analysis

Patients were more likely to have generalised epileptiform discharges compared with relatives and controls (17/35 patients, 2/42 relatives, 0/40 controls; chi-squared with Fisher's exact test,

one-sided $p<0.0001$ Bonferroni corrected in both instances), but there was no significant difference in the proportion of relatives with generalised epileptiform discharges compared with normal controls ($p = 0.27$ uncorrected). There were no significant differences between any pair of groups in the proportions of subjects with focal discharges, positive photoparoxysmal response or normal variants.

Graph theoretic metrics (Figure 1, Table 2)

Mean degree (K) differed between the groups only in the 6–9 Hz band (Kruskall-Wallis $p = 0.0064$, Bonferroni corrected for five frequency bands). Subsequent comparison of group pairs revealed that K was higher in the patients than normal controls (Mann-Whitney $p = 0.0008$, Bonferroni corrected for three between-group comparisons); in relatives, K was higher than healthy controls and lower than patients but did not differ significantly from either group. Degree distribution variance (D) showed a difference between the three groups only in the 6–9 Hz band ($p = 0.0005$, Bonferroni corrected for five frequency bands). Examining paired comparisons between groups, D was higher in patients and relatives than in normals in this band ($p = 0.0005$ and $p = 0.0009$ respectively, Bonferroni corrected). Clustering coefficient ($\hat{C}$) differed between the three groups only in the 6–9 Hz band ($p = 0.0018$, Bonferroni corrected). $\hat{C}$ was greater in the patients and relatives than in normal controls ($p = 0.0025$ and $p = 0.0013$ respectively, both Bonferroni corrected). There were no differences between groups for $\hat{L}$. There were no other significant differences or trends between groups in any other frequency band, comparing controls, patients and relatives. In particular, there were no differences between patient and relative groups in any frequency band for any measure.

Discussion

In this study we show that brain network topology, as inferred from scalp EEG, differs between normal subjects and patients with IGE. Moreover, we show that brain network topology differs between normal subjects and unaffected first-degree relatives of people with IGE – and that unaffected relatives and patients have similar networks. Although it is conceivable that EEG network features in the patients may differ from normal subjects as a result of antiepileptic drug treatment, the unaffected relatives were not taking medication. We conclude that brain network topology may be a component of an inherited endophenotype of IGE, and not dependent on medication effects.

We have previously reviewed in detail the literature describing brain networks in epilepsy using a wide range of approaches, not only graph theory [18]. We are not aware of prior literature examining brain network data from unaffected relatives of patients with IGE; however there is a small published literature examining brain networks of patients with IGE, using graph theory methods, in comparison with normal controls. A small study examined interictal MEG in five adults with absence epilepsy and five matched controls [19]. Using coherence as the measure of interaction between channels, the authors found that average node strength, clustering coefficient, and global efficiency were all greater in patients than normal controls; these findings would be in keeping with ours. A group of 26 adults with IGE characterised by generalized tonic-clonic seizures was compared with 26 normal controls using fMRI and DTI [20]. The brain was parcellated into a large number of nodes, and connectivity between all pairs of nodes estimated from both datasets. The results were somewhat inconsistent between methods, but a decrease in small worldness and a decrease in clustering coefficient were found comparing

Table 1. Clinical characteristics of the patients.

Gender	Age	Syndrome	Age of onset (years)	Seizures and frequency	Time since last seizure	Medications (total daily dose mg)	EEG	MRI
M	26	GTCS	5	GTCS 1/month	2 weeks	Sodium Valproate 1600, Topiramate 200, Lamotrigine 100	GSW	Normal
M	25	GTCS	11	GTCS 3/month	3 weeks	Sodium Valproate 300	GSW	Normal
F	45	GTCS	2	SF	36 years	(none)	Normal	N/A
M	31	GTCS	8	GTCS 6/year	1 month	Sodium Valproate 2000, Zonisamide 250, Levetiracetam 500, Lamotrigine 100	GSW, Ph+	N/A
F	18	JAE	7	GTCS 1/month, Abs SF	1 week	Ethosuximide 250, Lamotrigine 600	GSW	Normal
F	20	GTCS	0.5	SF	9 years	(none)	Normal	N/A
M	49	GTCS	26	SF	1 year	(none)	GSW	Normal
F	21	JAE	10	SF	4 years	Lamotrigine 400, Ethosuximide 500	GSW	Normal
F	20	JME	13	MJ weekly, GTCS SF	1 week	Sodium Valproate 1000	GSW	Normal
M	59	JME	14	SF	10 years	(none)	GSW	N/A
F	19	GTCS	15	GTCS 4/year	3 months	Levetiracetam 2000	GSW	Normal
F	28	Unclassified	20	SF	7 years	Carbamazepine 200	Normal	Normal
F	23	CAE	8	SF	6 years	Sodium Valproate 800, Lamotrigine 25	GSW	Normal
M	48	JME	17	SF	5 years	Sodium Valproate 1500, Topiramate 200, Carbamazepine 600	GSW, PSW	N/A
F	32	CAE	4	GTCS SF, Abs weekly	1 weeks	(none)	GSW	N/A
M	30	Unclassified	11	SF	3 years	(none)	Normal	N/A
F	28	JME	15	SF	13 years	Sodium Valproate 1400	PSW	N/A
F	41	JME	11	GTCS rare, MJ weekly	1 week	Levetiracetam 1000, Lamotrigine 500, Zonisamide 200	GSW, PSW	N/A
M	45	CAE	3	SF	2 years	Sodium Valproate 1400, Levetiracetam 2000	GSW	N/A
M	31	Unclassified	8	SF	10 years	Sodium Valproate 400	Normal	Normal
M	27	Unclassified	16	SF	10 years	Carbamazepine 1200	Normal	N/A
F	39	GTCS	22	SF	10 years	Carbamazepine 200	GSW	Normal
M	28	CAE	4	SF	5 years	Sodium Valproate 600, Levetiracetam 750, Lamotrigine 250	GSW	N/A
F	18	JME	15	MJ SF, GTCS 1/month	4 months	Levetiracetam 1000	GSW	N/A
F	36	GTCS	21	GTCS 2/year	2 months	Levetiracetam 1750	GSW, Ph+	Normal
F	43	CAE	7	SF	10 years	(none)	GSW	N/A
M	28	GTCS	8	SF	1 year	Sodium Valproate 400	GSW	N/A
F	53	GTCS	3	GTCS SF, Abs daily	1 day	(none)	GSW, Ph+	Normal
F	33	JAE	12	GTCS 3/year	4 months	Topiramate 400	GSW, Ph+	Normal
F	55	GTCS	16	SF	25 years	(none)	Normal	N/A
M	26	CAE	5	SF	8 years	(none)	GSW	N/A
F	47	JAE	11	Abs daily, GTCS SF	1 day	Levetiracetam 2000	PSW	Normal
M	25	JME	14	GTCS 5/year, MJ weekly	1 week	Valproate	GSW	Normal
F	20	JME	15	MJ 2/month	2 weeks	Lamotrigine 400, Levetiracetam 1500	GSW	Normal
F	21	Absences with eyelid myoclonia	6	Abs daily, MJ weekly	1 day	Lamotrigine 500	PSW	N/A

CAE childhood absence epilepsy, GTCS generalised tonic clonic seizures only, JAE juvenile absence epilepsy, JME juvenile myoclonic epilepsy, MJ myoclonic jerks, Abs absences, Ph + Photosensitivity; GSW generalised spike and wave, PSW polyspike and wave; SF Seizure Free; N/a not available.

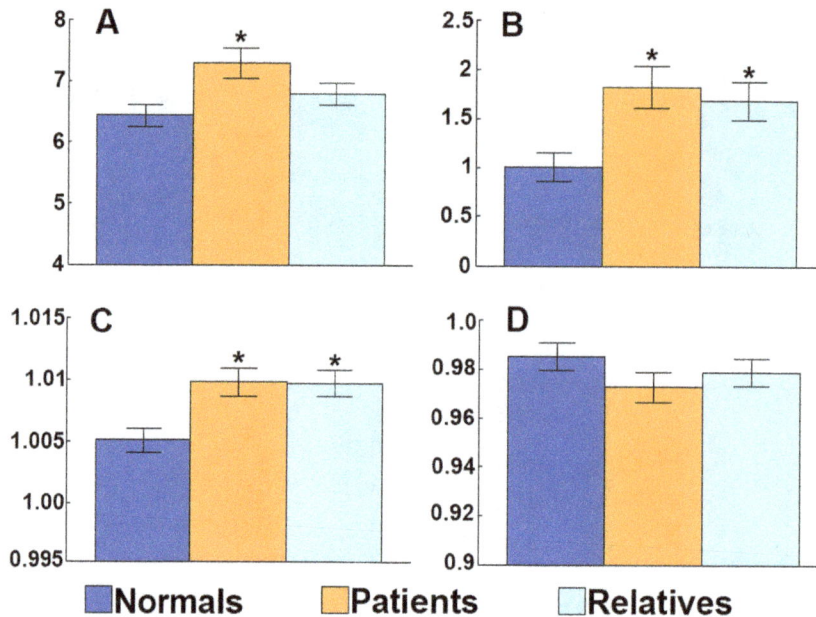

Figure 1. An abnormal EEG network topology is an endophenotype of IGE, present in patients and first-degree relatives. Group means +/- standard error of the mean are shown for: (A) mean degree K, (B) mean degree variance D, (C) clustering coefficient $\hat{C}$, and (D) normalised path length $\hat{L}$, in the 6–9 Hz band. Normal controls (dark blue), patients with IGE (orange), and first-degree relatives of patients with IGE (light blue). * = $p<0.05$ Bonferroni corrected compared with normal controls.

patients with normals. A further study also used DTI to compare brain networks in 18 children with childhood absence epilepsy with 18 matched normal controls [21]. This study found that the network connection strength, clustering coefficient, local efficiency and global efficiency were decreased in the patients, and the characteristic path length increased. Although some of these findings are contradictory to our findings and those of [19], at the current time, it is extremely difficult to reconcile results found with MRI methods with those found using EEG/MEG.

Animal models of childhood absence epilepsy (CAE) show abnormalities in a complex brain network comprising a combination of a focal cortical region which drives the onset of generalised seizure discharges in thalamocortical networks, and an abnormality of anterior transcallosal pathways [22,23]; this transcallosal abnormality has also been found in human juvenile myoclonic epilepsy (JME) [24], hence there is a justification to propose that large-scale brain network abnormalities are a feature of IGE. A large study of recent-onset IGE demonstrated 34–49% failed to achieve 12-month remission with first-line antiepileptic drugs [25], indicating an urgent need for better treatment based on improved mechanistic understanding of IGE. This improved understanding is likely to emerge from detailed phenotyping, genotyping, and the development of explanatory models. It seems likely that seizures emerge in large-scale brain networks through the interaction between brain network structure and the dynamics of the brain regions which constitute the network nodes [26]. We introduce the term "brain network ictogenicity" to describe the likelihood seizures will emerge from a brain network. In this study, we show that one contributor to brain network ictogenicity – network structure – is abnormal in IGE patients compared with healthy controls, and that a similar abnormality is observed in the unaffected relatives of the patients. We propose that our findings in the current study contribute to a more detailed phenotype of IGE and have implications for future genetic studies.

Fundamental to our approach is to identify a brain network endophenotype of IGE. An endophenotype is a heritable trait which is a component of a disorder or associated with high liability to develop the disorder. An endophenotype may be present in family members who do not have the disease, hence increasing the power of genetic studies, and its inheritance is likely to be simpler than the full disorder [6]. This concept has been extensively exploited in other common brain disorders with complex inheritance, such as schizophrenia [27]. Given the universal availability of EEG, and that GSW is a cardinal feature of IGE, EEG is an obvious place to look for an IGE endophenotype. It has been shown that 0.5% of unaffected adults and 1.8% of unaffected children under 16 yrs may show GSW [28,29]. Unaffected first-degree relatives of patients with IGE show a much higher prevalence of GSW: 8–40% of unaffected siblings under 16 yrs had GSW when awake and up to 72% when asleep [30,31]; but only 6–9% of unaffected siblings over 16 yrs had GSW [31,32]. Therefore GSW may be an endophenotype of limited usefulness in adults, since, if IGE is explained by complex inheritance, at least 50% of first-degree relatives of patients with IGE should share one or more genes contributing to the IGE phenotype.

Conventional expert EEG review of our subjects revealed GSW in 49% of patients, 5% of relatives and zero controls; these findings are expected, and suggest that our cohort is unexceptional. Finding GSW in some "unaffected" relatives might suggest the possibility that some relatives in fact have unsuspected epilepsy. Although we concede this is possible, our detailed assessment of the relatives did not reveal any evidence of symptomatic seizures in any of the unaffected relatives group; post hoc exclusion of the two relatives with GSW does not alter the effects found.

Measures of EEG network topology differed between groups, revealing strong similarities between brain networks of patients and first degree relatives. For networks inferred from EEG band-pass filtered in the 6–9 Hz band, both the mean degree and mean degree variance was lower in normals than either patients or

Table 2. Summary of effects found comparing three groups (normal controls, patients, relatives).

Measure	Comparison	1–5 Hz Uncorr.	1–5 Hz Bonferroni corrected	6–9 Hz Uncorr.	6–9 Hz Bonferroni corrected	10–11 Hz Uncorr.	10–11 Hz Bonferroni corrected	12–19 Hz Uncorr.	12–19 Hz Bonferroni corrected	21–70 Hz Uncorr.	21–70 Hz Bonferroni corrected
Mean degree	difference between groups	0.9513		0.0013	0.0064	0.9321		0.5501		0.5435	
Mean degree	normals vs patients			0.0003	0.0008						
Mean degree	normals vs relatives			0.0514							
Mean degree	relatives vs patients			0.0718							
Mean degree variance	difference between groups	0.8795		0.0001	0.0005	0.8533		0.6280		0.0441	0.2206.
Mean degree variance	normals vs patients			0.0002	0.0005						
Mean degree variance	normals vs relatives			0.0003	0.0009						
Mean degree variance	relatives vs patients			0.5947							
Clustering coefficient	difference between groups	0.9003		0.0004	0.0018	0.7291		0.5370		0.1315	
Clustering coefficient	normals vs patients			0.0008	0.0025						
Clustering coefficient	normals vs relatives			0.0004	0.0013						
Clustering coefficient	relatives vs patients			0.8780							
Characteristic path length	difference between groups	0.5920		0.0814		0.4343		0.3798		0.8177	
Characteristic path length	normals vs patients										
Characteristic path length	normals vs relatives										
Characteristic path length	relatives vs patients										

For details of Bonferroni correction see Methods. Uncorr = uncorrected.

relatives. This indicates that the variability in the number of connections per network node is greater in patients and relatives, revealing the existence of a brain network endophenotype characterised by both unusually overconnected brain regions (hubs) and underconnected brain regions.

Comparison of epilepsy patients taking antiepileptic drugs with unmedicated normal controls introduces the potential confound that effects found may be due to the drugs and not due to the disease. We cannot exclude this possibility in our study. However, the relatives were unmedicated, therefore the comparison of relatives with controls does not suffer this confound.

Our network analyses were carried out in "sensor space" – that is, networks were constructed which described the interactions between activities at the EEG electrodes, rather than the interactions between the brain sources which generated these activities. The limited spatial sampling of routine clinical EEG would not readily permit source reconstruction, but future studies should attempt to identify the origins of these network properties in the brain.

We chose to examine weighted graphs, in contrast to some studies (eg. [33]) which have examined unweighted graphs. An unweighted graph is produced by choosing a threshold for edge weight, and assigning the value of an edge as either zero or one according to this threshold. As has been discussed in detail elsewhere [34], there are limitations to either approach. One practical limitation in our data is that our networks have only 19 nodes, therefore the range of possible network degree is limited; the consequence of this is that defining an unweighted network using a high threshold (or low network degree) would have the consequence that many networks will fall apart into disconnected components and therefore could not be validly compared; whereas using a low threshold (or high network degree) would have the outcome that the networks would tend to be fully connected (ie. every possible edge is present) therefore there would be very limited possibility to identify any difference between networks. Given these limitations, we argue that using a weighted unthresholded approach is preferable. Furthermore, some studies have compared between groups the weights of individual edges; we chose here to examine global properties, but have also examined for differences in individual edge strength finding no differences that survived Bonferroni correction.

There is an inherent problem in work of this kind, which may be described as the problem of reducing bias due to common sources of EEG activity seen at more than one scalp electrode, and which encompasses both the selection of reference electrode and consideration of the effect of volume conduction in selection of the method to determine interaction between EEG timeseries. The problem of common sources is well-known and does not have a single optimal solution [35] [36] [37]. We chose here to use an average reference, and to use a measure of interaction between EEG timeseries, PLF, which detects synchronization at zero phase lag. Note that previous work shows this combination of measure and reference is able to detect real differences in synchronization [37]; we are currently examining alternative measures of synchronization which may be less sensitive to volume conduction.

An important consideration in any experimental work is whether results are reliable and can be reproduced. An important strength of our study is the sample size: we have 117 subjects, and detected very large effect sizes, which is a strong defence against error. However, an important question is whether results are stable if a different epoch of EEG data were chosen from each subject. The difficulty of identifying artefact-free EEG data epochs of 20 s from every subject should not be underestimated – EEG is highly prone to movement, blink and other artefacts – and we chose to identify artefact-free epochs rather than clean the data using artefact removal tools. Hence, we were not able to find more than one suitable epoch for every subject. Nonetheless, post hoc, we sought to examine the stability of our findings by dividing the single epoch from each subject into two equal non-overlapping epochs of half the length (which we labelled epoch 1 and epoch 2). We repeated an identical analysis for both epochs from all subjects: in the analysis of the full 20 s epoch, we report five pairwise comparisons that reached significance using Bonferroni correction; using epoch 1 for every subject, the same 5 comparisons remained significant; using the epoch 2, three of the five comparisons remained significant and two were at the level of strong trend (and were significant without Bonferroni correction). Furthermore, the comparison between patients and relatives of mean degree, degree distribution variance, and clustering coefficient revealed no differences using the full 20 s epoch, and also revealed no differences using either epoch 1 or epoch 2. Therefore, our findings are reproducible within two non-overlapping epochs of EEG data. Nonetheless, we recognise that the reliability of our findings needs to be established in an independent dataset.

It is not yet established whether individual syndromes of IGE are entirely unrelated, with no shared aetiologic, genetic or mechanistic factors, or represent a continuum or set of overlapping disorders with important shared pathophysiology. We recognise in this context a divergence of views between those who seek to identify individual syndromes on the basis of highly detailed phenotyping, and those who seek common aetiological and mechanistic factors across the range of common IGE syndromes, as we do here. In this study, we specifically seek shared factors between families and between different IGE syndromes, hypothesising that there are likely to be shared genetic and mechanistic factors between different IGE syndromes [38] [39,40]. We note this approach has been highly successful in recent genetic studies, which have identified recurrent chromosomal microdeletions as the most frequent identifiable genetic factor associated with all the common IGE syndromes studied here [41–43]. For example, the most frequently identified microdeletions each accounted for patients with at least three of the four common IGE syndromes included in our study here [42]: Microdeletions at 15q11.2 were identified in patients with JME, JAE, CAE and GTCS; microdeletions at16p13.11 were found in JME, CAE and GTCS; and microdeletions at 15q13.3 were found in JAE, JME and CAE. We argue that these genetic findings strongly support our argument that a similar brain network endophenotype might be found across the range of common IGE syndromes.

In summary, we show here for the first time the existence of a brain network endophenotype of IGE, present in relatives and patients. We propose that our findings have significant implications for the current mechanistic understanding of IGE, and for future phenotyping and genetics studies.

Acknowledgments

We are grateful for the expert assistance of Mrs Devyani Amin (Chief EEG Technician) and her team.

Author Contributions

Conceived and designed the experiments: FAC WW THBF RDCE LN JRT MPR. Performed the experiments: FAC. Analyzed the data: FAC WW THBF RDCE JRT. Contributed reagents/materials/analysis tools: RDCE LN JRT. Wrote the paper: FAC WW THBF RDCE LN JRT MPR.

References

1. Jallon P, Latour P (2005) Epidemiology of idiopathic generalized epilepsies. Epilepsia 46 Suppl 9: 10–14.
2. Helbig I, Scheffer IE, Mulley JC, Berkovic SF (2008) Navigating the channels and beyond: unravelling the genetics of the epilepsies. Lancet Neurol 7: 231–245.
3. Pal DK, Strug LJ, Greenberg DA (2008) Evaluating candidate genes in common epilepsies and the nature of evidence. Epilepsia 49: 386–392.
4. Richardson M (2010) Current themes in neuroimaging of epilepsy: brain networks, dynamic phenomena, and clinical relevance. Clin Neurophysiol 121: 1153–1175.
5. Bullmore E, Sporns O (2009) Complex brain networks: graph theoretical analysis of structural and functional systems. Nat Rev Neurosci 10: 186–198.
6. Gottesman II, Gould TD (2003) The endophenotype concept in psychiatry: etymology and strategic intentions. Am J Psychiatry 160: 636–645.
7. Smit DJ, Stam CJ, Posthuma D, Boomsma DI, de Geus EJ (2008) Heritability of "small-world" networks in the brain: a graph theoretical analysis of resting-state EEG functional connectivity. Hum Brain Mapp 29: 1368–1378.
8. Smit DJ, Boersma M, van Beijsterveldt CE, Posthuma D, Boomsma DI, et al. (2010) Endophenotypes in a dynamically connected brain. Behav Genet 40: 167–177.
9. Power JD, Fair DA, Schlaggar BL, Petersen SE (2010) The development of human functional brain networks. Neuron 67: 735–748.
10. Tuunainen A, Nousiainen U, Pilke A, Mervaala E, Partanen J, et al. (1995) Spectral EEG during short-term discontinuation of antiepileptic medication in partial epilepsy. Epilepsia 36: 817–823.
11. Shackman AJ, McMenamin BW, Maxwell JS, Greischar LL, Davidson RJ (2010) Identifying robust and sensitive frequency bands for interrogating neural oscillations. Neuroimage 51: 1319–1333.
12. Chowdhury FA, Elwes RDC, Koutroumanidis M, Morris RG, Nashef L, et al. (in press) Impaired cognitive function in IGE and unaffected family members: an epilepsy endophenotype. Epilepsia.
13. Delorme A, Makeig S (2004) EEGLAB: an open source toolbox for analysis of single-trial EEG dynamics including independent component analysis. J Neurosci Methods 134: 9–21.
14. Rubinov M, Sporns O (2010) Complex network measures of brain connectivity: uses and interpretations. Neuroimage 52: 1059–1069.
15. Tass P, Rosenblum MG, Weule J, Kurths J, Pikovsky A, et al. (1998) Detection of n:m phase locking from noisy data: application to magnetoencephalography. Phys Rev Lett 81: 3291–3294.
16. Stam CJ, de Haan W, Daffertshofer A, Jones BF, Manshanden I, et al. (2009) Graph theoretical analysis of magnetoencephalographic functional connectivity in Alzheimer's disease. Brain 132: 213–224.
17. Stam CJ, Jones BF, Nolte G, Breakspear M, Scheltens P (2007) Small-world networks and functional connectivity in Alzheimer's disease. Cereb Cortex 17: 92–99.
18. Richardson MP (2012) Large scale brain models of epilepsy: dynamics meets connectomics. J Neurol Neurosurg Psychiatry 83: 1238–1248.
19. Chavez M, Valencia M, Navarro V, Latora V, Martinerie J (2010) Functional modularity of background activities in normal and epileptic brain networks. Phys Rev Lett 104: 118701.
20. Zhang Z, Liao W, Chen H, Mantini D, Ding JR, et al. (2011) Altered functional-structural coupling of large-scale brain networks in idiopathic generalized epilepsy. Brain 134: 2912–2928.
21. Xue K, Luo C, Zhang D, Yang T, Li J, et al. (2014) Diffusion tensor tractography reveals disrupted structural connectivity in childhood absence epilepsy. Epilepsy Res 108: 125–138.
22. Meeren H, van Luijtelaar G, Lopes da Silva F, Coenen A (2005) Evolving concepts on the pathophysiology of absence seizures: the cortical focus theory. Arch Neurol 62: 371–376.
23. Chahboune H, Mishra AM, DeSalvo MN, Staib LH, Purcaro M, et al. (2009) DTI abnormalities in anterior corpus callosum of rats with spike-wave epilepsy. Neuroimage 47: 459–466.
24. O'Muircheartaigh J, Vollmar C, Barker GJ, Kumari V, Symms MR, et al. (2011) Focal structural changes and cognitive dysfunction in juvenile myoclonic epilepsy. Neurology 76: 34–40.
25. Marson A, Jacoby A, Johnson A, Kim L, Gamble C, et al. (2005) Immediate versus deferred antiepileptic drug treatment for early epilepsy and single seizures: a randomised controlled trial. Lancet 365: 2007–2013.
26. Terry JR, Benjamin O, Richardson MP (2012) Seizure generation: The role of nodes and networks. Epilepsia 53: e166–169.
27. Allen AJ, Griss ME, Folley BS, Hawkins KA, Pearlson GD (2009) Endophenotypes in schizophrenia: a selective review. Schizophr Res 109: 24–37.
28. Gregory RP, Oates T, Merry RT (1993) Electroencephalogram epileptiform abnormalities in candidates for aircrew training. Electroencephalogr Clin Neurophysiol 86: 75–77.
29. Gerken H, Doose H (1973) On the genetics of EEG-anomalies in childhood 3. Spikes and waves. Neuropadiatrie 4: 88–97.
30. Degen R, Degen HE, Roth C (1990) Some genetic aspects of idiopathic and symptomatic absence seizures: waking and sleep EEGs in siblings. Epilepsia 31: 784–794.
31. Doose H, Baier WK (1987) Genetic factors in epilepsies with primarily generalised minor seizures. Neuropaediatrics 18 (Suppl 1): 1–64.
32. Jayalakshmi SS, Mohandas S, Sailaja S, Borgohain R (2006) Clinical and electroencephalographic study of first-degree relatives and probands with juvenile myoclonic epilepsy. Seizure 15: 177–183.
33. Quraan MA, McCormick C, Cohn M, Valiante TA, McAndrews MP (2013) Altered resting state brain dynamics in temporal lobe epilepsy can be observed in spectral power, functional connectivity and graph theory metrics. PLoS One 8: e68609.
34. van Wijk BC, Stam CJ, Daffertshofer A (2010) Comparing brain networks of different size and connectivity density using graph theory. PLoS One 5: e13701.
35. Guevara R, Velazquez JL, Nenadovic V, Wennberg R, Senjanovic G, et al. (2005) Phase synchronization measurements using electroencephalographic recordings: what can we really say about neuronal synchrony? Neuroinformatics 3: 301–314.
36. Peraza LR, Asghar AU, Green G, Halliday DM (2012) Volume conduction effects in brain network inference from electroencephalographic recordings using phase lag index. J Neurosci Methods 207: 189–199.
37. Stam CJ, Nolte G, Daffertshofer A (2007) Phase lag index: assessment of functional connectivity from multi channel EEG and MEG with diminished bias from common sources. Hum Brain Mapp 28: 1178–1193.
38. Andermann F, Berkovic SF (2001) Idiopathic generalized epilepsy with generalized and other seizures in adolescence. Epilepsia 42: 317–320.
39. Blumenfeld H (2005) Cellular and network mechanisms of spike-wave seizures. Epilepsia 46 Suppl 9: 21–33.
40. Motelow JE, Blumenfeld H (2009) Functional neuroimaging of spike-wave seizures. Methods Mol Biol 489: 189–209.
41. Helbig I, Mefford HC, Sharp AJ, Guipponi M, Fichera M, et al. (2009) 15q13.3 microdeletions increase risk of idiopathic generalized epilepsy. Nat Genet 41: 160–162.
42. de Kovel CG, Trucks H, Helbig I, Mefford HC, Baker C, et al. (2010) Recurrent microdeletions at 15q11.2 and 16p13.11 predispose to idiopathic generalized epilepsies. Brain 133: 23–32.
43. Dibbens LM, Mullen S, Helbig I, Mefford HC, Bayly MA, et al. (2009) Familial and sporadic 15q13.3 microdeletions in idiopathic generalized epilepsy: precedent for disorders with complex inheritance. Hum Mol Genet 18: 3626–3631.

22

White and Grey Matter Changes in the Language Network during Healthy Aging

Yanhui Yang[1,2◊], Bohan Dai[3,4◊], Peter Howell[5], Xianling Wang[6], Kuncheng Li[1,2,7]*, Chunming Lu[3,4]*

1 Department of Radiology, Xuanwu Hospital, Capital Medical University, Beijing, P.R. China, 2 Key Laboratory for Neurodegenerative Diseases, Ministry of Education, Beijing, P.R. China, 3 State Key Laboratory of Cognitive Neuroscience and Learning & IDG/McGovern Institute for Brain Research, Beijing Normal University, Beijing, P.R. China, 4 Center for Collaboration and Innovation in Brain and Learning Sciences, Beijing Normal University, Beijing, P.R. China, 5 Division of Psychology and Language Sciences, University College London, London, United Kingdom, 6 Department of Neurology, Xuanwu Hospital, Capital Medical University, Beijing, P.R. China, 7 Beijing Key laboratory of Magnetic Resonance Imaging and Brain Informatics, Beijing, P.R. China

Abstract

Neural structures change with age but there is no consensus on the exact processes involved. This study tested the hypothesis that white and grey matter in the language network changes during aging according to a "last in, first out" process. The fractional anisotropy (FA) of white matter and cortical thickness of grey matter were measured in 36 participants whose ages ranged from 55 to 79 years. Within the language network, the dorsal pathway connecting the mid-to-posterior superior temporal cortex (STC) and the inferior frontal cortex (IFC) was affected more by aging in both FA and thickness than the other dorsal pathway connecting the STC with the premotor cortex and the ventral pathway connecting the mid-to-anterior STC with the ventral IFC. These results were independently validated in a second group of 20 participants whose ages ranged from 50 to 73 years. The pathway that is most affected during aging matures later than the other two pathways (which are present at birth). The results are interpreted as showing that the neural structures which mature later are affected more than those that mature earlier, supporting the "last in, first out" theory.

Editor: Thomas Arendt, University of Leipzig, Germany

Funding: This work was supported by the National Natural Science Foundation of China (31270023), the Fund of Capital Medical University (No. 11JL24), the National Basic Research Program of China (973 Program; 2012CB720704), the Fundamental Research Funds for the Central Universities, the Beijing Higher Education Young Elite Teacher Project, and the Open Research Fund of the State Key Laboratory of Cognitive Neuroscience and Learning. The funders had no role in study design, data collection and analysis, decision to publish, or preparation of the manuscript.

* Email: luchunming@bnu.edu.cn (CL); cjr.likuncheng@vip.163.com (KL)

◊ These authors contributed equally to this work.

Introduction

Dealing with the effects of healthy aging is one of the biggest challenges facing the world today. Studies have shown that aging brings with it significant changes in white and grey matter (WM and GM) architecture that serve various functions [1,2]. The neural changes that happen during aging have been explained by the "last in, first out" (LIFO) theoretical principle [3,4]. Studies have shown that the late-myelinating neocortical regions are most vulnerable to aging and aging-related disease, whereas the primary motor and sensory regions that myelinate early are more resistant to these changes, only being affected at later ages [5,6]. Consistent with this, a recent large-scale longitudinal volume examination of both neural development and aging confirmed that cortices that develop late are especially vulnerable to atrophy in aging [7]. However, there is also evidence showing that aging-related WM change occurs in specific fiber bundles that do not follow LIFO [8–10]. Thus, alternative principles such as "first in, first out" (FIFO) are also plausible. According to FIFO, the neural structures that mature earlier would be the first to be affected after maturity.

It is well known that myelination can markedly increase speed of signal transmission, which is important for the integration of information across the highly distributed neural networks that underlie higher cognitive functions such as memory, executive functions, and language. Aging is associated with reduction of length of myelinated axons, which might have a marked impact on those higher cognitive brain functions that are most susceptible to these changes [3]. Here aging-related neural structure changes in the language network were examined as this has received little attention.

It is well established that areas of the brain that deal with language are connected by: 1) A ventral pathway between the mid-to-anterior superior temporal cortex (STC) and the ventral inferior frontal cortex (IFC) and insula traversing the extreme capsule; and 2) Two dorsal pathways passing via the arcuate fasciculus and the superior longitudinal fasciculus (SLF). One of these two pathways connects the mid-to-posterior STC (Wernicke's area) with the premotor cortex, and the other one connects Wernicke's area with the IFC (Broca's area) via the premotor cortex [11–14]. Recent evidence has shown that the ventral pathway is present at birth as is the dorsal pathway that connects the STC and the premotor cortex [15]. However, the dorsal pathway that connects the STC and the IFC is not detectable in newborns [15] and appears to mature late [16].

A cross-sectional design was used to examine how the neural structures for language that mature at different ages are affected during healthy aging. Participants' ages covered a 24-year range (from 50 to 70+ years). Two independent groups of participants were recruited. The data from the second group were used to validate the results obtained from the first group. Both fractional anisotropy (FA) of WM fibers and cortical thickness of GM were examined to establish the relationship between WM and GM changes during aging. LIFO would predict that neural structures that lie in the dorsal pathway connecting the STC with the IFC would be affected more than those that lie in the other two pathways during aging, whereas FIFO would predict the opposite pattern.

Methods

Participants

Two groups of right-handed native Mandarin speakers were recruited. The first group included thirty-six participants whose ages ranged from 55 to 79 years (Mean = 63 years, S.D. = 6.34, 16 females). The second group included twenty participants whose ages ranged from 50 to 73 years (Mean = 61 years, S.D. = 7.23, 9 females). The large age range made correlation analysis between age and neural structure indexes feasible. All participants had hearing loss within age-appropriate ranges, and eyesight deterioration was corrected by glasses. The amount of education participants received ranged from 3 to 17 years (Mean = 10 years, S.D. = 3.28) for the first group and from 8 to 14 years (Mean = 12 years, S.D. = 1.97) for the second group. In order to exclude potential cognitive impairment, all participants were assessed by the Mini Mental State Examination (MMSE) [17]. The MMSE scores indicated that the cognitive functions of these participants were all within the normal range (group one: from 24 to 30, Mean = 28, S.D. = 1.61; group two: from 28 to 30, Mean = 29, S.D. = 0.74). Additional clinical assessment also showed that no participant had cognitive or neurological problems. All participants were right-handed, as assessed by the Edinburgh Handedness Inventory [18].

Ethics Statement

Written informed consent was obtained from each participant. The study protocol was in compliance with the Code of Ethics of the World Medical Association (Declaration of Helsinki) and was approved by the Research Ethics Committee of Xuanwu Hospital, Capital Medical University.

Imaging data acquisition

Imaging data were acquired from all participants on a Siemens TRIO 3T scanner at Xuanwu Hospital. Participants lay supine within the scanner with their head secured with foam padding. Structural images were obtained first from each participant with a high resolution T1-weighted MP-RAGE sequence. Then, the DTI images were obtained using an echo planar imaging (EPI) sequence. The scanning parameters are given in the Supporting Information (Text S1).

Imaging data analysis

The two groups were not compared directly because the scanning parameters differed. Regions-of-interest (ROIs) identified from the whole-brain analyses of the first group were examined in the data from the second group.

Analyses of group one

DTI data analysis. All DTI images were processed following the TBSS pipeline which is part of the FMRIB Software Library (FSL, http://www.fmrib.ox.ac.uk/fsl). Briefly, images were preprocessed to correct for motion and eddy current distortion, and the diffusion tensors were fitted to each voxel. The measure of FA was derived voxel-wise. The TBSS registration then nonlinearly transformed the FA images using the FMRIB58_FA standard space image (http://www.fmrib.ox.ac.uk/fsl/data/FMRIB58_FA.html) as the target, and the tract skeletonization process was subsequently performed using a threshold FA of 0.2 to exclude non-WM voxels. The final WM skeleton is a representation of the WM tract geometry common to the entire group of participants.

Whole-brain FA skeletons were regressed with age using a general linear model (GLM) method. Sex and education were included as covariates. Statistical parametric maps were thresholded at a voxel-wise level of $P<0.05$ (corrected by Monte Carlo simulation method, individual voxel $P<0.01$, cluster size$>$ 13 mm^3). The Monte Carlo simulation used the 3dCustSim program of AFNI (Analysis of Functional NeuroImages, see http://afni.nimh.nih.gov/pub/dist/doc/program_help/3dClustSim.html) on the WM skeleton image [19,20].

Cortical thickness analysis. Cortical surface reconstruction and thickness measurements were performed using the FreeSurfer toolkit (http://surfer.nmr.mgh.harvard.edu/). Briefly, the structural image data of each participant were motion-corrected and the volume data were obtained. Cerebral GM/WM was then segmented and the GM/WM boundaries were estimated [21]. Topological defects at the GM/WM boundaries were corrected [22]. The boundaries were then used in a deformable surface algorithm designed to find the pial surface with submillimeter precision [23]. Cortical thickness measurements were obtained by calculating the distance between the GM/WM boundary and pial surface at each of approximately 160,000 points (per hemisphere) across the cortical mantle [23].

The surface representing the GM/WM border was "inflated" [24], differences among individuals in the depth of gyri and sulci were normalized, and each participant's reconstructed brain was then morphed and registered to an average spherical surface representation that optimally aligned sulcal and gyral features across participants [24,25]. Thickness measures were then mapped to the inflated surface of each participant's reconstructed brain [24]. The data were smoothed on the surface using an iterative nearest-neighbor averaging procedure with a full width at half maximum of 10 mm. The data were then resampled into a common spherical coordinate system [25]. Further details of the method are available elsewhere [21,23,24,26,27].

A surface map was generated by regressing the cortical thickness with age using a GLM method ($P<0.05$, corrected by Monte Carlo simulation method on the segmented GM image, individual voxel $P<0.01$, cluster size$>$ 100 mm^2). Sex and education were included as covariates.

ROI validation of the aging-related neural changes. Because the correlation in the whole-brain analysis might be slightly above threshold in one region but slightly below threshold in another region, it was possible that this would lead to spurious difference in correlations among regions. In order to address this issue, a regression analysis was conducted on the WM/GM regions, where whole-brain analysis showed significant results, to test for differences in age correlations across regions. The analysis was conducted using IBM SPSS software (version 20, http://www.ibm.com/software/analytics/spss/).

The analysis involved the following steps. First, two groups of ROIs were selected: 1) Brain regions where significant correlations with age in WM/GM were found in the whole-brain analysis (see *Results*); 2) Two brain regions in the ventral pathway were selected as controls that mature earlier than the target dorsal pathway. The first control region was a WM control region in the extreme capsule underlying the anterior STC [EC-STC, x, y, z = -43, -5, -24 in Montreal Neurological Institute (MNI) template, radius = 3 mm]. This was located according to ICBM-DTI-81 atlas [28,29] that is distributed with FSL software. The second control region was a GM control region in the anterior STC (x, y, z = -49, -5, -24 in MNI template, radius = 3 mm) located according to the spherical coordinate system in Freesurfer [25]. Cortical thickness or FA values were then extracted from these ROIs for each participant, and transformed into Fisher's z-values. Then a regression analysis was conducted, in which all WM ROIs and the interactions between these WM ROIs were included as independent variables (see *Results*), and age was the dependent variable. A similar analysis was conducted on the GM ROIs. Finally, the results were corrected at $P<0.05$ level using a false discovery rate (FDR) method (FDR toolbox, http://www-personal.umich.edu/~nichols/FDR/, running under MatLab, http://www.mathworks.cn/products/matlab/). It was hypothesized that if LIFO applies, the ROIs that lie in the dorsal language pathway connecting the STC with the IFC should make a significant contribution to the change with age, but the ROIs that lie in the other two language pathways should not. FIFO predicts the opposite pattern.

Consistency among WM/GM changes. To establish whether different brain regions showed similar patterns of neural change with age, the WM ROIs were correlated with each other. The same procedure was conducted on the GM ROIs. The results were corrected at $P<0.05$ level using the FDR method. It was hypothesized that the control WM/GM ROIs would show different patterns of neural changes with age to those seen in the target ROIs. That is, the neural structural changes in the control ROIs would neither correlate significantly with those seen in the target ROIs nor with age.

Consistency between WM and GM changes. Correlations between each WM ROI and each GM ROI were computed to examine the consistency between WM and GM changes with age. The results were corrected at $P<0.05$ level according to the FDR method.

The following additional analyses were conducted in order to further elucidate the relationship between WM and GM changes and to specify which pathways were most affected during aging. First, FA values from all WM ROIs and cortical thickness from all GM ROIs (except for the control ROIs) were averaged separately to generate a grand-averaged FA value (GA-FA) and a grand-averaged cortical thickness value (GA-thickness). The correlation between GA-FA and GA-thickness was computed to examine the general relationship between GM and WM. Second, FA values from WM ROIs in the left (except for the control ROI of the EC-STC) and right hemispheres were averaged separately to generate a left FA value (L-FA) and a right FA value (R-FA). The L-FA and R-FA were correlated to the GA-thickness in order to distinguish the relationship between GM and WM changes in the left and right hemisphere respectively. Third, the ROIs that might be distinctive for, or have a close relationship with, the late-maturing fibers underlying the left IFC, were combined to generate the anterior part (L-A-FA) of the dorsal pathway. The ROIs in the temporal-parietal association cortex were considered as the posterior part (L-P-FA) of the dorsal pathway (see *Results*). L-A-FA and L-P-FA were correlated to GA-thickness to determine the roles of the two parts of the dorsal pathway. In order to confirm the correlation analysis, a regression analysis was conducted. In

this analysis, the GA-thickness was predicted by the L-A, R-FA, L-A-FA, L-P-FA, and interactions between L-A-FA and L-P-FA.

In order to further confirm the relationship between L-FA, R-FA, L-A-FA, L-P-FA and age, an additional regression analysis was conducted that used age as the dependent variable.

Re-examination of the neural changes in group two

In order to validate the results obtained from group one, the ROIs selected from this group were used as masks to extract both FA and cortical thickness for group two. The analysis procedures outlined above were conducted using group one's ROIs with group two's data.

Results

Whole-brain DTI results

In accord with the expectations, there were two brain regions along the late-maturing dorsal pathway that connects the STC with the IFC that showed significant negative correlation with age: One underlies the IFC and precentral gyrus (SLF-IFC/Prg), and the other one underlies the temporal-parietal association cortex (SLF-TP). In addition to these, significant negative correlations were also found in the bilateral inferior fronto-occipital fasciculus underlying the IFC (IFOF-IFC), right forceps minor underlying the medial frontal cortex (FM-MeFC), and the body of the corpus callosum (bCC). Table 1 and Figure 1A summarize these results.

No significant positive correlations were found in either the left or right hemisphere, nor in the extreme capsule of the ventral pathway.

Whole-brain cortical thickness results

Two brain regions along the late-maturing dorsal pathway correlated negatively with age. One was located in the left IFC (pars triangularis, BA47) and the other in the precentral gyrus (Prg, BA4). No significant positive correlations were found (Table 1 and Figure 1B). These results confirmed the DTI results, indicating that brain regions along the dorsal pathway that connects the STC with the IFC showed significant decline of cortical thickness with age, particularly the part that extends to the IFC.

ROI validation of the aging-related neural changes

The first regression analysis included all WM ROIs and their interactions (Left: SLF-IFC/Prg × SLF-TP, SLF-IFC/Prg × IFOF-IFC, SLF-TP × IFOF-IFC, SLF-IFC/Prg × SLF-TP× IFOF-IFC; Right: IFOF-IFC × FM-MeFC) as independent variables. The resultant regression model ($F_{(2,35)} = 32.873$, $P< 0.001$) showed that the left SLF-IFC/Prg ($\beta = -0.368$, $P = 0.026$) and IFOF-IFC ($\beta = -0.498$, $P = 0.003$) accounted for almost 67% of the variance over age ($R^2 = 0.666$). No other variables made significant contributions. The second regression analysis included all GM ROIs and their interactions (IFC, Prg and IFC × Prg). The resultant regression model ($F_{(2,35)} = 13.795$, $P<0.001$) showed that the IFC ($\beta = -0.447$, $P = 0.003$) and Prg ($\beta = -0.369$, $P = 0.011$) accounted for 46% of the variance with age ($R^2 = 0.455$). No other variables made significant contributions. These results indicated that neural changes in both GM and WM of the dorsal pathway connecting the STC with the IFC made significant contributions to the variance with age compared to those in other anatomical positions.

Consistency among WM/GM changes

There was a high level of consistency in the pattern of neural changes among the targeted WM/GM ROIs, but no such

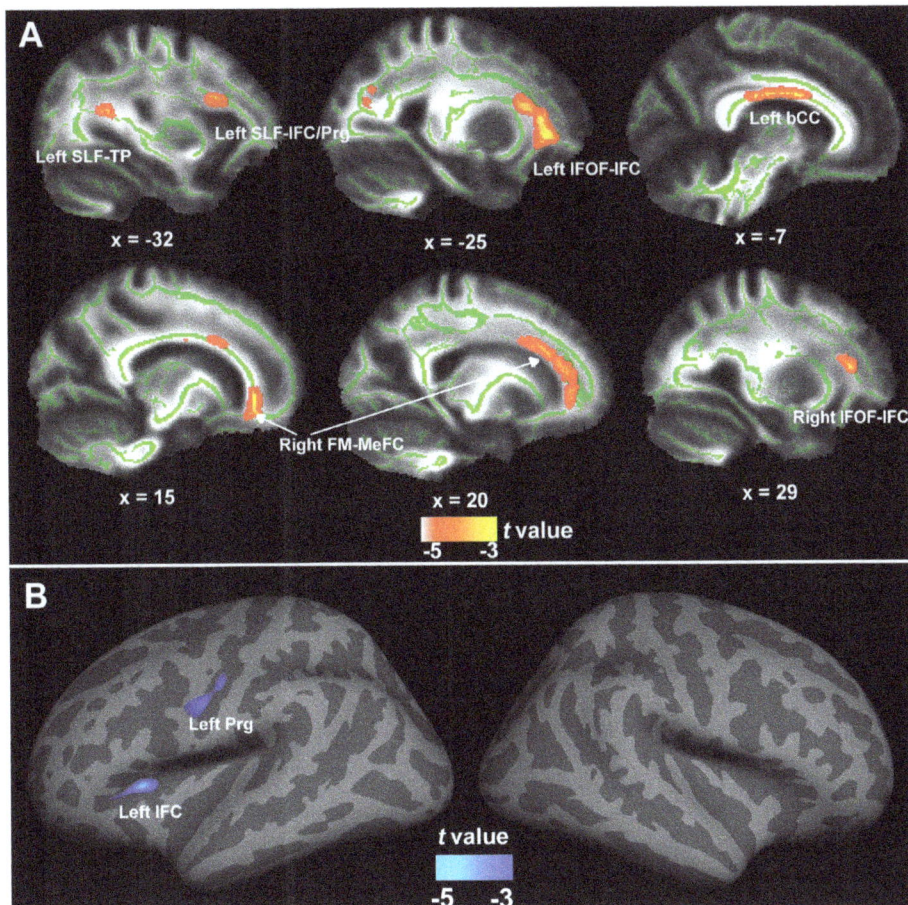

Figure 1. Neural structural changes with age in Group 1. (A) shows FA changes. Note that the skeletonized results are "thickened" to help visualization. Left SLF-IFC/Prg, left superior longitudinal fasciculus underlying the inferior frontal cortex and precentral gyrus; Left SLF-TP, left superior longitudinal fasciculus underlying the temporal-parietal association cortex; Left and right IFOF-IFC, left and right inferior fronto-occipital fasciculus underlying the inferior frontal cortex; Right FM-MeFC, right forceps minor underlying the medial frontal cortex; Left bCC, left body of corpus callosum. (B) shows cortical thickness changes. The colored blobs (blue for cortical thickness, red for FA) indicate brain areas that correlated negatively with age. Left IFC, left inferior frontal cortex; Left Prg, left precentral gyrus. No positive correlations were found.

Table 1. Brain regions showing significant correlations with age in group one.

Brain regions	Position			t-value	Volume (mm³/mm²)
	x	y	z		
White matter (FA) changes					
Left inferior fronto-occipital fasciculus underlying the inferior frontal cortex	−25	33	8	−7.36	634
Left superior longitudinal fasciculus underlying the inferior frontal cortex and precentral gyrus	−32	15	22	−5.88	142
Left superior longitudinal fasciculus underlying the temporal-parietal association cortex	−31	−47	16	−4.185	139
Left body of corpus callosum	−7	3	26	−5.164	465
Right inferior fronto-occipital fasciculus underlying the inferior frontal cortex	29	31	12	−6.704	213
Right Forceps minor underlying the medial frontal cortex	15	34	−4	−5.491	154
	20	21	29	−3.656	153
Grey matter (cortical thickness) changes					
Left inferior frontal cortex (pars triangularis, BA47)	−31	21	12	−3.199	165
Left precentral gyrus (BA4)	−43	−14	29	−2.614	331

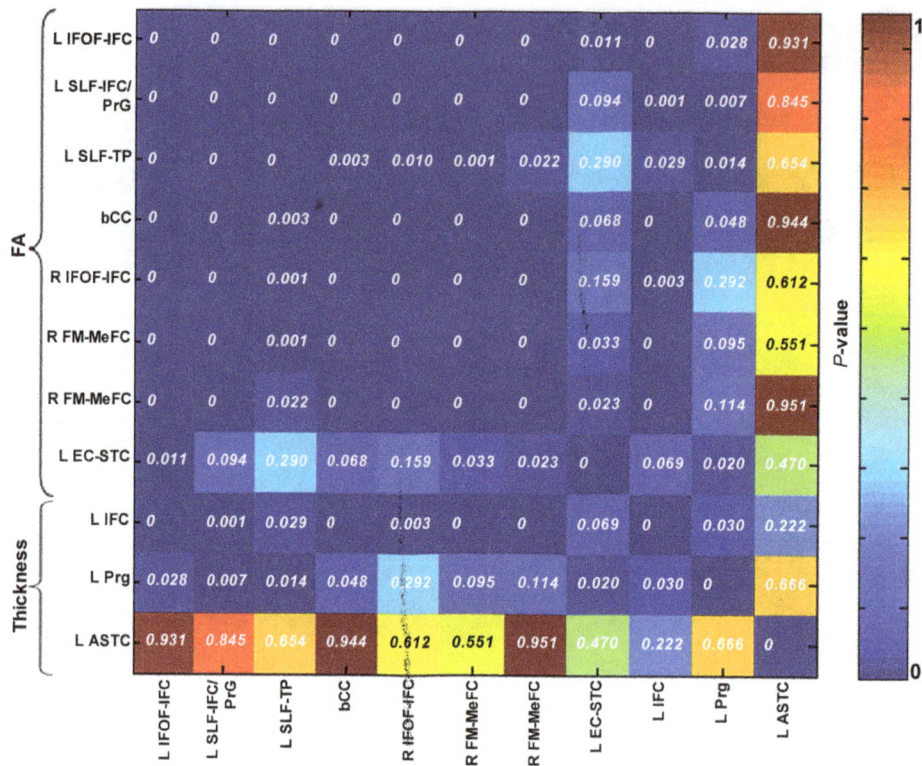

Figure 2. Consistency among WM/GM and between WM and GM matter changes in Group 1. The correlation matrix among all ROIs, including both GM and WM matter, are given.

consistency between the target ROIs and the control ROIs ($P < 0.05$) (Figure 2).

Consistency between WM and GM changes

As Figure 2 shows, FA of all WM ROIs except for the SLF-TP ($r = 0.364$, $P = 0.029$) showed significant positive correlations with cortical thickness of the IFC ($P<0.05$), but, only FA of the SLF-IFC/Prg and SLF-TP correlated significantly with cortical thickness of the Prg ($r = 0.442$, $P = 0.007$; $r = 0.405$, $P = 0.014$). These results indicated that the change of FA value in the SLF-IFC/Prg was more closely related to the change of cortical thickness than other regions.

An additional analysis showed that GA-FA (averaged from all WM ROIs except for the control ROI of EC-STC) and GA-thickness (averaged from the IFC and Prg) correlated significantly with each other ($r = 0.586$, $P<0.001$), but neither showed significant correlation with the control ROIs (between GA-FA and STC: $r = 0.008$, $P = 0.964$; between GA-thickness and EC-STC: $r = 0.385$, $P = 0.02$ after FDR correction). Consequently, further correlation analyses were not conducted. The regression analysis was conducted next.

The regression analysis included L-A-FA (averaged from the SLF-IFC/Prg and IFOF-IFC), L-P-FA (i.e., the SLF-TP), R-FA (averaged from the right IFOF-IFC and FM-MeFC), bCC, and the control ROI of EC-STC as independent variables, and GA-thickness was the dependent variable. The regression model ($F_{(1, 34)} = 18.301$, $P<0.001$) showed that the L-A-FA ($\beta = 0.592$, $P<0.001$) accounted for 35% of the GA-thickness variance ($R^2 = 0.35$), whereas other WM ROIs did not make significant contributions (Figure 3A). Additional regression analysis using age as the dependent variable showed that the L-A-FA ($\beta = -0.815$,

$P<0.001$) accounted for about 65% of the variance with age ($R^2 = 0.654$, $F_{(1, 34)} = 67.143$, $P<0.001$), whereas other variables did not make significant contributions (Figure 3B).

Together, these results indicated that the dorsal pathway that connects the STC with the IFC showed significant aging-related change in both GM and WM, whereas the ventral pathway and the dorsal pathway connecting the STC with the premotor cortex (i.e., no extension to the IFC) did not. Overall the results supported the LIFO account.

Re-examination of the neural changes in group two

Results of whole-brain and ROI analyses for group two were provided in the Text S1, Table S1, and Figure S1 and S2. Most importantly, the neural changes (i.e., those in the late maturing dorsal pathway) of group one were examined next using group one's ROIs on FA/cortical thickness for participants in group two. The results showed that the regression analysis that used the L-A-FA, L-P-FA, R-FA and their interactions as the independent variables, and age as the dependent variables, showed significant contributions of the L-A-FA ($\beta = -0.669$, $P = 0.001$) to the variance with age ($F_{(1, 18)} = 14.553$, $P = 0.001$) which accounted for about 45% of the variance with age ($R^2 = 0.447$) (Figure 3C). No other variables made significant contributions. These results suggest that the L-A-FA made significant contribution to the variance with age, whereas the L-P-FA and the control ROI of EC-STC did not.

Discussion

This study addressed the theoretical issue about how neural structures that mature at different ages are affected during healthy

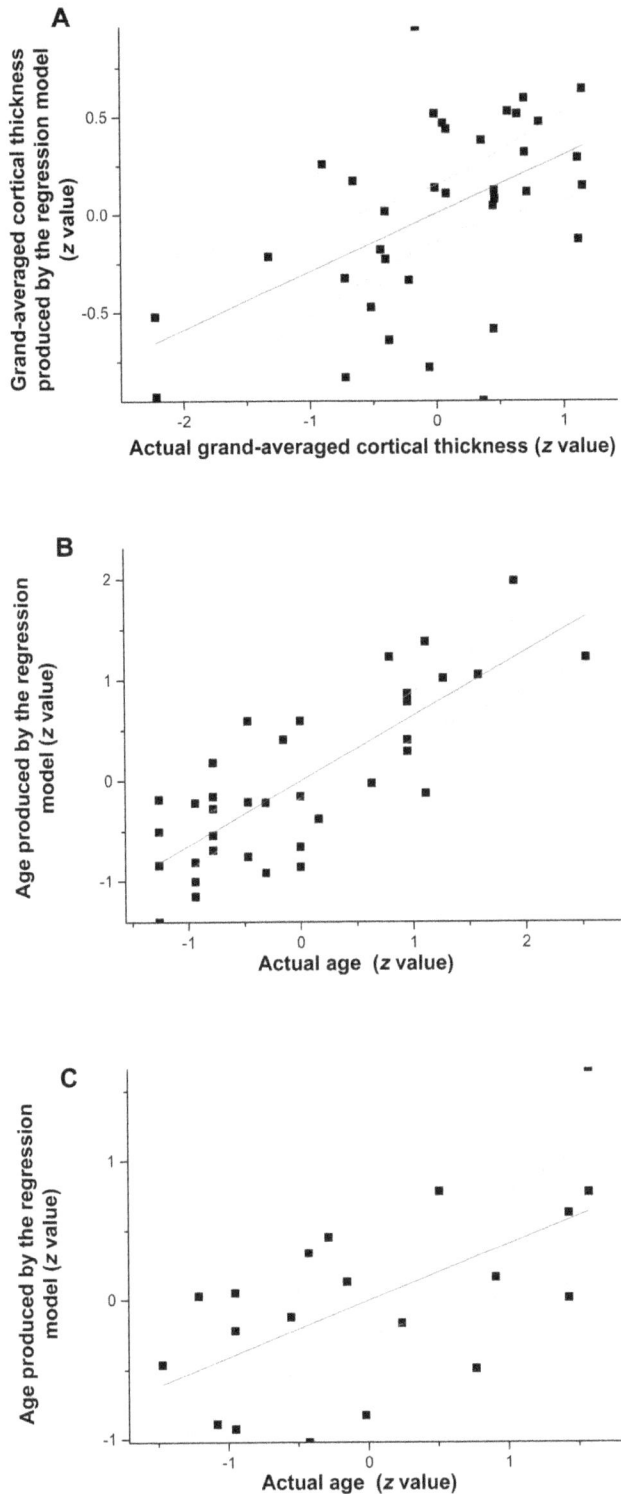

Figure 3. Linear regression fit results. (A) shows fitting result when using grand-averaged cortical thickness as the dependent variable in Group 1. (B) shows fitting result when using age as the dependent variable in Group 1. (C) Re-examination of Group 1's ROI in Group 2's data. Age is the dependent variable. Note that the red line is the linear fit result, whereas the green lines are the confidence internal (95%). For all three panels, the x-axis corresponds to the actual age or cortical thickness, whereas the y-axis corresponds to the age or cortical thickness produced by the regression model.

aging. While LIFO predicts that the neural structures that mature later would be affected more than those that mature earlier, alternative theories such as FIFO predict the opposite pattern. In this study, the results for both groups showed that one of the dorsal language pathways, the one connected by the SLF/arcuate fasciculus between the mid-to-posterior STC and the IFC, was affected more by age with regards to both WM fibers and GM cortical thickness than the other dorsal pathway, the one connecting the STC with the premotor cortex, or the ventral pathway that connects the mid-to-anterior STC with the ventral IFC. These results indicated that the influence of aging on the neural structures serving language is selective, and different neural structures are affected at different stages of aging. Corresponding with this finding, previous evidence has shown that the dorsal and ventral pathways also mature at different ages [15]. While both the ventral pathway connecting the mid-to-anterior STC with the ventral IFC and the dorsal pathway connecting the mid-to-posterior STC and the premotor cortex are clearly present at birth, the other dorsal pathway connecting the STC and the IFC is not [15,16,30]. Thus, the present findings suggested that the neural structures which mature later may be affected more than those that mature earlier, supporting the LIFO account of aging for these structures [31].

The above findings were validated in several additional analyses. First, no significant correlations with age were found in the extreme capsule of the ventral pathway. In order to confirm this, two areas in the ventral pathway were selected and WM and GM were obtained (EC-STC for WM and STC for GM). The results did not show any significant correlations between GM/WM and age in these brain areas, either. Second, the brain areas that correlated significantly with age were highly consistent with each other, but not with the control areas which did not correlate significantly with age, in each group's data. These results further indicated that the affected neural structures were driven by similar underlying biological mechanisms and they were distinct from other unaffected neural structures.

The results showed that only FA of the left anterior part of the dorsal pathway (i.e., the part that is specific to the dorsal pathway connecting the STC and the IFC) correlated significantly with cortical thickness in the left IFC and premotor cortex. Meanwhile, FA at this position was also able to account for a large percent of the variance of age as indicated in the regression analysis. Moreover, the close association between the anterior part of the dorsal fiber tract and the cortical thickness/age were replicated in a second independent group of participants. These results help to elucidate the changes in GM and WM during aging, in that they suggest that both WM and GM are affected in ways that are consistent with the LIFO principle for aging.

There is much evidence showing various neural structural change as aging occurs [1,2], but most of these studies have examined the corpus callosum [4]. One of the robust findings from these studies is that changes in neural structure associated with aging seem to be restricted to the frontal part of the brain, suggesting an anterior-posterior gradient [32–34]. Developmental studies have shown that frontal and temporal association areas are the last ones to myelinate [35]. Together the aging and developmental findings are consistent with the assumption that the brain areas that mature last during development tend to decline first during aging. The current results extend this principle to a large-scale neural network corresponding to a high-level cognitive function (i.e., language).

Bartzokis [3] proposed that oligodendrocytes could be one of the mechanisms that underlie the LIFO of aging. Oligodendrocytes produce myelin and changes in myelinization are crucial for human brain development. The axons in the association brain areas myelinate late. It is estimated that the development of these axons reaches its peak at around the fourth decade of life and continue up to the end of the fifth decade of life [10,36]. The late-differentiating oligodendrocytes cannot produce the same myelin thickness per axon segment as earlier-myelinating oligodendrocytes. The thinner, later-myelinating sheaths are more susceptible to functional impairment and destruction. Thus, later-myelinating neurons of the association areas may be more susceptible to myelin breakdown than earlier-myelinating neurons in the primary motor and visual areas. In addition, this process causes a slow-progressive disruption of neural-impulse transmission that degrades the temporal synchrony of widely distributed neural networks underlying normal brain function. The primary result is large-scale network "disconnection". The present study provided imaging evidence that is consistent with this proposition.

There are several limitations in this study. First, this study did not include younger age ranges and thus could not examine the trajectory of FA and cortical thickness below fifty years of age [37]. Other studies that have examined younger age groups have shown that the development of WM in the prefrontal, temporal, and parietal areas myelinate late and this continues until the end of the fifth decade of life. Other evidence shows that development of WM peaks at around the fourth decade of life [10,36]. Moreover, studies have shown decline of both density of GM [38] and FA of WM [10,36] after age fifty. Thus, it seems that normal aging and late development might partly overlap in some brain areas. Further studies are required to test the development-loss relationship in different brain areas. Second, this study only examined FA of WM and cortical thickness of GM. Future studies are needed to consider whether the development, or aging, process varies with different indexes since different index of neural structures might reflect different aspects of development or aging [39]. Finally, although a cross-sectional design can cover a large age-range, the results need to be addressed using a longitudinal design.

In many countries, the proportion of people aged over 60 years is growing faster than any other age group and this has become a major challenge. There is still much to be learned about the underlying biochemical mechanism of GM/WM changes during aging. In particular, it appears likely that genetic factors may play additional roles in this process. Future studies are needed to

quantify the relationship between neural structure changes and the biochemical and genetic factors and how they relate to cognitive functions such as language. Furthermore, intervention approaches may be developed that are designed to delay the aging process.

Supporting Information

Figure S1 Neural structural changes with age in Group 2. (A) shows FA changes. Note that the skeletonized results are "thickened" to help visualization. Left SLF_Prg, left superior longitudinal fasciculus underlying the precentral gyrus; Left SLF_TP, left superior longitudinal fasciculus underlying the temporal-parietal association cortex; Left FM-MeFC, left forceps minor/uncinate fasciculus near the medial frontal cortex (BA10/32); Right SLF-CC, right superior longitudinal fasciculus/anterior corona radiate underlying the cingulate cortex; Right ATR-CC, anterior thalamic radiation close to the cingulate cortex (BA32). (B) shows cortical thickness changes. The colored blobs (blue for cortical thickness, red for FA) indicate brain areas that showed significant negative correlations with age. No positive correlations were found. Left MFC, left middle frontal gyrus (BA10); Left TP, left inferior parietal gyrus (BA39).

Figure S2 Consistency among WM/GM and between WM and GM matter changes in Group 2. The correlation matrix among all ROIs, including both GM and WM matter, are given.

Table S1 Brain regions showing significant correlations with age for Group 2.

Text S1 Imaging data acquisition and results for Group 2.

Author Contributions

Conceived and designed the experiments: CL KL PH. Performed the experiments: YY BD XW. Analyzed the data: YY BD CL. Wrote the paper: CL PH KL YY BD.

References

1. Wen W, Zhu W, He Y, Kochan NA, Reppermund S, et al. (2011) Discrete neuroanatomical networks are associated with specific cognitive abilities in old age. J Neurosci 31: 1204–1212.
2. Kantarci K, Senjem ML, Avula R, Zhang B, Samikoglu AR, et al. (2011) Diffusion tensor imaging and cognitive function in older adults with no dementia. Neurology 77: 26–34.
3. Bartzokis G (2004) Age-related myelin breakdown: a developmental model of cognitive decline and Alzheimer's disease. Neurobiology of Aging 25: 5–18; author reply 49–62.
4. Sullivan EV, Rohlfing T, Pfefferbaum A (2010) Longitudinal study of callosal microstructure in the normal adult aging brain using quantitative DTI fiber tracking. Dev Neuropsychol 35: 233–256.
5. Hedden T, Gabrieli JD (2004) Insights into the ageing mind: a view from cognitive neuroscience. Nat Rev Neurosci 5: 87–96.
6. Kochunov P, Williamson DE, Lancaster J, Fox P, Cornell J, et al. (2012) Fractional anisotropy of water diffusion in cerebral white matter across the lifespan. Neurobiol Aging 33: 9–20.
7. Tamnes CK, Walhovd KB, Dale AM, Ostby Y, Grydeland H, et al. (2013) Brain development and aging: overlapping and unique patterns of change. Neuro-image 68: 63–74.
8. Madden DJ, Whiting WL, Huettel SA, White LE, MacFall JR, et al. (2004) Diffusion tensor imaging of adult age differences in cerebral white matter: relation to response time. Neuroimage 21: 1174–1181.
9. Salat DH, Tuch DS, Hevelone ND, Fischl B, Corkin S, et al. (2005) Age-related changes in prefrontal white matter measured by diffusion tensor imaging. Annals of the New York Academy of Sciences 1064: 37–49.
10. Westlye LT, Walhovd KB, Dale AM, Bjornerud A, Due-Tonnessen P, et al. (2010) Life-span changes of the human brain white matter: diffusion tensor imaging (DTI) and volumetry. Cereb Cortex 20: 2055–2068.
11. Dehaene-Lambertz G, Hertz-Pannier L, Dubois J, Meriaux S, Roche A, et al. (2006) Functional organization of perisylvian activation during presentation of sentences in preverbal infants. Proc Natl Acad Sci U S A 103: 14240–14245.
12. Saur D, Kreher BW, Schnell S, Kummerer D, Kellmeyer P, et al. (2008) Ventral and dorsal pathways for language. Proceedings of the National Academy of Sciences of the United States of America 105: 18035–18040.
13. Friederici AD, Bahlmann J, Heim S, Schubotz RI, Anwander A (2006) The brain differentiates human and non-human grammars: functional localization and structural connectivity. Proc Natl Acad Sci U S A 103: 2458–2463.
14. Anwander A, Tittgemeyer M, von Cramon DY, Friederici AD, Knosche TR (2007) Connectivity-Based Parcellation of Broca's Area. Cereb Cortex 17: 816–825.
15. Perani D, Saccuman MC, Scifo P, Awander A, Spada D, et al. (2011) Neural language networks at birth. Proceedings of the National Academy of Sciences 108: 16056–16061.
16. Dubois J, Dehaene-Lambertz G, Perrin M, Mangin JF, Cointepas Y, et al. (2008) Asynchrony of the early maturation of white matter bundles in healthy infants: quantitative landmarks revealed noninvasively by diffusion tensor imaging. Hum Brain Mapp 29: 14–27.

17. Folstein MF, Folstein SE, McHugh PR (1975) "Mini-mental state". A practical method for grading the cognitive state of patients for the clinician. J Psychiatr Res 12: 189–198.
18. Oldfield RC (1971) The assessment and analysis of handedness: the Edinburgh inventory. Neuropsychologia 9: 97–113.
19. Xiong J, Gao JH, Lancaster JL, Fox PT (1995) Clustered pixels analysis for functional MRI activation studies of the human brain. Hum Brain Mapp 3: 287–301.
20. Forman SD, Cohen JD, Fitzgerald M, Eddy WF, Mintun MA, et al. (1995) Improved assessment of significant activation in functional magnetic resonance imaging (fMRI): use of a cluster-size threshold. Magnetic Resonance in Medicine 33: 636–647.
21. Dale AM, Fischl B, Sereno MI (1999) Cortical surface-based analysis. I. Segmentation and surface reconstruction. NeuroImage 9: 179–194.
22. Fischl B, Liu A, Dale AM (2001) Automated manifold surgery: constructing geometrically accurate and topologically correct models of the human cerebral cortex. IEEE Transactions on Medical Imaging 20: 70–80.
23. Fischl B, Dale AM (2000) Measuring the thickness of the human cerebral cortex from magnetic resonance images. Proceedings of the National Academy of Sciences of the United States of America 97: 11050–11055.
24. Fischl B, Sereno MI, Dale AM (1999) Cortical surface-based analysis. II: Inflation, flattening, and a surface-based coordinate system. NeuroImage 9: 195–207.
25. Fischl B, Sereno MI, Tootell RB, Dale AM (1999) High-resolution intersubject averaging and a coordinate system for the cortical surface. Human Brain Mapping 8: 272–284.
26. Kuperberg GR, Broome MR, McGuire PK, David AS, Eddy M, et al. (2003) Regionally localized thinning of the cerebral cortex in schizophrenia. Archives of General Psychiatry 60: 878–888.
27. Salat DH, Buckner RL, Snyder AZ, Greve DN, Desikan RS, et al. (2004) Thinning of the cerebral cortex in aging. Cerebral Cortex 14: 721–730.
28. Mori S, Oishi K, Jiang H, Jiang L, Li X, et al. (2008) Stereotaxic white matter atlas based on diffusion tensor imaging in an ICBM template. Neuroimage 40: 570–582.
29. Oishi K, Zilles K, Amunts K, Faria A, Jiang H, et al. (2008) Human brain white matter atlas: identification and assignment of common anatomical structures in superficial white matter. Neuroimage 43: 447–457.
30. Dubois J, Hertz-Pannier L, Dehaene-Lambertz G, Cointepas Y, Le Bihan D (2006) Assessment of the early organization and maturation of infants' cerebral white matter fiber bundles: a feasibility study using quantitative diffusion tensor imaging and tractography. NeuroImage 30: 1121–1132.
31. Davis SW, Dennis NA, Buchler NG, White LE, Madden DJ, et al. (2009) Assessing the effects of age on long white matter tracts using diffusion tensor tractography. NeuroImage 46: 530–541.
32. Pfefferbaum A, Rosenbloom MJ, Adalsteinsson E, Sullivan EV (2007) Diffusion tensor imaging with quantitative fibre tracking in HIV infection and alcoholism comorbidity: synergistic white matter damage. Brain 130: 48–64.
33. Sullivan EV, Pfefferbaum A, Adalsteinsson E, Swan GE, Carmelli D (2002) Differential rates of regional brain change in callosal and ventricular size: a 4-year longitudinal MRI study of elderly men. Cereb Cortex 12: 438–445.
34. Sullivan EV, Rohlfing T, Pfefferbaum A (2010) Quantitative fiber tracking of lateral and interhemispheric white matter systems in normal aging: relations to timed performance. Neurobiology of Aging 31: 464–481.
35. Hill J, Inder T, Neil J, Dierker D, Harwell J, et al. (2010) Similar patterns of cortical expansion during human development and evolution. Proc Natl Acad Sci U S A 107: 13135–13140.
36. Lebel C, Gee M, Camicioli R, Wieler M, Martin W, et al. (2012) Diffusion tensor imaging of white matter tract evolution over the lifespan. Neuroimage 60: 340–352.
37. Bartzokis G (2004) Age-related myelin breakdown: a developmental model of cognitive decline and Alzheimer's disease. Neurobiology of Aging 25: 5–18.
38. Sowell ER, Peterson BS, Thompson PM, Welcome SE, Henkenius AL, et al. (2003) Mapping cortical change across the human life span. Nat Neurosci 6: 309–315.
39. Bartzokis G, Lu PH, Heydari P, Couvrette A, Lee GJ, et al. (2012) Multimodal magnetic resonance imaging assessment of white matter aging trajectories over the lifespan of healthy individuals. Biol Psychiatry 72: 1026–1034.

23

Identifying the Core Components of Emotional Intelligence: Evidence from Amplitude of Low-Frequency Fluctuations during Resting State

Weigang Pan⊋, **Ting Wang**⊋, **Xiangpeng Wang, Glenn Hitchman, Lijun Wang, Antao Chen***

Key Laboratory of Cognition and Personality (Ministry of Education), Faculty of Psychology, Southwest University, Chongqing, China

Abstract

Emotional intelligence (EI) is a multi-faceted construct consisting of our ability to perceive, monitor, regulate and use emotions. Despite much attention being paid to the neural substrates of EI, little is known of the spontaneous brain activity associated with EI during resting state. We used resting-state fMRI to investigate the association between the amplitude of low-frequency fluctuations (ALFFs) and EI in a large sample of young, healthy adults. We found that EI was significantly associated with ALFFs in key nodes of two networks: the social emotional processing network (the fusiform gyrus, right superior orbital frontal gyrus, left inferior frontal gyrus and left inferior parietal lobule) and the cognitive control network (the bilateral pre-SMA, cerebellum and right precuneus). These findings suggest that the neural correlates of EI involve several brain regions in two crucial networks, which reflect the core components of EI: emotion perception and emotional control.

Editor: Xi-Nian Zuo, Institute of Psychology, Chinese Academy of Sciences, China

Funding: This study was supported by "the National Natural Science Foundation of China" (31170980, 81271477) to W. Pan and A. Chen, the Foundation for the Author of National Excellent Doctoral Dissertation of PR China (201107) to A. Chen, the New Century Excellent Talents in University (NCET-10698), and the Fundamental Research Funds for the Central Universities (SWU1009001, SWU1309351) to A. Chen and research fellow. Study design and data collection were supported by "the National Natural Science Foundation of China" (31170980, 81271477). Data analysis, preparation of the manuscript and decision to publish was supported by the Foundation for the Author of National Excellent Doctoral Dissertation of PR China (201107), the New Century Excellent Talents in University (NCET-110698), and the Fundamental Research Funds for the Central Universities (SWU1009001, SWU1309351).

Competing Interests: The authors have declared that no competing interests exist.

* Email: xscat@swu.edu.cn

⊋ These authors contributed equally to this work.

Introduction

Emotional intelligence (EI) is the capacity to process emotional information accurately and effectively, including the ability to monitor one's own and others' feelings and emotions, discriminate among them and use this information to guide one's thinking and actions [1]. There is an increasing body of evidence indicating that EI plays a critical role in daily life. Research has shown that EI can predict successful social interactions [2], job performance [3], mental health [4] and emotional well-being [5]. In contrast, impaired or deficient EI has been linked to certain symptoms, such as substance abuse disorder [6], anxiety and depression [7,8].

EI is generally considered as a multidimensional construct [1,9,10]. Most conceptualizations of this construct address one or more of the following basic components: (i) the ability to be aware of and express emotions; (ii) the ability to be aware of others' feelings; (iii) the ability to manage and regulate emotions; (iv) the ability to realistically and flexibly cope with the immediate situation; and (v) the ability to generate positive affect in order to be sufficiently self-motivated to achieve personal goals [11]. In short, EI includes the ability to engage in sophisticated information processing about one's own and others' emotions and the ability to use this information as a

guide to thinking and behavior [12]. Accordingly, the emotional processing and executive control may be two core processes associated with EI.

Previous neuroimaging studies suggested that the various aspects of EI were supported by separate neural substrates. The social cognition network (SCN) facilitates the understanding of others' feelings, thoughts or desires [13–15]. The SCN includes the medial prefrontal cortex (mPFC) and the superior temporal sulcus (STS), which show altered activity during face recognition and mental state attribution [14], and the temporoparietal junction (TPJ), which is associated with the process of inferring temporary states such as the goals, intentions, and desires of other people [15]. In addition, the inferior frontal gyrus (IFG), amygdala, anterior cingulate cortex, and anterior insula are also important portions of the SCN [14]. From the perspective of large-scale networks, the salience network (with key nodes of anterior insula and anterior cingulate cortex) and central executive network (with key nodes of dorsolateral prefrontal cortex and posterior parietal cortex) were considered to be two key networks in cognition [16]. Another critical network related to EI is the emotion processing network. Leppänen and Nelson suggested that the neural systems that are involved in processing emotional signals from faces include the amygdala, orbitofrontal

Table 1. Means and SDs of WLEIS total and subscale scores.

	EI-total	SEA	OEA	ROE	UOE
Mean	83.20	21.53	21.08	19.73	20.86
SD	14.73	4.53	4.73	5.04	3.80

cortex (OFC), fusiform gyrus and posterior STS [17]. In addition, the anterior insula and anterior cingulate cortex in the salience network were activated in emotional processing [18]. A recent review revealed that the process of experience and perception of emotion involved in broadly distributed functional networks, such as the salience network, executive network and default mode work [19,20]. Structural or anatomical imaging studies (e.g., voxel-based morphometry and diffusion tensor imaging) have found more direct relations between EI and regions in the social emotional processing networks, such as the ventromedial prefrontal cortex, STS, insula and fusiform gyrus [21–23]. Additionally, the top-down control network involving fronto-parietal and cingulo-opercular control networks [24–27] have been linked to control of emotional expression. Specially, the fronto-parietal component seems to initiate and adjust control, while the cingulo-opercular component provides stable set-maintenance, and both are connected to the cerebellar error-network [25,27]. A psychophysiological interactions analysis indicated that volitional regulation of emotions produced distributed alterations in connectivity between visual, attention control, and default networks [28]. Several voxel-based morphometry studies found that some regions in the top-down control network were linked to EI, such as the frontal and inferior parietal areas, precuneus and cerebellum [23,29]. A resting state functional connectivity (RSFC) study found that total trait EI was positively correlated with RSFC between the mPFC and the precuneus, as well as between the left anterior insula and the middle part of the right dorsolateral prefrontal cortex [30].

Although previous studies mainly focused on structural or anatomical neuroimaging to investigate the EI-related brain regions and networks, it is necessary to pay more attention to explore the underlying spontaneous brain activity related to EI. The spontaneous fluctuations in the blood oxygen level dependent (BOLD) signal reveal the intrinsic functional architecture of the brain and relate to extrinsic task performance [31,32]. Moreover, the absence of demanding cognitive activities and instructions makes it more straightforward to compare brain activity across groups that may differ in behavioral performances [33]. Therefore, the task-free resting state spontaneous activity has a unique advantage to investigate the underlying neural basis of EI. The amplitude of spontaneous low-frequency fluctuations (ALFFs) are widely used for measurement of the spontaneous fluctuations in brain activity [34–36]. The ALFF has been suggested to reflect the intensity of regional spontaneous brain activity [34,37]. It has been proved to correlate with task-evoked BOLD responses and is also found to have robust predictive value for behavior [32]. Specially, ALFF has been reported to be associated with cognitive processing abilities (e.g., conceptual processing capacity; object color knowledge performance) [35,38] and personality traits [39,40]. Furthermore, ALFF was considered as promising potential biomarkers of mental disease or disorders, such as bipolar disorder [41], amnestic mild cognitive impairment [42],

PTSD [33] and Parkinson's disease [43]. These findings suggest that ALFF may be an effective indicator to reflect EI-related spontaneous regional brain activity.

To our knowledge, no study has yet investigated the relationship between the resting state fMRI indicator of ALFF and EI. Thus, in the present study, we explored the ALFFs of resting state fMRI signals to elucidate the intrinsic neural basis of EI. As mentioned previously, EI is a multidimensional construct and includes the ability to understand one's own and others' emotions and the ability to regulate and manage emotions. These different processes may involve in emotional information processing and advanced executive control function of the brain. Therefore, we hypothesized that EI might be linked to several brain regions or networks, such as emotion processing networks, cognitive control networks, salience networks or default mode networks.

Methods

Ethics statements

The procedure of this study was approved by the Ethics Committee of the Southwest University. Written informed consent was obtained from all participants. They were informed that the experiment was completely voluntary and they can quit at any time during the experiment. Two of the participants are less than 18 years old, so written informed consent was obtained from their parents on behalf of them.

Participants

One hundred and seventy participants were recruited to take part in this study. Seven of them exhibited excessive head motion and two failed to register to the standard Montreal Neurological Institute (MNI) space in data preprocessing and thus were excluded. Finally, one hundred and sixty-one individuals were included in the formal analysis. All the participants were healthy, right-handed college students (91 females and 70 males; 19.40 ± 1.28 years old, range: 17–25 years old) with no history of neurological or psychiatric disorders. Each participant was required to complete the emotional intelligence scale immediately after the rest-state scanning.

Emotional intelligence scale

All the participants completed the Chinese version of the Wong and Law Emotional Intelligence Scale (WLEIS), a 16-item self-report questionnaire designed to measure trait EI [44]. The scale has been demonstrated to be reliable and valid to assess Chinese trait EI [10,45–47]. The WLEIS is comprised of four subscales: (a) self-emotion appraisal (SEA), (b) others' emotion appraisal (OEA), (c) regulation of emotion (ROE), and (d) use of emotion (UOE) [44]. Examples of WLEIS items are as follows: "I have good understanding of my own emotions" (SEA); "I always know my friends' emotions from their behavior." (OEA); "I have good control of my own emotions." (ROE); "I always encourage myself to try my best." (UOE) [44]. All the responses were made on 7-point Likert-type scales (from 1: strongly disagree, to 7: strongly agree). In the present study, the internal consistency reliabilities (Cronbach αs) of the total scale and four subscales were 0.92, 0.84, 0.92, 0.70 and 0.90, respectively.

Image acquisition

MRI data were obtained using a 3.0 Tesla Siemens Trio scanner (Siemens Medical, Erlangen, Germany) in Southwest University, China. First, high-resolution anatomical images were acquired sagittally with the following parameters: 128 slices, 2530/3.39 ms (TR/TE), 1.33 mm (thickness), 256*256 mm (FOV), 1100 ms (inversion time), 7° (flip angle). In addition, an echoplanar imaging sequence was used to collect resting state functional images, and the acquisition parameters were: 33 axial slices; slice thickness, 3 mm; repetition time (TR), 2 s; echo time (TE), 30 ms; image matrix, 64*64; flip angle, 90°; field of view (FOV), 200*200 mm; and 240 volumes. During the resting state scanning, participants were instructed to lay still with eyes closed, and not to think of anything in particular.

Data preprocessing

The anatomical and functional image preprocessing was performed using SPM8 (Wellcome Department of Conitive Nurology, London, UK, SPM8; http://www.fil.ion.ucl.ac.uk/spm) and Data Processing Assistant for Resting-State fMRI (DPARSF) [48]. The first 10 volumes of the functional images were discarded to ensure the signals approached a dynamic equilibrium. Then, slice timing was used to correct slice order, and head motion correction was performed to estimate and

modify the head movements. Seven participants exhibited head motion >2 mm maximum translation and/or 2° rotation throughout the course of scans, so they did not go into the formal data analysis. Then, each participant's anatomical image was coregistered to the mean functional image and was subsequently segmented. Next, the segmented data was used to normalize all the functional images into standard MNI space in 3*3*3 mm voxel sizes. The normalized images were spatially smoothed with an 8-mm full-width at half maximum (FWHM). After the linear trends were removed, the images were temporally band-pass filtered (0.01–0.08 Hz) to reduce low-frequency drift and high-frequency noise [49].

ALFF analysis

ALFF analysis [34] was performed using the Resting-State fMRI Data Analysis Toolkit (REST 1.8) [50]. According to Zang et al. [34], the time series was transformed to a frequency domain with a fast Fourier transform (FFT) and the power spectrum was then obtained. The obtained power spectrum was square-rooted and averaged across 0.01–0.08 Hz at each voxel, and this averaged square root was taken as the ALFF. The ALFF value of each voxel in the brain was extracted as the sum of amplitudes within the low-frequency range (0.01–0.08 Hz) [35,38]. To reduce the global volume effects of variability across the participants, the ALFF maps were divided by whole brain mean ALFF values. Because low-frequency fluctuations are sensitive to signals in the gray matter [38], we calculated ALFFs only in the gray mask. Following the methods of Wang et al. [35] and Wei et al. [38], we included voxels with a probability

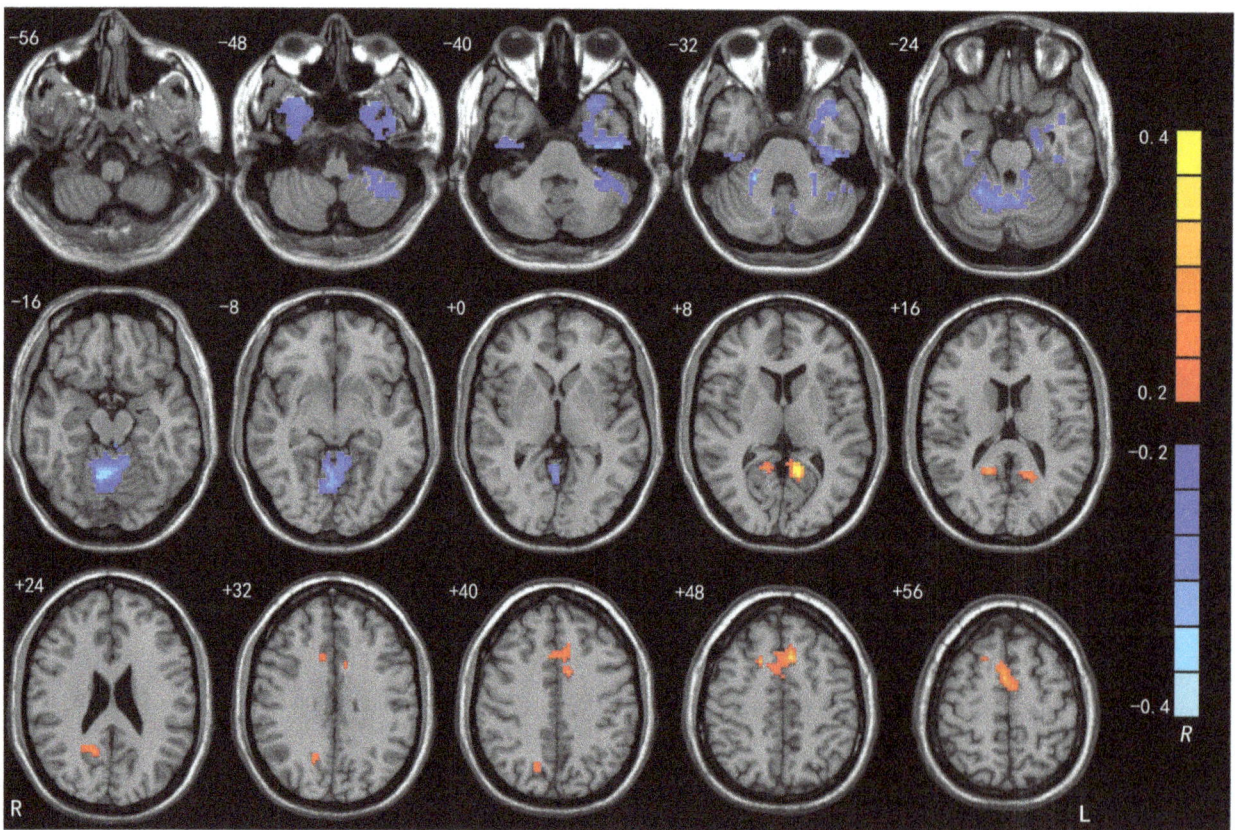

Figure 1. Brain regions which exhibited significant correlations between ALFFs and WLEIS total scores. Color bars represent R values. The results are shown with $p<0.05$ (corrected).

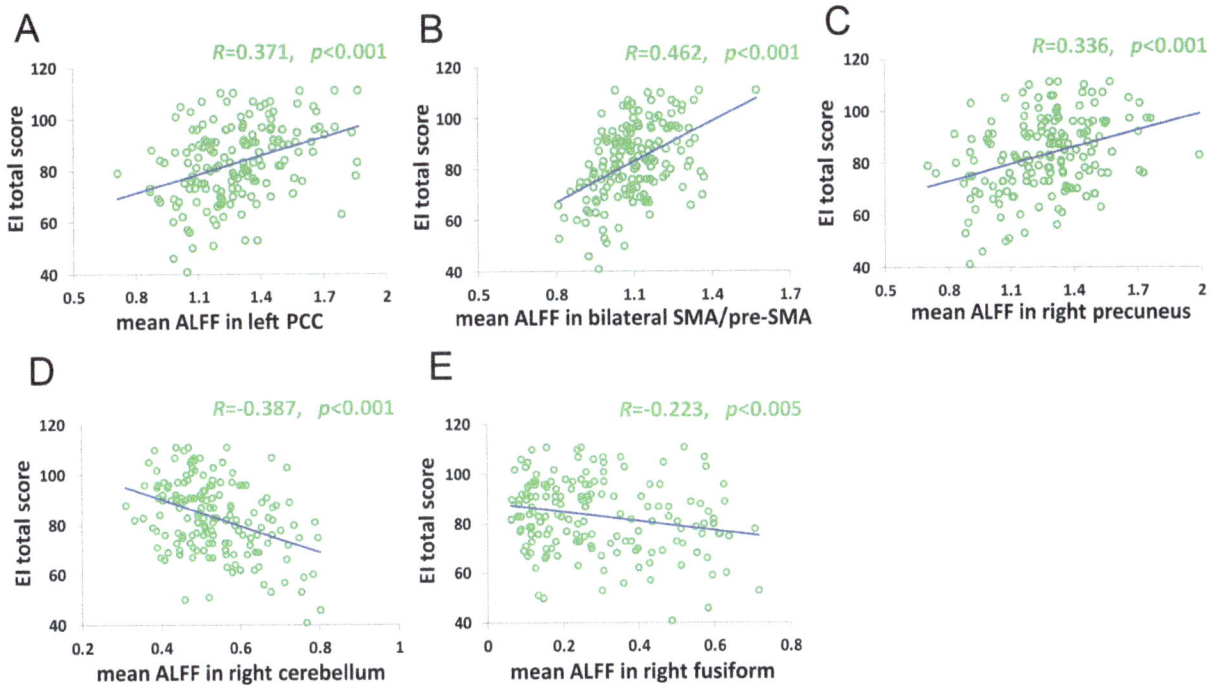

Figure 2. Scatter plots of the relationships between WLEIS total score and mean ALFF values in the significant clusters. A, B, C, D and E showed significant correlations between EI total score and mean ALFFs in left PCC, bilateral SMA/pre-SMA, right precuneus, right cerebellum and right fusiform gyrus, respectively.

higher than 0.4 in the SPM8 template onto the gray matter mask, and finally there were 53,464 voxels (1,443,528 mm^3) in the gray matter mask.

ALFF-EI correlation analysis

A multiple regression analysis was conducted to examine the correlations between the mean ALFF values and the EI scores. We included gender and age as nuisance covariates in this analysis. Because there is no agreed conclusion about the gender effect on EI [51,52], we also performed the analysis without regressing out gender. We found these results were similar (for additional details about the effect of gender on EI, see Text S1 in File S1). We performed further analysis to examine the moderator role of gender on the relationship between ALFF and EI and found the moderating effect of gender was not significant. To control for Type I errors, AlphaSim was used for multiple comparisons correction. A threshold of corrected cluster $p < 0.05$ (single voxel $p < 0.01$, cluster size $\geq 1,647$ mm^3) was set.

Results

Behavioral data

The means and standard deviations of WLEIS total score and scores on its four subscales are presented in Table 1. Pearson correlation analysis showed that the correlations among the four subscales ranged from 0.432 to 0.641 (ps < 0.001) and the correlations between each subscale and the total score ranged from 0.765 to 0.852 (ps < 0.001).

EI-related brain regions

We performed regression analysis to explore the correlations between the brain's regional spontaneous activity and EI. As shown in Figure 1, Figure 2 and Table 2, EI total scores were positively correlated with ALFFs in the left PCC ($r_{peak} = 0.38$, $r_{cluster} = 0.37$, ps < 0.001), bilateral SMA (mainly the pre-SMA; $r_{peak} = 0.37$, $r_{cluster} = 0.46$, ps < 0.001) and right precuneus ($r_{peak} = 0.29$, $r_{cluster} = 0.34$, ps < 0.001), and negatively correlated with ALFFs in the right cerebellum ($r_{peak} = -0.41$, $r_{cluster} = -0.39$, ps < 0.001) and right fusiform gyrus ($r_{peak} = -0.29$, $p < 0.001$; $r_{cluster} = -0.22$, $p < 0.005$).

Within the subscales of the WLEIS, the following associations were found. As shown in Table 2, ALFFs in the SMA/pre-SMA, cerebellum, fusiform gyrus, right precuneus, left PCC and temporal pole (TP) were significantly associated with most subscales of WLEIS. Whereas, the right superior orbital frontal cortex (OFC) and left supramarginal gyrus (SMG) were merely correlated with ROE and the left inferior parietal lobule (IPL) and left IFG were only correlated with OEA. Specially, the SMA/pre-SMA, precuneus, PCC, SMG, IPL and IFG were positively correlated with EI, but the fusiform gyrus, OFC and TP were negatively correlated with EI. All significant correlations were set at the threshold of corrected cluster $p < 0.05$ (single voxel $p < 0.01$, cluster size $\geq 1,647$ mm^3).

Discussion

In the present study, we performed ALFF-EI correlation analysis to investigate the neural basis of EI. Our results indicated that inter-individual differences in EI were reflected in the ALFFs during resting state. As expected, EI was linked with some regions that are known to be involved in social and emotional information processing to understand emotions of self and others, such as the fusiform gyrus, right superior orbital frontal gyrus, left inferior frontal gyrus and left inferior parietal lobule. Additionally, some regions in the top-down control network, such as the bilateral pre-SMA, cerebellum and right precuneus were associated with EI, which may contribute to the control of emotional expression.

Table 2. Regions in which ALFFs were significantly related with WLEIS in the whole-brain analysis.

Brain regions	BA	Peak MNI coordinates			Peak R	No. of voxels
		x	y	z		
EI-total						
L PCC	29	−9	−51	6	0.38	74
B SMA/pre-SMA	6/8	−6	21	51	0.37	272
R precuneus	31/7	18	−54	18	0.29	96
R cerebellum		3	−60	−3	−0.41	1601
R fusiform/temporal pole	37/38	36	15	−48	−0.29	192
SEA						
L PCC	29	−9	−51	6	0.37	61
R precuneus	31/7	15	−57	27	0.32	135
B SMA/pre-SMA	6/8	6	9	54	0.28	91
L cerebellum		−15	−36	−30	−0.39	743
L fusiform	37	−39	−24	−30	−0.37	558
R temporal pole	38	33	18	−48	−0.27	156
R fusiform	37	42	−27	−33	−0.27	113
OEA						
L inferior parietal lobule	40	−54	−39	54	0.39	80
L inferior frontal gyrus	44/45	−36	39	12	0.33	61
R cerebellum		33	−72	−24	−0.35	551
L cerebellum		−51	−69	−33	−0.31	271
L fusiform	37	−30	−18	−39	−0.26	121
ROE						
B SMA/pre-SMA	6/8	−6	21	51	0.42	245
L supramarginal gyrus	40	−54	−24	18	0.36	63
R cerebellum		9	−57	−18	−0.34	285
R superior orbital frontal gyrus	11	12	45	−27	−0.32	85
UOE						
B SMA/pre-SMA	6/8	−9	18	51	0.30	122
R precuneus	31/7	21	−51	18	0.29	83
R cerebellum		9	−57	−18	−0.39	679
L temporal pole	38/20	−36	15	−30	−0.36	622
R temporal pole	38/28	39	18	−30	−0.35	77
R fusiform	37	33	−24	−27	−0.29	78

Note: The threshold was set at $p<0.05$ (AlphaSim corrected). BA = Brodmann area; B = bilateral; R = right; L = left; SEA = self-emotion appraisal; OEA = others' emotion appraisal; ROE = regulation of emotion; UOE = use of emotion. All of the correlation coefficients were significant at the level of $p<0.001$.

EI-related brain regions in the social emotional processing network

We found ALFFs in the fusiform gyrus were negatively correlated with EI total, SEA, OEA and UOE scores and ALFFs in the superior OFC were negatively correlated with ROE score. These results indicated that people with high EI showed low spontaneous neural activities in these brain regions. The fusiform gyrus and OFC are core parts of the emotional processing network [17]. The fusiform gyrus is a face-sensitive region [53]. Specially, the activity in this area is enhanced in response to fearful as compared with neutral facial expressions [17,54]. The OFC is also critical for perceptual processing of emotional signals from faces [17]. Furthermore, OFC has been linked to the experience of anger [55], as well as to aggression [19]. The fusiform gyrus can send visual information to the amygdala and OFC and receive feedback from them [17]. This neural circuit may provide the basis of facial expression cognition and contribute to the understanding and regulation of emotions according to others' feedback in interpersonal communications. It is worth noting that ALFFs in the fusiform gyrus and OFC were negatively related to EI. Given that the fusiform gyrus and OFC, like the amygdala, were associated with negative emotion processing, we suppose that people with low EI would experience more negative emotions. This speculation is in accordance with the finding that impaired or deficient EI was linked to anxiety and depression [7,8]. These results may contribute to our understanding on the mechanism of susceptibility of depression and social maladjustment of people with low EI. However, further work is required to confirm the mechanism by which the fusiform gyrus, OFC and EI are linked.

In this study, there was a significant positive relationship between OEA score and ALFFs in the IFG and IPL. The IFG and IPL are important parts of the mirror neuron system [56,57]. There is a "mirror" system in the brain such that the same areas are activated when we observe another person experiencing an emotion as when we experience the same emotion ourselves, so we can experience the emotional states of another person [58]. A lot of research revealed the mirror system's role in social cognition and its contribution to understanding the actions and intentions of other individuals [59,60]. In line with these findings, our results showed that increased spontaneous brain activity in the IFG and IPL was associated with higher OEA. The IFG and IPL are important nodes of the social cognition network [14,15,61]. Posterior regions of the IFG are involved in emotional judgement and might have a role in top-down aspects of emotion recognition [62]. By contrast, the IPL might play a role in high-level mental state inference, such as understanding others' behavior in terms of internal beliefs, feelings, goals, and intentions [15,61].

Taken together, we provide evidence that EI was significantly associated with ALFFs in certain regions in the social emotional processing network, which is involved in understanding the emotions of self and others.

EI-related brain regions in the cognitive control network

Our results showed a significant positive correlation between EI total, ROE and UOE scores and ALFFs in the bilateral SMA/pre-SMA. By contrast, EI total and four subscales were negatively correlated to ALFFs in the cerebellum. ALFFs in the right precuneus were positively associated with EI total, SEA and UOE scores. The SMA/pre-SMA, cerebellum and precuneus are key nodes of the cognitive control network [24–27]. The SMA/pre-SMA is known to be involved in the processing of task switching [63] and response inhibition [64,65]. Moreover, the pre-SMA was found to be associated with the control of action [66] and response selection [67]. The pre-SMA was also involved in appraisal and expression of negative emotion [68] and emotional conflict detection [69]. Specially, reappraisal, a cognitive strategy of regulating negative emotions, was reliably associated with activation in the pre-SMA [68,70]. These findings demonstrate the cognitive and behavioral control functions of the pre-SMA in emotional processing. It is consistent with our finding that increased spontaneous activity in pre-SMA was associated with higher ability of ROE and UOE. We speculate that the activity of the pre-SMA may be conducive to emotional control (to express or inhibit emotion) in complicated interpersonal interactions and further improving the ability of emotional regulation and use.

The cerebellum has neuroanatomical associations with SMA/pre-SMA [71–73].The traditional view of cerebellar function is that it is purely involved in motor control and coordination [74]. However, increasing studies suggest that the cerebellum also contributes to cognitive processing and emotional control [72,73,75,76]. A repetitive transcranial magnetic stimulation study found that the inhibition of cerebellar function would lead to increased negative mood as a result of impaired emotion regulation [77]. A meta-analysis suggested that the cerebellum does not play a domain-specific role in social cognition, but most probably provides domain-general executive and semantic support [78]. Besides the social cognition function, the cerebellum is also activated in negative emotion processing, such as anger [79]. Interestingly, the cerebellar activations associated with negative emotions occurred concomitantly with activations of mirror neuron domains, suggesting that the

potential role of the cerebellum in control of emotions may be particularly relevant for goal-directed behavior that is required for observing and reacting to another person's negative expressions [80]. In the present study, we found ALFFs in the cerebellum were negatively linked to EI, indicating that low spontaneous activity in cerebellum was related to high EI. This finding is partly consistent with the structural imaging result that the right cerebellum was negatively correlated to the intrapersonal factor of EI [23]. However, it is difficult to interpret why spontaneous activity in cerebellum was negatively related to EI. Because of the multiple functions of brain regions, we suppose that pre-SMA might mainly involve in emotion regulation and control, while the cerebellum tends to be active in negative emotion processing. Future studies should further explore the relationship between the activity in the cerebellum and EI.

The precuneus is in the fronto-parietal control network and is involved in initiating and adjusting control [25,27]. In our study, the precuneus was positively associated with EI total and UOE scores. This result partly fits with previous evidence that the total EI was positively correlated with RSFC between the mPFC and the precuneus [30]. Moreover, the precuneus was also found to be involved in the processes of emotional regulation [81] and emotional awareness [82]. The ability of emotional awareness and regulation may further improve the efficiency of using emotions. It is worth noting that the SMA/pre-SMA, cerebellum and precuneus are not independent but functionally connected in a larger network [25,27].

This study may have some limitations. First, the subjects in this study were young college students with high educational backgrounds. Their EI may be higher than the average population. Future studies might use more representative samples to test our findings. Second, although these results provide insight into the neural bases of EI, they only revealed EI-related brain regions, and we do not know whether they work together or independently. Furthermore, a framework that relies on domain general, distributed structure–function mappings emerges recently [83]. Some studies in social cognitive neuroscience revealed that a specific mental activity or trait may involve several domain general networks, such as salience network, central executive network, dorsal attention network and default mode network [20,83,84]. Thus, future research may investigate how these networks functionally associate with EI.

In summary, we examined whether individual differences in the amplitude of spontaneous low-frequency fluctuations (ALFFs) during resting state were predictive of variations in EI. We found that several brain regions were significantly associated with EI, including the bilateral fusiform gyrus, right superior OFC, left IFG and left IPL that belong to the social emotional processing network and the bilateral pre-SMA, cerebellum and right precuneus that are in the top-down control network. These regions are involved in understanding and controlling emotions. These findings provide additional evidence of individual differences in brain spontaneous activity linked to EI and deepen our understanding on the core components of EI.

Supporting Information

File S1 Contains the following files: Text S1. The effect of gender on EI. Table S1. Regions in which ALFF significantly related to WLEIS in the whole-brain analysis. Figure S1. Brain regions exhibited significant correlations between ALFF and WLEIS total score. Figure S2. The common brain regions of Figure 1 and Figure S1.

Author Contributions

Conceived and designed the experiments: WP TW AC. Performed the experiments: TW. Analyzed the data: WP XW. Contributed reagents/materials/analysis tools: TW. Wrote the paper: WP TW GH LW AC.

References

1. Salovey P, Mayer JD (1990) Emotional intelligence. Imagination, cognition and personality 9: 185–211.
2. Lopes PN, Salovey P, Côté S, Beers M, Petty RE (2005) Emotion regulation abilities and the quality of social interaction. Emotion 5: 113–118.
3. O'Boyle EH, Humphrey RH, Pollack JM, Hawver TH, Story PA (2011) The relation between emotional intelligence and job performance: A meta-analysis. Journal of Organizational Behavior 32: 788–818.
4. Davis SK, Humphrey N (2012) Emotional intelligence predicts adolescent mental health beyond personality and cognitive ability. Personality and Individual Differences 52: 144–149.
5. Schutte NS, Malouff JM, Simunek M, McKenley J, Hollander S (2002) Characteristic emotional intelligence and emotional well-being. Cognition & Emotion 16: 769–785.
6. Hertel J, Schütz A, Lammers CH (2009) Emotional intelligence and mental disorder. Journal of Clinical Psychology 65: 942–954.
7. Fernandez-Berrocal P, Alcaide R, Extremera N, Pizarro D (2006) The role of emotional intelligence in anxiety and depression among adolescents. Individual Differences Research 4: 16–27.
8. Lizeretti NP, Extremera N (2011) Emotional intelligence and clinical symptoms in outpatients with generalized anxiety disorder (GAD). Psychiatric quarterly 82: 253–260.
9. Bar-On R, Brown J, Kirkcaldy BD, Thome E (2000) Emotional expression and implications for occupational stress; an application of the Emotional Quotient Inventory (EQ-i). Personality and individual differences 28: 1107–1118.
10. Law K, Wong C, Song L (2004) The construct and criterion validity of emotional intelligence and its potential utility for management studies. The Journal of applied psychology 89: 483–496.
11. Bar-On R, Tranel D, Denburg NL, Bechara A (2003) Exploring the neurological substrate of emotional and social intelligence. Brain 126: 1790–1800.
12. Mayer JD, Salovey P, Caruso DR (2008) Emotional Intelligence: New Ability or Eclectic Traits? American Psychologist 63: 503–517.
13. Adolphs R (2009) The social brain: neural basis of social knowledge. Annual Review of Psychology 60: 693–716.
14. Blakemore S-J (2008) The social brain in adolescence. Nature Reviews Neuroscience 9: 267–277.
15. Van Overwalle F (2009) Social cognition and the brain: A meta-analysis. Human brain mapping 30: 829–858.
16. Bressler SL, Menon V (2010) Large-scale brain networks in cognition: emerging methods and principles. Trends in cognitive sciences 14: 277–290.
17. Leppänen JM, Nelson CA (2009) Tuning the developing brain to social signals of emotions. Nature Reviews Neuroscience 10: 37–47.
18. Taylor KS, Seminowicz DA, Davis KD (2009) Two systems of resting state connectivity between the insula and cingulate cortex. Human Brain Mapping 30: 2731–2745.
19. Lindquist KA, Wager TD, Kober H, Bliss-Moreau E, Barrett LF (2012) The brain basis of emotion: a meta-analytic review. Behavioral and Brain Sciences 35: 121–143.
20. Lindquist KA, Barrett LF (2012) A functional architecture of the human brain: emerging insights from the science of emotion. Trends in cognitive sciences 16: 533–540.
21. Killgore WD, Weber M, Schwab ZJ, DelDonno SR, Kipman M, et al. (2012) Gray matter correlates of Trait and Ability models of emotional intelligence. NeuroReport 23: 551–555.
22. Takeuchi H, Taki Y, Sassa Y, Hashizume H, Sekiguchi A, et al. (2013) White matter structures associated with emotional intelligence: Evidence from diffusion tensor imaging. Human Brain Mapping 34: 1025–1034.
23. Takeuchi H, Taki Y, Sassa Y, Hashizume H, Sekiguchi A, et al. (2011) Regional gray matter density associated with emotional intelligence: Evidence from voxel-based morphometry. Human brain mapping 32: 1497–1510.
24. Cole MW, Schneider W (2007) The cognitive control network: Integrated cortical regions with dissociable functions. Neuroimage 37: 343–360.
25. Dosenbach NU, Fair DA, Cohen AL, Schlaggar BL, Petersen SE (2008) A dual-networks architecture of top-down control. Trends in cognitive sciences 12: 99–105.
26. Niendam TA, Laird AR, Ray KL, Dean YM, Glahn DC, et al. (2012) Meta-analytic evidence for a superordinate cognitive control network subserving diverse executive functions. Cognitive, Affective, & Behavioral Neuroscience 12: 241–268.
27. Power JD, Petersen SE (2013) Control-related systems in the human brain. Current opinion in neurobiology 23: 223–228.
28. Sripada C, Angstadt M, Kessler D, Phan KL, Liberzon I, et al. (2014) Volitional regulation of emotions produces distributed alterations in connectivity between visual, attention control, and default networks. NeuroImage 89: 110–121.
29. Koven NS, Roth RM, Garlinghouse MA, Flashman LA, Saykin AJ (2011) Regional gray matter correlates of perceived emotional intelligence. Social cognitive and affective neuroscience 6: 582–590.
30. Takeuchi H, Taki Y, Nouchi R, Sekiguchi A, Hashizume H, et al. (2013) Resting state functional connectivity associated with trait emotional intelligence. NeuroImage 83: 318–328.
31. Fox MD, Raichle ME (2007) Spontaneous fluctuations in brain activity observed with functional magnetic resonance imaging. Nature Reviews Neuroscience 8: 700–711.
32. Mennes M, Zuo X-N, Kelly C, Di Martino A, Zang Y-F, et al. (2011) Linking inter-individual differences in neural activation and behavior to intrinsic brain dynamics. NeuroImage 54: 2950–2959.
33. Xie B, Qiu M-G, Zhang Y, Zhang J-N, Li M, et al. (2013) Alterations in the cortical thickness and the amplitude of low-frequency fluctuation in patients with post-traumatic stress disorder. Brain Research 1490: 225–232.
34. Zang Y, He Y, Zhu C, Cao Q, Sui M, et al. (2007) Altered baseline brain activity in children with ADHD revealed by resting-state functional MRI. Brain & development 29: 83–91.
35. Wang X, Han Z, He Y, Caramazza A, Song L, et al. (2013) Where color rests: Spontaneous brain activity of bilateral fusiform and lingual regions predicts object color knowledge performance. NeuroImage 76: 252–263.
36. Zuo X-N, Di Martino A, Kelly C, Shehzad ZE, Gee DG, et al. (2010) The oscillating brain: complex and reliable. NeuroImage 49: 1432–1445.
37. Zou Q-H, Zhu C-Z, Yang Y, Zuo X-N, Long X-Y, et al. (2008) An improved approach to detection of amplitude of low-frequency fluctuation (ALFF) for resting-state fMRI: fractional ALFF. Journal of Neuroscience Methods 172: 137–141.
38. Wei T, Liang X, He Y, Zang Y, Han Z, et al. (2012) Predicting conceptual processing capacity from spontaneous neuronal activity of the left middle temporal gyrus. The Journal of Neuroscience 32: 481–489.
39. Kunisato Y, Okamoto Y, Okada G, Aoyama S, Nishiyama Y, et al. (2011) Personality traits and the amplitude of spontaneous low-frequency oscillations during resting state. Neuroscience Letters 492: 109–113.
40. Wei L, Duan X, Zheng C, Wang S, Gao Q, et al. (2014) Specific frequency bands of amplitude low-frequency oscillation encodes personality. Human Brain Mapping 35: 331–339.
41. Xu K, Liu H, Li H, Tang Y, Womer F, et al. (2014) Amplitude of low-frequency fluctuations in bipolar disorder: A resting state fMRI study. Journal of affective disorders 152: 237–242.
42. Han Y, Wang J, Zhao Z, Min B, Lu J, et al. (2011) Frequency-dependent changes in the amplitude of low-frequency fluctuations in amnestic mild cognitive impairment: a resting-state fMRI study. Neuroimage 55: 287–295.
43. Zhang J, Wei L, Hu X, Zhang Y, Zhou D, et al. (2013) Specific frequency band of amplitude low-frequency fluctuation predicts Parkinson's disease. Behavioural Brain Research 252: 18–23.
44. Wong C-S, Law KS (2002) The effects of leader and follower emotional intelligence on performance and attitude: An exploratory study. The Leadership Quarterly 13: 243–274.
45. Law KS, Wong C-S, Song LJ (2004) The construct and criterion validity of emotional intelligence and its potential utility for management studies. Journal of Applied Psychology 89: 483–496.
46. Ng K-M, Wang C, Zalaquett CP, Bodenhorn N (2007) A confirmatory factor analysis of the Wong and Law Emotional Intelligence Scale in a sample of international college students. International Journal for the Advancement of Counselling 29: 173–185.
47. Shi J, Wang L (2007) Validation of emotional intelligence scale in Chinese university students. Personality and Individual Differences 43: 377–387.
48. Yan C-G, Zang Y-F (2010) DPARSF: A MATLAB Toolbox for "Pipeline" Data Analysis of Resting-State fMRI. Frontiers in systems neuroscience 4: 1–7.
49. Biswal B, Zerrin Yetkin F, Haughton VM, Hyde JS (1995) Functional connectivity in the motor cortex of resting human brain using echo-planar mri. Magnetic resonance in medicine 34: 537–541.
50. Song X-W, Dong Z-Y, Long X-Y, Li S-F, Zuo X-N, et al. (2011) REST: a toolkit for resting-state functional magnetic resonance imaging data processing. PloS one 6: e25031.
51. Craig A, Tran Y, Hermens G, Williams L, Kemp A, et al. (2009) Psychological and neural correlates of emotional intelligence in a large sample of adult males and females. Personality and Individual Differences 46: 111–115.
52. Petrides K, Furnham A (2000) Gender differences in measured and self-estimated trait emotional intelligence. Sex roles 42: 449–461.
53. Kanwisher N, Yovel G (2006) The fusiform face area: a cortical region specialized for the perception of faces. Philosophical Transactions of the Royal Society B: Biological Sciences 361: 2109–2128.

54. Morris JS, Friston KJ, Büchel C, Frith CD, Young AW, et al. (1998) A neuromodulatory role for the human amygdala in processing emotional facial expressions. Brain 121: 47–57.

55. Vytal K, Hamann S (2010) Neuroimaging support for discrete neural correlates of basic emotions: a voxel-based meta-analysis. Journal of Cognitive Neuroscience 22: 2864–2885.

56. Kilner JM, Neal A, Weiskopf N, Friston KJ, Frith CD (2009) Evidence of mirror neurons in human inferior frontal gyrus. The Journal of Neuroscience 29: 10153–10159.

57. Pelphrey KA, Carter EJ (2008) Brain mechanisms for social perception. Annals of the New York Academy of Sciences 1145: 283–299.

58. Frith CD, Frith U (2006) The neural basis of mentalizing. Neuron 50: 531–534.

59. Rizzolatti G, Sinigaglia C (2010) The functional role of the parieto-frontal mirror circuit: interpretations and misinterpretations. Nature Reviews Neuroscience 11: 264–274.

60. Iacoboni M, Dapretto M (2006) The mirror neuron system and the consequences of its dysfunction. Nature Reviews Neuroscience 7: 942–951.

61. Ochsner KN (2008) The social-emotional processing stream: five core constructs and their translational potential for schizophrenia and beyond. Biological psychiatry 64: 48–61.

62. Nakamura K, Kawashima R, Ito K, Sugiura M, Kato T, et al. (1999) Activation of the right inferior frontal cortex during assessment of facial emotion. Journal of Neurophysiology 82: 1610–1614.

63. Crone EA, Wendelken C, Donohue SE, Bunge SA (2006) Neural evidence for dissociable components of task-switching. Cerebral Cortex 16: 475–486.

64. Aron AR, Poldrack RA (2006) Cortical and subcortical contributions to Stop signal response inhibition: role of the subthalamic nucleus. The Journal of Neuroscience 26: 2424–2433.

65. Duann J-R, Ide JS, Luo X, Li C-sR (2009) Functional connectivity delineates distinct roles of the inferior frontal cortex and presupplementary motor area in stop signal inhibition. The Journal of Neuroscience 29: 10171–10179.

66. Nachev P, Wydell H, O'Neill K, Husain M, Kennard C (2007) The role of the pre-supplementary motor area in the control of action. Neuroimage 36: T155–T163.

67. Nachev P, Kennard C, Husain M (2008) Functional role of the supplementary and pre-supplementary motor areas. Nature Reviews Neuroscience 9: 856–869.

68. Etkin A, Egner T, Kalisch R (2011) Emotional processing in anterior cingulate and medial prefrontal cortex. Trends in cognitive sciences 15: 85–93.

69. Jarcho JM, Fox NA, Pine DS, Etkin A, Leibenluft E, et al. (2013) The neural correlates of emotion-based cognitive control in adults with early childhood behavioral inhibition. Biological psychology 92: 306–314.

70. Kalisch R (2009) The functional neuroanatomy of reappraisal: time matters. Neuroscience & Biobehavioral Reviews 33: 1215–1226.

71. Akkal D, Dum RP, Strick PL (2007) Supplementary motor area and presupplementary motor area: targets of basal ganglia and cerebellar output. The Journal of Neuroscience 27: 10659–10673.

72. Bostan AC, Dum RP, Strick PL (2013) Cerebellar networks with the cerebral cortex and basal ganglia. Trends in cognitive sciences 17: 241–254.

73. Strick PL, Dum RP, Fiez JA (2009) Cerebellum and nonmotor function. Annual review of neuroscience 32: 413–434.

74. Kornhuber HH (1971) Motor functions of cerebellum and basal ganglia: the cerebellocortical saccadic (ballistic) clock, the cerebellonuclear hold regulator, and the basal ganglia ramp (voluntary speed smooth movement) generator. Kybernetik 8: 157–162.

75. Schmahmann JD (2010) The role of the cerebellum in cognition and emotion: personal reflections since 1982 on the dysmetria of thought hypothesis, and its historical evolution from theory to therapy. Neuropsychology review 20: 236–260.

76. Schmahmann JD, Caplan D (2006) Cognition, emotion and the cerebellum. Brain 129: 290–292.

77. Schutter DJ, van Honk J (2009) The cerebellum in emotion regulation: a repetitive transcranial magnetic stimulation study. The Cerebellum 8: 28–34.

78. Van Overwalle F, Baetens K, Mariën P, Vandekerckhove M (2014) Social cognition and the cerebellum: A meta-analysis of over 350 fMRI studies. NeuroImage 86: 554–572.

79. Park J-Y, Gu B-M, Kang D-H, Shin Y-W, Choi C-H, et al. (2010) Integration of cross-modal emotional information in the human brain: an fMRI study. Cortex 46: 161–169.

80. Schraa-Tam CK, Rietdijk WJ, Verbeke WJ, Dietvorst RC, van den Berg WE, et al. (2012) fMRI activities in the emotional cerebellum: a preference for negative stimuli and goal-directed behavior. The Cerebellum 11: 233–245.

81. Koenigsberg HW, Fan J, Ochsner KN, Liu X, Guise K, et al. (2010) Neural correlates of using distancing to regulate emotional responses to social situations. Neuropsychologia 48: 1813–1822.

82. van der Velde J, Servaas MN, Goerlich KS, Bruggeman R, Horton P, et al. (2013) Neural correlates of alexithymia: A meta-analysis of emotion processing studies. Neuroscience & Biobehavioral Reviews 37: 1774–1785.

83. Barrett LF, Satpute AB (2013) Large-scale brain networks in affective and social neuroscience: towards an integrative functional architecture of the brain. Current Opinion in Neurobiology 23: 361–372.

84. Satpute AB, Shu J, Weber J, Roy M, Ochsner KN (2013) The functional neural architecture of self-reports of affective experience. Biological psychiatry 73: 631–638.

24

Functional Cortical Network in Alpha Band Correlates with Social Bargaining

Pablo Billeke[1,2,3]*, **Francisco Zamorano**[1,2,3], **Mario Chavez**[5], **Diego Cosmelli**[2,4], **Francisco Aboitiz**[2,3]

1 División Neurociencia de la Conducta, Centro de Investigación en Complejidad Social (CICS), Facultad de Gobierno, Universidad del Desarrollo, Santiago, Chile, **2** Centro Interdisciplinario de Neurociencias, Pontificia Universidad Católica de Chile, Santiago, Chile, **3** Departamento de Psiquiatría, Escuela de Medicina, Pontificia Universidad Católica de Chile, Santiago, Chile, **4** Escuela de Psicología, Pontificia Universidad Católica de Chile, Santiago, Chile, **5** CNRS UMR-7225, Hôpital de la Salpêtrière, Paris, France

Abstract

Solving demanding tasks requires fast and flexible coordination among different brain areas. Everyday examples of this are the social dilemmas in which goals tend to clash, requiring one to weigh alternative courses of action in limited time. In spite of this fact, there are few studies that directly address the dynamics of flexible brain network integration during social interaction. To study the preceding, we carried out EEG recordings while subjects played a repeated version of the Ultimatum Game in both human (social) and computer (non-social) conditions. We found phase synchrony (inter-site-phase-clustering) modulation in alpha band that was specific to the human condition and independent of power modulation. The strength and patterns of the inter-site-phase-clustering of the cortical networks were also modulated, and these modulations were mainly in frontal and parietal regions. Moreover, changes in the individuals' alpha network structure correlated with the risk of the offers made only in social conditions. This correlation was independent of changes in power and inter-site-phase-clustering strength. Our results indicate that, when subjects believe they are participating in a social interaction, a specific modulation of functional cortical networks in alpha band takes place, suggesting that phase synchrony of alpha oscillations could serve as a mechanism by which different brain areas flexibly interact in order to adapt ongoing behavior in socially demanding contexts.

Editor: Sam Doesburg, Hospital for Sick Children, Canada

Funding: This work was supported by CONICYT [Grant number 791220014 to PB], Project "Anillo en Complejidad Social" [SOC-1101 to PB, DC and FZ] and by the Millennium Center for the Neuroscience of Memory, Chile [NC10-001-F], which is developed with funds from the Innovation for Competitivity from the Ministry for Economics, Fomentation and Tourism, Chile. MC is partially supported by the EU-LASAGNE Project [Contract no.318132 (STREP)]. The funders had no role in study design, data collection and analysis, decision to publish, or preparation of the manuscript.

Competing Interests: The authors have declared that no competing interests exist.

* Email: pbilleke@udd.cl

Introduction

In daily life, we spend an great deal of time dealing with social dilemmas [1]. A crucial characteristic of such situations is that goals that tend to clash can co-exist with the consequence of making an analytical approach non-trivial [2]. Naturally, then, when people face social dilemmas, several cognitive processes must be recruited. Neurobiological studies have identified several brain areas which underlie different functions supporting our capacity to maintain a social interaction and solve social dilemmas [3,4]. Rather than having specific and isolated functions, it has been proposed that these areas work as a network which requires a rapid, efficient, adaptive interaction among them and with other domain-general networks [5,6]. Thus social processing, like empathy [7] and imitation [8], has been shown to generate an increase in the connectivity among different brain areas. In spite of this evidence, it remains unknown whether specific changes in functional connectivity of the brain networks are related to social behavior. Indeed, a recent study shows that flexible organization in connectivity patterns of fronto-parietal network is related to our capacity to adapt our cognitive resources according to the task demands [9]. Thus, we hypothesize that during social interactions, a particular functional reorganization of brain functional connec-

tivity takes place, and that this reorganization is reflected in the dynamics of the cortical networks as estimated by inter-site-phase-clustering between brain sources.

Empirical studies have led to the hypothesis that functional neural assemblies are largely distributed and linked to form a web-like structure in the brain [10]. Within this framework, brain regions are conceived as partitioned into a collection of modules, representing functional units that are separable from -but related to- the functions of other modules. Detecting the modular brain structure may be crucial to understanding the structural and functional properties of neural systems during social interactions. To evaluate this possibility, we used Graph Theory analysis of the electroencephalographic (EEG) activity of human subjects while they played a standard behavioral economics game that recreates a social dilemma of bargaining, namely the repeated version of the Ultimatum Game (Figure 1) [11,12]. The game involves two players, namely the proposer and the responder. The proposer makes an offer as to how to split a certain amount of money between the two players. The responder can either accept or reject the offer. If the offer is accepted, the money is split as proposed, but if it is rejected, neither player receives any money. Crucially, during this repeated interaction, proposers have to predict the most probable behavior of the responders to estimate the risk of

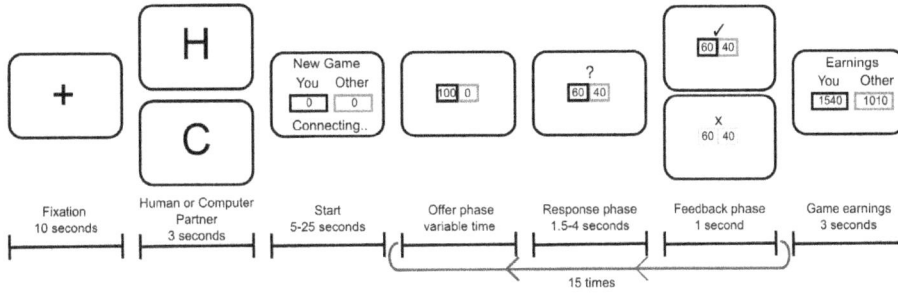

Figure 1. Timeline of a game. Proposers (black box) and responders (gray box, computational simulations, see Methods) played a repeated Ultimatum Game. The proposer makes an offer on how to split 100 Chilean pesos between the responder and himself/herself (offer phase). The responder decides to either accept or reject it (response phase). If the responder accepts the offer, the money is split as proposed, and if he/she rejects it, the money is lost. The response is shown on the screen during 1 s (feedback phase). Each game consists of 15 offers. At the beginning of each game, the proposer sees a cue that indicates if his/her partner is a human ("H") or computer ("PC").

their actions and adapt their own behavior accordingly [13]. To make this behavioral prediction, it is necessary to recruit brain networks that participate in social processing to figure out the other players' intentions (e.i., Mentalizing) [14].

Methods

Twenty-five individuals (11 women) participated for monetary compensation after online recruitment. Seventeen subject data were originally recollected for the control task of a previous work [15]. All the analyses presented here are new. All participants were right-handed Spanish speakers, aged from 20 to 37 years (M = 25.31, SEM = 0.71). All participants had normal or corrected-to-normal vision, no color-vision deficiency, no history of neurological diseases, and no current psychiatric diagnosis or psychotropic prescriptions. All participants provided their written informed consent to participate in this study and the Ethics Committee of the Pontificia Universidad Católica de Chile approved the experimental protocol. All experiments were performed at the Cognitive Neuroscience Laboratory of the Department of Psychiatry of the University.

Task

Participants played as proposers in a repeated version of the Ultimatum Game (see Figure 1). Subjects believed they were playing either with a human partner or a computer partner, but they were actually always playing with a computational simulation (see below). Participants began their participation by reading on-screen instructions describing the game. At the beginning of each game, participants watched the fixation cross (10 seconds, fixation phase). Then, a signal on the screen indicated whether the game was against a computer ("PC") or a human ("H") partner. Each game consisted of 15 rounds and each participant played as a proposer 32 times with different simulated responders (16 human games and 16 computer games, randomly distributed). For computer games, the experimenter explained to the participant that the computer simulation assigned a probability to accept the offer given the amount of money offered (a direct relation), and that this probability could change between different games but not during a game with the same computer partner. Importantly, the simulation used in human and computer games was the same. Each trial had three phases as follows: In the first (offer phase, variable duration), the proposer had to make the offer. In the second (anticipation phase, 1.5–4 seconds), the proposer waited for the response of the partner. In the last phase (feedback phase, 1 second), the response was revealed to the proposer. At the end of

each game, the earnings each player had made in the game were revealed. After the set of games concluded, the experimenter interviewed each participant individually in order to check whether they had understood the game correctly. The amount of money each participant received depended on his/her performance in one of the 32 games chosen randomly, and ranged from 6,000 to 12,000 Chilean pesos, 12 to 24 USD approximately.

Simulation

Simulations used in the tasks were based on a mixed logistic modeling of 33 people playing as receptors with other people (for more details see [13]). Using this model, we were able to create different virtual players. All participants played with the same simulated partners. Specifically, the simulation algorithm assigns a probability to reject or accept the offer given the following two equations:

for round (x) = 1,

$$logit(R_x) = (b_0 + r_0^i) + (b_1 + r_1^i)O_x$$

and for round (x) >1,

$$logit(R_x) =$$
$$(b_0 + r_0^i) + (b_1 + r_1^i)O_x + (b_2 + r_2^i)\Delta O_x + b_2 \text{Pr}_x + b_3 \Delta O_x \text{Pr}_x$$

where $logit(R_x)$ is the logit transform of the probability of rejection for the round x, O_x the offer, ΔO_x the change of offer in relation to the preceding offer, and PR_x the preceding response. The coefficients for each regressor were composed by a population parameter (b_y) and a random effect for each simulated responder (r_y^i, y = regressor and i = simulated partner). The simulation and experimental setting generated a credible human interaction for the following reasons: (1) The distributions of acceptances and rejections, and the offering behaviors related to a rejection in the simulation game were similar to those obtained in a real human game [13], suggesting that simulated responders elicited comparable behaviors in proposers. (2) During post hoc interviews, experimenters asked participants whether they believed that they had played against a human counterpart. All participants indicated that they actually believed that they had played against another human and that they felt the human games different from the computer games. We used the *logit(R_x)* to the quantification of the risk per each offer made.

Electrophysiological Recordings

Continuous EEG recordings were obtained with a 40-electrode NuAmps EEG System (Compumedics Neuroscan). All impedances were kept below 5 kΩ. Electrode impedance was retested during pauses to ensure stable values throughout the experiment. All electrodes were referenced to averaged mastoids during acquisition and the signal was digitized at 1 kHz. Electro-oculogram was obtained with four electrodes with both vertical and horizontal bipolar derivation. All recordings were acquired using Scan 4.3 (Compumedics Neuroscan) and stored for off-line treatment. At the end of each session, electrode position and head points were digitalized using a 3D tracking system (Polhemus Isotrak).

EEG Data Analysis

EEG signals were preprocessed using a 0.1–100 Hz band-pass Butterworth filter (third-order, forward and reverse filtering). Eye blinks were identified by a threshold criterion of ±100 µV, and their contribution was removed from each dataset using principal component analysis by singular value decomposition and spatial filter transform using Scan 4.3 (Compumedics Neuroscan). Other remaining artifacts (e.g., muscular artifacts) were detected by visual inspection of the signal and the trials that contained them were removed. After this procedure, we obtained 424 ± 33 artifact-free trials across the subjects. Time frequency (TF) distributions were obtained by means of the wavelet transform, between -1.5 and 1.5s. We displayed the result only for -1 to 1 s over the segmented signals to avoid edged artifact. A signal x(t) was convolved with a complex Morlet's wavelet function defined as $w(t,f_0) = Ae^{-t^2/2\sigma_t^2}e^{i2\pi f_0 t}$. Wavelets were normalized and thus $A = (\sigma_t\sqrt{\pi})^{-1/2}$ the width of each wavelet function $m = f_o/\sigma_t$ was chosen to be 7; where $\sigma_f = \frac{1}{2}\pi\sigma_t$. TF contents was represented as the energy of the convolved signal: $E(t,f_o) = |w(t,f_o)\otimes x(t)|^2$. Thus, we obtained the phase and amplitude per each temporal bin (in steps of 10 ms) and frequency (from 4 to 30 Hz in step of 1 Hz). We used for analysis only the 90 riskiest and the 90 safest offers per subject and condition, in order to ensure equal number of trials for statistical comparison. For all power spectrum analysis, we used the dB of power related to a baseline during the fixation phase (ten seconds at the beginning of each game, Figure 1).

Source Estimations

The neural current density time series at each elementary brain location was estimated by applying a weighted minimum norm estimate inverse solution [16] with unconstrained dipole orientations in single-trials. A tessellated cortical mesh template surface derived from the default anatomy of the Montreal Neurological Institute (MNI/Colin27) wrapped to the individual head shape (using ~300 headpoints per subject) was used as a brain model to estimate the current source distribution. We defined 3×390 sources constrained to the segmented cortical surface (3 orthogonal sources at each spatial location, avoiding deep and basal structures since the sensitivity of the EEG signal to the activity of those structures is poor), and computed a three-layer (scalp, inner skull, outer skull) boundary element conductivity model and the physical forward model [17]. The measured electrode level data $X(t) = [x_1(t), \cdots, x_{n\_electrode}(t)]$ is assumed to be linearly related to a set of cortical sources $Y(t) = [y_1(t), \cdots, y_{m\_source}(t)]$ and additive noise $N(t) : X(t) = LY(t) + N(t)$, where L is the physical forward

model. The inverse solution was then derived as $Y(t) = WX(t) = RL^T(LRL^T + \lambda^2 C)^{-1}X(t)$ where W is the inverse operator, R and C are the source and noise covariances respectively, the superscript T indicates the matrix transpose, and λ^2 is the regularization parameter. R was the identity matrix that was modified to implement depth-weighing (weighing exponent: 0.8 [18]), The regularization parameter λ was set to 1/3. To estimate cortical activity at the cortical sources, the recorded raw EEG time series at the sensors x(t) were multiplied by the inverse operator W to yield the estimated source current, as a function of time, at the cortical surface: $Y(t) = WX(t)$. Since this is a linear transformation, it does not modify the spectral content of the underlying sources. It is therefore possible to undertake time–frequency analysis on the source space directly. Finally, we reduced the number of sources by keeping a single source at each spatial location that pointed into the direction of maximal variance. To this end, we applied a principal component analysis to covariance matrix obtained from the 3 orthogonal time series estimated at each source location. This resulted in a single filter for each spatial location that was then applied to the complex valued data to derive frequency specific single trial source estimates. Since we used a small number of electrodes (40) and no individual anatomy for head model calculation, the spatial precision of the source estimations are limited. In order to minimize the possibility of erroneous results we only present source estimations if there are both statistically significant differences at the electrode level and the differences at the source levels survive a multiple comparison correction.

Functional Network

We consider the functional links in brain signals defined via the phase-locking value (PLV) computed between all pairs of electrodes or brain sources [19]. The PLV measures the inter-site-phase-clustering. To compute the PLVs, we used a complex Morlet's wavelet function of 7 cycles. By means of this complex wavelet transform, an instantaneous phase $\phi_i^{tr}(t,f)$ is obtained for each frequency component of signals i (electrodes or sources) at each trial (tr). The PLV between any pair of signals (i,k) is inversely related to the variability of phase differences across trials:

$$PLV_{ik}(t,f) = \frac{1}{N_{tr}}\left|\sum_{tr=1}^{N_{tr}} \exp^{j(\phi_i^{tr}(t,f) - \phi_k^{tr}(t,f))}\right|$$

where N_{tr} is the total number of trials. If the phase difference varies little across trials, its distribution is concentrated around a preferred value and PLV<1. In contrast, under the null hypothesis of a uniformity of phase distribution, PLV values are close to zero. Finally, to assess whether two different nodes are functionally connected, we calculated the significance probability of the PLVs by a Rayleigh test of uniformity of phase. According to this test, the significance of a PLV determined from N_{tr} can be calculated as $p = \exp^{(-N_{tr}PLV^2)}$ [20]. To correct for multiple testing, the False Discovery Rate (FDR, q<0.05) method was applied to each matrix of PLVs. In the construction of the networks, a functional connection between two brain sites was assumed as an undirected and weighted edge (functional connectivity strength between node $w_{ij} = PLV_{ij}$, for significant links and $w_{ij} = 0$ otherwise). We calculated the strength of inter-site-phase-clustering for each node (electrode or source) as the sum of all significant PLVs of that node.

Network partitions

To partition the functional networks in modules, we used a random walk-based algorithm [21]. This data-driven approach is based on the intuition that a random walker on a graph tends to remain into densely connected subsets corresponding to modules. To find the modular structure, the algorithm starts with a partition in which each node in the network is the sole member of a module. Modules are then merged by an agglomerative approach based on a hierarchical clustering method. At each step the algorithm evaluates the quality of partition Q, which compares the abundance of edges lying inside each community with respect to a null model. The modularity of a given partition is defined as, $Q = \sum_{s=1}^{M} \left[l_s/L - (k_s/2L)^2 \right]$ where M is the number of modules, L is the total number of connections in the network, l_s is the number of connections between vertices in module s, and k_s is the sum of the degrees of the vertices in modules. The partition that maximizes Q is considered as the partition that better captures the modular structure of the network. Further details can be found in [22,23].

To evaluate the agreement between community structures we use the Rand index [24], which is a traditional criterion for comparison of different results provided by classifiers and clustering algorithms, including partitions with different numbers of classes or clusters. For two partitions P and P', the Rand index is defined as $R = \dfrac{(a+d)}{(a+b+c+d)}$; where a is the number of pairs of data objects belonging to the same class in P and to the same class in P', b is the number of pairs of data objects belonging to the same class in P and to different classes in P', c is the number of pairs of data objects belonging to different classes in P and to the same class in P', and d is number of pairs of data objects belonging to different classes in P and to different classes in P'. The Rand index has a straightforward interpretation as a percentage of agreement between the two partitions and it yields values between 0 (if the two partitions are randomly drawn) and 1 (for identical partition structures).

Statistical analysis

For pair comparison and correlation, we used non-parametric tests (Wilcoxon and Spearman correlation). For multiple regressions, we used robust linear regression. To correct for multiple comparisons in time-frequency chart and sources, we used the Cluster-based permutation test for the EEG data [25]. In the latter method, clusters of significant areas were defined by pooling neighboring sites (in the time-frequency chart) that showed the same effect (p<0.05). The cluster-level statistics was computed as the sum of the statistics of all sites within the corresponding cluster. We evaluated the cluster-level significance under the permutation distribution of the cluster that had the largest cluster-level statistics. The permutation distribution was obtained by randomly permuting the original data. After each permutation, the original statistical test was computed (e.g., Wilcoxon), and the cluster-level statistics of the largest cluster resulting was used for the permutation distribution. After 1,000 permutations, the cluster-level significance for each observed cluster was estimated as the proportion of elements of the permutation distribution greater than the cluster-level statistics of the corresponding cluster.

Software

All behavioral statistical analyses were performed in R. The EEG signal processing was implemented in MATLAB using in-house scripts (LAN toolbox, available online at http://lantoolbox. wikispaces.com/, e.g. [26]). For the source estimation and head model, we used the BrainStorm [27] and openMEEG toolboxes [28].

Results

Behavior

Subjects in both human (HGs) and computer games (CGs) made comparable offers in the amount of money (HG = $42.5; CG = $42.3, Chilean pesos; Wilcoxon signed rank test; p = 0.78) and risk (measured as the logit of the probability to acceptance; HG = 0.89; CG = 0.86; p = 0.9). Like in our previous work, we found a strategic difference between HGs and CGs given by the evolution of the offer risk during a game. In CGs there was a stronger correlation between the offer risk and the round number (Spaerman's rho = 0.88, p<2e−16) than that of HG (rho = 0.61, p = 0.01), giving a difference in the interaction between conditions (HG and CG) and round number in the robust linear regression (Table 1). These results suggest that subjects use a learning strategy in CGs but a bargaining strategy in HGs [15].

EEG

We explored the oscillatory brain activity related to the anticipation of the other's response. We calculated the risk for each offer and compared the 90 riskiest with the 90 safest offers per subject. To explore changes in the global dynamics we first compared the overall power and inter-site-phase-clustering strength (by means of PLV) between risky and safe offers per condition, at the electrode level. For this, we explored for changes in the sum of the inter-site-phase-clustering strength or power across all electrodes. First we defined a time-window of interest (0 to 1 second after the subject made the offer) and calculated a repeated measure ANOVA. In this analysis we found that the interaction between conditions (Human and Computer games), offer risk (risky vs. safe offer) and frequency band (theta, 4–7 Hz, alpha, 8–12 Hz, beta 13–25 Hz) was significant ($F_2 = 3.25$, p = 0.0406, Table S1 in File S1). Then, we explored the entire time-frequency chart and, in those regions where we found significant modulations, we explored their topographies and the electrodes that showed significant effect (Figure 2).

Over occipital electrodes, we found a significant drop in alpha power before the subject made the offer in both HGs and CGs (main effect: 8–10 Hz; −0.8 to −0.2 s; O1 and O2 electrodes; Figure 2A–B). After the subjects made the offer and before they received the response (anticipatory phase), we found a drop in alpha band power over left posterior temporo-parietal electrodes only in HGs (main effect: 9–12 Hz; 0.5 to 1 s; TP8 electrode; Figure 2A, upper panel, Wilcoxon rank sum test and cluster based permutation test, p<0.01). During this anticipatory phase, we also found an increase of the alpha inter-site-phase-clustering strength prior to the difference in power (main effect: 7–10 Hz; 0.2 to 0.4 s; FC3, C3, CP3 and Pz electrode; Figure 2A, lower panel, note that the inter-site-phase-clustering strength was calculated based on all possible electrode pairs). This synchrony increase was mainly in risky offers made during HG (7–10 Hz, Figure 2C). Notably, we did not find any difference in inter-site-phase-clustering between risky and safe offers made during CGs (Figure 2B–D).

Since the volumetric conduction of distal sources can spuriously generate synchrony at the electrode level, we carried out the same analysis using both the current source density (CSD) at the electrode level and source reconstruction at cortical level. CSD analysis replicates the difference between human and computer games shown in Figure 2 (See Figure S1 in File S1). For source reconstruction, we calculated the electrical activity in 390 source nodes over the cortex (Figure 3A), avoiding subcortical structures where the sensitivity of EEG is poor. Then, we calculated the strength of inter-site-phase-clustering for each node in alpha band (7–10 Hz, where we found the main modulation at the electrode

Table 1. Model of the risk of offers.

	Scope	Std. Error	T-value	p-value
(Intercept)	0.3747	0.1136	3.2976	0.00002
Round	0.1021	0.0125	8.1701	0.00000001
Human Games	0.3101	0.1607	1.9296	0.06
Round×Human Games	−0.0686	0.0177	−3.8813	0.0006
degree of freedom = 26				

level), and found differences in the medial parietal and frontal nodes between safe and risky offers for HGs but not for CGs (Figure 3B). In order to evaluate if the strength change reflects a change in functional network, we calculated the community structure of the networks at group and individual levels for both conditions at cortical source level (see Methods).

In agreement with the above result, we found that the community structure changed between risky and safe offers in HGs but not in CGs, at group levels, in frontal and parietal regions (Figure 3C). We obtained seven communities per condition except for safe offers in HGs in which we obtained six. We found a bilateral module in dorsolateral prefrontal cortex, which was conserved across conditions (light-blue in Figure 3C). We observed two modules in inferior frontal gyrus and fronto-polar regions, which were joined only in safe offers in HGs (blue and red in Figure 3C). We also found a central module in sensory-motor cortex, which was greater especially in the left hemisphere in risky offers in HGs (Green). Finally, we detected one medial and two lateral modules in parietal and occipital regions, which changed in risky offers in HGs in comparison with the other conditions.

In order to evaluate whether this differential functional organization is specifically related to social interaction, we computed the individual differences in community structure between risky and safe offer networks using the rand index (at the cortical source level). Interestingly, the difference in community structure was significantly correlated with the differences in the risk of the offer only in HGs (rho = −0.44, p = 0.02), but not in CGs (rho = 0.2, p = 0.2). Indeed, using robust linear regression, the interaction between conditions (HGs and CGs) and risk differences was significant (t_{46} = −2.05, p = 0.045) even after correcting by power and inter-site-phase-clustering strength differences between risky and safe offers (Table 2). This indicates that functional network activation was specifically related to the behavior during HGs (t_{44} = −2.42, p = 0.02) independently of change of strength of inter-site-phase-clustering (p = 0.99) and possible influences of changes in power (p = 0.04, Table 2).

Discussion

It has been proposed that the complex and flexible behaviors that sustain human social interactions rely on the dynamic modulation of patterns of interaction among specialized large-scale brain systems [29]. Here, we explored such specific modulations of patterns in brain connectivity during two types of interaction. Crucially, we used two tasks that were exactly the same except by the context instructed to the subject (human *vs* computer partners), and we found a significant modulation in alpha power and inter-site-phase-clustering, depending on the social context. A recent work has shown that inter-site-phase-clustering in alpha band at the electrode level correlates with the activity of fronto-parietal networks [30]. In that work, using

concomitant EEG and fMRI recordings during rest, the authors found that the inter-site-phase-clustering of alpha band was specifically correlated with the BOLD signal of frontal pole, inferior parietal lobe and medial parietal lobe [30]. Interestingly, the activity of fronto-parietal networks is specifically correlated to alpha band, and does not show correlation with other frequency bands [30]. This specific correlation includes the anterior prefrontal cortex and the medial parietal cortex where we found inter-site-phase-clustering strength modulation at source level. Although other studies have found a correlation between alpha inter-site-phase-clustering with default mode network (see [31]), our results are in accordance with the correlation with fronto-parietal regions (compared Figure 2B with Figure 1 in [30]), and match the hypothesis that the fronto-parietal network participates in cognitive control, especially in a trial-by-trial high adaptive control situation [32]. Moreover, evidence from intracortical recording in monkeys, shows the existence of a prefronto-parietal network that shows phase synchrony at in 5–10 Hz [33]. This network increases its inter-site-phase-clustering strength during the anticipation of top-down controlled processes [33]. Indeed, cognitive control is highly required to solve difficult social situations like the dilemmas recreated by game theory tasks such as the one used here [34]. In the same line, it has been proposed that cognitive control is necessary for humans to develop pro-social behavior like mutual cooperation [35]. Thus, the increase in phase synchrony that we found probably reflects the higher cognitive demands required by the expectation of the partner's behavior in a repeated interaction with humans (e.g., integrating the other's intention, the previous interactions and the future consequences) than that required in a computer interaction.

An important limitation of our work concerns the interpretation of functional connectivity using EEG. Volume conduction may cause spurious connectivity by the fact that activity in one source can be represented in multiple measurement points [36]. In order to lessen erroneous results, we explored the synchrony in both electrode and source reconstruction levels, and studied global dynamics rather that local modulations. Additionally, our results indicated that inter-site-phase-clustering changes were dissociated from power changes, which argues against possible volume conduction effects. Finally, behavior was significantly related to network dynamics independently of its overall inter-site-phase-clustering strength and power.

It has been proposed that alpha power shows a negative correlation with cortical activity [37–40]. Alpha power has shown a negative correlation with the dorsal attention network and a positive correlation with the cingulo-opercular network, with no relation to the fronto-pariental network [41]. Works in focused attention suggest that phase locking during the processing of a stimulus can occur with concomitant amplitude reduction [42]. Additionally, it seems that oscillatory alpha activity operates in a phasic manner [43,44]. Thus, the phase of pre-stimulus alpha

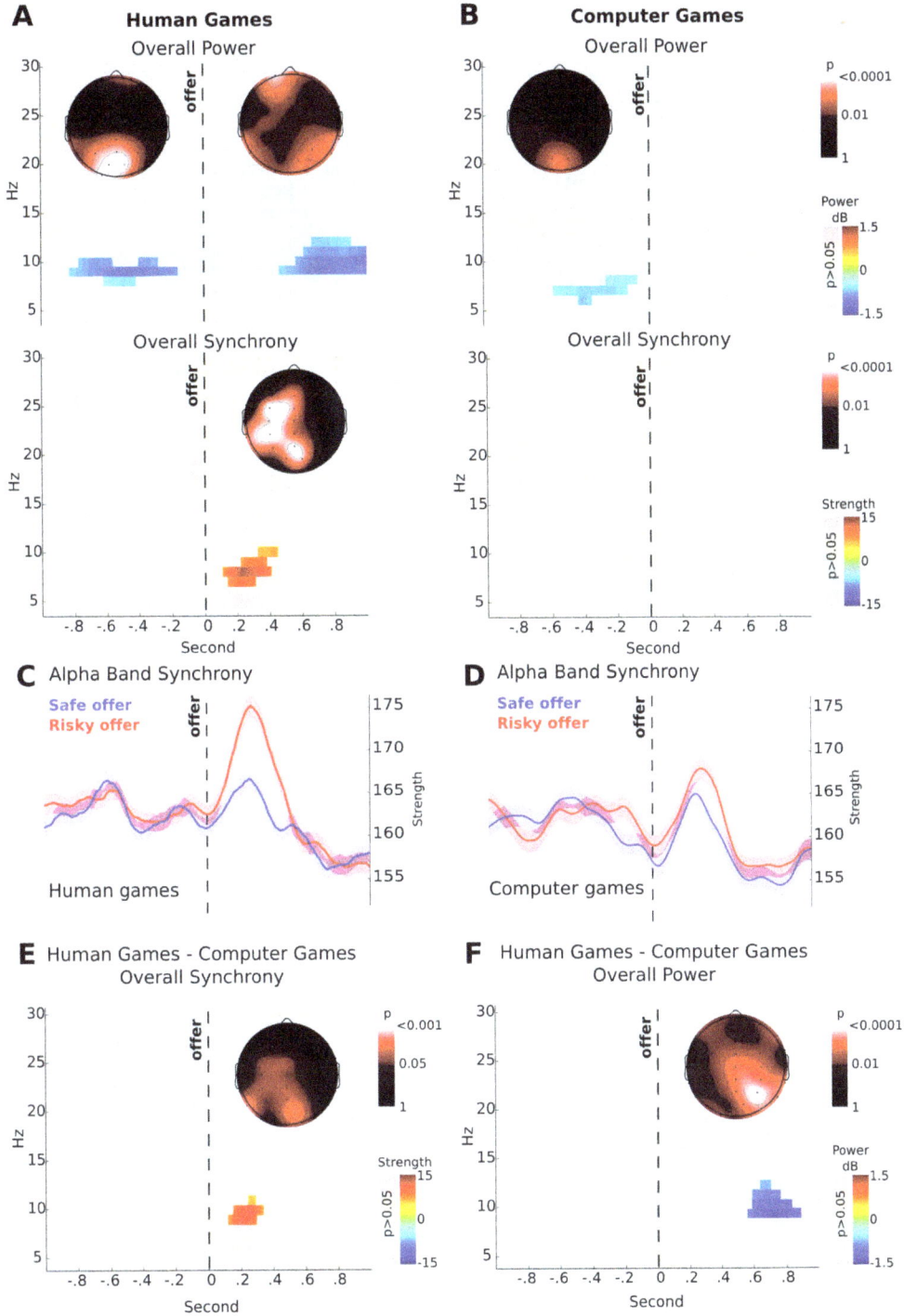

Figure 2. Scalp levels. A, B, Time-frequency charts of the difference between risky and save offers in human (**A**) and computer games (**B**). The upper panel shows differences in the overall power (dB) and the lower panel in strength of synchrony (inter-site-phase-clustering). **C, D** Inter-site-phase-clustering strength in alpha band (7–10 Hz) in safe (blue) and risky (red) offer in human (**C**) and computer (**D**) games. Areas represent the standard error of means. **E, F,** Difference between human and computer games in overall power (**E**) and synchrony (**F**). **A–F,** The non-significant areas are overshadowed and for each significant area, the scalp distribution of p-values is shown. Time-frequency charts and time line plots show the mean of the power or the sum of inter-site-phase-clustering strengths across all electrodes, and the topographic plots show the distribution of the significant time-frequency windows highlighted.

oscillations modulates visual detection [45]. Following this evidence, it has been proposed that alpha oscillation works as a pulsed inhibition and that its synchronized activity could have a important role in the change of network activity in the brain [46–

48]. In our experiment, alpha inter-site-phase-clustering modulation was temporally dissociated from power modulation (Figure 2). Using the same task but only considering games among actual human partners, we have previously shown that the power

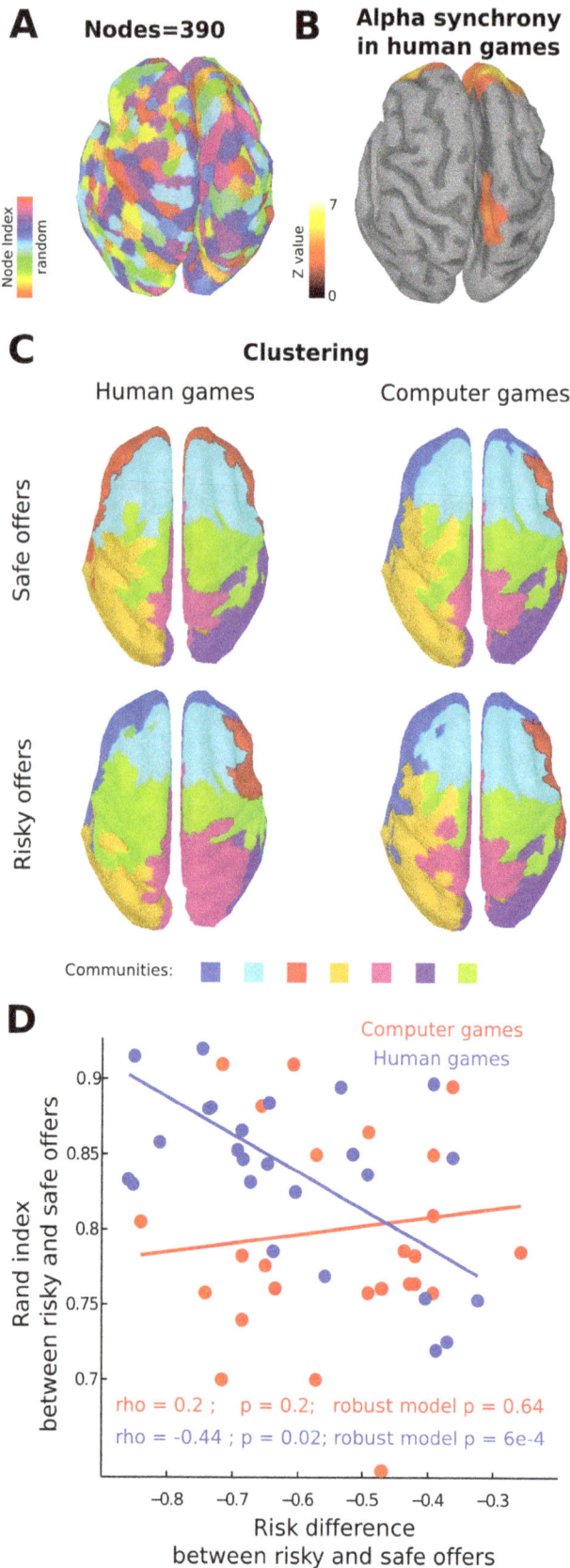

Figure 3. Source level. A, Cortical areas that represent each node in the global network (colors represent node indexes in random order). B, Areas where the synchrony (inter-site-phase-clustering) differences between risky and safe offers in human game were significant (FDR, q<0.05). C, Community structure of the population networks by conditions (colors represent de community index). Note that there are no main variations between risky and safe offers in the computer game, while there is a notorious variation in human games. D, Correlation between the differences in the risk of the offers made (logit of the probability to acceptance, risky offers – safe offers) and the change of the community structure per each subject. Note that only in human games there is a significant correlation. Blue depicts human games and red computer games.

modulation in alpha is associated with the risk of the offer in a temporo-parietal region compatible with social processing areas (such as the temporo-parietal junction and superior temporal sulcus), and the entropy of the offer in regions syndicated as part of the cingulo-opercular network [13]. Altogether, this evidence is compatible with a functional dissociation between phase and power modulation in the alpha band measure over the scalp [49].

Since cognitive control processes necessary to solve social dilemmas require flexible long-range communication and integration among brain areas [5], we finally explored changes in the cortical network structure using graph theory analysis. At the population level, the community structure between risky and safe offers did not differ in games with computer partners. Interestingly, in human games the community structure was different between conditions mainly in prefrontal and parietal cortex. Although a one-to-one assignment of anatomical brain regions to the retrieved modules is difficult to define, our results reveal an overlap between the modules and some well-known functional areas of the brain. The modules in inferior frontal gyrus are compatible with the frontal parts of the fronto-parietal control network [50]. As we mentioned above, cognitive control is an essential process that enables us to carry out social interaction [34]. In childhood, prefrontal cortex maturation correlates with both impulse control and cooperative behavior in social contexts [51]. In addition, alterations in cognitive control are an important factor underlying social impairments of several psychiatric diseases such as schizophrenia [52,53] and depression [54,55]. The notorious differences in frontal and parietal modules in HGs may therefore reflect the behavioral control required to carry out a social bargaining. Across the HGs, people tended to change less their offers, as if expecting that the others would also change their behaviors (Table 1, and [15]). Thus on the first rounds, people can tolerate rejection and do not change their behavior in order to obtain more acceptances on the later rounds [15,56]. However, to maintain this strategy, a greater cognitive control is required. In accordance with this interpretation, we found a specific correlation in HGs, where people who presented less difference between high-risk and low-risk offers showed a greater functional network differentiation (Figure 3D).

The functional networks that we found also include a central module in sensory-motor cortex. This module is compatible with the source of mu rhythms [57] whose power decreases (also called suppression or local desynchronization) has been related to mirror system activity during social games [58], motor coordination between humans [59] and the imagination of social interactions [60]. Moreover, recent work has shown that power in alpha range over sensory motor cortex is related to facial emotion recognition and it is negatively correlated with connectivity of the motor sensory cortex with other cortical areas [61]. In our experiment we found that the main modulation of global alpha synchrony was temporally dissociated from power modulation (Figure 2). However, the change in power was related to the community structure and not to the overall synchrony as the robust linear model shows

Table 2. Model of the difference in modularity between risky and safe offer (Rand Index).

	Scope	Std. Error.	T-value	p-value
(Intercept)	0.8329	0.0539	15.4663	0
Risk diff.	0.0639	0.0939	0.6801	0.5008
Strength diff.	0	0.0003	−0.0093	0.9926
Power diff.	0.5665	0,268	2.1138	0.0415
Human Games	−0.128	0.0711	−1.7992	0.0804
Risk diff.×Human Games	−0.2923	0.1203	−2.4295	0.0202
degree of freedom = 44				

(Table 2). This most likely reflects that the relations between phase synchrony and power is specific for each cortical area. Due to the low spatial resolution of our source reconstructions, we cannot accurately test these local differences. Finally, the spatial variations of the modules in lateral parietal region could be related to attentional and control networks that present nodes in this region [62,63]. Thus, the variation of community structure over these networks could reflect flexible changes in attentional and control processing during social interactions.

In conclusion, our results complement evidence that shows that during social interaction, humans establish flexible global interactions among different brain regions [6]. More specifically, we show that changes in the functional network in alpha band range takes place during social interaction, which could reflect cognitive control requirements to maintain an ongoing bargaining. Inter-site-phase-clustering (phase synchrony) of alpha oscillations could therefore serve as a mechanism by which cognitive control areas exert modulation over and receive information from social specialized brain areas in order to adapt behavior to current demands and changing social contexts.

Supporting Information

File S1 Supporting information. Table S1 in File S1. Analysis of variance of the modulation of the overall inter-site-phase-clustering strength by the conditions (human and computer games), offer risk (risky and safe offers) and frequency band (theta, alpha and beta). **Figure S1 in File S1.** Alpha band (7–10 Hz) inter-site-phase-clustering strength difference between safe and risky offers in human (red line) and computer (blue line) games. In the upper panel, inter-site-phase-clustering was calculated over voltage data reference to linking mastoids. In the lower panel, inter-site-phase-clustering was calculated over current source density (CSD). Grey areas indicate significant differences between human and computer games (p<0.05, cluster-corrected).

Acknowledgments

We want to thank Matías Morales and Marina Flores for proofreading the manuscript.

Author Contributions

Conceived and designed the experiments: PB DC FA. Performed the experiments: PB FZ. Analyzed the data: PB FZ MC. Contributed reagents/materials/analysis tools: PB FZ MC. Wrote the paper: PB MC DC FA.

References

1. Batson C (1990) How social an animal? The human capacity for caring. Am Psychol 45: 336–346. doi:10.1037/0003-066X.45.3.336.
2. Humphrey N (1976) The Social Function of intellect. In: Hinde PPGB& RA, editor. Growing points in ethology. Cambridge, England: Cambridge University Press.
3. Adolphs R (2009) The social brain: neural basis of social knowledge. Annu Rev Psychol 60: 693–716. doi:10.1146/annurev.psych.60.110707.163514.
4. Rilling JK, Sanfey AG (2011) The neuroscience of social decision-making. Annu Rev Psychol 62: 23–48. doi:10.1146/annurev.psych.121208.131647.
5. Kennedy DP, Adolphs R (2012) The social brain in psychiatric and neurological disorders. Trends Cogn Sci 16: 559–572. doi:10.1016/j.tics.2012.09.006.
6. Barrett LF, Satpute AB (2013) Large-scale brain networks in affective and social neuroscience: towards an integrative functional architecture of the brain. Curr Opin Neurobiol 23: 361–372. doi:10.1016/j.conb.2012.12.012.
7. Betti V, Zappasodi F, Rossini PM, Aglioti SM, Tecchio F (2009) Synchronous with your feelings: sensorimotor gamma band and empathy for pain. J Neurosci 29: 12384–12392. doi:10.1523/JNEUROSCI.2759-09.2009.
8. Dumas G, Nadel J, Soussignan R, Martinerie J, Garnero L (2010) Inter-brain synchronization during social interaction. PLoS One 5: e12166. doi:10.1371/journal.pone.0012166.
9. Cole MW, Reynolds JR, Power JD, Repovs G, Anticevic A, et al. (2013) Multi-task connectivity reveals flexible hubs for adaptive task control. Nat Neurosci 16. doi:10.1038/nn.3470.
10. Varela F, Lachaux JP, Rodriguez E, Martinerie J (2001) The brainweb: phase synchronization and large-scale integration. Nat Rev Neurosci 2: 229–239. doi:10.1038/35067550.
11. Güth W, Schmittberger R, Schwarze B (1982) An experimental analysis of ultimatum bargaining. J Econ Behav Organ 3: 367–388. doi:10.1016/0167-2681(82)90011-7.
12. Slembeck T (1999) Reputations and Fairness in Bargaining Experimental Evidence from a Repeated Ultimatum Game. Discuss Pap Dep Econ Univ St Gall 9904: 29.
13. Billeke P, Zamorano F, Cosmelli D, Aboitiz F (2013) Oscillatory Brain Activity Correlates with Risk Perception and Predicts Social Decisions. Cereb Cortex 23: 2872–2883. doi:10.1093/cercor/bhs269.
14. Koster-Hale J, Saxe R (2013) Theory of Mind: A Neural Prediction Problem. Neuron 79: 836–848. doi:10.1016/j.neuron.2013.08.020.
15. Billeke P, Zamorano F, López T, Rodriguez C, Cosmelli D, et al. (2014) Someone has to Give In: Theta Oscillations Correlate with Adaptive Behavior in Social Bargaining. Soc Cogn Affect Neurosci in press. doi:10.1093/scan/nsu012.
16. Baillet S, Mosher JC, Leahy RM (2001) Electromagnetic brain mapping. IEEE Signal Process Mag 18: 14–30.
17. Clerc M, Gramfort A, Olivi E, Papadopoulo T (2010) The symmetric BEM: bringing in more variables for better accuracy. In: Supek S, Sušac A, editors. 17th International Conference on Biomagnetism Advances in Biomagnetism – Biomag2010. Dubrovnik (Croatia): Springer Berlin Heidelberg, Vol. 28. 109–112. doi:10.1007/978-3-642-12197-5_21.
18. Lin F-H, Witzel T, Ahlfors SP, Stufflebeam SM, Belliveau JW, et al. (2006) Assessing and improving the spatial accuracy in MEG source localization by depth-weighted minimum-norm estimates. Neuroimage 31: 160–171. doi:10.1016/j.neuroimage.2005.11.054.
19. Lachaux JP, Rodriguez E, Martinerie J, Varela FJ (1999) Measuring phase synchrony in brain signals. Hum Brain Mapp 8: 194–208.

20. Fisher N (1995) Statistical analysis of circular data. Cambridge University Press.

21. Pons P, Latapy M (2005) Computing communities in large networks using random walks (long version). J Graph Algorith Appl 10: 191–218.

22. Newman MEJ (2006) Modularity and community structure in networks. Proc Natl Acad Sci U S A 103: 8577–8582. doi:10.1073/pnas.0601602103.

23. Valencia M, Pastor M a, Fernández-Seara M a, Artieda J, Martinerie J, et al. (2009) Complex modular structure of large-scale brain networks. Chaos 19: 023119. doi:10.1063/1.3129783.

24. Rand WM (1971) Objective Criteria for the Evaluation of Clustering Methods. J Am Stat Assoc 66: 846–850.

25. Maris E, Oostenveld R (2007) Nonparametric statistical testing of EEG- and MEG-data. J Neurosci Methods 164: 177–190. doi:10.1016/j.jneumeth.2007.03.024.

26. Zamorano F, Billeke P, Hurtado JM, López V, Carrasco X, et al. (2014) Temporal Constraints of Behavioral Inhibition: Relevance of Inter-stimulus Interval in a Go-Nogo Task. PLoS One 9: e87232. doi:10.1371/journal.pone.0087232.

27. Tadel F, Baillet S, Mosher JC, Pantazis D, Leahy RM (2011) Brainstorm: a user-friendly application for MEG/EEG analysis. Comput Intell Neurosci 2011: 879716. doi:10.1155/2011/879716.

28. Gramfort A, Papadopoulo T, Olivi E, Clerc M (2011) Forward field computation with OpenMEEG. Comput Intell Neurosci 2011: 923703. doi:10.1155/2011/923703.

29. Cocchi L, Zalesky A, Fornito A, Mattingley JB (2013) Dynamic cooperation and competition between brain systems during cognitive control. Trends Cogn Sci 17: 493–501. doi:10.1016/j.tics.2013.08.006.

30. Sadaghiani S, Scheeringa R, Lehongre K, Morillon B, Giraud A-L, et al. (2012) Alpha-Band Phase Synchrony Is Related To Activity in the Fronto-Parietal Adaptive Control Network. J Neurosci 32: 14305–14310. doi:10.1523/JNEUROSCI.1358-12.2012.

31. Jann K, Dierks T, Boesch C, Kottlow M, Strik W, et al. (2009) BOLD correlates of EEG alpha phase-locking and the fMRI default mode network. Neuroimage 45: 903–916. doi:10.1016/j.neuroimage.2009.01.001.

32. Dosenbach NUF, Fair D a, Cohen AL, Schlaggar BL, Petersen SE (2008) A dual-networks architecture of top-down control. Trends Cogn Sci 12: 99–105. doi:10.1016/j.tics.2008.01.001.

33. Phillips JM, Vinck M, Everling S, Womelsdorf T (2013) A Long-Range Fronto-Parietal 5- to 10-Hz Network Predicts "Top-Down" Controlled Guidance in a Task-Switch Paradigm. Cereb Cortex. doi:10.1093/cercor/bht050.

34. Declerck CH, Boone C, Emonds G (2013) When do people cooperate? The neuroeconomics of prosocial decision making. Brain Cogn 81: 95–117. doi:10.1016/j.bandc.2012.09.009.

35. Stevens JR, Hauser MD (2004) Why be nice? Psychological constraints on the evolution of cooperation. Trends Cogn Sci 8: 60–65. doi:10.1016/j.tics.2003.12.003.

36. Haufe S, Nikulin V V, Müller K-R, Nolte G (2013) A critical assessment of connectivity measures for EEG data: a simulation study. Neuroimage 64: 120–133. doi:10.1016/j.neuroimage.2012.09.036.

37. Gonçalves SI, de Munck JC, Pouwels PJW, Schoonhoven R, Kuijer JP a, et al. (2006) Correlating the alpha rhythm to BOLD using simultaneous EEG/fMRI: inter-subject variability. Neuroimage 30: 203–213. doi:10.1016/j.neuroimage.2005.09.062.

38. Laufs H, Kleinschmidt a, Beyerle a, Eger E, Salek-Haddadi a, et al. (2003) EEG-correlated fMRI of human alpha activity. Neuroimage 19: 1463–1476. doi:10.1016/S1053-8119(03)00286-6.

39. Laufs H, Holt JL, Elfont R, Krams M, Paul JS, et al. (2006) Where the BOLD signal goes when alpha EEG leaves. Neuroimage 31: 1408–1418. doi:10.1016/j.neuroimage.2006.02.002.

40. Cosmelli D, López V, Lachaux J-P, López-Calderón J, Renault B, et al. (2011) Shifting visual attention away from fixation is specifically associated with alpha band activity over ipsilateral parietal regions. Psychophysiology 48: 312–322. doi:10.1111/j.1469-8986.2010.01066.x.

41. Sadaghiani S, Scheeringa R, Lehongre K, Morillon B, Giraud A-L, et al. (2010) Intrinsic connectivity networks, alpha oscillations, and tonic alertness: a simultaneous electroencephalography/functional magnetic resonance imaging study. J Neurosci 30: 10243–10250. doi:10.1523/JNEUROSCI.1004-10.2010.

42. Hanslmayr S, Klimesch W, Sauseng P, Gruber W, Doppelmayr M, et al. (2005) Visual discrimination performance is related to decreased alpha amplitude but increased phase locking. Neurosci Lett 375: 64–68. doi:10.1016/j.neulet.2004.10.092.

43. Varela F, Toro A, John ER, Schwartz E (1981) Perceptual framing and cortical alpha rhythm. Neuropsychologia 19: 675–686.

44. VanRullen R, Koch C (2003) Is perception discrete or continuous? Trends Cogn Sci 7: 207–213. doi:10.1016/S1364-6613(03)00095-0.

45. Busch N a, Dubois J, VanRullen R (2009) The phase of ongoing EEG oscillations predicts visual perception. J Neurosci 29: 7869–7876. doi:10.1523/JNEUROSCI.0113-09.2009.

46. Jensen O, Mazaheri A (2010) Shaping functional architecture by oscillatory alpha activity: gating by inhibition. Front Hum Neurosci 4: 186. doi:10.3389/fnhum.2010.00186.

47. Mazaheri A, Jensen O (2010) Rhythmic pulsing: linking ongoing brain activity with evoked responses. Front Hum Neurosci 4: 177. doi:10.3389/fnhum.2010.00177.

48. Klimesch W (2012) Alpha-band oscillations, attention, and controlled access to stored information. Trends Cogn Sci 16: 606–617. doi:10.1016/j.tics.2012.10.007.

49. Palva S, Palva JM (2011) Functional roles of alpha-band phase synchronization in local and large-scale cortical networks. Front Psychol 2: 204. doi:10.3389/fpsyg.2011.00204.

50. Power JDD, Cohen ALL, Nelson SMM, Wig GSS, Barnes KAA, et al. (2011) Functional Network Organization of the Human Brain. Neuron 72: 665–678. doi:10.1016/j.neuron.2011.09.006.

51. Steinbeis N, Bernhardt BC, Singer T (2012) Impulse Control and Underlying Functions of the Left DLPFC Mediate Age-Related and Age-Independent Individual Differences in Strategic Social Behavior. Neuron 73: 1040–1051. doi:10.1016/j.neuron.2011.12.027.

52. Couture SM, Granholm EL, Fish SC (2011) A path model investigation of neurocognition, theory of mind, social competence, negative symptoms and real-world functioning in schizophrenia. Schizophr Res 125: 152–160. doi:10.1016/j.schres.2010.09.020.

53. Billeke P, Aboitiz F (2013) Social Cognition in Schizophrenia: From Social Stimuli Processing to Social Engagement. Front Psychiatry 4: 1–12. doi:10.3389/fpsyt.2013.00004.

54. Cusi AM, Nazarov A, Holshausen K, Macqueen GM, McKinnon MC (2012) Systematic review of the neural basis of social cognition in patients with mood disorders. J Psychiatry Neurosci 37: 154–169. doi:10.1503/jpn.100179.

55. Billeke P, Boardman S, Doraiswamy PM (2013) Social cognition in major depressive disorder: A new paradigm? Transl Neurosci 4: 437–447. doi:10.2478/s13380-013-0147-9.

56. Avrahami J, Güth W, Hertwig R, Kareev Y, Otsubo H (2013) Learning (not) to yield: An experimental study of evolving ultimatum game behavior. J Socio Econ 47: 47–54. doi:10.1016/j.socec.2013.08.009.

57. Arroyo S, Lesser RP, Gordon B, Uematsu S, Jackson D, et al. (1993) Functional significance of the mu rhythm of human cortex: an electrophysiologic study with subdural electrodes. Electroencephalogr Clin Neurophysiol 87: 76–87. doi:10.1016/0013-4694(93)90114-B.

58. Perry A, Stein L, Bentin S (2011) Motor and attentional mechanisms involved in social interaction–evidence from mu and alpha EEG suppression. Neuroimage 58: 895–904. doi:10.1016/j.neuroimage.2011.06.060.

59. Naeem M, Prasad G, Watson DR, Kelso J a S (2012) Functional dissociation of brain rhythms in social coordination. Clin Neurophysiol 123: 1789–1797. doi:10.1016/j.clinph.2012.02.065.

60. Vanderwert RE, Fox N a, Ferrari PF (2013) The mirror mechanism and mu rhythm in social development. Neurosci Lett 540: 15–20. doi:10.1016/j.neulet.2012.10.006.

61. Popov T, Miller G a., Rockstroh B, Weisz N (2013) Modulation of α power and functional connectivity during facial affect recognition. J Neurosci 33: 6018–6026. doi:10.1523/JNEUROSCI.2763-12.2013.

62. Smith SM, Fox PT, Miller KL, Glahn DC, Fox PM, et al. (2009) Correspondence of the brain's functional architecture during activation and rest. Proc Natl Acad Sci U S A 106: 13040–13045. doi:10.1073/pnas.0905267106.

63. Corbetta M, Shulman GL (2002) Control of goal-directed and stimulus-driven attention in the brain. Nat Rev Neurosci 3: 201–215. doi:10.1038/nrn755.

25

Re-Evaluation of the AASHTO-Flexible Pavement Design Equation with Neural Network Modeling

Mesut Tiğdemir*

Department of Civil Engineering, Süleyman Demirel University, Engineering Faculty, Isparta, Turkey

Abstract

Here we establish that equivalent single-axle loads values can be estimated using artificial neural networks without the complex design equality of American Association of State Highway and Transportation Officials (AASHTO). More importantly, we find that the neural network model gives the coefficients to be able to obtain the actual load values using the AASHTO design values. Thus, those design traffic values that might result in deterioration can be better calculated using the neural networks model than with the AASHTO design equation. The artificial neural network method is used for this purpose. The existing AASHTO flexible pavement design equation does not currently predict the pavement performance of the strategic highway research program (Long Term Pavement Performance studies) test sections very accurately, and typically over-estimates the number of equivalent single axle loads needed to cause a measured loss of the present serviceability index. Here we aimed to demonstrate that the proposed neural network model can more accurately represent the loads values data, compared against the performance of the AASHTO formula. It is concluded that the neural network may be an appropriate tool for the development of databased-nonparametric models of pavement performance.

Editor: Wen-Bo Du, Beihang University, China

Funding: The author has no support or funding to report.

Competing Interests: The author has declared that no competing interests exist.

* Email: mesuttigdemir@sdu.edu.tr

Introduction

The AASHO road test was probably the most significant piece of pavement research performed in the 20th century. The results of the AASHO road test have served as the basis for nearly all subsequent pavement designs used in the original construction of the interstate highway system (IHS) after 1961. When considering the overall performance of HIS pavements, we find that most of the pavements have lasted the expected 20 years while carrying traffic volumes far in excess of those predicted at the time of design [1].

The AASHO road test, possibly the largest and most successful controlled civil engineering experiment ever undertaken, was conducted about 50 years ago. The results of the study are still widely used across the world. Significant results from this road test still govern pavement design worldwide, including in areas such as: (a) equivalent single-axle loads (ESALs); (b) the serviceability–performance concept; (c) effects of layer thickness and strength; and (d) effectiveness of dowels and joint spacing. In addition, AASHO road test also changed the way that pavement research is conduct by illustrating the power of factorial experiments, high-quality data, and statistical analysis [2].

The American Association of State Highway Officials (AASHO) road test at Ottawa, Illinois provided the basis for calculating the required pavement thickness. Models were developed that related

pavement performance, vehicle loadings, the strength of roadbed soils, and the pavement structure. Equation 1 is the AASHTO equation used for design purposes. The purpose of the AASHTO model in the pavement thickness design process is to calculate the required structural number (SN). This is the strength of the pavement that must be constructed to carry the mixed vehicle loads over the roadbed soil, while providing satisfactory serviceability during the design period. Knowing the SN, the pavement layer thickness or overlay thickness can be calculated [3].

Vehicle loads are expressed in 18-kip equivalent single axle loads (18-kip ESAL). This information is normally generated by the district planning office.

$$\log_{10}(W_{18}) = Z_R * S_0 + 9.36 * \log_{10}(SN + 1) - 0.20$$
$$+ \frac{\log_{10}\left[\dfrac{\Delta PSI}{4.2 - 1.5}\right]}{0.40 + \dfrac{1094}{(SN + 1)^{5.19}}} + 2.32 * \log_{10}(MR) - 8.07 \quad (1)$$

The unknown to be determined is:

SN = Structural number required inches.

The inputs include the variables:

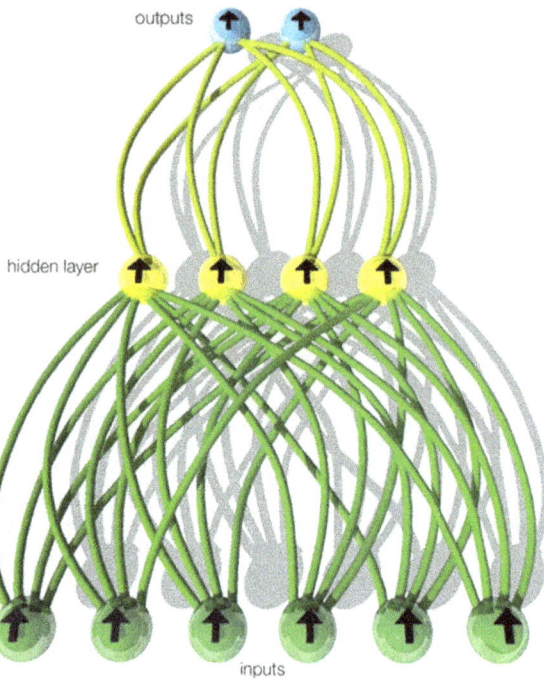

© 2010 Encyclopædia Britannica, Inc.

Figure 1. A simple feed-forward neural network [15].

W_{18} = Accumulated 18-kip ESAL over the life of the project.

Z_R = Standard normal deviate.

M_R = Resilient modulus psi

The inputs include the constants:

S_O = Standard deviation.

ΔPSI = Change in serviceability.

In the strategic highway research program (SHRP) project [4], as the equation was being used for research rather than design, a 50% reliability was selected as appropriate for mean predictions. At 50% reliability ZR = 0, and this term drops out of the equation. Equation 1 was used to predict the total KESALs (1000 ESALs) required to cause the observed losses in PSI.

Resilient moduli for the subgrade (Mr) were estimated based on the procedure provided in the 1986 guide. It should be noted that this procedure does not consider seasonal effects, so the subgrade moduli were not entirely consistent. However, the differences in magnitudes that would have occurred from seasonal adjustments would not have made significant differences to the results. Historical traffic data provided by the State Highway Agencies (SHAs) were used for the traffic data (W) in these calculations. The cumulative KESALs for each section were divided by the number of years since the test section was opened to traffic to obtain average values per year. This allowed extrapolation of an addition one or two year beyond 1989, to estimate a traffic level associated with the date of performance monitoring activities. Most of the monitoring data used were obtained in 1990 or 1991.

Banan and Hjelmstad [5] re-examined the AASHO road-test data, using adaptive random partitioning neural-network model developed by Banan and Hjelmstad (1995), and show that neural network model can represent the data far better than the AASHO formula. They conclude that the neural network may be an appropriate tool for the development of data-based models of pavement performance in the future.

In the report of FHWA-HRT-06-109, Souza et al. [6] presents an analysis between the international roughness index (IRI) and the standard deviation of longitudinal roughness (s), as well as a neural network study developed to predict the critical level of roughness. Using suitable software, the IRI and s values were computed for every longitudinal pavement profile measured. The neural network could forecast the IRI with an extremely high correlation factor ($R^2 = 0.99$).

Ozgan used the artificial neural network method to model the Marshall Stability (MS) of asphalt concrete under varying temperature and exposure times [7]. Alavi et al., derived a high-precision model to predict the flow number of dense asphalt mixtures using a generalized regression neural network and

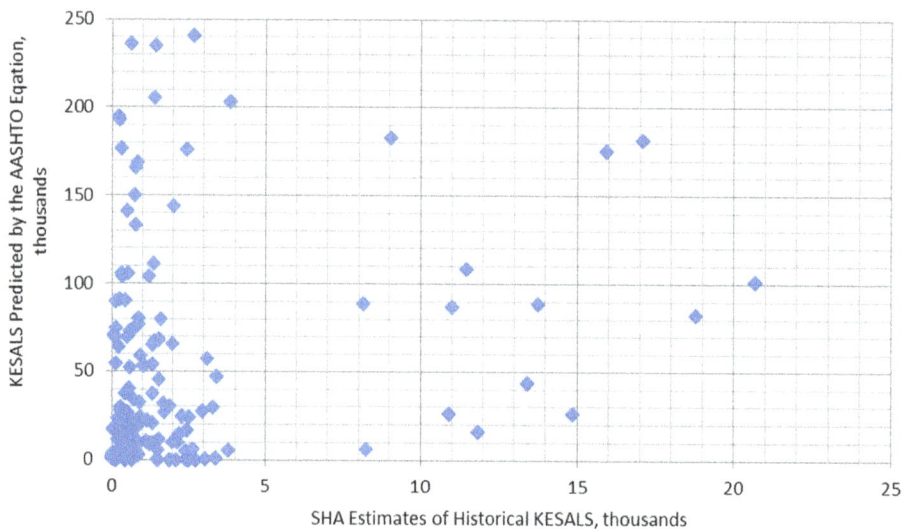

Figure 2. SHA Estimates of Historical Traffic Versus AASHTO Predicted Traffic.

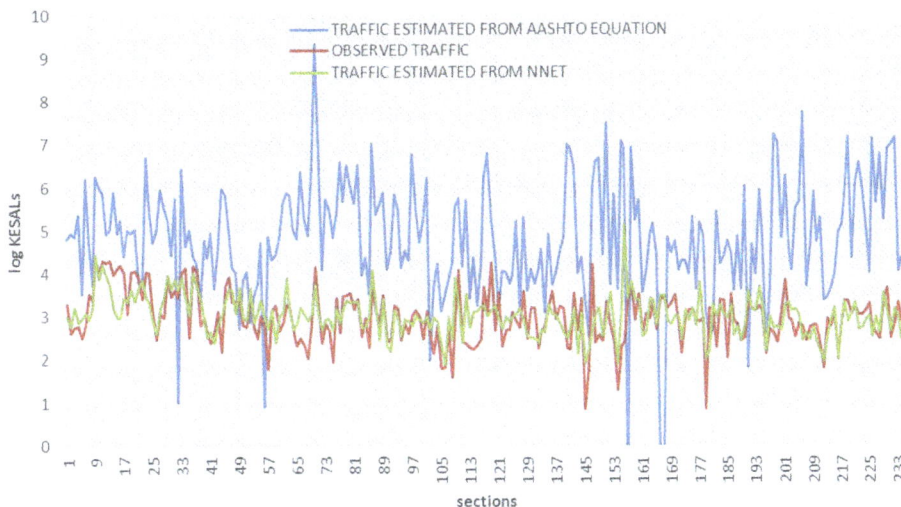

Figure 3. Predicted KESALs values by AASHTO equation, NNET model, and the relations of them to the observed values.

multiple regression-based analyses [8]. Kok and et al., aimed to model the complex modulus of base and styrene–butadiene–styrene (SBS) modified bitumens by using artificial neural networks (ANNs). They used the variants of the Levenberg–Marquardt, scaled conjugate gradient and Pola-Ribiere conjugate gradient algorithms [9]. Wu and et al., studied the computation of the stress intensity factors at the crack tip for pavement crack propagation analysis using a neural network approach based on semi-analytical finite element analysis [10]. Kok and et al., studied to model the complex modulus of styrene–butadiene–styrene modified bitumen samples by different methods using artificial neural networks [11].

The principal goal of this study was to relate the design life of the pavements obtained from the AASHTO equation, which is known worldwide, with the observed life in terms of equivalent single-axle loads.

Methods

A neural network is a massively parallel distributed processor that has a natural propensity for storing experiential knowledge and making it available for use. It resembles the brain in two respects [12]:

1. Knowledge is acquired by the network through a learning process.
2. Interconnection strengths known as synaptic weights are used to store the knowledge.

At its most basic, learning is a process by which the free parameters (i.e., synaptic weights and bias levels) of a neural network are adapted through a continuing process of stimulation by the environment in which the network is embedded. The type of learning is determined by the manner in which the parameter changes take place. In a general sense, the learning process may be classified as [13]: Learning with a teacher (also referred to as supervised learning); or learning without a teacher (also referred to as unsupervised learning).

Learning is thus a development from the simple Delta rule in which extra hidden layers (layers additional to the input and output layers, not connected externally) are added. The network topology is constrained to be feed-forward (i.e., loop-free); generally connections are allowed from the input layer to the first (and possibly only) hidden layer; from the first hidden layer to the second, and so no until progressing from the last hidden layer to the output layer (Figure 1) [14–15].

The hidden layer learns to recode (or to provide a representation for) the inputs. More than one hidden layer can be used. This architecture is more powerful than single-layer networks as it can be shown that any mapping can be learned, given two hidden layers (of units). The units are generally more complex than those in the original perceptron and their input/output graph can be summarized as the function:

$$Y = \frac{1}{1 + e^{(-k*(\sum W_{in}*X_{in}))}} \qquad (2)$$

The weight change rule is a development of the perceptron learning rule. Weights are changed by an amount proportional to the error at that unit multiplied by the output of the unit feeding into the weight.

Running such a network consists of several components, including: Forward pass, where the outputs are calculated and the error at the output units calculated; backward pass, where the output unit error is used to alter weights on the output units. Subsequently, the errors at the hidden nodes are calculated (by back-propagating the error at the output units through the weights), and the weights on the hidden nodes are altered accordingly.

For each data pair to be learned a forward pass and backwards pass is performed. This is repeated until the error is acceptably low.

Table 1. Regression coefficients for the different network architectures.

NETWORK	LOOP	NEURON	R	NEURON	R	NEURON	R
FEED FORWARD BACKPROP.	1000	5	0.744	10	0.923	20	0.968
CASCADE FORWARD BACKPROP.			0.785		0.886		0.972
ELMAN BACKPROP.			0.707		0.699		0.688

training:Levenberg-Marquardt, performance: mean squared error.

Comparisons of Predicted Versus Observed Traffic

With data from 244 general pavement studies (GPS)-I and GPS-2 of in-service flexible pavement test sections across the USA, the Long Term Pavement Performance (LTPP) database offers an unprecedented opportunity for evaluating the ways in which flexible pavements are designed and their associated performance. In these analyses of the SHRP LTPP database, all efforts were concentrated on evaluating the AASHTO pavement design equation and the suitability of the data collected from these test sections for use in such evaluations. From these evaluations, it has been established that the existing AASHTO flexible pavement design equation does not accurately predict the pavement performance of the SHRP LTPP test sections, and unfortunately, generally predicts many more ESALs needed to cause a measured loss of present serviceability index (PSI) than the pavements had actually experienced. Many explanations have been identified. Although modifications have been made over the years to expand the inference space of these design equations, any such modifications cannot be without their own limitations [4].

From SHRP long-term pavement performance (LTPP) studies, it is evident that environmental properties such as rainfall, freezing index, and freeze-thaw cycles have a greater impact on pavement performance than that accommodated by the AASHTO flexible pavement design equation.

Figure 2 provides a plot of predicted KESALs versus those estimated by the SHA's throughout 1989 and extrapolated through 1991. As can be seen, the traffic predicted by the AASHTO equation is consistently much higher than the estimates of historical traffic provided by the SHAs. Only nine of the 244 predictions were lower than the estimates of the state highway agencies. Almost half of the estimates (in 112 sections) predicted traffic levels 100-fold greater than the SHA estimates (Figure 3). Note that the average ratio (8770) and standard deviation (51,800) are distorted by several sections where this ratio exceeded 100,000. This extreme lack of fit of the design equation to the in-service data is not entirely due to the shortcomings of the equation itself. Limitation of the input data are also believed to have contributed to the apparent differences between predicted and estimated ESALs. The future availability of ESALs estimates that would include some years of measured data, plus higher [resent serviceability index values should allow a somewhat more accurate evaluation of the deficiencies in the equation itself.

Prediction of the observed traffic (KESALs) using neural networks

In this study, different network architectures have been employed to model the database. The regression coefficients were given in Table 1 for the output of KESALs estimated by the AASHTO pavement equation. As a result of the comparison of the network architectures, the feed forward-back propagation network architecture was chosen for this study.

The previously described AASHTO road test database was initially analyzed using the feed-forward/back-propagation neural network modeling system with the objective of finding an NN model as a function of the available input parameters. A single output layer for the KESALs value was used. The input layer consisted of 7 data neurons as follows:

- Input 1: rain = average annual rain fall
- Input 2: avg32 = average annual number of days below 32 F (0 C)
- Input 3: drainage coefficient (m) = $(1.2 - 0.006*\text{average rain}) * (1.2 - 0.006*\% - 200)$

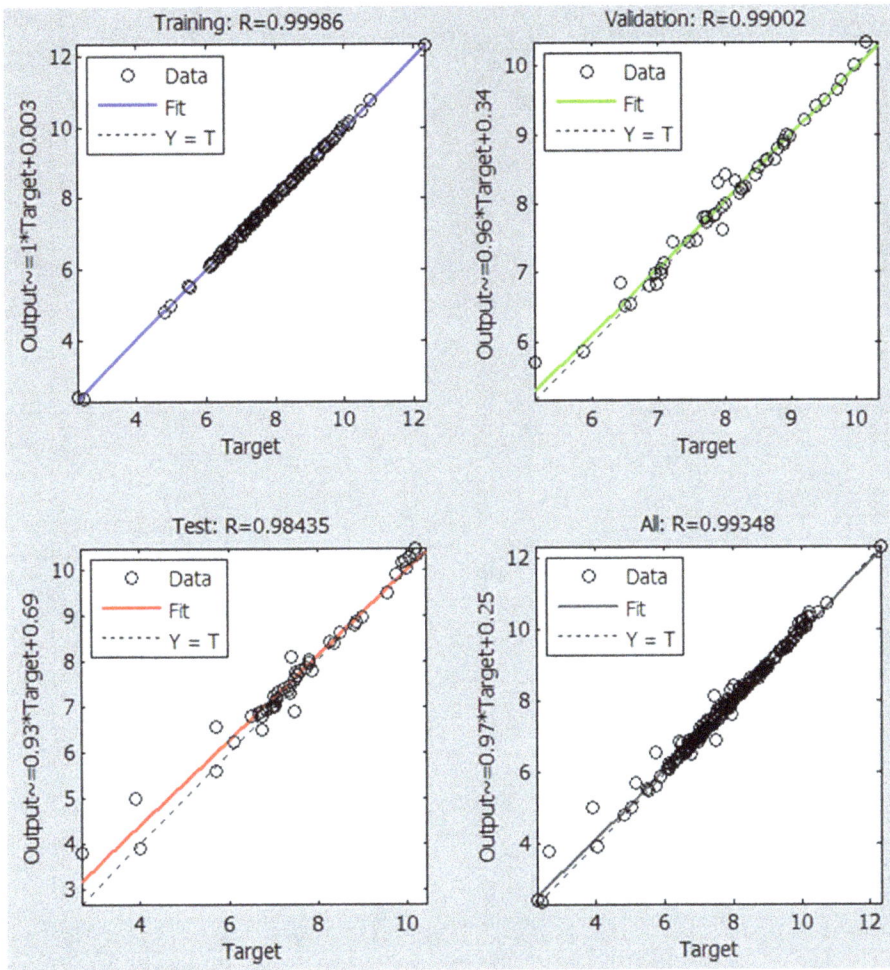

Figure 4. Regression plot of KESALs predictions for target (AASHTO Equation produced) with model output of ANN (7 inputs).

– Input 4: observed PSI loss = (initial PSI) − (calculated PSI)

– Input 5: back-calculated mr = [(fwd load)*0.2792)/(deflection at 60″) * 60]

– Input 6:SN = .44*AC+.34*BBB+.23*NBBB+m*(.14*UBB+.07*SUBB+.15*SS)

Asphalt (AC), Bit Bound Base (BBB), Non Bit Bound Base(NBBB), Unbound Base(UBB), Sub-base (SUBB), Stab-Subgrade (SS)

– Input 7: The subgrade type = Gravel, Sand, Silt, Clay, Silty Clay, Rock

The subgrade type was divided into 6 types according to the unified soil classification system (SUCS), plus rock foundation. The following codes were attributed to input of the subgrade type: Gravel = 1; Sand = 2; Silt = 3; Clay = 4; Silty Clay = 5; and Rock = 6.

Two neural network models have been employed. In the first model, KESALs predicted by the AASHTO equation as log10(KESALs)AASHTO was used as the output. In order to obtain the AASHTO KESALs traffic value without using the

design equation, the first neural network model was developed. Owing to the large differentiation between the observed and AASHTO KESALs, in the second model, the output was chosen to be the observed KESALs values. However, the model was not able to present the database as expected. Hence, the output was accepted as the ratio of logarithmic KESALs by AASHTO to logarithmic observed KESALs value.

Because of an absence of rain data for some sections, 234 of a total of 244 sections were employed for modeling. The training data-set, comprising 164 random sections of 234 available (70%), was initially chosen for the learning stage. The NN model produced excellent results, as illustrated in Figure 4, which shows the training targets (predicted KESALs by AASHTO equation) and the network outputs (computed KESALs values). The correlation coefficient for the training stage was high ($R^2 = 0.999$). Of the remaining 30% of the data-set, 15% of the sections were used to validate the model and another 15% were used to test the model. Predictions were good despite a higher dispersion than in the learning stage. The correlation coefficient for the validation stage was $R^2 = 0.990$.

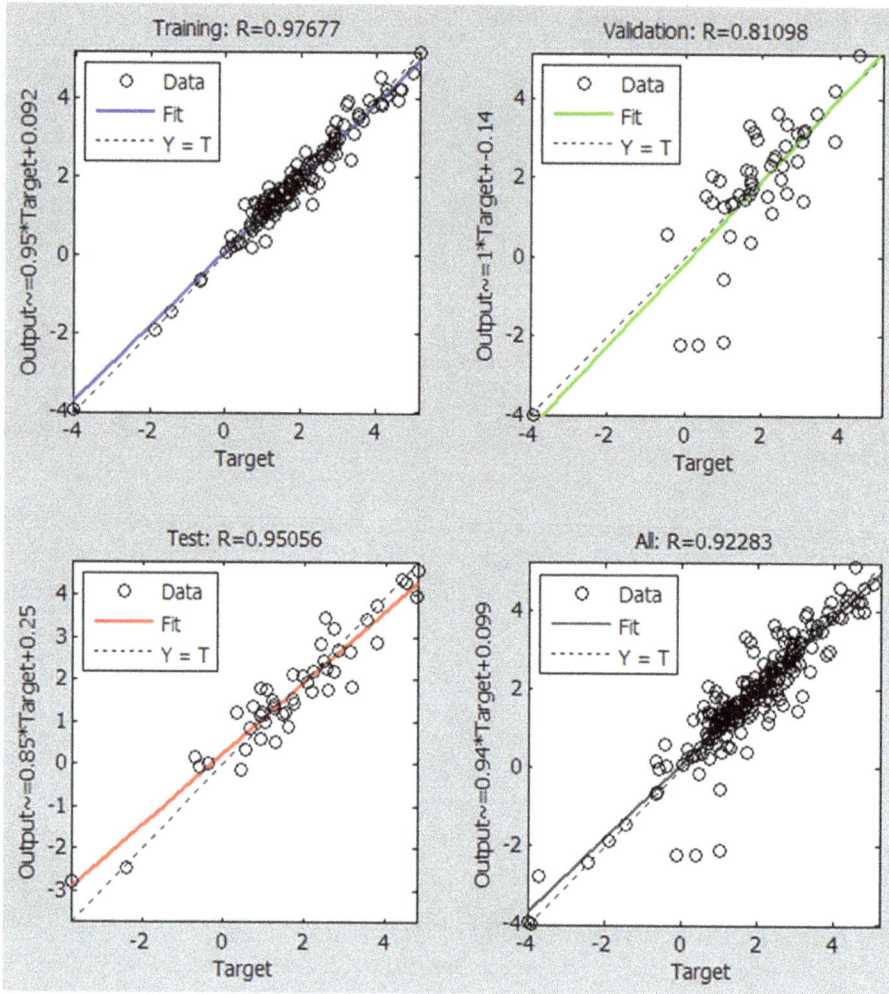

Figure 5. Regression plot of KESALs ratio (log10[AASHTO/actual KESALs]) predictions for target with model output of ANN (7 inputs).

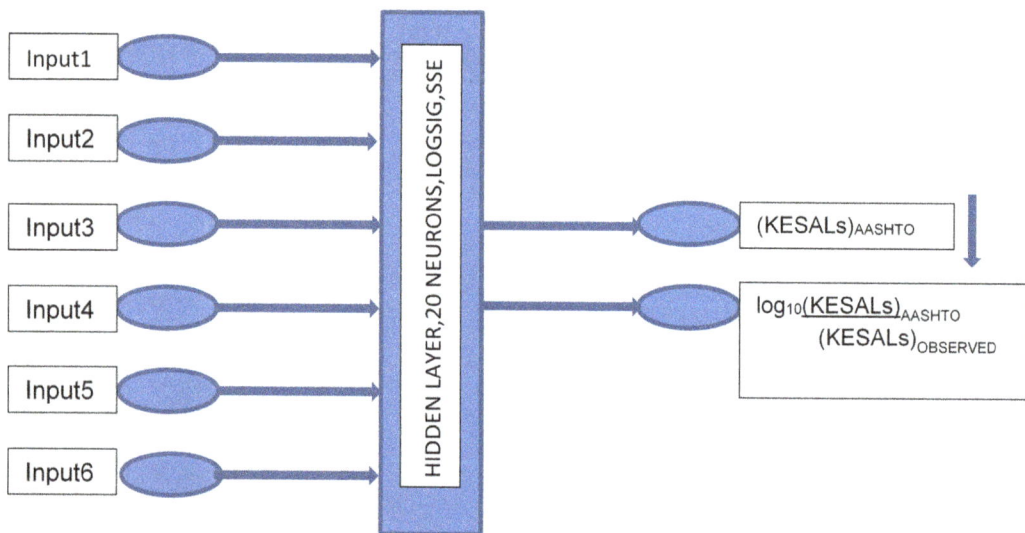

Figure 6. The proposed NN model combined of the NN1 and NN2 models.

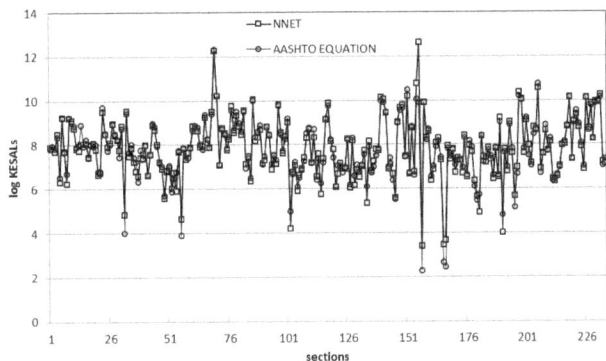

Figure 7. AASHTO equation modeling with neural networks (correlation of 0.97).

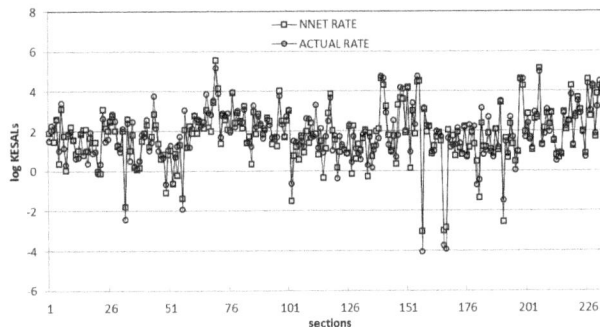

Figure 8. The ratio of KESALsAASHTO to KESALsOBSERVED modeling with neural networks (correlation of 0.94).

In the second model, the output was chosen to be the logarithmic ratio of KESALs calculated by the AASHTO design equation to observed values. The inputs were the same as the first model of 7 inputs. The training, the validation, and the test databases were the same as used above. The results are shown in Figure 5. With this model, for inputs of road test data, the output will be given as the ratio of calculated KESALs to those observed, and the observed value may therefore be predicted as follows:

The output of NN model:

$$M = \log_{10} \frac{(KESALs)_{AASHTO}}{(KESALSs)_{OBSERVED}} \quad (3)$$

This neural network model can easily give the KESALs value without using the AASHTO complex pavement design equation. At the same time, the model gives the ratio M, hence the observed values can be predicted as:

$$(KESALs)_{OBSERVED} = \frac{(KESALs)_{AASHTO}}{10^M} \quad (4)$$

Here, based on the previous two NN models, a new combined model that contains two outputs is proposed. The inputs are the same as in previous studies. The first output is the KESALs predicted by the AASHTO design equation. This value is estimated by the combined NN model using the inputs of road test data. In parallel, the second output of the model is estimated as the logarithmic ratio of the KESALs by the AASHTO equation to observed KESALs. Thus, the observed KESALs may be estimated using Equation 4. Figure 6 shows the proposed combined NN model. Scatter plots between targets and estimations by the NN model are given for both output 1 (i.e., KESALs obtained using the AASHTO design equation) and output 2 (i.e., the logarithmic ratio between predicted and observed KESALs) with correlations of 0.97 and 0.94, respectively (Figure 7, 8).

The developed NN model first predicts the output value of the AASHTO design equation and, second, gives the ratio of this estimated value to the actual observed value. Using this ratio, the actual KESALs value may be estimated.

A sensitivity analysis was performed to determine the relative contribution of each input parameters to the estimation of the output. The outputs are KESALs and the ratio of estimated KESALs to observed KESALs. This analysis have been performed for the change of +10% of all inputs' individually for the twenty sections. The inputs of the delta-PSI, the MR, and the SN give the most relative contribution to the estimation of outputs (Figure 9).

Prediction of KESALs Using Multivariate Statistical Models

The seven inputs of the same road test database were used to attempt to assess the performance of the established statistical models for predicting the actual KESALs, as well as those predicted using the AASHTO equation. The multivariate linear models were tested. The results of the database statistical analyses are given in Table 2–3. No correlation could be found ($R^2 = 0.23$) of the linear model for observed KESALs values. Whereas the correlation is about $R^2 = 0.68$ for predicted KESALs using the AASHTO equation. The stepwise analysis was employed to model the database. The results show highly significant (P<0.0001) inputs on the outputs as the delta-PSI, MR, and the SN values according to the statistical significance (P, 2 tail) analysis, as seen before in the sensitivity analysis.

Conclusions

In this paper, databased mathematical-neural network models of long-term pavement performance studies have been obtained by re-evaluating the AASHO road-test data.

Two neural network models have been developed based on the feed-forward/back-propagation algorithm and their performances compared to the KESALs predicted using the AASHO formula.

Neural network and multivariate statistics regression were used to an attempt to model the computed and predicted KESALs values. Of the 244 pavement sections, 234 sections were selected to achieve the aims of this study.

A complete set of average annual rain fall, average annual number of days below 32°F (0°C), drainage coefficients, observed PSI loss, back-calculated resilient moduli for the subgrade, structural numbers, and the subgrade types (Gravel, Sand, Silt, Clay, SiltyClay, Rock) were used for the prediction of the KESALs, using the AASHTO equation as well as those obtained from observed values.

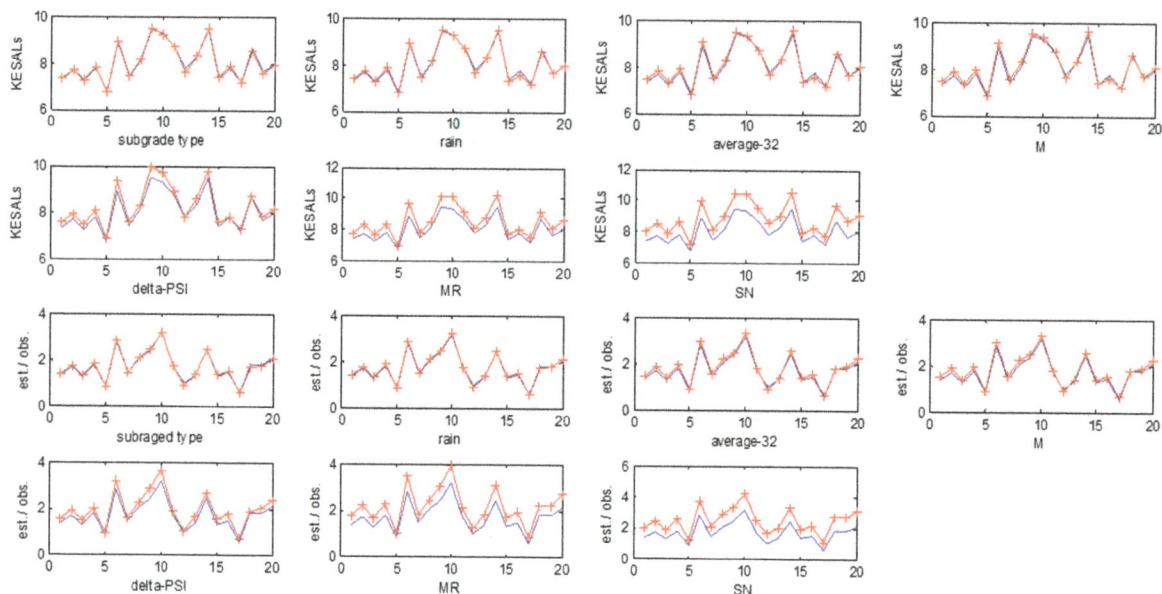

Figure 9. The sensitivity analysis of relative contributions of each input parameters to the outputs.

An extremely accurate model using neural network modeling method was developed.

This NN model gave coefficient of correlations of 0.999 and 0.976 during the training stage, in models 1 and 2, respectively. Whereas it was not possible to model the data using multivariate linear statistic models with a coefficient of correlation of 0.68.

The neural network proved to be an extremely powerful tool for predicting KESALS (both predicted and observed). Similar NN models may be developed for other databases of LTPP's GPS program to include other types of pavement structures.

Throughout this paper, the database has been studied in order to re-evaluate the model for equivalent single-axle loads to cause the observed losses in PSI using the database presented in AASHO road test.

We found that the AASHO equation does not represent the cumulative equivalent single-axle loads. Significant discrepancies between the AASHO-predicted KESALS and the observed values have been modeled using the neural networks.

It has been shown that a local approximation feed-forward/back-propagation neural network can model the pavement performance data for the entire input domain better than a global approximation, such as the AASHTO formula.

The neural network method was used to build a nonparametric model for pavement performance using the road test data and its performance was compared with the AASHTO model.

In this study, NN design method for flexible pavements is proposed as a replacement for the AASHTO classical design equation.

This new model can represent the data much more accurately than the AASHTO formula. The AASHTO design overestimates ESALs whereas the proposed new model does not.

KESAL values can be estimated using artificial neural networks without the complex design equality of AASHTO. More importantly, the NN model gives the transfer coefficient from the AASHTO design estimation output to actual KESAL values occurred in test sections.

Thus, the design traffic values that can cause deterioration can be calculated more accurately using the NN model than with the AASHTO design equation.

Table 2. Statistical analysis of the database.

Effect	Coefficient	Std Error	Std Coef	Tolerance	t	P(2 Tail)
CONSTANT	3,944	0,191	0,000	,	20,697	0,000
AVG32	0,002	0,001	0,072	0,835	1,745	0,082
DELTAPSI	1,335	0,111	0,479	0,886	11,981	0,000
MR	0,000	0,000	0,366	0,995	9,696	0,000
SN	0,428	0,032	0,520	0,939	13,392	0,000

Dep Var: KESALS N: 234 Multiple R: 0,822 squared multiple R: 0,676.
Adjusted squared multiple R: 0,670 Standard error of estimate: 0,791.

Table 3. Analysis of Variance.

Source	Sum-of-Squares	df	Mean-Square	F-ratio	P
Regression	298,208	4	74,552	119,195	0,000
Residual	143,232	229	0,625		

Author Contributions

Analyzed the data: MT. Contributed reagents/materials/analysis tools: MT. Wrote the paper: MT.

References

1. Hallin JP, Teng TP, Scofield LA, Von Quintus HL (2007) Pavement Design in the Post-AASHO road test Era. E-C118, s.l.: Transportation Research Board, Transportation Research Circular, pp. 1–16.
2. Hudson WR, Monismith CL, Shook JF, Finn FN, Skok Jr EL (2007) AASHO road test Effect on Pavement Design and Evaluation After 50 Years. E-C118, s.l.: Transportation Research Board, Transportation Research Circular, pp. 17–30.
3. Flexible Pavement Design Manual (2008) Florida: Florida Department of Transportation. 183p.
4. Evaluation of the AASHTO Design Equations and Recommend Improvements (1994). Washington DC: Strategic Highway Research Program. SHRP-P-394. 214p.
5. Banan MR, Hjelmstad KD (1996) Neural Networks And Aasho Road Test. Journal of Transportation Engineering 122 (5), pp. 358–366.
6. Souza RO, Neto SD, Farias MM (2006) Improving Pavements With Long-Term Pavement Performance: Products for Today and Tomorrow. Statistical analysis between roughness indices and roughness Prediction model using neural networks. s.l.: FHWA.
7. Ozgan E (2011) Artificial neural network based modelling of the Marshall Stability of asphalt concrete. Expert Systems with Applications 38(5), 6025–6030. doi:10.1016/j.eswa.2010.11.018
8. Alavi AH, Ameri M, Gandomi AH, Mirzahosseini MR (2011) Formulation of flow number of asphalt mixes using a hybrid computational method. Construction and Building Materials 25(3), 1338–1355. doi:10.1016/j.conbuildmat.2010.09.010
9. Kok BV, Yilmaz M, Sengoz B, Sengur A, Avci E (2010) Investigation of complex modulus of base and SBS modified bitumen with artificial neural networks. Expert Systems with Applications 37(12), 7775–7780. doi:10.1016/j.eswa.2010.04.063
10. Wu Z, Hu S, Zhou F (2014) Prediction of stress intensity factors in pavement cracking with neural networks based on semi-analytical FEA. Expert Systems with Applications 41(4), 1021–1030. doi:10.1016/j.eswa.2013.07.063
11. Kök BV, Yilmaz M, Çakiroğlu M, Kuloğlu N, Şengür A (2013) Neural network modeling of SBS modified bitumen produced with different methods. Fuel 106, 265–270. doi:10.1016/j.fuel.2012.12.073
12. HAYKIN Simon (1999) Neural Networks: A Comprehensive Foundation. s.l.: Englewood Cliffs, NJ: Prentice-Hall.
13. Feedforward Neural Networks. Available: http://media.wiley.com/product_data/excerpt/19/04713491/0471349119.pdf. Accessed 2014 Oct 28.
14. Smith, Prof. Leslie. An Introduction to Neural Networks. Available: http://www.cs.stir.ac.uk/~lss/NNIntro/InvSlides.html#algs. Accessed 2014 Oct 28.
15. Feedforward control: feedforward neural network - Britannica Online Encyclopedia. Encyclopædia Britannica, Inc. Available: http://www.britannica.com/EBchecked/media/56311/A-simple-feedforward-neural-network-In-a-simple-feedforward-neural. Accessed 2014 Oct 28.

Permissions

List of Contributors

Junqi Chen
Department of Rehabilitation, The Third Affiliated Hospital of Southern Medical University, Guangzhou, China

Jizhou Wang
The First Clinical Medical School, Southern Medical University, Guangzhou, China

Yong Huang and Shanshan Qu
School of Traditional Chinese Medicine, Southern Medical University, Guangzhou, China

Xinsheng Lai, Chunzhi Tang and Junjun Yang
School of Acupuncture and Rehabilitation, Guangzhou University of Traditional Chinese Medicine, Guangzhou, China

Junxian Wu
Department of Acupuncture and Moxibustion, Shantou Central Hospital, Shantou, China

Tongjun Zeng
The First People's Hospital of Shunde, Foshan, China

Yangyang Zhang, Shuchen Guan, Xiaolong Hong and Xianchun Li
School of Psychology and Cognitive Science, East China Normal University, Shanghai, P. R. China

Yang Hu and Zhaoxin Wang
Institute of Cognitive Neuroscience, East China Normal University, Shanghai, P. R. China

Anne Bolwerk and Christian Maihöfner
Department of Neurology, University Hospital Erlangen, Erlangen, Germany
Department of Physiology and Pathophysiology, Friedrich-Alexander-University Erlangen-Nürnberg, Erlangen, Germany

Jessica Mack-Andrick
Education Department of the Museums in Nuremberg, Nuremberg, Germany

Frieder R. Lang
Institute of Psychogerontology, Friedrich-Alexander- University Erlangen-Nürnberg, Nuremberg, Germany

Arnd Dörfler
Department of Neuroradiology, University Hospital Erlangen, Erlangen, Germany

Yu Qian
Nonlinear Research Institute, Baoji University of Arts and Sciences, Baoji, China
Center for Systems Biology, Soochow University, Suzhou, China
State Key Laboratory of Theoretical Physics, Institute of Theoretical Physics, Chinese Academy of Sciences, Beijing, China

Chen Niu, Ming Zhang, Zhigang Min, Netra Rana, Qiuli Zhang and Min Li
Department of Medical Imaging, First Affiliated Hospital of Xi'an Jiaotong University, Xi'an, Shaanxi-Province, P. R. China

Xin Liu and Pan Lin
Institute of Biomedical Engineering, Xi'an Jiaotong University, Xi'an, Shaanxi-Province, P.R. China

Norma Naima Rüther
Institute of Cognitive Neuroscience, Dept. of Neuropsychology, Ruhr University Bochum, Bochum, Germany
International Graduate School of Neuroscience, Ruhr University Bochum, Bochum, Germany

Marco Tettamanti
Division Neuroscience, San Raffaele Scientific Institute, Milano, Italy
Department of Nuclear Medicine, San Raffaele Scientific Institute, Milano, Italy

Stefano F. Cappa
Department of Nuclear Medicine, San Raffaele Scientific Institute, Milano, Italy
Faculty of Psychology, Vita-Salute San Raffaele University, Milano, Italy

Christian Bellebaum
Institute of Experimental Psychology, Heinrich Heine University Düsseldorf, Düsseldorf, Germany

Nicola Bertolino and Francesco Ghielmetti
Health Department, Carlo Besta Neurological Institute, Milan, Italy

Stefania Ferraro, Anna Nigri and Maria Grazia Bruzzone
Neuro-Radiology Department, Carlo Besta Neurological Institute, Milan, Italy

Jing Shang, Yajing Meng, Hongru Zhu, Changjian Qiu and Wei Zhang
Mental Health Center, Department of Psychiatry, West China Hospital of Sichuan University, Chengdu, Sichuan, People's Republic of China

Qiyong Gong
Huaxi MR Research Center (HMRRC), Department of Radiology, West China Hospital of Sichuan University, Chengdu, Sichuan, People's Republic of China

Su Lui
Huaxi MR Research Center (HMRRC), Department of Radiology, West China Hospital of Sichuan University, Chengdu, Sichuan, People's Republic of China
Radiology Department of the Second Affiliated Hospital, Wenzhou Medical University, Wenzhou, Zhejiang, People's Republic of China

Wei Liao
Center for Cognition and Brain Disorders (CCBD), Hangzhou Normal University, Hangzhou, Zhejiang, People's Republic of China

Ágnes Melinda Kovács, György Gergely and Gergely Csibra
Cognitive Development Centre, Central European University, Budapest, Hungary

Simone Kühn
Max Planck Institute for Human Development, Center for Lifespan Psychology, Berlin, Germany

Marcel Brass
Department of Experimental Psychology and Ghent Institute of Functional and Metabolic Imaging, Ghent University, Ghent, Belgium
Behavioural Science Institute, Radboud University, Nijmegen, The Netherlands

Huixin Qin, Jun Ma and Chunni Wang
Department of Physics, Lanzhou University of Technology, Lanzhou, China

Ying Wu
School of Aerospace, Xian Jiaotong University, Xian, China

Vipul Lugade and Li-Shan Chou
Department of Human Physiology, University of Oregon, Eugene, Oregon, United States of America

Victor Lin
Rehabilitation Medicine Associates of Eugene-Springfield, P.C., Eugene, Oregon, United States of America

Arthur Farley
Department of Computer and Information Sciences, University of Oregon, Eugene, Oregon, United States of America

Jorge Arrubla and Desmond H. Y. Tse
Institute of Neuroscience and Medicine 4, INM 4, Forschungszentrum Jülich, Jülich, Germany

Christin Amkreutz
Institute of Neuroscience and Medicine 4, INM 4, Forschungszentrum Jülich, Jülich, Germany
Department of Psychiatry, Psychotherapy and Psychosomatics, RWTH Aachen University, Aachen, Germany

Irene Neuner
Institute of Neuroscience and Medicine 4, INM 4, Forschungszentrum Jülich, Jülich, Germany
Department of Psychiatry, Psychotherapy and Psychosomatics, RWTH Aachen University, Aachen, Germany
JARA – BRAIN – Translational Medicine, RWTH Aachen University, Aachen, Germany

N. Jon Shah
Institute of Neuroscience and Medicine 4, INM 4, Forschungszentrum Jülich, Jülich, Germany
JARA – BRAIN – Translational Medicine, RWTH Aachen University, Aachen, Germany
Department of Neurology, RWTH Aachen University, Aachen, Germany

Xingyi Ge and Nadia Naffakh
Institut Pasteur, Unité de Génétique Moléculaire des Virus à ARN, Département de Virologie, Paris, France
CNRS, URA3015, Paris, France

Université Paris Diderot, Sorbonne Paris Cité, Unité de Génétique Moléculaire des Virus à ARN, Paris, France

Emmanuel dos Santos Afonso
Institut Pasteur, Unité de Génétique Moléculaire des Virus à ARN, Département de Virologie, Paris, France
CNRS, URA3015, Paris, France
Université Paris Diderot, Sorbonne Paris Cité, Unité de Génétique Moléculaire des Virus à ARN, Paris, France
Promega France, Charbonniéres-les-Bains, France

Marie-Anne Rameix-Welti and Elyanne Gault
Institut Pasteur, Unité de Génétique Moléculaire des Virus à ARN, Département de Virologie, Paris, France
CNRS, URA3015, Paris, France
Université Paris Diderot, Sorbonne Paris Cité, Unité de Génétique Moléculaire des Virus à ARN, Paris, France
Université Versailles Saint-Quentin-en-Yvelines, Guyancourt, France

Martin Schwemmle and Geoffrey Chase
Department of Virology, Institute for Medical Microbiology and Hygiene, University of Freiburg, Germany

Didier Picard
Département de Biologie Cellulaire, Université de Genève, Genève, Switzerland

Francisco Gomez and Damien Lesenfants
Coma Science Group, Cyclotron Research Centre, University of Liège, Liège, Belgium

Enrico Amico
Coma Science Group, Cyclotron Research Centre, University of Liège, Liège, Belgium
Faculty of Psychology and Educational Sciences, Department of Data Analysis, Ghent University, Ghent, Belgium

Steven Laureys
Coma Science Group, Cyclotron Research Centre, University of Liège, Liège, Belgium
Department of Neurology, University of Liège, Liège, Belgium

Pierre Boveroux
Coma Science Group, Cyclotron Research Centre, University of Liège, Liège, Belgium
Department of Anesthesia and Intensive Care Medicine, CHU Sart Tilman Hospital, University of Liège, Liège, Belgium

Vincent Bonhomme
Coma Science Group, Cyclotron Research Centre, University of Liège, Liège, Belgium
Department of Anesthesia and Intensive Care Medicine, CHU Sart Tilman Hospital, University of Liège, Liège, Belgium
Department of Anesthesia and Intensive Care Medicine, CHR Citadelle, University of Liège, Liège, Belgium

Audrey Vanhaudenhuyse
Coma Science Group, Cyclotron Research Centre, University of Liège, Liège, Belgium
Department of Algology and Palliative Care, CHU Sart Tilman Hospital, University of Liège, Liège, Belgium

Daniele Marinazzo
Faculty of Psychology and Educational Sciences, Department of Data Analysis, Ghent University, Ghent, Belgium

Jean-François Brichant
Department of Anesthesia and Intensive Care Medicine, CHU Sart Tilman Hospital, University of Liège, Liège, Belgium

Carol Di Perri
Department of Neuroradiology, National Neurological Institute C. Mondino, Pavia, Italy

Leonid L. Moroz
Department of Molecular & Integrative Physiology, University of Illinois, Urbana, Illinois, United States of America
The Whitney Laboratory for Marine Bioscience, University of Florida, St. Augustine, Florida, United States of America

Nathan G. Hatcher
Department of Molecular & Integrative Physiology, University of Illinois, Urbana, Illinois, United States of America
Merck & Co., Inc., West Point, Pennsylvania, United States of America

Rhanor Gillette
Department of Molecular & Integrative Physiology, University of Illinois, Urbana, Illinois, United States of America
The Neuroscience Program, University of Illinois, Urbana, Illinois, United States of America

Keiko Hirayama
The Neuroscience Program, University of Illinois, Urbana, Illinois, United States of America Wolfram Inc., Champaign, Illinois, United States of America

Xinyu Zhao
Department of Neuroscience and Waisman Center, School of Medicine and Public Health, University of Wisconsin, Madison, Wisconsin, United States of America

Weixiang Guo
Department of Neuroscience and Waisman Center, School of Medicine and Public Health, University of Wisconsin, Madison, Wisconsin, United States of America,
State Key Laboratory of Molecular Developmental Biology, Institute of Genetics and Developmental Biology, Chinese Academy of Sciences, Beijing, China

Keita Tsujimura, Kinichi Nakashima and Koichiro Irie
Department of Stem Cell Biology and Medicine, Graduate School of Medical Sciences, Kyushu University, Fukuoka, Japan

Maky Otsuka I. and Katsuhide Igarashi
Life Science Tokyo Advanced Research center (L-StaR), Hoshi University School of Pharmacy and Pharmaceutical Science, Tokyo, Japan

Berna Güroğlu, Geert-Jan Will and Eveline A. Crone
Institute of Psychology, Leiden University, Leiden, the Netherlands
Leiden Institute for Brain and Cognition (LIBC), Leiden University, Leiden, the Netherlands

Wenliang Zhu
Institute of Clinical Pharmacology, the Second Affiliated Hospital of Harbin Medical University, Harbin, China

Xuan Kan
Department of Otolaryngology, the Second Affiliated Hospital of Harbin Medical University, Harbin, China

Rolando Berlinguer-Palmini, Patrick Degenaar and Kamyar Merhan
School of Electric and Electronic Engineering – Institute of Neuroscience, Newcastle University, Newcastle, United Kingdom

Arianna Dilaghi, Flavio Moroni, Alessio Masi, Maria Sili, Roberto Narducci and Guido Mannaioni
Department of Neuroscience, Psychology, Drug Research and Child Health Section of Pharmacology and Toxicology, University of Florence, Florence, Italy

Antonio Schettini, Tania Scartabelli and Elisa Landucci
Department of Health Science, Section of Clinical Pharmacology and Oncology, University of Florence, Florence, Italy

Brian McGovern
Institute of Biomedical Engineering, Imperial College, London, United Kingdom

Pleun Maskaant
Tyndall National Institute of Technology, Cork, Ireland

Hong-Ying Zhang, Wen-Xin Chen and Jing-Tao Wu
Department of Radiology, Subei People's Hospital of Jiangsu Province, Yangzhou University, Yangzhou, China

Yun Jiao
Jiangsu Key Laboratory of Molecular and Functional Imaging, Southeast University, Nanjing, China

Yao Xu
Department of Neurology, Subei People's Hospital of Jiangsu Province, Yangzhou University, Yangzhou, China

Xiang-Rong Zhang
Department of Psychiatry, Zhongda Hospital, Southeast University, Nanjing, China

Fahmida A. Chowdhury and Mark P. Richardson
1 Institute of Psychiatry, Psychology and Neuroscience, King's College London, London, United Kingdom, 2 Centre for Epilepsy, King's College Hospital, London, United Kingdom

Robert D. C. Elwes and Lina Nashef
Centre for Epilepsy, King's College Hospital, London, United Kingdom

Wessel Woldman and John R. Terry
College of Engineering, Mathematics and Physical Sciences, University of Exeter, Exeter, United Kingdom

Thomas H. B. FitzGerald
Institute of Psychiatry, Psychology and Neuroscience, King's College London, London, United Kingdom
Wellcome Trust Centre for Neuroimaging, UCL, London, United Kingdom

Yanhui Yang
Department of Radiology, Xuanwu Hospital, Capital Medical University, Beijing, P.R. China
Key Laboratory for Neurodegenerative Diseases, Ministry of Education, Beijing, P.R. China

Chunming Lu and Bohan Dai
State Key Laboratory of Cognitive Neuroscience and Learning & IDG/McGovern Institute for Brain Research, Beijing Normal University, Beijing, P.R. China
Center for Collaboration and Innovation in Brain and Learning Sciences, Beijing Normal University, Beijing, P.R. China

Peter Howell
Division of Psychology and Language Sciences, University College London, London, United Kingdom

Xianling Wang
Department of Neurology, Xuanwu Hospital, Capital Medical University, Beijing, P.R. China

Kuncheng Li
Department of Radiology, Xuanwu Hospital, Capital Medical University, Beijing, P.R. China

Key Laboratory for Neurodegenerative Diseases, Ministry of Education, Beijing, P.R. China
Beijing Key laboratory of Magnetic Resonance Imaging and Brain Informatics, Beijing, P.R. China

Weigang Pan, Ting Wang, Xiangpeng Wang, Glenn Hitchman, Lijun Wang and Antao Chen
Key Laboratory of Cognition and Personality (Ministry of Education), Faculty of Psychology, Southwest University, Chongqing, China

Pablo Billeke and Francisco Zamorano
División Neurociencia de la Conducta, Centro de Investigación en Complejidad Social (CICS), Facultad de Gobierno, Universidad del Desarrollo, Santiago, Chile
Centro Interdisciplinario de Neurociencias, Pontificia Universidad Católica de Chile, Santiago, Chile
Departamento de Psiquiatría, Escuela de Medicina, Pontificia Universidad Católica de Chile, Santiago, Chile

Francisco Aboitiz
Centro Interdisciplinario de Neurociencias, Pontificia Universidad Católica de Chile, Santiago, Chile
Departamento de Psiquiatría, Escuela de Medicina, Pontificia Universidad Católica de Chile, Santiago, Chile

Diego Cosmelli
Centro Interdisciplinario de Neurociencias, Pontificia Universidad Católica de Chile, Santiago, Chile
Escuela de Psicología, Pontificia Universidad Católica de Chile, Santiago, Chile

Mario Chavez
CNRS UMR-7225, Hôpital de la Salpêtriére, Paris, France

Mesut Tiğdemir
Department of Civil Engineering, Süleyman Demirel University, Engineering Faculty, Isparta, Turkey

Index

www.ingramcontent.com/pod-product-compliance
Lightning Source LLC
Chambersburg PA
CBHW082040190326
41458CB00010B/3419